DR.
SUSAN
LOVE'S
BREAST
BOOK

DR. SUSAN LOVE'S BREAST BOOK

FIFTH EDITION

SUSAN M. LOVE, M.D.

with Karen Lindsey

A MERLOYD LAWRENCE BOOK
DA CAPO LIFELONG

Set in 11.5 point Fairfield LH Light by the Perseus Books Group

Library of Congress Cataloging-in-Publication Data
Love, Susan M.
    Dr. Susan Love's breast book / Susan M. Love, with Karen Lindsey.—5th ed., 1st Da Capo Press ed.
        p. cm.
    "A Merloyd Lawrence Book"—
    Includes bibliographical references and index.
    ISBN 978-0-7382-1359-0 (alk. paper)
    1. Breast—Diseases—Popular works. 2. Breast—Cancer—Popular works. I. Lindsey, Karen, 1944– II. Title. III. Title: Breast book. IV. Title: Doctor Susan Love's breast book.

RG491.L68 2010
618.1'9—dc22

                                                                            2010021598

A Merloyd Lawrence Book
Published by Da Capo Press
A Member of the Perseus Books Group
www.dacapopress.com

Da Capo Press books are available at special discounts for bulk purchases in the U.S. by corporations, institutions, and other organizations. For more information, please contact the Special Markets Department at the Perseus Books Group, 2300 Chestnut Street, Philadelphia, PA 19103 or call (800) 810-4145, extension 5000 or e-mail special.markets@perseusbooks.com.

7 8 9 10

To Carolina Hinestrosa and all the women
who have died from breast cancer or its treatment,
that this disease can end with us.

Contents

Acknowledgments

Every five years I sit down to completely revamp the *Breast Book* and think to myself, I just cannot do this alone! The good news is that I don't have to: I have had lots of help in the past year and a half, and I am very grateful for it. Breast cancer has become immensely complicated since I wrote the first edition. It has been critically important to read everything I can get my hands on, and even more to touch base with friends and acquaintances who are in the thick of research and patient care. Their generous support is what makes this book valuable. I especially want to mention Judi Hirschfield-Bartek, Dixie Mills, and Sherry Goldman, who read through the fourth edition, highlighting areas that needed updating. Drafts of the fifth edition were read and commented on by Judi Hirschfield-Bartek, Sherry Goldman, Lisa Bailey, Ellen Mahoney, Dixie Mills, Shelly Hwang, Ben Anderson, Eric Halvorson, Steven Cummings, Karla Kerlikowske, Leslie Bernstein, Nicki DeBruhl, Larry Bassett, Judy Garber, Carol Fabian, Steve Narod, Thea Tlsty, Sanford Barsky, Dan Hayes, Craig Henderson, Silvana Martino, Lisa Weissmann, Mary Ann Rose, Irene Gage, Susan Pierce, Musa Mayer, Marlene McCarthy, and Hester Hill.

The other important experts are the women who have shared their experiences with me. They include not only the survivors I have met and talked to over the past years but my Facebook friends, who always responded right away when I would post an urgent request for real-life stories to illustrate a point. I promised anonymity, but you know who you are.

I appreciate all the help, but any errors are mine alone.

Then there are the people in my life who facilitate the work and pitch in when needed. My major activity currently is the Dr. Susan Love Research Foundation, and the team there has been terrific. Our wonderful board of directors: Kate McLean, Helene Brown, Nina Gomez, Meribeth Brand, Karen Duval, and Melissa Wayne, and until recently P. Kay Coleman and Pamela Hearn. Their continual support is critical to our mission. I want to specifically name Naz Sykes, the wonderful executive director whose hard work and dedication has taken our efforts to eradicate breast cancer to new heights; Dixie Mills, who was always there to pick up the slack and has contributed significantly to this edition; the Army of Women team of Hedi Jalon and Leah Wilcox, and most significantly Dakota Katona, my assistant, who not only keeps my calendar and makes sure I know where I am going but also keyed in a whole chapter when I needed an electronic version ASAP. Sade Osilaja is the newest member of the team and is already adding a great new perspective. Tinh Nguyen has been indispensible in assisting with research and filling in where and whenever needed. He and our wonderful premed students—Alex Preston, Tiffany Yanase, Bill Wu, and Sarah-Michelle Lahti—spent a whole day getting the references into shape when I could not bear to look at them another minute.

It is remarkable to me that we have had the same core team working on this book since the first edition. Karen Lindsey continues to be a great cowriter, even when her questions asking for clarification drive me crazy. She is always right. Merloyd Lawrence is the wonderful, patient editor who makes sure it all falls together and makes sense. The final steps of this edition involved Karen in the Netherlands and me in Egypt and then Shanghai, but with Merloyd's steady hand we managed to get it all done. Then there is Marcia Williams, whose artwork is such a help in demonstrating the concepts I am trying to explain. I point her in a direction and she always gets it and always comes back with something better than I had expected. My agent, Sidney Kramer, has never wavered in his enthusiasm for this book through all of the editions.

And Jill Kneerim's gentle guidance and cheerleading makes sure I stay on track.

This book and these acknowledgments have tracked my life over the past twenty-five years. The first edition was conceived before my daughter, who nonetheless beat it to being born. She is now finishing college and is a great writer in her own right, not to mention the light of her mothers' lives. And my dear wife, Helen, has put up with "Dr. Susan Love's GD Breast Book" over the more than twenty-seven years of our life together. To her I owe all my love and gratitude: You are the wind beneath my sails. And to all the women with breast cancer who share their stories with me on-line and in person, it is for you that I continue to do this work!

Introduction

In the introduction to the fourth edition of this book, I likened it to a software upgrade. But this fifth edition goes much farther: it represents a shift in the paradigm we use to think about the breast and its problems. A slow revolution, you could say, and a good example of how these things happen.

In science we come up with hypotheses or stories that we use to explain our observations and pull them together into a framework that can be used to direct future research and treatment. The first edition of this book was written to explain what was then a new paradigm—that the most lethal part of breast cancer was the cells that may have already gotten out into other parts of the body before diagnosis. The addition of hormone therapy and then chemotherapy to the initial treatment of the disease was an exciting result of this new way of thinking and established the limitations of extensive surgery as the sole approach. The result has been a definite improvement in overall survival for many women with breast cancer.

This paradigm, however, assumed that all breast cancers are the same and should be treated the same and that the more aggressive tumors require more aggressive treatments. This led to high-dose chemotherapy and stem cell rescue in an effort to kill every cancer cell, whether it is hiding somewhere or not. While this approach resonated with newly diagnosed women who were willing to do whatever it took to cure their disease, it was ultimately shown not to be any better than regular dose chemotherapy. The first crack in the hypothesis.

Observations in the laboratory by scientists like my friend Mina Bissell started to suggest that cancer cells might be influenced by their surroundings, while clinically doctors were noting that some cancers were sensitive to hormones while others weren't, and further that some cancers had different molecular patterns that seemed to define their behavior. Add this to the observations that even with the best screening the reduction in deaths from breast cancer was stuck at 30 percent, and the stage was set for a new story.

This edition has been completely reorganized and rewritten to present the data with the perspective of the current hypothesis, which is based on two new understandings from basic science. First, all breast cancers are not the same. There are at least five or six different molecular subtypes and each probably develops from a different step in the evolution of a tumor stem cell. That observation alone leads to the need to determine which subtype a woman has and then to personalize the treatment to match. This means better results and also ensures we are not treating women with drugs that won't benefit them (and may even harm them). While this is still a work in progress, I have tried to explain throughout the book how we figure it out and where I think it is going.

The second big shift is the realization that cancer cells do not function in isolation. You need more than a mutated cell to get actual cancer. You need it to be in a local environment, a sort of neighborhood, that nourishes it. A bad cell in a good neighborhood will most of the time stay dormant. But if the neighborhood changes, there is likely to be trouble. This innovative understanding gives us a whole new way to think about risk factors, screening, and treatment. Without abandoning the goal to kill as many cancer cells as possible, we can also try to improve the neighborhood with lifestyle changes, as I discuss at length in Chapter 18. The result is an improvement not only in survival but also in quality of life.

This new paradigm explains a lot and will carry us forward for many years. I don't guarantee that it will be the ultimate answer, but the new insights and successes we are having in treatment and the leads for prevention are unmistakable. We can figure out what causes the bad cell or we can make sure that we maintain a good neighborhood.

It is an exciting time, and I hope the new edition reflects this shift in thinking. Unfortunately it makes understanding *your* cancer more difficult and the decision making more complicated. I try to give you tools to understand what the decisions are and what information you need to make them. This information too will change, so check the website—www.drsusanloveresearch foundation.org—for the latest news.

My goal is still to stop this disease once and for all, and for that I need to know the cause. I describe my new efforts toward encouraging this approach in the epilogue. We can be the generation that stops breast cancer, but it will take all of us, an Army of Women!

Part One

THE HEALTHY BREAST AND COMMON PROBLEMS

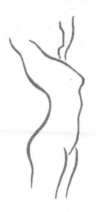

Chapter 1

THE BREAST AND ITS DEVELOPMENT

Is THERE SUCH A THING AS A "NORMAL" BREAST? MEDICALLY speaking, yes: a normal breast is one capable of producing milk. Beyond that, no. The range of size and shape of breasts is wide and individual. Most of us haven't seen many other women's breasts, and we've all grown up with the image of "ideal" breasts that permeates our society. But few of us fit that image, and there's no reason we should. Breasts can be very large or very small, and in most women one breast is slightly larger than the other. It is not uncommon, and perfectly normal, to have a cup-size difference. Breast size is genetically determined and depends chiefly on the percentage of fat to other tissue in the breasts. Usually about a third of the breast is composed of fat tissue; the rest is milk ducts and supportive fibrous tissue (Figure 1.1). The amount of fat varies as you gain or lose weight; the amount of breast tissue remains constant. A "flat-chested" woman's breasts will grow as she gains weight, just as her stomach and thighs do; so if she loses the weight, she'll also lose her larger breasts. (This is actually a block to weight loss for many women, since the

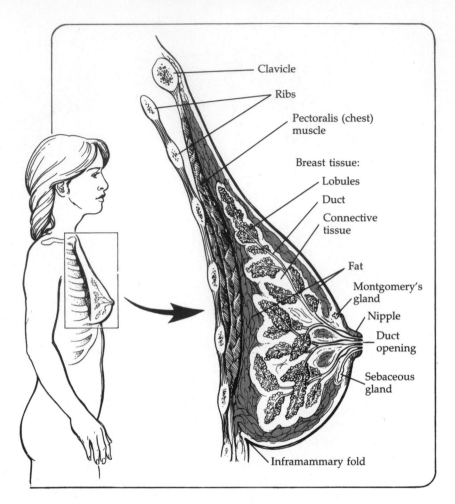

Clavicle
Ribs
Pectoralis (chest) muscle
Breast tissue:
Lobules
Duct
Connective tissue
Fat
Montgomery's gland
Nipple
Duct opening
Sebaceous gland
Inframammary fold

Figure 1.1

weight seems to leave the breasts first; they hate the effect on the breasts so much that they decide to go off the diet.) A normal breast of any cup size can produce enough milk to feed a baby, and breast size has nothing to do with vulnerability to breast cancer or other breast disease. Very large breasts can be physically uncomfortable, and, like very small or very uneven breasts, they can be emotionally uncomfortable as well. We'll consider this at length in Chapter 2.

The breast itself is usually tear-shaped (Figure 1.2). There's breast tissue from the collarbone all the way down to the last few

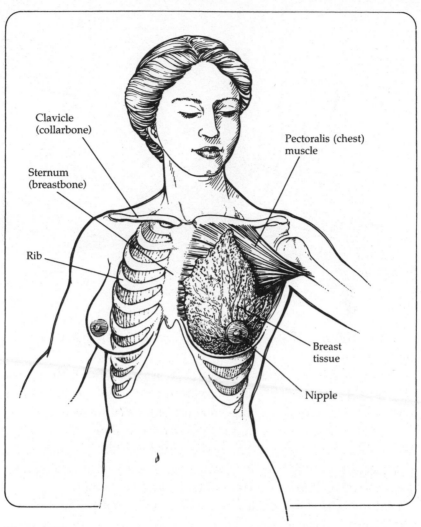

Clavicle
(collarbone)

Sternum
(breastbone)

Rib

Pectoralis (chest)
muscle

Breast
tissue

Nipple

Figure 1.2

ribs, and from the breastbone in the middle of the chest to the back of the armpit. Your ribs lie behind your breast, and sometimes they may feel hard and lumpy. When I was in medical school, I embarrassed myself horribly when I found a "lump" in my breast and frantically ran to one of the older doctors to find out if I had cancer. I found out I had a rib.

Often there's a ridge of fat at the bottom of the breast—the inframammary ridge (Figure 1.3). This ridge is perfectly normal, the

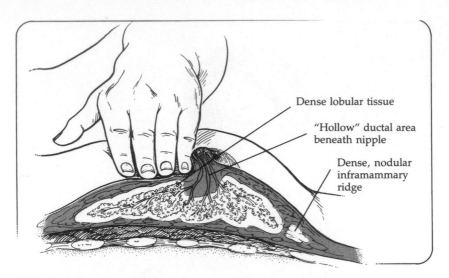

Dense lobular tissue

"Hollow" ductal area beneath nipple

Dense, nodular inframammary ridge

Figure 1.3

result of the fact that we walk upright and our breasts fold over themselves.

The areola is the darker area of the breast surrounding the nipple (Figure 1.4). Its size and shape vary from woman to woman, and its color varies according to complexion. In blondes it tends to be pink, in brunettes it's browner, and in dark-skinned people it's brown to black. In most women it gets darker after the first pregnancy. Its color also changes during the various stages of sexual arousal and orgasm as well as with some types of oral contraceptives.

Many women find their nipples don't face front; they stick out slightly toward the armpits. There's a reason for this. Picture yourself holding a baby you're about to nurse. The baby's head is held in the crook of your arm—a nipple pointing to the side is comfortably close to the baby's mouth (Figure 1.5).

There are hair follicles around the nipple, so most women have at least some nipple hair. It's perfectly natural, and you can ignore it. If you don't like it, you can shave it off, pluck it out, use electrolysis, or get rid of it any sensible way you want—it's just like leg or armpit hair except softer. You may also notice little bumps around the areola that look like goose pimples. These are known as Montgomery's glands. The nipple also has sebaceous glands, which I'll talk about later on in this chapter.

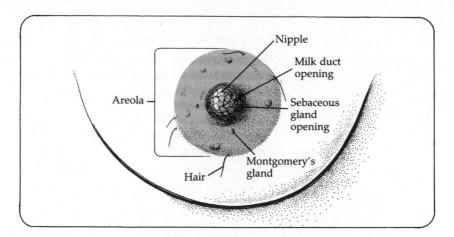

Figure 1.4

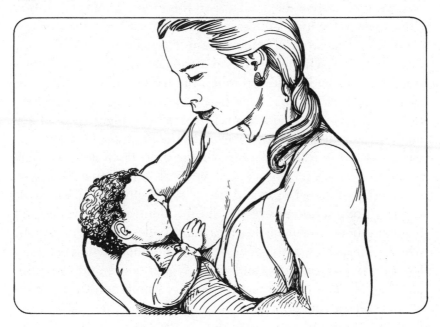

Figure 1.5

Sometimes nipples are "shy": when they're stimulated they re-treat into themselves and become temporarily inverted. This is nothing to worry about; it has no effect on milk supply, breast-feeding, sexual pleasure, or anything else. Nipples that newly be-come permanently inverted could be an early sign of cancer and needs to be investigated.

The tissue inside the breast is sandwiched between layers of fat, behind which is the chest muscle. The fat has some give to it, which is why we bounce. The breast tissue is firm and rubbery. A patient once told me while I was operating on her under local anesthetic that she thought the breast was constructed like a woman—soft and pliant on the outside, and tough underneath. The breast also has its share of the connective tissue that holds the entire body together. This material creates a solid structure—like gelatin—in which the other kinds of tissues are loosely set. This is sometimes called the stroma.

Like the rest of the body, the breast has arteries, veins, and nerves. As you probably know, the arteries carry blood rich with oxygen and fuel to the cells, while the veins carry the depleted blood full of carbon dioxide back to the lungs. There is another, almost parallel, network of vessels called the lymphatic system (or *lymphatics*) that works like recyclers or filters for helping the body fight infection. The job of this network is to collect the debris from the cells and strain it through the lymph nodes found scattered in nests throughout the body; they then send the filtered fluid back into the bloodstream to be reused (Figure 1.6). They do more than just recycle, however. In the process of filtering the unnecessary fluid, they identify what is in it. If there is anything threatening—a bacterial cell, a piece of suture material, or a virus—they hold on to it and use it to develop an immune response. They send cells to the site to identify the invader and make antibodies to fight it. The lymph nodes will be important when I discuss breast cancer later in the book. It is crucial to identify which lymphatics and which lymph nodes drain a particular area of the breast so that the correct lymph nodes can be removed and examined for signs of cancer.

There's very little muscle in the breast. The areola has a bit of muscle, which is why it contracts and stands out with cold, sexual stimulation, and, of course, breast-feeding. This too makes sense: if the nipple stands out, it's easier for the baby's mouth to get a good grip on it. There are also tiny muscles around the lobules that help deliver milk, as we will see later in this chapter. The major muscles in the area are behind the breasts—the pectorals. Because there is so little muscle inside the breasts, the idea that you

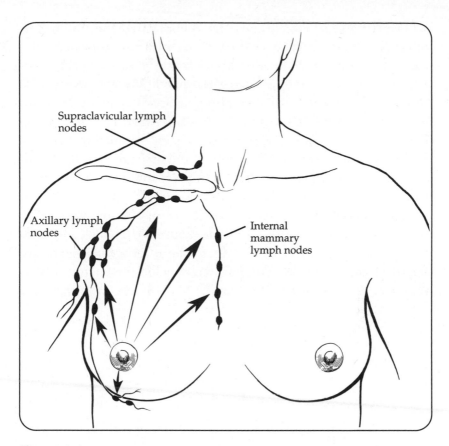

Figure 1.6

can grow larger breasts through exercise is false. You can grow stronger pectorals—as bodybuilders do—but all this means is that your breasts will rest on an expanded chest.

THE PARTS OF THE BREAST:
AN INTERACTIVE COMMUNITY

During most of my career the critical component of the breast was thought to be the system of milk ducts that are responsible for lactation, with everything else just along for the ride. Yet there has been little research on the anatomy of the breast ducts. So I have devoted much of my own research to the subject.

Over the years my studies[1] have confirmed the findings of other researchers.[2] When we try to insert a tiny tube (called a cannula) into the milk duct openings from the surface of the nipple, we find that there are between five and eight openings,[3,4] (Figure 1.7) (Figure 1.8). Examining a breast that has been removed and cut across the nipple reveals between 15 and 22 duct-like structures.[5,6] This puzzle has not been completely resolved, but recent work suggests that some of the ducts meet together inside the breast before they exit the nipple, thus sharing an opening while others exit the nipple separately (Figure 1.9). In addition, some of what appear to be ducts may be something else: little glands that make a sebaceous material—a white, oily substance—and join with the milk duct. These sebaceous glands are found all over the body. We don't know what they're for, or why there are so many around the nipple. My own theory is that they

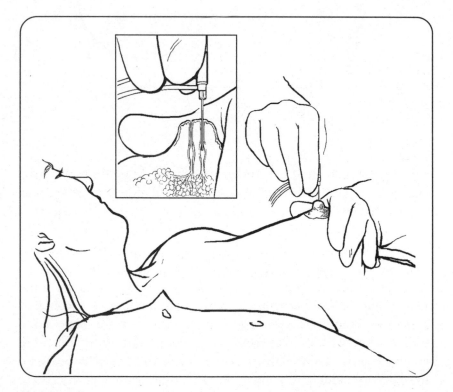

Figure 1.7

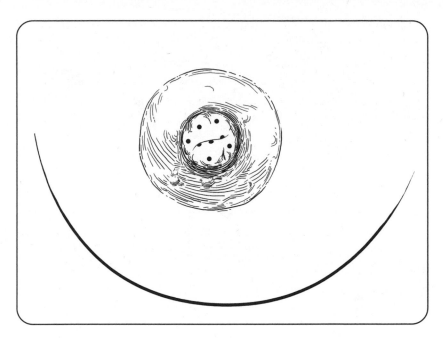

Figure 1.8

provide a coating that protects the skin—sort of your own little skin care system. The nipple, designed to be sucked on, is especially vulnerable to getting chapped and sore, so having a lot of these glands makes sense.

My colleagues and I studied the anatomy of the breast beyond the nipple, using both cadavers and breasts that had been removed by mastectomy (with the patients' permission). We learned that the duct opening in the nipple leads into the breast in a straight line for a very short distance—only about a centimeter (less than one-half inch). There's a little sphincter muscle here that prevents milk from squirting out when a breast-feeding woman is not nursing her baby. Behind that is a little antechamber called the *lactiferous sinus*. From there, the ductal system, like a tree, breaks up into little branches that go to the back of the breast. These branches are the ducts. Leafing out at the end of each branch are the lobules, which make the breast milk and then send it through the

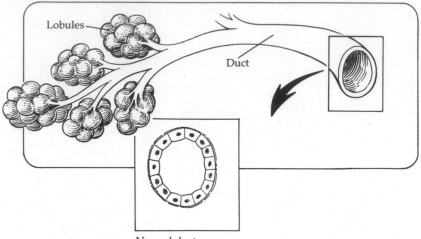

Normal duct

Figure 1.9

ducts to the nipple (Figure 1.9). Each ductal system is independent of all the others; each creates milk separately. They coexist, but they don't connect with one another. Each ductal system is fully lined or "tiled" by a single layer of small cells that completely coat the inside of the whole structure from nipple to the very last branch closest to the chest wall. Breast cancer is thought to arise from changes in these lining cells, as we will see later (Figure 1.9). If we could selectively remove these lining cells from the inside of the ductal system after women finish breast-feeding, we believe we could eliminate breast cancer.

That was where the story ended in the fourth edition of this book. However, recent studies have shown that it isn't quite so simple. It turns out that the cells living around the ducts and lobules—fat cells, fibrous cells, and white blood cells—are as specialized and important as the ductal and lobular cells that line the inside of each ductal system. The cells all influence each other in a complex community that creates the breast's versatility, allowing it to go from the resting state to pregnancy and milk production

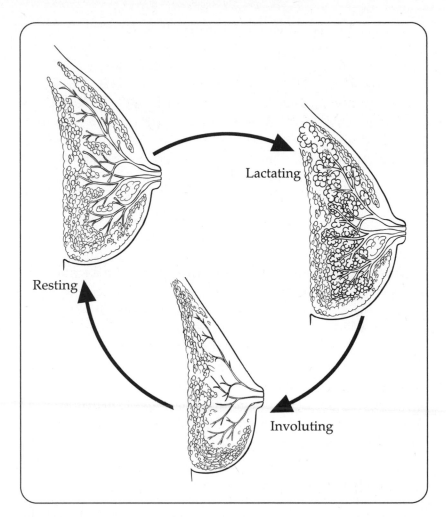

Figure 1.10

and back to the resting state (Figure 1.10). As the exact mechanism for this is currently a topic of much research, I won't go into the theories now (you'll have to wait for the next edition). But we do know that when this interaction goes awry, it probably produces the environment that promotes cancer development and growth (see Chapter 4).[7]

How the Breast Develops

To understand how the breast typically develops, we need to know what it's for. The breast is an integral part of a woman's reproductive system. Indeed, it defines our biological class: mammals derive their name from the fact that they have mammary glands and feed their young at their breasts. Different mammals have different numbers and sizes of breasts, but human females are the only ones to develop full breasts long before they are needed to feed their young. We are also the only animals who are actively sexual when we're not fertile. This suggests that our breasts have the important secondary function of contributing to sensual pleasure.

Though as Simone de Beauvoir wrote, women have traditionally been thought of as "the other," biologically we're the norm. The genitalia of all embryos are female—even of those programmed to be male. When the hormones produced at the direction of the Y chromosome prompt the fetus, it starts to develop male genitalia. If the testes are destroyed early in fetal development, the male fetus will develop breasts and retain female genitalia. It makes sense to suggest that the basis of "mankind" is, in fact, woman. To me that is confirmed by the fact that men have rudimentary nipples.

Early Development

Human breast tissue begins to develop remarkably early—in the sixth week of fetal life. It forms across a line known as the milk ridge, which runs from the armpit down to just below the breast (Figure 1.11). So you already have breast tissue and even little ducts at birth, and that tissue is already sensitive to hormones (your mother's sex hormones circulate through the placenta). Infants may even have nipple discharge. This "witch's milk," as it's called, goes away in a couple of weeks, since the infant is no longer getting the mother's hormones. Between 80 and 90 percent of all infants of both genders have this discharge on the second or third day after birth.

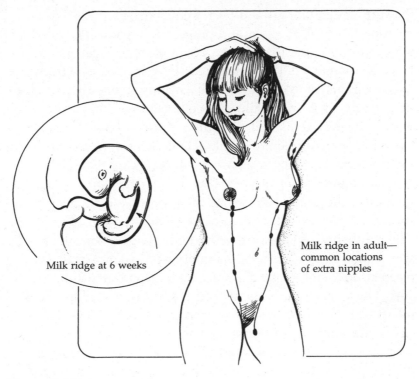

Milk ridge at 6 weeks

Milk ridge in adult—
common locations
of extra nipples

Figure 1.11

Puberty

After early infancy, not much happens to the breast until puberty
(Figure 1.12). The breast is one of the only organs that is not fully
developed at birth. This means it needs stem cells—cells capable
of turning into other cells. They're sort of great-grandmother pro-
genitor cells that can morph into various types of cells as needed,
such as duct cells or lobular cells. The stem cells are not limited
to this period of development, as they will be needed later to help
the breast create milk and then again to reconstitute the resting
breast when the feeding days are over. A current hypothesis pos-
tulates that these cells can become mutated and initiate cancer
(see Chapter 4).[8]

Although we are not sure which component of the breast is
the first to hear the call of hormones at puberty, we do know that

the surrounding fibrous and fat tissue changes in response to increasing levels of estrogen and progesterone, and the tiny ducts grow into this tissue like roots. Some of the ducts get started first and take up much of the breast area. They secrete something that tells other ducts to stay out of their territory so that they will have room to grow later when they are called to make milk. As a result some ductal systems will take up a third or half of the breast while others may be quite small.[9] The lobules don't develop until the girl starts ovulating and having full cycles.

From a girl's point of view, this breast development happens soon after the pubic hair begins to grow. (Typically her periods start a year or two after her breasts begin growing.) They begin with a little bud of breast tissue under the nipple—it can be itchy and sometimes a bit sore. The breasts expand until they've reached their full growth, usually by the time menstruation begins. The first tiny breasts can be confusing to children and to their parents as well. One of my patients was an eleven-year-old girl whose mother had breast cancer. The girl had what her parents were sure was a lump under her nipple, and feared that she too had cancer. It was very unlikely at that age, and my examination showed it to be simply the beginning of her breast development, so I was able to reassure them. Of course if you come

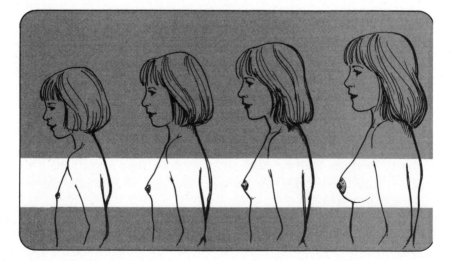

Figure 1.12

across something you find suspicious, have it checked out. But if you're told it should be biopsied or removed, get a second and third opinion. If newly forming breast tissue is removed, it won't grow back and the child will never have that breast.

The rate at which breasts grow varies greatly from girl to girl; some start off very flat-chested and end up with large breasts; others have large breasts at an early age. Often one breast grows more quickly than the other. (We'll consider this and other variations in breast development in Chapter 2.)

Sometimes, because of their hormonal development, adolescent boys develop a condition called *gynecomastia*—which translates to "breasts like a woman." This can be in one breast or both. For obvious reasons, the boys' reactions don't parallel the ambivalence felt by developing girls—for boys, breast development is uniformly embarrassing. I remember my seventh grade boyfriend was so humiliated by it that he paid another boy to push him into the swimming pool so he wouldn't have to take off his shirt to swim or explain to the other kids why he was swimming with his shirt on. I occasionally had patients suffering from gynecomastia. Their mental anguish, as well as their acute embarrassment at having to show me their chest, was really disheartening to see. Fortunately the condition usually regresses on its own in about 18 months; if it doesn't, it can easily be helped through surgery.

The Menstruating Years

A girl's initial breast development is followed by the establishment of the menstrual cycle. Hormones play a crucial part in this development, as they do in all aspects of reproductive growth. On the ovary are follicles with eggs encased in their developmental sacs (Figure 1.13). These, stimulated by FSH (follicle-stimulating hormone) in the pituitary gland, produce estrogen. The resulting high levels of estrogen in the blood tell the pituitary to turn off the FSH and start secreting LH (luteinizing hormone). When the estrogen and LH are both at their peak, you ovulate—the follicle bursts and releases its egg into the fallopian tube.

The follicle is now an empty sac, but it still has a job to do: it becomes the *corpus luteum* and starts producing progesterone, which prepares the lining of the uterus for pregnancy ("progesterone"

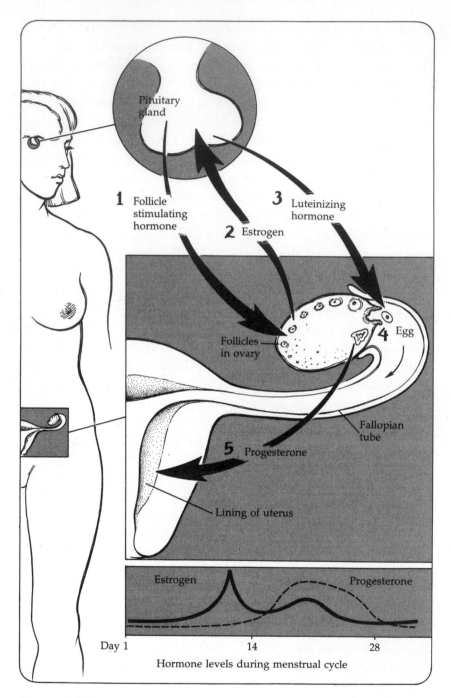

Figure 1.13

means "pro-pregnancy"). Usually the egg doesn't get fertilized. Then the progesterone level falls off, the lining of the uterus is shed, and you start all over again. If the egg is fertilized, the corpus luteum starts to produce HCG (human choriogonadotropin), which maintains the progesterone level until the placenta takes over producing it, and you're pregnant.

Throughout this monthly process, the cyclical hormones have been busily preparing the breast for a potential pregnancy. The progesterone produced by the corpus luteum is essential for the lobules to develop at the ends of the ducts, like leaves on a tree. These undoubtedly also affect the tissue surrounding the ducts and lobules.

Breast development of the early reproductive years is considered to go on from age 15 to 25. The years from 25 to 40 are considered the mature reproductive years, the years of cyclical activity. At this point most menstrual cycles are ovulatory and the breast, along with the rest of the body, has become pretty used to menstruation. As the hormones stimulate the breast, we experience a familiar cyclical pattern of swelling, nodularity, pain, and tenderness. This pattern, which continues up to 40 years of reproductive life, gives the breast ample opportunity for minor changes to occur, resulting in many of the common benign problems that women frequently experience (see Chapter 3).

Breast-Feeding

The ultimate purpose of the breast is to make milk, and so a woman's breast doesn't reach its full potential until she's been through a nine-month pregnancy. This stage of the breast's development becomes evident soon after conception. Even before she misses her period, a woman may notice that her breasts are unusually tender or her nipples are unusually sore. I have had a few patients complaining of strange breast pain that turned out to be an early sign of pregnancy.

Breasts enlarge rapidly and become very firm during pregnancy. The Montgomery's glands become darker and more prominent, and the areola darkens. The nipples become larger and more erect, preparing themselves for future milk production (Figure 1.14).

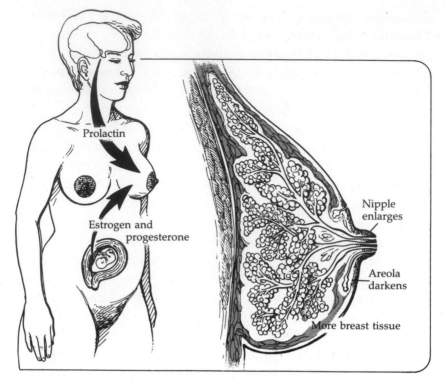

Figure 1.14

The development of the breast into a milk-producing machine is orchestrated by several hormones, including estrogen, progesterone, prolactin, and oxytocin. Meanwhile, other hormones are at work—insulin, thyroid, and cortisol, as well as background nutritional hormones. As with development, both the ductal system and its surrounding stroma take part in the lactational process. The lobules actually make the milk, and in the process of pregnancy they go from type 1 lobules (immature structures thought to be more susceptible to carcinogenesis) to mature type 4, which form by the end of the nine months and stay for lactation. These take part of the food the pregnant woman eats and remanufacture it into part of the baby's milk.

Once the baby is born and the placenta has been delivered, the woman's estrogen and progesterone levels plummet, while prolactin levels first remain high and then begin a slow decline.

This is the sign for the breasts to begin producing milk. The milk, however, doesn't come right away, and for three to five days the breasts make another liquid, a sort of premilk called *colostrum,* which the baby can drink while waiting for the milk to come in. Colostrum is filled with antibodies that help the infant fight off infection.

While some milk is sucked out by the baby, some simply gushes into the baby's mouth, squeezed out by the tiny muscles lining the lobules. The mother experiences this as letdown: her milk is literally being let down inside her breasts. The other surprise to most new parents is that the milk comes out of many holes in the nipple—like a watering can. As noted above, these holes are the openings of the six to nine milk duct systems.

If a new mother is not producing milk within a week of the baby's birth, something is wrong and a clinician should be consulted. Aside from deliberate attempts to inhibit milk, several things can prevent breasts from producing it. There might be a problem in the woman's pituitary gland—she may have bled into it, or it may be otherwise damaged, compromising her body's ability to produce the necessary prolactin and oxytocin (Figure 1.15). Sometimes the milk comes into the breast but can't get out. This is caused by damage to the duct system, usually by surgery around the nipple or perhaps by breast reduction surgery or insertion of implants (see Chapter 2). Sometimes the ducts can be unblocked but often they can't, and in that case the baby will have to be bottle-fed. (The breast milk is reabsorbed into the mother's body.) Sometimes the baby has a problem coordinating tongue motions, or the shape of a woman's nipples makes it hard for the baby to latch on. Insufficient milk needs to be evaluated by a clinician expert in breast-feeding: a pediatrician, family doctor, or lactation consultant.

After the mother stops breast-feeding, prolactin levels decline gradually and she continues to have some secretions for two or three months and sometimes even a year or two.

Breast-feeding has some contraceptive effect, but only in the first three or four months—and even then, it's important to realize that it isn't 100 percent effective. Many a pregnancy has occurred during breast-feeding.

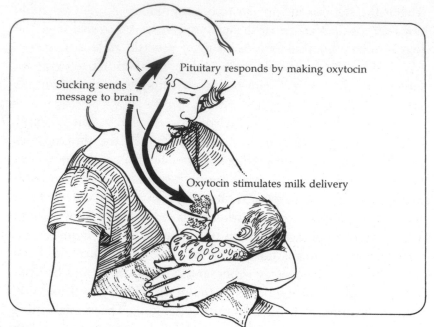

Pituitary responds by making oxytocin

Sucking sends
message to brain

Oxytocin stimulates milk delivery

Figure 1.15

Some women have too little milk. In most cases this can be alleviated by feeding more often—a feeding every two hours generally helps. If such a rigorous schedule proves impossible for you, it may be time to stop breast-feeding and turn to formula—or at least combine breast- and bottle-feeding. Sometimes even frequent feeding doesn't help. For some reason, the woman's body simply doesn't make enough milk, no matter what she does. Many women feel guilty when this happens, as though they've failed in their "motherly duties." They haven't—it's a biological idiosyncrasy, not a personal flaw.

What are the advantages of breast-feeding? Probably the most important is the nutritional composition of breast milk. It's tailor-made for the human baby's needs—it has the perfect combination of water, protein, carbohydrates (mainly lactose), immunoglobin (which helps create immunity against disease), lots of cholesterol (which, though unhealthy for adults, is great for babies), and vitamins and minerals. Cow's milk, on the other hand, is tailor-made for the needs of baby cows, which are obviously different from those of the human baby.

Formula is our attempt to modify cow's milk to make it as close as possible to human milk. We've done a pretty impressive job, but it's not perfect. For one thing, cow's milk isn't as digestible as human milk. It takes a baby four hours to digest formula, and only two to digest human milk. Further, no formula has been able to duplicate the immunity-providing properties of colostrum.

Breast-feeding also creates a unique bonding between mother and infant, which some psychologists feel is essential to the child's later well-being. While there are plenty of emotionally healthy people who were bottle-fed and many neurotics who were breast-fed, the particular bonding created by breast-feeding can't be wholly duplicated in bottle-feeding. On the other hand, breast-feeding can create difficulties for the mother that may compete with the advantages to the child—difficulties that proselytizers for breast-feeding sometimes underrate. Breast-feeding every two or three hours may be very difficult for a woman who has a job outside her home, and it's not always that easy for the woman at home who has primary responsibility for raising other children and doing housework. Sometimes a combination of breast-feeding and bottle-feeding (using either formula or breast milk expressed or pumped by the mother at an earlier time) can be a wise compromise (Figure 1.16).

Lactation can cause other problems, even for the mother combining breast and bottle feeding. Oxytocin, the hormone that causes breast milk to flow, can be produced by emotional as well as direct physical responses to the baby, and many mothers find to their embarrassment that milk suddenly begins to flow when they think about the baby. A surgeon colleague of mine decided to stop breast-feeding when an image of her baby came to her during an operation and milk started dripping onto her patient.

There are also women whose eating habits or medications can make breast-feeding a problem. It's true that the baby will consume, through your milk, everything you consume, and many women really cherish their cups of coffee or their evening martinis. It's probably safest to remain drug- and alcohol-free while breast-feeding. For some women this is easy; for others, it's not. Some mothers are on medication for chronic health problems, and some (though certainly not all) medication will harm a breast-feeding

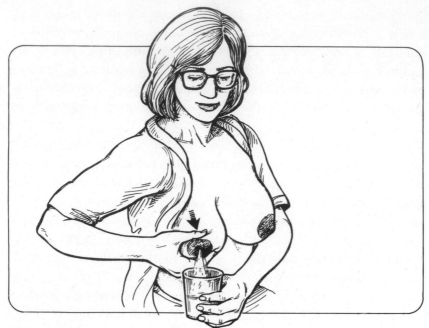

Figure 1.16

baby. Sacrificing your own health or comfort may not be the best thing for *either* you or your child.

Involution

After the baby has been weaned, a new stage begins. The milk-producing cells die off (a process known as involution) and the stem cells get to work making a new resting gland, complete with ducts and lobules and ready for the next pregnancy. Women who have never been pregnant continue to have type 1 lobules, but those who have gone through the full nine months have the more mature type 2 or type 3 lobules. As I explained earlier in this chapter, the mature lobules are less vulnerable to cancer, which may help explain why early pregnancy decreases the risk of breast cancer.

Menopause

We've got the menstruating years figured out, but our understanding of the process is a little fuzzier when we come to the end of the fertile years. The standard line in the textbooks is that when you run out of eggs and you're no longer ovulating, your body stops making estrogen. This causes your FSH (follicle-stimulating hormone) to go up as your pituitary tries to kick-start the ovary into producing more eggs. When that doesn't work, everything just shuts down.

Yet often the symptoms of perimenopause (right before menopause)—breast tenderness, headaches, increased vaginal lubrication—are symptoms of high, not low, estrogen. Sometimes your estrogen levels are high and your progesterone is low, and you might get symptoms of PMS (premenstrual syndrome), while other times your estrogen levels shift and you get hot flashes. Then for several months you're back to normal. So the common explanation is wrong: your symptoms aren't due to low estrogen. They're caused by fluctuations of high and low estrogen.

Sometimes doctors test FSH levels in the blood to decide whether you are in menopause. The problem is that just as estrogen and progesterone fluctuate widely, so does FSH. It could be high at one time and low a month later. If you've stopped menstruating for several months, the FSH tests might be a little more useful for determining if you've really gone into menopause. But even then, it's not 100 percent accurate. One study found that 20 percent of women who had no period for three months started having their cycles again.[10] Breast cancer patients who were thrown into menopause by their chemotherapy treatments missed three or four months of periods, showed high FSH levels—and then got their periods back. There's no foolproof test to determine menopause. The only way we can really do that is the good old-fashioned way. If you haven't menstruated for a year, you're considered menopausal. However, don't assume you're totally out of the woods even then. Some women will get another period after the magic year has passed. If this happens, you should consult with your health care provider. Getting a period after a year should be distinguished from postmenopausal bleeding, which can be a symptom of endometrial cancer.

THE ROLE OF THE OVARY

Throughout most of medical history we have not really understood the ovary. And because we haven't grasped the full complexity of this intricate organ, doctors have assumed that after menopause, when it is no longer capable of making eggs, the ovary shrivels, dries up, and becomes completely useless.

But egg making isn't the ovary's whole function anymore than reproduction is a woman's whole function. The ovary is more than just an egg sac. It's an endocrine organ—one that produces hormones. And it produces them before, during, and after menopause. With menopause, the ovary goes through a shift. It changes from a follicle-rich producer of estrogen and progesterone into a stromal-rich producer of estrogen and the male hormone androgen. Stroma is the glue or background tissue in which eggs are embedded. In youth, you have more eggs and less stroma. As time goes on, you have fewer and fewer eggs and more and more stroma. In its hormonal dance with the hypothalamus and pituitary, the postmenopausal ovary continues to respond to the call of the pituitary. It responds to high levels of FSH and LH (luteinizing hormone) with increased production of testosterone as well as lower levels of estrone and estradiol (two forms of estrogen) and androstenedione (a hormone precursor).[11,12] The hormonal dance doesn't end; the band just strikes up a different tune (Figure 1.17).

Testosterone, of course, is a male hormone. But don't panic: you're not going to grow a beard even if few hairs pop out on your chin. Every human being produces both male and female hormones; the proportion differs according to gender. Much of a woman's testosterone and androstenedione is converted to estrone throughout the body by an enzyme called aromatase. This continued production of hormones varies from one woman to the next and may explain some of the individual differences in symptoms after menopause. It also explains why women who have both ovaries removed surgically, losing all of these hormones, have worse symptoms of menopause and increased vulnerability to cardiovascular disease and osteoporosis.[13]

What all this tells us is that the ovaries have more than one function. Reproduction is their most dramatic task, but it isn't the only one. These organs have as much to do with maintaining the woman's own life as they do with her role in bringing other lives into the world. A former medical colleague of mine, Bill Parker,

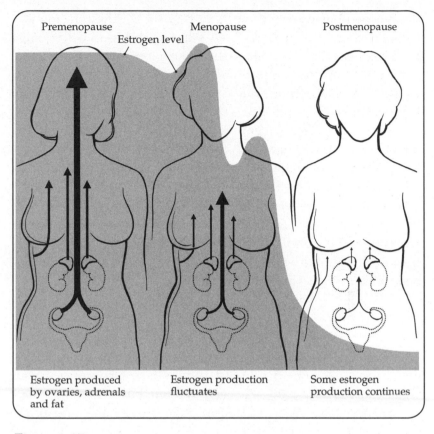

Figure 1.17

confirmed the important postmenopausal role of the ovary when he demonstrated that women who had their ovaries removed preventatively during hysterectomy had an overall *increase* in mortality compared to women who kept their ovaries—even though they had less breast and ovarian cancer.[14] The menopausal ovary is neither failing nor useless. It's simply beginning to shift from its reproductive to its maintenance function. It's doing in midlife exactly what many people do—changing careers.

And what about the breasts? Clearly menopause is the ultimate involution—the breasts get the message that they will not be called into active duty again and can finally rest. But nothing is ever that simple. Different women have different levels of hormones after menopause, depending on several factors. If a woman has reached menopause through surgery such as hysterectomy or through chemotherapy, her body's hormone levels will change more dramatically than if she goes through it naturally. Even in the latter case, however, some women naturally have higher levels of estrogen or testosterone, which causes increased vulnerability to breast cancer. We have observed, for example, that women with osteoporosis have 60 percent less breast cancer than women with normal bone density have; this is probably due to natural estrogen levels. If you have relatively high levels of estrogen in your body after menopause, you will have good bones and bad breasts; if your estrogen levels are lower, you will have good breasts and bad bones. These differences in residual hormonal stimulation may be reflected in the stroma and appear more dense on a mammogram than do those of a woman whose breasts totally retired and become mostly ducts suspended in fat.

SYNTHETIC HORMONES

Giving women hormones (estrogen and usually progestins) can create hormone-sensitive breast tumors (see Chapter 5). Also, women on postmenopausal hormones often, but not always, experience an increase in breast density, known to be a risk factor for breast cancer (see Chapter 6).

Yet not every woman who takes hormones after menopause gets breast cancer. It is likely that some women are more sensitive to postmenopausal hormones than others. Which ones and why remains a subject of much research. Recent studies suggest that mammographic breast density (see Chapter 9) may give us a hint. Karla Kerlikowske showed that postmenopausal women who had dense breasts on mammograms had a higher risk of cancer than those with fatty breasts.[15]

In addition, recent studies have shown that breast tissue itself has the enzyme aromatase, which can convert testosterone and androstenedione into estrogen. This means that estrogen levels in the breast may indeed be higher than those in the rest of the body after menopause and may explain the estrogen-sensitive cancers that can occur at this age. Our increasing understanding of the postmenopausal breast's response to hormones will give us further insight into the cause of breast cancer after menopause.

BRAS

In our society breasts and their coverings have become almost a fetish. The bra, a relatively recent invention, became popular in the 1920s as a replacement for the uncomfortable and often mutilating corsets of the nineteenth century. Wearing a bra is neither physically harmful nor medically necessary. Many of my large-breasted patients feel more comfortable wearing a bra, especially if they engage in athletic activities. As one patient said, "These babies need all the support they can get!"

Many women, however, find bras uncomfortable. Interestingly, I had one patient who got a rash underneath her breasts when she didn't wear a bra and her breasts sagged, and another who had very sensitive skin and got a rash when she *did* wear a bra, because of the elastic, the stitching, and the metal hooks (she switched to camisoles). Except for the women who find bras especially comfortable or uncomfortable, the decision to wear or not wear one is purely aesthetic—or emotional.

For some women, bras are a necessity created by society. One of my patients told me she enjoyed going without a bra, but, she said, "Men made nasty and degrading comments as I walked down the street." Another patient, a high school teacher, felt obligated to wear a bra to work, although she described it as "a ritual object, like a dog collar . . . I take it off immediately after work."

But some others like the uplift and the different contours a bra provides. A woman quoted in *Breasts* said she was "crazy about bras—I think of them as jewelry."[16] She and others find them sexy and enjoy incorporating them into their lovemaking rituals.

A popular belief maintains that wearing a bra strengthens your breasts and prevents sagging. But you sag because of the proportion of fat and tissue in your breasts, and no bra changes that. All a bra can do is hold your breasts up while you are wearing it. Furthermore, breast-feeding and lactation increase the size of the breasts, and when the tissue returns to its normal size the skin is stretched out and saggy. As I noted earlier, except for the small muscles of the areola and lobules, the muscles are behind your breast—and are unaffected by whether or not you wear a bra. If you've been wearing a bra regularly and decide to give it up, you may find that your breasts hurt for a while. Don't be alarmed. The connective tissue in which the ducts and lobules are suspended is suddenly being strained. It's the same tissue that hurts when you jog or run. Once your body adjusts to not wearing a bra, the pain will go away.

No type of bra is better or worse for you in terms of health. Some of my patients who wear underwire bras have been told they can get cancer from them. This is total nonsense. It makes no difference medically whether your bra has wires or not, opens in the front or back, is padded or not padded, is made of nylon, cotton, or any other material, or gives much support or little support. The only time I'd recommend a bra for medical reasons is after breast surgery. Then the pull from a hanging breast can cause more pain, slow the healing of the wound, and create larger scars. For this purpose, I suggest a firmer (but not underwire) bra rather than a lighter bra during the immediate postoperative period.

Otherwise, if you enjoy a bra for esthetic, sexual, or comfort reasons, by all means wear one. If you don't enjoy it, and job or social pressures don't force you into it, don't bother. Medically, it's all the same.

BREAST SENSITIVITY

Breasts are very sensitive—as you'll notice if you get hit in the breasts. But if you've been told that a breast injury leads to cancer, ignore it. All a bruised breast causes is temporary pain. Nor will scar tissue that may result from an injury to the breast cause cancer. Breast sensitivity changes during the menstrual cycle. During the first two weeks of the cycle the breasts are less sensitive; they are very sensitive around ovulation and after and less sensitive again during menstruation. There are also changes during the larger development process. There's little sensitivity before puberty, much sensitivity after puberty, and extreme sensitivity during pregnancy and perimenopause. After menopause, the sensitivity diminishes but never fully vanishes. As in most aspects of the normal breast, sensitivity varies greatly among women.

Breasts also vary greatly in their sensitivity to sexual stimuli. Physiologic changes in the breasts are an integral part of female sexual response. In the excitement phase the nipples harden and become more erect, the breasts plump up, and the areola swells. In the plateau just before orgasm breasts, nipples, and areola get larger still, peaking with the orgasm and then gradually subsiding. For most women, breast stimulation contributes to sexual pleasure. Many who enjoy having their breasts stroked or sucked by their lovers have been told that this can lead to cancer. It can't. Breasts, after all, are made to be suckled, and your body won't punish you because it's a lover rather than a baby doing it. Some women's breasts are so erogenous that breast stimulation alone can bring them to orgasm; others find breast stimulation uninteresting or even unpleasant. Neither extreme is more "normal." Different people have different sexual needs and respond to different sexual stimuli. Patients have asked me whether a lack of sexual responsiveness around their breasts means something is wrong with them. It doesn't. There is an unfortunate tradition in our culture to label as "frigid" women whose sexual needs don't correspond to those of their (usually) male partners. Ironically, the converse of this persists in our supposedly liberated era: a woman who is easily sexually stimulated is seen as a "slut." All such stereotypes are unfortunate and destructive. If your breasts contribute to your sexual pleasure, enjoy it. If not, focus on what you do like and don't worry.

GETTING ACQUAINTED WITH YOUR BREASTS

Babies, as yet unconditioned by social inhibitions, are wiser than their elders. Watch a baby gleefully playing with its toes. We smile at this but often stop smiling when the baby's joyful self-discovery focuses on the genitals. Then children learn that body parts associated with sexuality are taboo. We need to reverse this process, to teach little children to respect and cherish their bodies. And as adults, we need to reclaim that lesson for ourselves.

This is as true for breasts as for any other part of the body. Little girls should be encouraged to know their breasts, so that when the changes of puberty come about, they can experience their growing breasts with comfort and pride, and continue to do so for the rest of their lives. Most of us have not been raised that way, however, and it's often hard for an adult woman to begin feeling comfortable with her breasts. Yet it's important to know what your breasts feel like and what to expect from them. No part of your body should be foreign to you (Figure 1.18).

There are two things to remember as you read this section. One is that breasts are a body part, just as elbows and ribs are, and there's nothing shameful about exploring them. The other is that for many women they are centers of erotic feeling, and in the process of exploring them you might experience some sexual arousal. So what? That's a perfectly reasonable response. We've finally come to realize that it's a bad idea to teach kids to be ashamed of their sexual feelings; rather, we need to help them understand and cherish them. Similarly, we need to give ourselves permission to feel the entire range of reactions—sexual and nonsexual—to our own bodies.

To begin getting acquainted with your breasts, look at them. Stand in front of a mirror and look at yourself. See how your breasts hang and get a sense of how they project. If you're young they'll tend to stick out; if you're older they'll tend to be droopier. Feel the inframammary ridge, where the breast folds over itself, and the underlying muscles, the pectorals. Look at your nipple—what color is it? Does it have hairs or little bumps on it? If so, that's perfectly normal. You might want to swing your arms around and watch how your breasts move, or don't move, with the motion. Put your hands on your hips; flex your muscles; stretch your arms up. How do your breasts look with each change of position?

It's important to do this without criticizing your appearance. You're not trying out for a *Playboy* centerfold; you're learning about your body. Forget everything you've learned about what breasts are supposed to look like. These are your breasts, and they look fine.

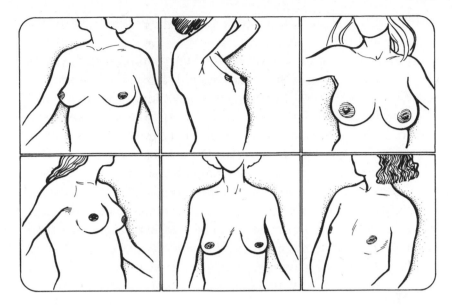

Figure 1.18

The next step is to feel your breasts. It's best to do this soaped up in the shower or bath. Your hands slip very easily over your skin. Put the hand of the side you want to explore behind your head. This shifts the breast tissue that's beneath your armpit to over your chest wall. Since the tissue is sandwiched between your skin and your chest bones you have good access to it. If you're very large-breasted you may want to do it lying down, in the bathtub, or even in bed. That allows you to roll on one side and then the other to shift the breast closer to your chest wall so you can get a better feel for it.

Breast tissue generally has a texture that is finely nodular or granular, like large seeds. A lot of this more or less bumpy feeling is caused by the normal fat that intermingles with the breast tissue. Lumpy breasts have inspired some of the most unfortunate misconceptions about our bodies. Often this lumpiness gets confused with actual breast lumps, as discussed in Chapter 3. But lumpiness itself often gets a bad press. Women have been told their lumpy breasts are symptoms of "fibrocystic disease" (see

Chapter 3) and have suffered from needless anxiety, fear, and even disfiguring surgery.

Lumpy breasts are caused by the way the breast tissue forms itself. In some women the breast tissue is fairly fine and thus not perceived as "lumpy." Others clearly have lumpy breasts, which can feel somewhat like cobblestone paving. Still others are somewhere between the extremes—just a bit nodular. There's nothing unusual about this—breasts vary as much as any other part of the body. Some women are tall and some short; some are fair-skinned and some dark; some have lumpier breasts and some have smoother breasts. There can even be differences within the same woman's breasts. Your breasts may be a little more nodular near your armpit or at the top, for example, and the pattern may be the same in both breasts or may occur only in one. You'll find, if you explore your breasts, that there's a general, fairly consistent pattern. It's important to get a sense of what your pattern is.

In the middle part of your chest you can feel your ribs. They jut out from your breastbone. If your ribs are very prominent or if you are thin or small-breasted, you may feel them under the breast tissue. Many women have congenital deformities in their ribs, which affect the flatness of the rib cage. This can show in different ways. When the ribs arch outward, a so-called chicken-breasted condition is produced. Then there's a sunken chest, in which the breastbone is depressed. Women can have either of these conditions and not realize it because their breasts camouflage their chest structure.

Another common variation in the rib cage occurs with scoliosis. Many women have minor scoliosis and never realize it. As you feel your breast tissue you may notice that your ribs are more prominent on one side or the other. This occurs because your back is not entirely straight. It has no real significance except that it can cause your ribs to be asymmetrical. Like the breasts, the rib cage is a little different in everyone, and it affects the feel of the breast area differently in different women.

Usually you'll feel more tissue up toward your armpit than in the middle of the breast. As I said earlier, the breast is really tear-shaped. The tissue toward the armpit is often the part that tends to get lumpier before your period and less lumpy after. There are lymph nodes in the armpits, as there are in many other parts of the body, and if you've had any sort of infection you might feel these nodes. The inframammary ridge, described earlier in this chapter, is an area of thickening, and the older you get, the thicker that area gets. It usually has some fat globules that are larger than in other areas. There's a hollow spot under the nipple, where the ducts join together to exit the nipple. Around this area is a ridge of tissue—shaped rather like the crater edge of a volcano.

All of this you can easily get to know with the pads of your fingers just by running your hand over your breast area, getting a sense of how it feels (see Figure 1.3). There's no point in grabbing at the breast. You won't get a good idea of its texture because you're pulling it forward into a big wad.

You can squeeze your nipple if you're curious about how it feels. Don't be surprised if there's some discharge—that's normal in many women. (If you're concerned about it, see Chapter 3.)

To become thoroughly acquainted with your breasts, explore them at different times of the month. Hormones affect your breasts and they'll feel different at different points in your menstrual cycle. It's interesting to be aware of these changes. Are they lumpier or more tender before your period? If you've had a hysterectomy but still have your ovaries, the hormone patterns continue: monitoring your breasts may help you know where you would have been in your menstrual cycle. If you're postmenopausal or if you've had your ovaries out and aren't taking hormones, the changes no longer occur. Your breast tissue in general will be less sore, less full, less lumpy. And if you take hormones, that too will affect your breasts (see Chapter 5). They often become enlarged and sore, although not necessarily firmer. Similarly, if you're on birth control pills, your breasts may respond to those hormonal changes by becoming more sore or less lumpy.

There's a good practical as well as psychological reason for knowing your breasts: such knowledge can help prevent needless biopsies. In our mobile era, you rarely have the same doctor all your life. If you've got a lump from something like silicone injections or scar tissue from a previous operation, your new doctor, who doesn't know your medical history, may well feel a biopsy is necessary. If you can say with conviction, "Yes, I know about that lump: it formed right after my operation 10 years ago, and it's been there ever since," the doctor will know the lump is okay. I've often been through this with patients. If a doctor thinks a lump is okay but the patient doesn't know whether or not it's been there a long while, the doctor has to assume it might be dangerous and will want to operate. If you know it's an old lump, your doctor won't have to worry.

If the doctor argues with you, argue back. Remember that you are a perfectly valid observer of your own body. You don't need to be a medical expert to know that you've had the same lump in the same place and it hasn't grown at all in 10 years. I had one eighty-year-old patient who came to me after her doctors insisted that she'd been wrong about a lump in her breast that looked trouble-some on her mammogram. Sexism and ageism can unite into a potent force, and obviously the doctors had decided that the "lit-tle old lady" didn't know what she was talking about when she told them her breast had been that way since her last child was born, 50 years earlier. They intimidated her, and she decided they must be right and had me do a biopsy. What I found was a con-genital condition, perfectly harmless, that she'd probably had all her life and noticed after breast-feeding. She knew her body in a way that her doctors couldn't.

Women with disabilities may have a more difficult time getting to know their bodies. Often they have less mobility and thus don't reach all areas of their bodies when they bathe. Some women use adaptive equipment to help them bathe—which is wonderful for its purpose but can't feel lumps, the way one's hand does. In such cases, more frequent physician examination is a good idea.

This process should start in adolescence. Its side benefits are marvelous—it teaches the girl to be comfortable with her own body, and it can be a pleasing rite of passage, a confirmation and exploration of her womanhood. Every woman should continue to explore her breasts periodically for the rest of her life, noting and embracing each change that all the stages of life entail in her breasts, as in the rest of her body. There is a powerful feeling that comes from knowing and becoming comfortable with your body—a feeling and a power that is yours alone and that no one can take from you.

This may all sound a bit like breast self-examination (BSE), but there's a crucial difference. In breast self-examination you're hunting for something. What I'm talking about is different— knowing your body, apart from anything ominous that may or may not occur there. For example, advocates of BSE tell you to examine your breasts once a month at the same time each month to see if there's a lump. What I'm suggesting, however, is that you check out your breasts at different times of the month to know how they feel at all times. Once you do know, you don't have to keep checking on a rigid schedule every month, unless that pleases you. (Do keep in mind that breasts, like the rest of your body, change over time, so it's worth exploring your breasts regularly, every couple of months, even after you feel fully acquainted with them. But again, this isn't on any particular timetable.)

The idea is to become familiar with your breasts as a significant part of your body, and to experience all their variations. Breast self-exam, on the other hand, has been set up as a way to monitor your breasts for cancer. Why am I making such a big point of this? I have very strong feelings about the concept of breast self-exam and its overuse. I think it alienates women from their breasts instead of making them more comfortable with them. It puts you in a position of examining yourself once a month to see if your breast has betrayed you. It pits you against your breast: can you find the tiniest lump that may be cancer?

Admittedly, breast cancer is scary. But setting up this alienation won't prevent it, and can cause its own set of problems. I get particularly alarmed when I hear people talk about teaching breast self-exam in the high schools. This takes young girls just developing breasts and, instead of teaching them to revel in their changing bodies, encourages them to see the breast as an enemy, something alien that has the ability to hurt them. It's a destructive way to define breasts.

Many women will stop me at this point and tell me that they or their friend found their cancer themselves. This is undoubtedly true: 80 percent of cancers not found on mammography are found by the woman herself. But when I ask these women to explain how they found the lump, I find that few actually did a formal breast self-exam, as seen on those shower cards you get from the American Cancer Society. More typically, the woman just rolled over in bed, or felt a lump while soaping up in the shower, or had it pointed out by a lover. This touching and knowing your body is what can help you find cancer, not the rigid routine outlined involved in BSE. (For more on BSE, see Chapter 9.)

Chapter 2

VARIATIONS IN DEVELOPMENT AND PLASTIC SURGERY

HEALTHY BREASTS COME IN MANY DIFFERENT SHAPES AND SIZES. There's nothing "abnormal" about large, small, or asymmetrical breasts, or about extra nipples.

Common variations in breast development fall into one of two categories: those that are obvious from birth and those that don't show themselves until puberty. The latter are far more frequent. (There are also variations due to accident or illness, the surgical remedies for which are essentially the same as those used for genetic variations.)

VARIATIONS APPARENT AT BIRTH

The most common variation to appear at birth is polymastia—an extra nipple or nipples. These can appear anywhere along the milk ridge (see Figure 1.11). Usually the milk ridge—a throwback to the days when we were animals with many nipples—regresses before birth, but in some people it remains throughout life. Between 1 and 5 percent of extra nipples are on women whose mothers also had extra nipples. Usually they're below the breast, and often women don't even know they're there, since they look like moles. When I would point out an extra nipple to a patient, it was usually the first time she'd been aware of it.

Extra nipples cause no problems and usually don't appear cosmetically unattractive. One patient was actually fond of her extra nipple. She told me that her husband had one too, and that's how they knew they were meant for each other! Men sometimes *do* have extra nipples, though as far as we know, less frequently than women do. This may be a result of some biological factor we don't yet know about, or it may simply be that men and their doctors don't notice the nipples because they're covered by chest hair.

Extra nipples don't cause any problems, though they may lactate if you breast-feed. There's nothing wrong with this, unless it causes you discomfort. A variation of the extra nipple is extra breast tissue without a nipple, most often under the armpit. It may feel like hard, cyst-like lumps that swell and hurt the way your breasts do when you menstruate. Like extra nipples, this extra breast tissue is often unnoticed by doctor and patient. One of my patients found that she had swelling under both armpits during her second pregnancy. It was probably caused by extra breast tissue and it went down after she finished lactating. The extra tissue is subject to all the problems of normally situated tissue. I have had patients with cysts, fibroadenomas, or even cancers in such tissue.

Unless the extra nipple or breast tissue causes you extreme physical discomfort or psychological distress, there's no need to worry about it. If it does bother you, it's easy to get rid of surgically. The nipple can be removed under local anesthetic in your doctor's office, and the extra breast tissue can be removed under either local or general anesthetic.

A much rarer condition is known as amastia—being born with a breast that has breast tissue but no nipple. It's usually associated with problems in the development of the chest bone and muscles, like scoliosis and rib deformities. Aside from whatever medical procedures you may need because of the associated problems, you might want to have a fake nipple created by a plastic surgeon, the same way a nipple is created during reconstruction after a mastectomy (see Chapter 15). The nipple can be created using skin from the breast and the areola can be tattooed on or created using a skin graft, commonly from the inner thigh. The skin becomes darker after it's grafted and, if it still doesn't match the color of your other nipple, it can be tattooed to a darker shade. Though this artificial nipple will look real, it won't feel completely like a real nipple. There is no erectile tissue, so it won't change as your other nipple does. It's usually constructed midway between erect and flat. It will have no sensation because it has no nerves. Because it won't have ducts, it can't produce milk. Its advantages are wholly cosmetic.

Some women have an underdeveloped breast on one side. This condition is sometimes called Poland's syndrome, and it involves not just the breast but also the pectoralis muscle and the ribs, as well as, in some cases, abnormalities of the hand. A woman with Poland's syndrome may have a small but very deformed breast. A patient of mine in Los Angeles was doubly unlucky. She had been born with Poland's syndrome and had a very undeveloped breast on one side. When she developed breast cancer in the good breast, she was anxious to have a lumpectomy rather than a mastectomy. She very much wanted to preserve her only functional breast.

There is another condition in which women have permanently inverted nipples (they grow in instead of out)—a congenital condition that usually doesn't manifest until puberty.

Various injuries can affect breast development. This may happen surgically or with trauma. If the nipple and breast bud are seriously injured before puberty, the potential adult breast is destroyed as well. Sometimes injuring the skin can limit future breast development. Most commonly this occurs as a result of a severe burn. The resulting scars are so tight that breast tissue cannot develop. In the past, some congenital conditions such as hemangiomas (birthmarks) were treated with radiation, which damaged the nipple and breast bud and prevented later growth. Any serious injury to the breast bud can cause such arrested development.

VARIATIONS APPEARING AT PUBERTY

Three basic variations appear when the breasts begin to develop: extremely large breasts, extremely small breasts, and asymmetrical breasts.

Very Large Breasts

Very large breasts can occur early in puberty—a condition known as "virginal hypertrophy." After the breasts begin to grow, the shut-off mechanism, whatever it is, forgets to do its job and the breasts keep on growing, becoming huge and greatly out of proportion to the rest of the body. Sometimes the condition runs in families. In very rare instances, virginal hypertrophy occurs in one breast and not the other. It's worth noting here that "large" is both subjective and variable. A five-foot-tall woman with a C cup is very large-breasted; a five-foot-eight woman with a C cup may not feel especially uncomfortable with her size. A five-foot-eight woman with a DD cup is likely to be very uncomfortable.

Large breasts have been a problem for a number of my patients. "I almost never wear a bathing suit," one patient told me, "because people stare at my breasts." Another, at 71, still "hunches over" when she walks to avoid having her breasts stared at.

Huge breasts can be very distressful to a teenage girl. She faces ridicule from her schoolmates, and—unlike the small-breasted girl—extreme physical discomfort as well. She may be unable to participate in sports, and she may have severe backache all the time. She usually needs a bra to hold the breasts in, but the bra, pulled down by the weight of the breasts, can dig painful ridges into her shoulders.

If the breasts cause this much discomfort, the girl may want to have reduction surgery done while she's still in her teens. (See later in this chapter.) The surgical trauma involved in breast reduction can interfere with the ability to breast-feed. For this reason, some mothers refuse to let their daughters have reduction surgery, urging them to wait until they've had children. Both mother and daughter must weigh the physical and emotional damage the girl will go through first. If she decides to have children, pregnancy may worsen her problem. When the breasts become engorged with milk, they become even larger and, in a woman with huge breasts, more uncomfortable. Though it's unfortunate that someone so young is faced with a decision that affects her whole life, it's important to realize that not having the surgery will also affect her life. Many girls of 15 or 16 are mature enough to make their own decisions if all the facts are carefully explained to them, including the possibility of bottle-feeding. In any case, the losses and gains of either choice are the girl's, and she should be given the right and the time to decide for herself what to do. She should be encouraged to talk to doctors, mothers of young children, and very large-breasted women; to read all the material she can find about the pros and cons of the procedure and of breast-feeding; and to make her decision only when she feels she is fully informed.

Not all problems with huge breasts appear right after puberty. Some comfortably large-breasted women find that their breasts have expanded considerably after pregnancy; others become uncomfortable after their breast size has increased with an overall weight gain or after menopause. Many surgeons are reluctant to operate in the latter case, preferring to wait till the woman has lost weight because of the increased risk of wound-healing complications. Sometimes, however, this can backfire psychologically. I've known women who were so depressed by their huge breasts that they compensated by overeating, thus intensifying both problems. In such cases, the pleasing appearance of their breasts created by reduction surgery can be a spur to continue their self-improvement.

In any case, the decision must be made by the individual woman; she's the one who lives with the problem and she's the one who can best judge its impact on her life. Some women with very large breasts don't mind them. One patient, who admits they cause her discomfort, nonetheless enjoys their size because, she says, "they feel feminine and sexy."

Very Small Breasts

The opposite problem is extreme flat-chestedness. Like "large-breasted," the notion of "small-breasted" is subjective and relative, and culturally determined. Some women, however, have breasts so small that their chests look like men's. This causes no physical or medical problems but can make a woman feel unattractive and sexless.

Because very small breasts can both feed babies and respond sexually, some women aren't bothered by them. Others are satisfied simply by wearing "falsies" or padded bras. Some want to have the breasts altered surgically. (I'll discuss this later in the chapter.)

Asymmetrical Breasts

In most women breasts develop unevenly to some degree. But in some they develop quite differently, resulting in severe asymmetry. For a woman who is bothered by this, plastic surgery can help achieve a reasonable match. Either the larger breast can be reduced or the smaller one augmented—or a combination of both can be done. It's important for the surgeon to discuss these options. Often we assume a woman will want her small breast made larger and fail to suggest the possibility of reducing the larger breast. What a woman decides will depend on the size of both breasts, the degree of asymmetry, and above all her own esthetic goals.

It's fortunate that plastic surgery techniques exist for women who want them. But don't assume that because you have atypical-looking breasts you have to get them altered. Many women are quite pleased with how their breasts look. Some women with large breasts feel, as did the patient I mentioned earlier, that their breasts are "feminine and sexy." Small breasts too have their advantages. One of my patients liked her small breasts because "they're unobtrusive, and they worked well during nursing. Occasionally some male person will intimate that they're less than optimal. That's his problem, not mine." Another liked her tiny breasts ("they're really just enlarged nipples") because they didn't get in her way when she engaged in sports. A patient with asymmetrical breasts said she used to feel self-conscious but had "come to terms with them" since she nursed her child.

And another patient tells a wonderful story about a friend of hers who had inverted nipples. "When I was 12 and my cousin was 14, we stood before the bathroom mirror and compared breasts. I noticed how different her nipples were; they didn't protrude the way mine did. We had this big discussion about whose were 'normal.' I was convinced mine were, but she insisted hers were, and since she was older and, I thought, more knowledge-able, I decided she must be right.

"After she graduated from college and was studying in Paris, she became ill and had to be hospitalized. The doctor who was ex-amining her asked if her nipples 'had always been like that.' That's how she learned that she had inverted nipples—and that mine were the normal ones!"

PLASTIC SURGERY

No operation is medically necessary in these cases. Still, it's good to know such operations are available. For a woman deeply un-happy with the way her breasts look, plastic surgery offers a solu-tion that can make a major psychological difference in her life. No operation will make you look "perfect" (whatever that is), but all of these procedures can help you feel more normal and more comfortable in your body.

If you're thinking about plastic surgery, you should ask yourself a few questions. The first and probably most important is, who wants the surgery? If you're content with your breasts but your mother or boyfriend or someone else is pressuring you into it, you probably shouldn't do it. It's your body, not theirs.

The second question is, how realistic are your expectations, and how clear an idea do you have about the kind of breasts you want? It is crucial that you and your surgeon have the same goal, and this requires good communication and reasonable expecta-tions that are spelled out in advance. Dr. John T. Heuston, a noted plastic surgeon, has written some wise words about reduc-tion surgery that can apply to all forms of cosmetic surgery for the breasts.[1] "The concept of an ideal operation," he writes, "carries with it the concept of an ideal breast. The surgeon seeks the best means to construct the breast form—but for whom? For him or her, or for the patient, or both?" As Heuston notes, there is no ob-jectively ideal breast; each of us has her own ideal. So you should have a clear sense of what size and shape of breast you want, and what your own goals are. The surgeon can't make your breasts ab-solutely perfect, but if your goals are fairly reasonable, they can come close to being met. If you do decide on plastic surgery, make sure you know the range of possible results. Some plastic surgeons like to "sell" their operation. If you're shown pictures of a surgeon's best results insist on seeing pictures of the average and worst results as well.

Once you know what you want, don't hesitate to shop around for the right plastic surgeon. You should choose someone you feel absolutely comfortable with and confident in. Above all, it should be someone who respects your ideal and doesn't seek to impose her or his ideal on you. The surgeon's "beautiful breast" and yours may be very dissimilar. Make sure you find someone who will construct *your* breast. And make sure you find someone who respects who you are, and why you're making your decision. If the surgeon you've approached acts insulting or condescending, even if that surgeon has a good reputation, go out and find someone with a more professional, more humane approach. It is also a good idea to find a surgeon who is board certified by the American Board of Plastic Surgery. This ensures that the surgeon has gone through good training and a rigorous certification process.

Of course, even if you have taken every precaution possible there's no guarantee that you'll be happy with your operation after it's done. But the odds are on your side. I've had very few patients who regretted having their breasts cosmetically altered, but I've had several who regretted not having it done. One of my Boston patients was an eighty-year-old woman with huge, uncomfortable breasts. When she was younger, she went to a surgeon to try and get her breasts reduced. He told her she shouldn't have the operation. She took his advice—those were the days when doctors were gods; you didn't question them—and since then had been uncomfortable and unhappy with her breasts. After we talked she decided to have the surgery done. She was very happy with her small breasts—and very sad about all the years she could have been this comfortable.

Another of my patients was a sophisticated career woman in her early thirties. During our first visit I noticed that her breasts were extremely asymmetrical, and after a few visits I asked her if she'd ever thought about plastic surgery. Her face lit up. "Can I really do that?" she asked me. I assured her that she could, and gave her a list of plastic surgeons. She didn't even wait till she got out of the building to call them; she found a phone booth downstairs, made an appointment, and had her implant within the month. She was absolutely delighted with it—but she needed me to suggest it and to give her "permission" to seek help for her asymmetry. Psychiatrist Sanford Gifford writes about a patient feeling she had "gained something lost in early puberty."[2] He observes that the degree of satisfaction is much greater among women who have had plastic surgery for their breasts than among those who have had face-lifts or nose jobs—they don't have the same unrealistic expectations. Often they're happier with their still imperfect breasts than the surgeon thinks they should be. For some reason people don't go into this kind of plastic surgery with the same dreams of impossible perfection they bring to facial surgery.

Interestingly, the first recorded breast surgery was done on a man with gynecomastia in A.D. 625.[3] Mammoplasty was not performed on a woman until over a thousand years later, in 1897—but we needn't feel too deprived. With the primitive state of surgery in the past, that poor man in the seventh century couldn't have had a comfortable time of it. Anyone contemplating plastic surgery today has much better options.

Good breast reduction techniques have now been with us for decades. Augmentation, as I mentioned earlier, is a much more recent procedure.

From a surgical standpoint the procedures are quite safe. They are often labeled "unnecessary surgery," and of course they *are* unnecessary in the sense that you won't die without them. But for many women the risk is well worth the chance of improved self-image and, in the case of large breasts, increased physical comfort.

Plastic surgery has always raised ethical concerns, especially for feminists. We have been told that we aren't right as we are, that we need to change our looks to please men or a particular man. Cosmetic surgery is often seen as a high-tech version of painful assaults on the body that women have experienced for centuries—like foot binding, corsets, genital mutilation. Rather than subjecting our bodies to procedures that carry the risk all surgery entails and may even cause other health problems, many activists in the women's health movement argue, we should change society's approach so that we don't feel the need to have "perfect" or "ideal" bodies. That's true, but it's hard to change emotions, and some women prefer to compromise with their utopian ideals and take advantage of plastic surgery.

Before we get into the various kinds of plastic surgery, there's a practical consideration you need to address: insurance. You'll want to check with your insurance company about what forms of plastic surgery it will or won't pay for. You'll also want to find out if the insurance company has a disclaimer or exclusion for coverage of future implant-related health problems (medical/surgical). You may have to shoulder the financial responsibility for the procedure yourself, and this often includes taking responsibility for the financial burden of any complications, hospitalizations, or future tests.

Breast Reduction

Most women come for this operation because they're embarrassed by their large breasts or because they have discomfort from neck and back pain. As with the other operations described in this chapter, a woman who is over 40 should have a mammogram to make sure there's no cancer.

It is important to think ahead of time about what size you want to be. Dr. William Shaw, a plastic surgeon and one of my former colleagues at UCLA, points out that it is difficult to be sure that the patient and the surgeon both have the same idea of what a B or C cup is. Cup size also depends greatly on the bra manufacturer. Victoria's Secret, for example, is notorious for overestimating cup size, whereas JC Penney somewhat underestimates. Dr. Shaw often asks patients to bring in pictures from magazines to be sure he knows what their expectations are. It's not always possible to get exactly the size you want, but a good surgeon can approximate it. There are a number of variations of the breast reduction operation, but all start with the same basic procedure.

The operation is usually done under general anesthesia and takes place the day you're admitted to the hospital. The procedure may be performed in an outpatient or 23-hour-stay setting. You will be given antibiotics prior to the operation in order to prevent infection. Often photographs are taken of your breasts to document how they looked before the surgery. The surgeon will have you stand up and then will mark out the planned operation on your chest. This is important because you will be lying on your back during the operation and it could be hard to determine the exact place to reposition your nipples. Your nipples can be either removed and grafted back, or left on breast tissue and moved up. Most doctors today prefer not to graft the nipples except in extremely large reductions, since they lose sensitivity if all the nerves are severed. They may also develop areas of lighter pigmentation, and there is no guarantee that they will heal onto the underlying tissue completely. The surgery may last up to four hours.

Most procedures involve some variation of what is known as the keyhole technique. The amount of tissue to be removed is determined (Figure 2.1), and the nipple is preserved on a small flap of tissue while the tissue to be removed is taken from above and from the sides. This allows the surgeon to elevate the nipple and bring the flaps of tissue together, giving both uplift and reduction. The resulting scars are below the breast in the inframammary fold and come right up the center to the nipple and around it. In recent years there has been a preference for shorter incisions under the breast. In some cases only a circular scar around the nipple is used—the so-called doughnut, or concentric, reduction pattern. It is important that you fully understand the way that your plastic surgeon plans to do the operation as well as what scars you can expect. That way there will be no surprises when the bandages are removed. The shorter scar techniques are typically reserved for minimal reductions, and may not be the best option if a lot of tissue is to be removed.

Patients experience pain the first day after the operation, but very little after that. You can go home the next morning, wearing a bra or some form of support. Surgeons vary as to whether or not they use drains; if they do, the drains usually come out after one day. The stitches are typically dissolvable, and you can go back to work within one to two weeks; in three to four weeks you can be

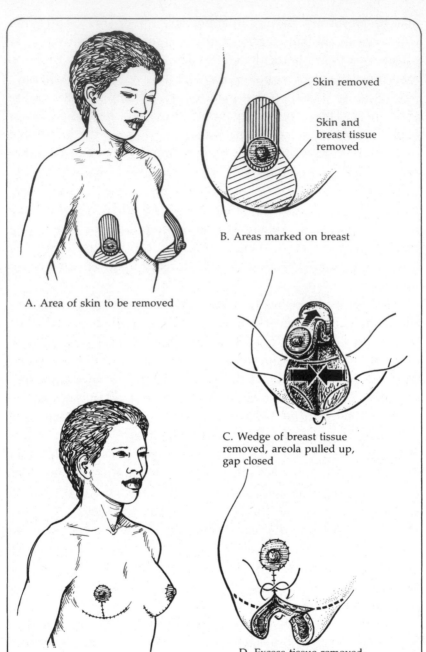

A. Area of skin to be removed

B. Areas marked on breast

Skin removed

Skin and breast tissue removed

C. Wedge of breast tissue removed, areola pulled up, gap closed

D. Excess tissue removed, skin closed with stitches

E. Post-operative appearance

Figure 2.1

playing tennis. After this surgery women consistently report satisfaction with the results, as well as a reduction in their symptoms prior to surgery.

Although women have a high level of satisfaction with the improvement in symptoms, breast reductions do have a risk of complications, including infection and bleeding, which can occur with any operation. There's a slight risk that you'll need blood transfusions, but it's very rare these days. If you're worried, however, give your own blood to the hospital two or three months in advance, and it will be there in case you need it. There's some danger of the operation interfering with the blood supply to the nipple and areola; if this happens the nipple and areola die and need to be artificially reconstructed. It's not a very great danger—it happens in less than 4 percent of operations. The larger your breasts are, the greater the danger. Reduction does not affect a woman's risk of cancer. Your ability to breast-feed will be decreased, but studies show that about half of women who have had reductions can still nurse their babies depending on the extent of the surgery.

Some of the erotic sensation in your nipples may be reduced, though for many women the increased relaxation actually makes sex more pleasurable after reduction surgery. Also, because the nerves in the nipple of the overlarge breast are so stretched out, the nipple is unlikely to have much sensitivity to begin with, and the loss of sensation—in terms of both sexual activity and breast-feeding—will probably go unnoticed. There's also a possibility of reduced sensitivity in the breast itself, although again this is minimal. There's no way to know in advance whether or not you'll experience reduced sensation, so you have to decide for yourself how important full sensation is, compared to whatever physical or emotional discomfort your large breasts create for you. In any case, you'll still retain most of your breast sensation. Some women develop increased sensitivity in their nipples, although this usually diminishes with time.

If you do decide to have reduction surgery, be aware that if you later gain weight, your breasts will probably also gain weight, just as they would without the surgery. This has happened to a number of my patients. One woman had her size 36EE breasts reduced to a 36B, but they ended up a 36D. With all of this, women undergoing breast reduction surgery are almost always happy they did.

Breast Augmentation

Although breast reduction surgery is generally well accepted by everyone as a reasonable operation, views of breast augmentation are more charged. I received criticisms from ardent feminists when the first edition of this book was published because I did not condemn this procedure. While there is some merit to this concern, it doesn't seem reasonable to me. First, it takes a very paternalistic—or maternalistic—view of what's best for other people. Second, some women have practical needs for bodies that society defines as ideal—like the young women I used to meet in my Los Angeles practice who were trying to succeed as actresses and models. Third, even for women whose needs are emotional rather than practical, the feelings are deeply ingrained—they can't just decide not to feel that way. Years of fighting an uphill battle against internalized social expectations can be as devastating as physical illness. A nose job, a face-lift, or a breast enlargement can make a major difference in a woman's life—and whether that would or wouldn't be the case in an ideal world is beside the point.

Not everyone who wants to alter her body is a bimbo. Over the years, I've had a range of patients who wanted their breasts augmented. Among them was a married gynecologist, a well-educated professional, not terribly young, who had silicone implants and said they had made a tremendous difference in her life, and that she'd do it again if she had to make the choice today. Another had gotten her implants in 1980 at the age of 40. "For the first time in my life I was proud of my figure," she told me. "I felt like a new woman." Perhaps it's a pity that society has made these women feel that way, and we can work to change the way we're taught to view our bodies. But meanwhile, we all have irrational feelings that deeply affect our lives, and nobody needs to be a martyr.

Silicone Implants

The societal pressures around breast augmentation have been made even worse with the controversies regarding the safety of silicone. The history of silicone implants is worth reviewing. In 1976 Congress told the FDA to regulate medical devices. At that time they decided that everything that was on the market prior to that time would be grandfathered in. Thus from 1976 to 1991 silicone implants could be marketed in the United States if they had been marketed prior to 1976, had a good safety record, or were substantially the same as those used before 1976. The assumption was that they were safe. In 1992 as a result of patient activism the FDA decided that appropriate studies to prove the safety of the implants had not been done, mostly because they had not been required. The implants were removed from the general market until their safety was proven. From 1992 to 2005 they could be used only for patients enrolled in research studies and women undergoing reconstruction. In 2005 the latest generation of silicone implants are approved for women undergoing breast reconstruction after mastectomy, and in 2006 they were approved for any woman over 22 desiring them for cosmetic purposes. While there has been much controversy about them during this time, the system worked. The correct studies were done and women again have access to a device that can be used for cosmetic reasons or reconstruction.

As you can see, silicone implants have been the source of much controversy since the first edition of this book came out. I don't mean to dismiss women's concerns about silicone implants. The biggest concern of the activists, however, remains unproven: the idea that the gel can cause an *autoimmune* disorder (a condition in which the immune system, once turned on, gets carried away and starts attacking the body and connective tissue). The most common of these are scleroderma, lupus, rheumatoid arthritis, dermatomyositis, and Sjorgen's syndrome. No studies have made any connections between the incidence of such diseases and silicone implants. A comprehensive review of over 15 epidemiological studies covering 4,000 women showed no increased risk of connective tissue diseases among women with breast implants.[4] So the fact that someone with implants gets such a disease doesn't mean there is a connection: they may simply be two unrelated facts in the woman's life.

Another concern was whether silicone implants increased the risk of breast cancer. The best study was in Los Angeles County, where over 3,000 women who had silicone implants were studied for a number of years, and their breast cancer rates compared to the expected incidence of breast cancer in LA.[5] Not only was there no increase in breast cancer in women with implants, but there appeared to be a possible decrease. This was substantiated by a second study in Alberta, Canada, in which 13,577 women with breast cancer were studied and only 41 of them had implants.[6] The researchers concluded that there was a lower risk of breast cancer in these women. This may be because plastic surgeons are less likely to put implants into women who are high risk for breast cancer. Women with implants also tend to be thinner and thus at lower risk. Interestingly, there are data in animals showing that silicone may protect against breast cancer. We have no idea at this point why this may be so. It does not, of course, suggest that women should run out and get implants as a way to protect them from breast cancer. But it certainly does suggest that silicone implants aren't the grave danger that they were once portrayed to be.

Implants can, however, interfere with how well mammograms can detect tumors in the breast. If you have implants it is important that you get your mammograms in a center specializing in breast imaging, since they can use special techniques to maximize the amount of breast visualized. MRI is another screening option for women with implants. (This is done differently than the MRI used to detect rupture, as we'll discuss below.) And certainly a woman should have any lump or change in her augmented breasts checked out.

There are more common problems that can happen with implants, which, though less serious than breast cancer, need to be considered. Silicone isn't the wholly inert substance it was once thought to be, and it always creates some reaction around it. Minuscule amounts of silicone will always leak. The reaction may be something that you'd never notice or be bothered by—the sort of thing that shows up only if the breast is biopsied. But it may be bothersome to some women.

Contracture—the formation of a thick, spherical scar tissue that causes the breast to be overly firm (Figure 2.2)—is a real possibility with most implants. Implants may be done either under

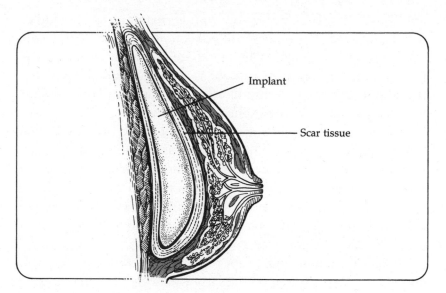

Figure 2.2

the muscle or between the muscle and the breast; both may undergo contracture. This occurs in 1–18 percent of cases in which the implant is under the muscle, and in 18–50 percent of cases in which it's between the muscle and breast. This firmness can be unnoticeable or it can feel like solid wood—or anything in between. Contracture can be painful, and it can change the appearance of the breast. It can happen to one implant and not the other, or may happen differently in the two implants, leaving one side higher than the other. Further, the incidence of contracture tends to increase over time. Thus results that still look great 5 to 10 years after the procedure may develop progressive distortion and contracture by 15 or 20 years. Another long-term problem can be rupture. Although some silicone always escapes from the surface of the implant, it does appear that the longer an implant is in place, the higher the chance for rupture. Some reports suggest that the rate of rupture is as high as 55 percent 10 to 15 years after surgery. As a result, some plastic surgeons recommend that implants be replaced every 10 years. Rupture is usually diagnosed by seeing a change in the size, shape, or consistency of the implant. It can also be detected through mammography coupled with ultrasound. The most sensitive tool, however, is MRI, which can show very accurately whether there has been a rupture and where. When gel implants rupture or leak, the bulk of the material stays together inside the fibrous scar capsule. Therefore the outside appearance may not change for some time.

The alternative to silicone is an implant filled with saline. This works similarly to silicone, except that saline—saltwater—is inside the silicone shell, instead of silicone gel. Saline implants are no more likely to leak than silicone, but when they do leak the saline becomes absorbed by the body fairly quickly, so that you realize suddenly that your breast has shrunk. Saline leakage won't cause any medical problems.

Saline has a somewhat less realistic feel than silicone. It's more like a bag of water, particularly when the covering tissue is thin.

Patients with saline implants have complained about problems of capsular contracture, poor aesthetic results, asymmetry, a fluid-like feeling in the breasts, and "rippling" of the breast skin surface due to rippling of the implant shell and capsule. These, however, are all part of the standard issues related to the use of implants; imperfect results occur sometimes. There are no known, specific, documented problems with the saline material itself, in contrast to gel material.

As noted earlier, women over 40 who are considering plastic surgery for their breasts should have a mammogram to rule out cancer. In addition, the surgeon should check for cysts that require needle aspiration (see Chapter 3). As one plastic surgeon put it, "You don't want to be sticking needles into the patient's breast when there's a silicone gel bag inside it." The plastic surgeon will also take a careful history.

The surgeon should show you pictures of breasts that have been augmented, including those with very visible scars, so you know both the best and the worst possible results of your operation. As with reductions, there are many pictures available on the Internet. You and the surgeon should also discuss what size you want your new breasts to be, and you need to be realistic about that—you may not have enough breast tissue to accommodate

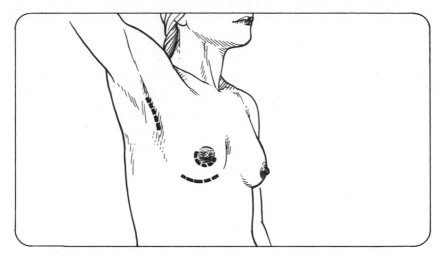

Figure 2.3

very large implants. Every augmentation should be appropriate for the size and build of the patient.

The operation can be done under either local or general anesthetic. The incision is made either through the armpit, underneath the breast, or around the areola (Figure 2.3). All of these have their proponents. As I have already pointed out, the implant can be placed under the breast tissue between the breast and the muscles or under the muscle (Figure 2.4). According to one of my plastic surgeon colleagues, putting the implant under the muscle has two disadvantages: a tendency for a flatter breast and the possibility of movement of the breast with the muscle. But it has two advantages: it seems to carry less risk of contracture and, even more important, it's less likely to hide a future cancer. Where the implant is placed is not merely a matter of choice. For some patients the result is better with the implant under the muscle, whereas for others it is better under the breast. Your plastic surgeon will help you through this process.

The operation is usually done on an outpatient basis; it takes about two hours or more, depending on whether or not the surgeon puts the implant under the muscle, which takes more time. You go home soon after the operation. The stitches are usually dissolvable. You'll be out of work for about two to five days, and shouldn't drive a car for a week. In three weeks you'll be able to jog or play tennis.

Side effects can include infection, which occurs in less than 1 percent of cases, and bleeding, which is equally rare. There may be permanent altering of sensation in the nipple or areola, which occurs in less than 2 percent of cases, and there is also a slight possibility of reduced sensation in the breast. There's also the possibility of visible scarring and contracture, both discussed earlier. And there is some possibility that lactation can be affected, unless the surgeon makes sure the scar is not next to the areola and no ducts are severed.

Implant rupture, as noted earlier, is a possible serious complication, though not a common one. It can occur through strenuous physical force or just spontaneously. Although this sounds like an emergency, it is not necessarily. Women live with ruptured silicone implants for years. If the implant is to be replaced the surgeon must try to take out all the silicone in a procedure known as *explantation*. This is tedious surgery, and it requires a surgeon experienced in the procedure.

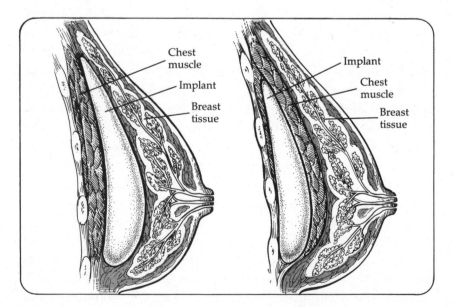

Figure 2.4

The safety studies give us a picture of how common these complications are in the first three years. It is estimated that one in five women who undergo augmentation will undergo an additional operation. Forty-two percent are for size or shape change and 33 percent are for leakage or deflation. For some women it is worth it to feel better about their bodies. This can be a problem over time. One woman on Facebook writes: "I had to have my implants replaced several times. I am thinking of removing them this fall." Her concerns have led her to think about the complexity of women's feelings about their breasts. "There is a real story to be passed on to the younger generation about the maintenance of and problems with breast implants. The breasts are such an integral part of the feminine and the nurturing. How are we nurturing ourselves?"

Luckily for women who want implants, plastic surgeons and manufacturers are now studying alternative materials to be used as fillers in breast implants in place of silicone or saline. There are new types of implants under study, including the "gummy bear" implant, where the silicone sticks together like a gummy bear candy and therefore should be less likely to leak. The critical point for any woman contemplating this surgery is to carefully investigate carefully the surgeon and approach ahead of time.

Surgery for Asymmetry

To correct major asymmetry, the doctor can use one of three procedures, and it's important for you to know which of the three you want. You can, as noted earlier, have an implant put in one, or you can have the other made smaller, or you can have a combination of both. Mastopexy, or breast lifting, is another procedure that may be useful in addressing breast asymmetry.

If your asymmetry results from Poland's syndrome or an injury, appropriate breast reconstruction (see Chapter 15) utilizing expanders, implants, or your own tissues can achieve a reasonable result. Unlike the situation of the woman with small but symmetrical breasts, the scars created in the area the tissue is taken from are likely to disturb you less than the asymmetry itself. The procedures used to reconstruct a breast after mastectomy are also a possibility (see Chapter 15).

When you're thinking of implants for asymmetry, keep in mind that exact matching is unlikely. If there's a difference in nipple and areola size, the implant operation will stretch the nipple and areola on the smaller breast. And since silicone has now been added under tight skin, the augmented breast will tend not to sag like a normal breast does as you age. Still, these differences are minor compared to the original asymmetry, and it's likely that you will be the only one to notice. Remember, you may need to have your implant replaced at some point, so be sure you know what size it is.

The Breast Lift

Some women are unhappy over the way their breasts sag as they age. Sagging breasts (known medically as ptosis) can be made firmer through an operation called a mastopexy, sometimes called "a face-lift for the breasts." A mastopexy can give your breasts up-lift but will not make them look like a twenty-year-old's. And it will leave scars—sometimes bad ones, depending on how your body usually scars. Like a face-lift, it won't last forever. Remember, you've got gravity and time working against you.

As with the other procedures we've considered, your plastic surgeon will take a very thorough medical history, and you should get a mammogram if you haven't had one recently. Be sure to get a full description of both the best and the worst possible results of a mastopexy and do an Internet search to find photos.

This operation usually involves removing excess skin and fat and elevating the nipple (Figure 2.5). If you're very large-breasted, you may want reduction surgery as well, especially since a mastopexy is less effective on very large breasts: gravity pulls them down further. If you're very small-breasted, you may want an augmentation, although augmentation mastopexy is one of the more difficult aesthetic breast procedures and you should seek a surgeon experienced in it. This procedure is difficult because you are trying to accomplish two seemingly opposite goals: on the one hand you are trying to make the breast larger (augmentation) whereas on the other hand you are trying to make the breast

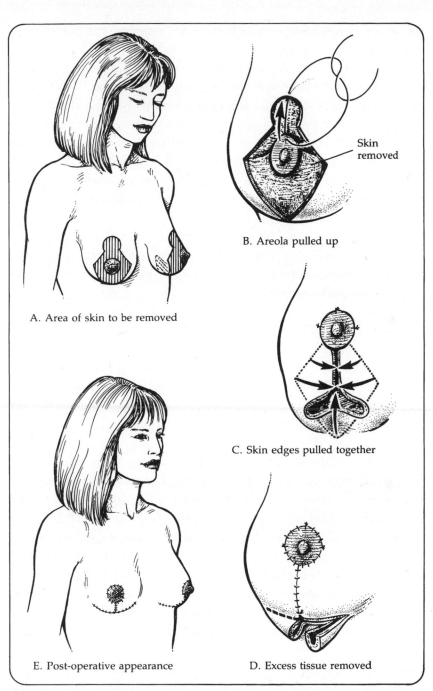

A. Area of skin to be removed

B. Areola pulled up

Skin removed

C. Skin edges pulled together

D. Excess tissue removed

E. Post-operative appearance

Figure 2.5

droop less (mastopexy). An experienced surgeon can find a balance that is right for you.

If your operation doesn't involve reduction or augmentation, it's a simpler procedure and can be done either in the hospital under general anesthesia or in the doctor's office with local anesthesia. Since insurance won't pay for it, most women prefer the latter. The operation lasts about two and a half hours; the stitches are usually dissolvable. By three weeks, you'll be able to participate in sports. You should wear a bra constantly for many weeks after surgery. Follow-up is minimal—three or four visits during the year after surgery.

You may experience some very slight loss of sensation in the nipple or areola. Other than that, there are no particular side effects to mastopexy, apart from the usual risks of any surgery such as bleeding and infection.

Inverted Nipples

There is an operation that can reverse nipple inversion. It's a simple procedure, usually done under local anesthetic with no intravenous medication, and you can go back to work the next day. The stitches may be dissolvable or may be removed in about two weeks.

Nipples are usually inverted because they are tethered down by scar or other tissue from birth. The surgeon will pull the nipple, stretch it, and make an incision, releasing the constricting tissue (Figure 2.6). There are a number of procedures, and each one has its advocates. If the inversion recurs, the operation can be redone. Sometimes the procedure causes a problem, since part of the nipple may scab and fall off because of the lack of blood supply.

This operation can make a psychological difference for teenagers, who often feel self-conscious about having inverted nipples. It definitely interferes with breast-feeding, but women with inverted nipples usually have difficulty with breast-feeding anyway.

If you are considering plastic surgery for your breasts, make sure you have all the information you need about risks, dangers, and reasonable expectations—and then do what you want. And

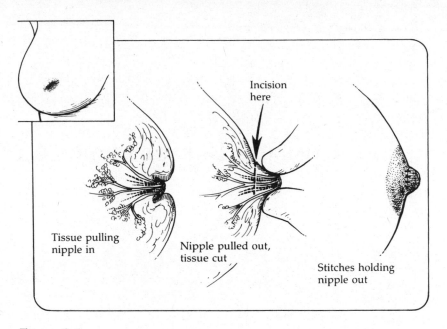

Incision here

Tissue pulling nipple in

Nipple pulled out, tissue cut

Stitches holding nipple out

Figure 2.6

don't let age deter you from the cosmetic surgery you desire. My eighty-year-old patient was delighted with her belated operation, and I've had many women in their fifties, sixties, and seventies who have had their breasts reduced or augmented. If your health is good enough to sustain surgery, it doesn't matter how old you are.

Chapter 3

COMMON BREAST PROBLEMS

IN THE FIRST EDITION OF THIS BOOK, I WROTE ABOUT THE common use of the term "fibrocystic disease," which doctors once used to describe a number of symptoms, often with no relation to each other: painful breasts, lumpy breasts, breasts that got swollen and firm before a woman's period. It seemed to me that "fibrocystic disease" meant "we don't know what is wrong with you but it isn't cancer so we are not going to pay attention to it." The term had no real meaning even though the symptoms were very real. So I began to call it a "garbage" term that lumps everything not related to breast cancer into one bucket (Figure 3.1). Luckily for us over the past 20 years, a few researchers have focused on benign (non-cancerous) breast problems and found that many of these conditions are related to various processes of reproductive life, with a spectrum that ranges from normal to aberration, and occasionally to disease. As the breasts develop, go through the changes of pregnancy and lactation, and finally wind down with involution, the potential for variations in timing, coordination, and resolution are enormous. These variations form the basis for most conditions that some consider benign breast disease.

Unfortunately, many doctors still tell women they have fibrocystic disease, as I discovered from the comments women have

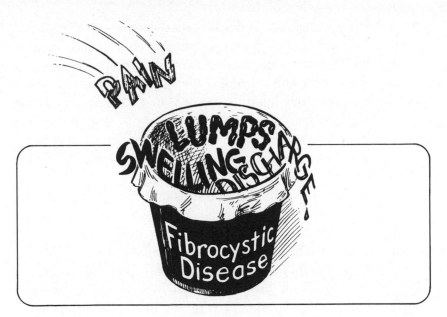

Figure 3.1

sent to me on Facebook. And some women, having been told this years ago, still believe they have it. This might be harmless, except that it keeps women from knowing precisely what their real condition is, and thus whether or not it needs to be treated. Further, most of the conditions called "fibrocystic disease" are simply the normal variations we considered in Chapter 2. They are not diseases, "fibrocystic" or otherwise.

In the following section I will describe the various kinds of benign breast problems that women experience and try to give you a better understanding of what is really going on and how, or even if, they should be treated.

LUMPS AND LUMPINESS

Lumpiness, as I explained in Chapter 1, isn't the same as having one dominant lump. It's a general pattern of many little lumps in both breasts, and it is usually perfectly normal. The distinction between "lumps" and "lumpiness" is important; confusing the two can cause a woman days and weeks of needless mental anguish.

Doctors who don't usually work with breast cancer—family practitioners and gynecologists—often get nervous about lumpy breasts and fear the lumps may be cancer. So your doctor may send you to a specialist—a surgeon or a breast specialist—to make sure you don't have a cancerous lump. If you or your doctor are uncertain about whether you've got a lump or just lumpy breasts, it's probably not a bad idea to check it out further. But understanding more about what a lump really is might make the trip to the specialist unnecessary.

Ellen Mahoney, a fellow breast surgeon, tells her patients to visualize what their breasts may be like inside—from butter to gravel to bubble wrap—and if it's the same all over, it's just the way they're made. The only area to be concerned about is the one that is different from all the rest. The most important thing to know about dominant lumps—benign or malignant—is that they're almost never subtle. They're not like little BB pellets. They're usually at least a centimeter or two, almost an inch, or the size of a grape. The lump will stick out prominently in the midst of the smaller lumps that constitute normal lumpiness. You'll know it's something different. In fact, that's why most breast cancers are found by the woman herself—the lumps are so clearly distinct from the rest of her breast tissue.

The obvious question here is, How do I know the BB-size thing isn't an early cancer? The answer is that you usually don't feel a malignant lump when it's small. The cancer has to grow to a large enough size for the body to begin to create a reaction to it—a fibrous, scar-like tissue forms around the cancer, and this, combined with the cancer itself, makes up the palpable lump. The body won't create that reaction when the cancer is tiny, and you won't feel the cancerous lump until the reaction is formed.

Although very large areas and multiple areas are rarely malignant, in this day and age it's easy enough to get an ultrasound test of the lump. Most breast surgeons have ultrasound in their offices and can check worrisome areas right there and, as always, if there is any question get a diagnostic mammogram as well.

There are three types of dominant lumps, two of which—cysts and fibroadenomas—are virtually harmless. It's the third type—the malignant lump—that you're worrying about when you have your lump examined by a health care provider. (I talk about cancerous lumps at length in Chapter 8.) It is important to remember that only about 1 in 12 palpable dominant lumps in premenopausal women is malignant. We often don't know the exact cause of any of the noncancerous lumps, though we do know they're somehow related to hormonal variations (see Chapter 1). Cysts and fibroadenomas form during a woman's menstruating years and are probably variations in the formation (fibroadenomas) and involution (cysts) that occur in the breast tissue at different times. Doctors have had a tendency to describe all nonmalignant lumps as cysts. They're not. A cyst is a distinct kind of lump.

CYSTS

A cyst typically occurs in women in their thirties, forties, and early fifties, and is most common in women approaching menopause. It rarely occurs in a younger woman or in a woman who's past menopause. However, I've had patients who don't follow that pattern—including a teenager and a woman who'd gone through menopause long ago and wasn't on artificial hormones. (As I said earlier, a woman taking estrogen to combat menopausal symptoms fools her body into thinking it's still premenopausal.) A gross (meaning "large," not "disgusting") cyst is a fluid-filled sac, like a large blister, which grows in breast tissue. It's smooth on the outside and ballotable—squishy—on the inside, so that if you push on it, you can feel that it's got fluid inside.

This, however, can be deceptive. Cysts *feel* like cysts only when they're close to the surface (Figure 3.2). Cysts that are deeply embedded in breast tissue tend to distend that tissue and push it forward, so that what you're feeling is the hard breast tissue, not the soft cyst. In these cases the cyst feels like a hard lump.

The classical cyst story goes something like this. A woman in her forties comes to a specialist and says, "I went to the gynecologist six weeks ago and everything was fine. I had a mammogram, and that was fine too. Then all of a sudden, in the shower last night, I found this lump in my breast, and I know it wasn't there before." So the doctor examines her and sure enough, there's a hard lump in her breast.

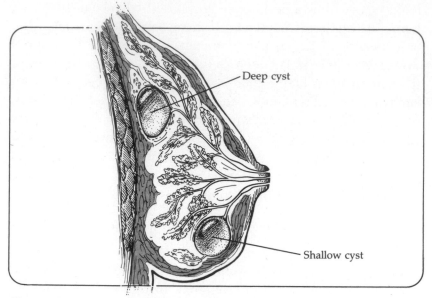

Figure 3.2

Because of its overnight appearance, the doctor is pretty sure it's a harmless cyst, but of course it's something the doctor—not to mention the patient—wants to be absolutely certain about: some cancers do seem to appear overnight. At this point the doctor has two options. If there's an ultrasound unit in the office, the lump can be imaged immediately to confirm the diagnosis. The ultrasound test works like radar or sonar. If you have a solid lump, the waves from the ultrasound will bounce back, showing a brighter spot with a dark shadow behind it. If it's a cyst, however, the sound waves will go right through it and there will be a black circle or oval without a shadow. (See Chapter 8 to read about mammograms and ultrasound techniques.)

The doctor can aspirate the cyst, once it's diagnosed, right there. If there's no ultrasound in the office and the lump is easily palpable, it too can be immediately aspirated. To do this, the doctor takes a tiny needle, like the kind used for insulin injections, and anesthetizes the sensitive skin over the lump. Then a larger needle—like the kind used to draw blood—is attached to a syringe and inserted into the breast through the skin and into

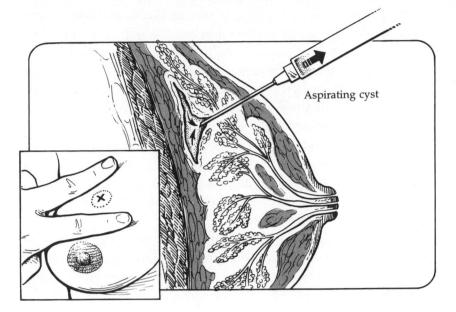

Figure 3.3

the cyst, where it draws out the fluid (Figure 3.3). The cyst col-
lapses like a punctured blister, and that's that. Though the
process sounds scary, it's usually almost painless. Most of the
nerves in the breast are in the skin, and that's been anes-
thetized. Some women with greater sensitivity to pain or especially sensitive breasts do find that it hurts, but most don't. The
only possible complications from aspirating a cyst are bruising
or bleeding into the cyst, neither of which is more than slightly
uncomfortable.

Another option is to arrange an ultrasound to be done at an
imaging center. If the area looks like a cyst, an aspiration can be
done under ultrasound guidance.

The fluid looks disgusting, but it's harmless. It can be almost
any color, but usually it's green, brown, or yellow. Sometimes the
fluid can even be milk. A breast-feeding woman can have a milk-
filled cyst, called a galactocele, which is treated like any other
cyst. The amount of fluid varies—from a few drops to as much as
a cup. One patient came to me with asymmetrical breasts; after I
aspirated her cyst, her breasts were the same size.

Usually a woman will get only one or two cysts in her entire life. But some get many at the same time, and they get them often. If a patient has recurring multiple cysts, she should be followed by a breast surgeon who has ultrasound and can monitor her and aspirate the cysts as needed. When a woman has multiple cysts, chances are she'll go on getting them until menopause—only rarely are they a onetime occurrence.

If cysts are harmless, why do we bother to image and/or aspirate them? Mostly because we need to be sure it is a cyst. You can't be absolutely certain a lump in the breast isn't cancer until you find out what it really is. Once they know it's a cyst, doctor and patient can both rest easy.

There are other ways of finding out you have a cyst—it may show up as an area of density on a routine mammogram, and then you can have an ultrasound test to see whether it's a cyst or a solid lump. If you've discovered a cyst through a mammogram and ultrasound and it doesn't worry you, don't bother having it aspirated—you already know it isn't cancer. Sometimes a cyst is painful, especially if it developed quickly. Aspirating it will usually relieve the pain.

Cysts are almost never malignant. There's a 1 percent incidence of cancer in cysts, and it's a seldom dangerous cancer called intracystic papillary carcinoma (Figure 3.4). It usually

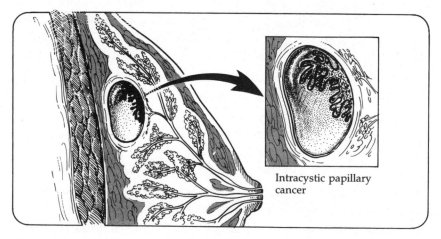

Intracystic papillary cancer

Figure 3.4

doesn't spread beyond the lining of the cyst, and unless there are specific irregularities in the cyst lining suggesting that it might be present, it's not worth risking surgical removal. If there are signs that cancer might be present in the cyst, I'd operate on it—never otherwise, and only if the ultrasound looks suspicious.

Sometimes a doctor will aspirate a cyst and won't get any fluid. This isn't a cause for panic. It can happen for a number of reasons. The lump may not be a cyst after all, but a nonmalignant solid lump like those discussed below. Or the doctor may have missed the middle of the cyst. The doctor tries to get the cyst between her or his fingers and then puncture it, but it's easy to miss the middle, especially in a small cyst. When this happened to me, I'd send the patient for ultrasound and let them aspirate it under direct vision. Operating on a cyst should only be a last resort.

Aspirating a cyst was once thought to be dangerous if someone had an unknown breast cancer; doctors believed the process of aspiration would spread the cancer over the needle's track. We now know that's completely untrue.[1] Any dominant lump should be aspirated before it's biopsied. It might be a cyst, and surgery can be avoided.

Cysts don't increase the risk of cancer. The real risk is mental rather than physical. A woman with frequent cysts is likely to feel a lump and shrug it off as just another cyst—only to learn later that it was a malignant growth. Every lump should be checked out to be sure it isn't dangerous.

FIBROADENOMAS

Another common nonmalignant lump is the fibroadenoma. These lesions come from lobules that are particularly sensitive to estrogen stimulation. They usually develop as the breasts are just getting used to hormonal cycling, during puberty and the teenage years. A fibroadenoma is a smooth, round lump that feels the way most people think a cyst should feel—it's smooth and hard, like a marble dropped into the breast tissue (Figure 3.5) where it can move around easily. It's often found near the nipple but can grow anywhere in the breast. It's also very distinct from the rest of the breast tissue. It can vary from a tiny 5 millimeters to a lemon-size

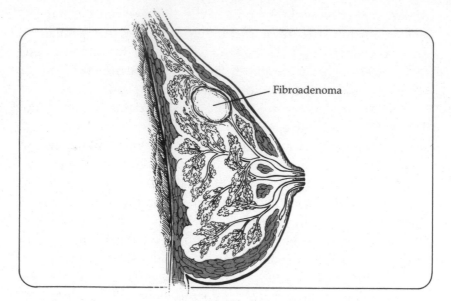

Fibroadenoma

Figure 3.5

5 centimeters. The largest are called, logically, "giant fibroadenomas." Generally fibroadenomas grow over a 12-month period to
around 2–3 centimeters (about the size of a marble to a large
grape) and then remain unchanged for several years. About 15
percent will go away on their own while only 5–10 percent continue to grow. Studies in women who were followed for up to 29
years found that the fibroadenoma shrank or disappeared in 16–
59 percent of cases. They concluded that a fibroadenoma would
probably disappear after five years in approximately 50 percent of
cases and after 15 years the rest of the time. [2]

A doctor can usually tell simply by feeling the lump that it's a
fibroadenoma; if a needle aspiration is done and no fluid comes
out, the doctor knows it isn't a cyst and is even more convinced
it's a fibroadenoma. The diagnosis can always be confirmed by doing a core biopsy (see Chapter 8) and sending the tissue off to the
lab just to make doubly sure. Fibroadenomas are usually distinct
on a mammogram or ultrasound test. They are harmless in themselves and don't need to be removed as long as we're sure they're
fibroadenomas.

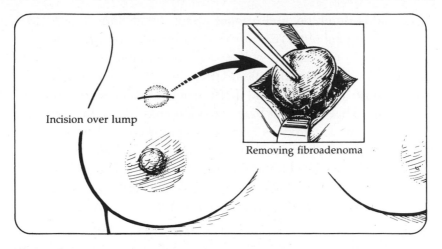

Incision over lump

Removing fibroadenoma

Figure 3.6

Since fibroadenomas develop at puberty, teenagers are more prone to have them and less likely to get breast cancer than are older women, so we might consider not removing them at all unless the woman desires it. In older women we tend to do a core biopsy of all fibroadenomas or simply remove them to be sure they're not cancer.

If the doctor and the patient want the fibroadenoma removed, it can be easily done under local anesthetic. The surgeon simply makes a small incision, finds the lump, and takes it out (Figure 3.6). (Some surgeons prefer to make a small incision around the nipple and then tunnel their way to the lump, to minimize scarring. I don't think this is a great idea because it's harder to find the lesion that way and may cause nipple numbness. If the doctor cuts over the fibroadenoma, it's easier to find and the scarring doesn't usually remain noticeable in most patients.) If your core biopsy proves that this is a fibroadenoma, there is no need to have it removed unless you want to. Some women remain nervous knowing there's a lump in their breasts, in which case it's reasonable to have it removed for their peace of mind. Another option has been developed that should appeal to many women: a minimally invasive procedure in which the fibroadenoma is frozen in place under ultrasound guidance. It is almost painless because the cold is numbing, and it takes about a half hour in a doctor's office. Within about a year or two the fibroadenoma disappears.[3]

Usually a woman has only one fibroadenoma; it's removed or treated, and she never gets another one. But some women get several over a lifetime—and a few women get many. It's not uncommon to have three or four fibroadenomas in one breast, or for fibroadenomas to grow as large as 4 centimeters (1.5 inches) in diameter. One of my patients had a fibroadenoma in her left breast, and I removed it. She returned a couple of years later with another one on the exact same spot in her other breast—a kind of mirror image. Occasionally a woman will have multiple fibroadenomas at once. After they are removed, more form. I had one woman with this problem and I must admit it is a difficult one. Obviously a surgeon can't keep removing them, but equally obviously a woman with this condition will be worried. One woman I talked to was told to have prophylactic mastectomies so the surgeon would not have to worry. This is pretty drastic for a benign condition that does not increase breast cancer risk. I'd generally recommend surgery only for the patient's needs, not for her doctor's peace of mind. It is probably more reasonable to monitor them with ultrasound and palpation and remove them only if they are growing.

Fibroadenomas shouldn't be confused with fibroids, which exist only in the uterus. There are similarities between the two conditions: in both cases, one section of glandular tissue becomes autonomous, growing like a ball in the midst of the rest of the tissue. But there's no other correlation—having one doesn't mean you're likely to get the other. In fact, they usually occur at different times in a woman's life: fibroids when you're heading toward menopause, fibroadenomas in your teens or early twenties.

However, fibroadenomas *can* occur at any age, up until menopause. As with cysts, you can get them after menopause if you're taking hormones that trick your body into thinking it's premenopausal. As we do more mammograms on "normal" women, we find more and more fibroadenomas in women in their sixties and seventies. Probably they've had them since their teens and simply, in those premammography days, didn't know about them. There are some very rare cancers that can look like fibroadenomas on a mammogram, so, in postmenopausal women, we usually do either a fine-needle aspiration, a core biopsy, or, if those don't give us the information, an excisional biopsy (removal of the whole lump), just to make sure it is a fibroadenoma.

Ellen Mahoney says, "I tell people it has to come out if it bothers you or if it grows. Following this rule, I have never missed the occasional indolent cancer. One of my patients had three in the same quadrant. A baseline was done and repeated in six months—two had grown. All were removed and all were cancer. Following this rule too, I have diagnosed some of the 2–3 millimeter tumors sitting next to fibroadenomas and stimulating them. I think there are two types of fibroadenomas: hamartomas, which rarely grow larger than 2.5 centimeters (like the sponge toys in the gelatin capsules), and others that may grow in response to a number of factors. I make sure I have a good measurement by ultrasound or by my little cloth tape measure, whichever is appropriate to the location."

There's also a rare cancer called cystosarcoma phylloides, or phylloides tumor (see Chapter 13), which is a cousin to a fibroadenoma. It is found in about 1 percent of the operations in which a surgeon is removing what is thought to be a fibroadenoma. It's usually a big lump—lemon-size or larger. Generally this is a relatively harmless cancer that doesn't tend to spread to other parts of the body. Some doctors will insist on removing all fibroadenomas on the theory that this cancer may be present. It's not a very sensible attitude, especially if a core biopsy has proven that the lump is a fibroadenoma, because of both the rarity and the lack of danger.

Finally, fibroadenomas themselves never turn into cancer. Rarely a cancer will arise in a fibroadenoma, but it won't be missed as long as you check the size at diagnosis and at six months and remove them if they are growing. If all is stable, size doesn't have to be checked again until there is a suspicion of change.

CANCER

The fear of cancer is, of course, the main reason we worry about any of these lumps. When you get a cyst aspirated or a fibroadenoma biopsied, it's chiefly to make sure there is no cancer.

It's reasonable to be afraid of getting breast cancer and to check out any suspicious lump. But remember that a dominant lump doesn't mean you have cancer. In premenopausal women there are 12 benign lumps for every malignant one. The statistics change dramatically in postmenopausal women who aren't taking hormones, not because they get that much more cancer but because they no longer get the lumps that come with hormonal changes—cysts and fibroadenomas. Yet even for postmenopausal women it's only a fifty-fifty chance that a lump is cancer. The main thing to remember is to be cautious but not frantic. Get it checked out. If it's cancer, you can start working on it; if it isn't, you can stop worrying.

What to Do If You Think You Have a Lump

If you have something that feels like it might be a lump, the first thing to do, obviously, is go to your doctor. If there is any question she will do an ultrasound or send you to a specialist for one. If you are over 35, you will have a mammogram to get additional information. The imaging may show evidence of a real lump. If it doesn't, an MRI may be ordered. If the examination and imaging don't give the surgeon the necessary clarification, it's wise to get a biopsy to find out what it is. In the past we were afraid of unnecessary surgery and didn't want to biopsy these "gray area" lumps. Now with the minimally invasive core biopsy (see Chapter 8), we can easily get an answer without surgery. These core biopsies can be done by a surgeon if the lump can be felt or seen on ultrasound or by a mammographer under imaging guidance. Find out who in your community has the most experience. In many places there are breast centers where you can have lumps evaluated by someone in the appropriate specialty.

It's important to stress one thing: if you're certain that something is wrong with your breast, get it biopsied, whatever the doctor's diagnosis. Often a woman is sure she has a lump, the doctor is sure she doesn't, and a year or two later a lump shows up on her mammogram. She believes the doctor was careless. Usually that's not the case. It's likely that the patient—who, after all, experiences her breast from both inside and outside, while the doctor can only experience the patient's breast from outside—has sensed something wrong and interpreted that in terms of the concept most familiar to her, a lump. I'm convinced that this is the basis of many of the malpractice suits that arise when a doctor "fails" to detect what later proves to be cancer. If you really feel something is wrong in your breast, insist on a biopsy. If you're wrong, you'll put your mind at rest—and if you're right, you may save your own life. It's a minor procedure with low risks and potentially high gains.

BREAST PAIN

Another common breast symptom is pain—frequently called either mastalgia or mastodynia (one is Latin, the other Greek, and they both translate to "breast pain"). It can run the gamut of a minor irritation a couple of days a month through permanent, nearly disabling agony, and everything in between. A study of 1,171 healthy premenopausal American women revealed that 69 percent suffered from regular discomfort, 36 percent had seen a doctor about their pain, and 11 percent experienced moderate to severe breast pain.[4] A study in a clinic in Cardiff, Wales, documented three main categories of breast pain: cyclical (pain related to the menstrual cycle), noncyclical ("trigger zone" pain), and pain that does not originate in the breast. Of these the most common by far is cyclical.[5]

The best way to determine which kind of pain you have is to keep a breast pain chart—a calendar where you mark every day whether your pain is severe, mild, or gone.[6] In addition, you mark the days of your period. Looking at this, you can easily determine whether your pain is premenstrual or variable (cyclical or noncyclical).

Cyclical Pain

We know that cyclical mastalgia is related to hormonal variations. The breasts are sensitive right before menstruation, then less sensitive once the period begins. For some women, tenderness begins at the time of ovulation and continues until their period, leaving only a couple of pain-free weeks during their cycle. For some, it's barely noticeable; others are in such pain they can't wear a T-shirt, lie on their stomach, or tolerate a hug. Sometimes it's only in one breast, and other times it radiates into the armpit and even down to the elbows, causing its poor victim to think she's got cancer spreading to her lymph nodes.

Understanding precisely the part hormones play in cyclical mastalgia is clouded by the fact that the relationship of women's hormonal cycles to the breast hasn't been that well researched. Hormones may also affect cyclical breast pain in a more subtle way—for example, as a result of stress. We know that stress can affect the menstrual cycle: you can miss your period or have a particularly heavy period, or an early or late period when you're under great stress, positive or negative. Similarly, your breast pain can increase or change pattern with the hormonal changes of stress. We also know that hormones vary at different points in your life and that the incidence of breast pain often follows these shifts. It's usually most intense in the teens and then again in the forties—at both ends of the fertile years. It almost always ends with menopause, though in some rare cases it lasts beyond menopause—perhaps because of the continuing estrogen production of the ovaries and breast tissue (see Chapter 1). And of course, if a postmenopausal woman is taking hormones, her body thinks she's still premenopausal and she's as likely to get breast pain as she was before.[7] We also know it's common in pregnant women; indeed, unusual breast pain can be an early sign of pregnancy.

The relation to hormones doesn't appear to be absolute. There must be other factors, since most often the pain is more severe in one breast than in the other, and a purely hormonal symptom would have to affect both equally. It appears to be caused by a combination of hormonal activity and something in the breast tissue that responds to that activity. More research needs to be done.

Breast pain is annoying but usually isn't unbearable; what can be unbearable is the fear that it's cancer. The best treatment, therefore, is reassurance. The study in Cardiff suggests that 85 percent of women with breast pain worry much more about the possibility of cancer than about the pain itself. Most of them, after appropriate exams and imaging, can be reassured that their problem has no relation to cancer, leading to emotional relief and the feeling that they can live with their pain. This study was repeated in Brazil to see if it was only Welsh women who responded to reassurance. Sure enough, Brazilian women also responded to reassurance with a success rate of 70.2 percent. Only 10–15 percent of the women had pain that was incapacitating and needed treatment.[8]

A wide variety of treatments have been proposed for cyclical breast pain. Some work and some don't. Many clinicians suggest stopping caffeine or taking vitamin E, despite studies showing that these approaches do not work. Sometimes they do this because their patients believe in it. One woman on Facebook who had benign lumps, for which she had surgery, later read in a magazine that caffeine caused "fibrocystic problems." She stopped drinking coffee and all caffeinated drinks, and she felt better. On her next visit to the doctor, she told him she'd given up caffeine. "Oh yes, that will do it," he responded. Logically, then, she was annoyed at him. "So why didn't he tell me this before??!!" she writes angrily. My guess is that he didn't tell her because he knew it wasn't true, and rather than discuss this with her, he just agreed with her. Her lumpiness was reduced and she felt better, so why argue? He would have had to take the time to explain that some lumpiness resolves itself, or that the earlier surgery had taken care of the problem.

Another woman, who also had benign lumps and breast pain, was also diagnosed with "fibrocystic disease." Her doctor further told her that she should have yearly mammograms, avoid caffeine, and "wear constrictive bras." Not surprisingly, none of this helped. Mammograms can help determine if lumps have grown, a bra can help keep painful breasts from jiggling, and avoiding caffeine can do nothing except perhaps make you less jittery so you don't worry as much. Only the bra can affect the pain, and then only minimally.

The belief in fibrocystic disease not only frightens women who don't have a disease but can confuse women who actually do. One woman, told that she had fibrocystic disease, "probably due to too much caffeine," stopped worrying about her lumps and "became lackadaisical about getting mammograms," until she realized one lump was growing larger. When she had it examined, they found cancer. "In retrospect," she says, "I should have had a biopsy of that lump much earlier."

Some physicians who believe the pain comes from water retention recommend diuretics (water pills). These give little relief. Others have tried everything from nonsteroidal anti-inflammatory drugs, ginseng tea, vitamin A, vitamin B complex, and antibiotics, to a firm support bra.

If you have breast pain, the first step is to get a good examination from a breast specialist or someone knowledgeable in the field who will take your symptoms and concerns seriously (this may take some searching). If you're over 40, have a mammogram. Once you know you don't have cancer you can decide whether you are able to live with your discomfort or want to explore further treatment. You may also want to look into Chinese herbs and acupuncture, which have been used for centuries in China. In some cases, herbs and acupuncture are used together; in others, the patient and/or practitioner prefer to use one or the other. They can also be used for noncyclical pain discussed later in this chapter.

Another possibility is the use of meditation and visualization techniques, such as those discussed in Chapter 18. A number of studies have shown that these techniques can be effective in reducing pain, and they may help relieve both cyclical and noncyclical breast pain.

If you are in your twenties, you may want to try the pill. Analgesics like aspirin, Tylenol, and ibuprofen can offer some relief, and wearing a firm bra will prevent bouncing breasts from increasing your discomfort.

A reasonable treatment plan for moderate to severe mastalgia has been proposed by the breast pain group in Wales. Although different women respond better to different drugs, this plan has ensured relief of pain in 70–80 percent of women when the regimen has been followed.[9] The first recommendation is evening primrose oil (a natural form of gamolenic acid) for women with moderate pain and for those who are taking oral contraceptives. It can be obtained in health food stores as tablets containing 500 milligrams of gamolenic acid. Six capsules should be taken twice a day. It has minor side effects. The reaction to therapy can take a while so a trial of treatment should last at least four months and be monitored by keeping a pain chart. This treatment has been shown to benefit 44–58 percent of women. If pain has decreased, evening primrose oil is continued for one to two months more and then discontinued. Many women will have long-lasting effects after discontinuing therapy.[10] But don't take it if you're pregnant or trying to get pregnant, as it can cause miscarriage.

If evening primrose doesn't work, the next step for treatment is hormonal. Danocrine (Danazol) and bromocriptine have been shown to have some benefit. If you are taking oral contraceptives, you should not use either drug; only women who are not taking oral contraceptives and are using adequate mechanical contraception or are not sexually active with men should use them. Again, these drugs should not be taken by pregnant women or those who are trying to get pregnant as they may cause birth defects. Danocrine is given at 200–300 milligrams per day and slowly reduced to 100 milligrams a day after relief of symptoms. Danocrine will relieve pain in 70–80 percent of women.[11] Side effects are common, including menstrual irregularities, leg cramps, weight gain, and decreased libido. The symptoms are related to the dose, and so the recommendation is to start with 200 milligrams a day for a month and, if the pain is diminished, to reduce it to 100 milligrams a day for the second month and then to stop. Few women need a longer course of therapy.

Bromocriptine inhibits the release of prolactin and has been shown to be effective in up to 65 percent of women treated for cyclical breast pain at doses of 5 milligrams a day. These results were demonstrated in a European multicenter randomized controlled trial.[12] Mild side effects such as nausea, dizziness, headaches, and irritability have been reported in 30 percent of women, and 10 percent complained of severe side effects. Most of these effects can be avoided by gradually increasing the dose, taking the drug with meals, and using the smallest amount necessary to get an effect. (See Figure 3.7 for an explanation of where the treatments described have their effects.) If bromocriptine is tried first and does not work, about 30 percent of women

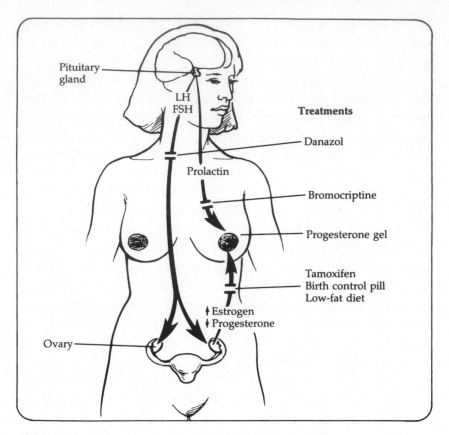

Figure 3.7

will respond to danocrine, and vice versa if danocrine is tried first. These two drugs are the only ones approved for the treatment of breast pain at this time. Other drugs have been shown to be effective but are not as yet approved for that purpose.

Tamoxifen is a selective estrogen receptor modulator (see Chapter 7). According to an English study, it's very good at relieving mastalgia (80–90 percent).[13] Side effects include hot flashes and menstrual irregularities. Luckily, it was shown to be just as effective at 10 milligrams per day as at 20 milligrams, and three months of treatment were just as good as six. A group in Minnesota reports using 10 milligrams for two months with good results and only a 30 percent recurrence rate.[14]

A nonmedicinal remedy, a low-fat diet, has been studied and shown to have some effect on cyclical mastalgia and hormone levels.[15]

A benign treatment for breast pain, like the prostaglandin inhibitors (ibuprofen) that work so well with menstrual cramps, would certainly be welcome. Until then, each woman will need to decide whether the side effects of drugs are worth the benefit to her.

Noncyclical Pain

Noncyclical pain is far less common than cyclical pain. It also feels a lot different. To begin with, it doesn't vary with your menstrual cycle—it's there and it stays there. It's also known as "trigger zone" breast pain because it's almost always in one specific area: you can point exactly to where it hurts. It's anatomical rather than hormonal—something in the breast tissue is causing it (although we usually don't know what). Sometimes it can be a sign of cancer, so it's always worth checking out with your doctor, especially if you are over 30.

One cause of noncyclical breast pain is trauma. A blow to the breast will obviously cause it to hurt, and a breast biopsy is likely to leave some pain (see Chapter 8). Many women get slight shooting or stabbing pains up to two years or more after a biopsy. And you're never quite perfect after any surgery—just as after breaking a leg you can always tell when it will rain. This kind of pain is usually pretty obvious: it's on the spot where your scar is. It's unpleasant, but it's nothing to worry about.

Often doctors simply don't know what causes noncyclical breast pain; they'll operate and remove the area, have the tissue studied, and find nothing abnormal. Unfortunately this doesn't relieve the pain.

Treatment for this kind of breast pain is more difficult than for cyclical breast pain. Again, start with a good exam, and, if you're over 35, a mammogram. If there's an obvious abnormality it can then be taken care of. For example, sometimes a gross cyst causing localized breast pain or tenderness can be cured by needle aspiration.

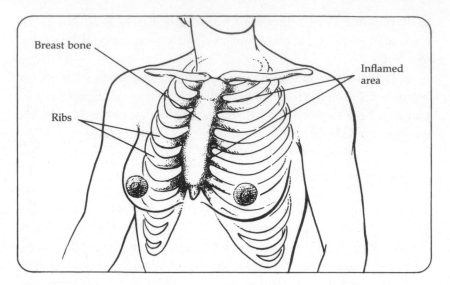

Figure 3.8

Since noncyclical pain is rarely caused by hormones, hormonal treatments are less likely to work. Some women, however, find relief with the kinds of treatments mentioned under cyclical breast pain. Sometimes, though not invariably, having a biopsy relieves the pain although we don't know why; you will experience pain for a while from the biopsy itself. A good test is for your doctor to inject some local anesthesia into the spot. If it gives relief, then surgery may work well; if not, then it probably isn't worth it.

Nonbreast-Origin Pain

This third category isn't really a form of breast pain, though that is how it feels to the patient. It's usually in the middle of the chest and doesn't change with your period. Most frequently it's arthritic pain—known as costochondritis—in the place where the ribs and breastbone connect (Figure 3.8).[16] When men get costochondritis they think it's a heart attack; when women get it, they think it's breast cancer. You can tell it's arthritis by pushing down on your breastbone where your ribs are—if it hurts a lot more, that's probably what you've got. Similarly, if you take a deep breath and the middle part of your breast hurts, it's probably arthritis. If you take aspirin or Motrin and it relieves the pain, it's probably arthritis, since they're anti-inflammatory agents and thus work especially effectively on conditions like arthritis. Having your doctor inject the spot with local anesthetic and steroids will relieve 90 percent of chest wall pain.[17]

You can also get nonbreast-origin pain from arthritis in the neck (a pinched nerve).[18] This pain can radiate down into the breast the way lower back arthritis goes into the legs. There's also a special kind of phlebitis (inflamed vein) that can occur in the breast, called Mondor's syndrome. It gives you a drawing sensation around the outer edge of your breast that extends down into your abdomen. Sometimes you can even feel a cord where it is most tender. None of these problems is serious. A nonbreast condition that appears in the breast area is treated as it would be in any other part of the body. That usually means, for the conditions just mentioned, aspirin or another anti-inflammatory agent. These pains are usually self-limited and will go away in time.

Cancer Concerns

How likely is any breast pain to be cancer? Cyclical pain has no relation to cancer, so don't worry. Noncyclical pain is rarely a sign of cancer, but it can be, so it's worth checking out. One of my patients discovered while she was traveling in Europe that her breast hurt when she lay on her stomach. Though she couldn't feel any lump, she had it checked when she came home and discovered she did indeed have a tiny cancer on the spot. About 5 percent of all target zone breast pain is cancer. So it's worth having your doctor check it—if only for the relief of being sure you aren't in the 5 percent.

BREAST INFECTIONS

Breast infections and nipple discharge are fairly uncommon and usually are not much more than a nuisance, but they can cause great anxiety to the woman who experiences them.

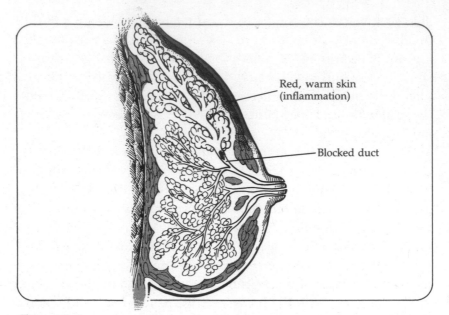

Red, warm skin
(inflammation)

Blocked duct

Figure 3.9

Lactational Mastitis

Lactational mastitis is the most common of these infections.[19] It occurs, as its name suggests, when the woman is breast-feeding. The breast is filled with milk, a medium that encourages the growth of bacteria. You've got a baby sucking and biting on your breast on a regular basis, causing cracks in the skin and introducing bacteria; it's really amazing that more nursing mothers don't get infections.

Probably it happens as seldom as it does because milk is always flowing through and flushing the bacteria out. However, sometimes when you're breast-feeding a duct will get blocked up with thick milk that doesn't flow very well. Then bacteria become trapped in the breast, the milk feeds them, and suddenly you've got a reddened, hot, and very painful breast (Figure 3.9).

Your doctor will probably suggest that you try to unblock the duct with massage and warm soaks; sometimes a doctor suggests heat (which liquefies the milk for better flow). If the infection persists, an ultrasound should be done to determine whether there is an area of infection that needs to be treated with antibiotics or an abscess that needs to be drained. Don't worry about the antibiotics affecting your nursing child. Your obstetrician will know which antibiotics are safe for children to ingest. Nor will the bacteria hurt the child, since they will be killed by the baby's stomach acid. It's actually good for you if the child goes on nursing. The sucking helps unblock the duct.

Antibiotics almost always get rid of infection, but in about 10 percent of cases an abscess forms, and antibiotics can't eliminate abscesses. An abscess, like a boil, is basically a collection of pus, which the doctor has to drain. This is usually done through a needle while the patient is having an ultrasound, and it may need to be repeated more than once. The pus can be sent to the lab to identify the bacteria and what drugs it is sensitive to so that the infection will be treated with the best antibiotic. Surgery is rarely done anymore, and only as a last resort.

Breast-feeding can continue during the infection and its treatment.

Nonlactational Mastitis

Mastitis can also occur in nonlactating women, especially in particular circumstances. For example, it may occur in women who've had lumpectomies followed by radiation, in women with diabetes, or in women whose immune systems are otherwise depressed. Such women are prone to infections either because some of the lymph nodes, which help fight infection, have been removed, or because their immune system is generally less strong than most people's. This type of infection will usually be a cellulitis—an infection of the skin—red, hot, and swollen all over rather than in one spot. It's generally accompanied by high fever and headache, both characteristics of a strep infection (staph infections, by contrast, are usually local). Your doctor will treat it with antibiotics, usually penicillin, and you may be briefly hospitalized.

Skin boils (or staph infections) can form on the breast, as they can on other parts of the body. If you're a carrier of staph and prone to infection as well—as in the case of diabetics—this is more likely to occur than in noncarriers or people less infection prone. It's also possible to get an abscess in the breast when you're not lactating and don't have any of the other risk factors, although this is unusual. Both cellulitis and these abscesses can mask cancer (as we'll discuss later), so, though such cancer is rare, if you've got one of these conditions it's important to have it checked out by a doctor.

Chronic Subareolar Abscess

The second most common breast infection—and it's rather infrequent—is the chronic subareolar abscess, which we don't understand very well, though there is some evidence that it is more common in smokers. Two theories about its cause demonstrate the fact that we also don't really understand the anatomy of the breast ducts and the nipples. One theory states that this infection is caused by ducts that become blocked with keratin and then become infected.[20] But Dr. Bruce Derrick at Temple University and Dr. Otto Sartorius put forth a different view, which I find more compelling.[21,22] As you'll recall from earlier in this chapter, there are little glands on the nipple, as well as ducts. These small, dead-ended glands can get infected, whether you're nursing or not. Bacteria from the skin or mouth of your child or lover get into the gland; thickened secretions block it so it can't drain well, and an infection forms. This is most common in women with inverted nipples, because their glands have narrower openings.

Whether the culprit in this condition is the ducts or the glands doesn't matter much to the patient. Either way, an abscess forms that can't drain through the usual exit and therefore tries to drain through the weakest part of the skin in the area—the border of the areola and the regular skin (Figure 3.10). The abscess is a red, hot, sore area on the border of the areola—like a boil. It looks and feels awful, and the frightened woman often thinks she's got breast cancer. She doesn't, and the infection doesn't affect her vulnerability to breast cancer.

If the infection is caught before an abscess forms, it may be helped by antibiotics and aspiration with a needle. But often it can't be and needs to be incised and drained. I think it's best to make the incision on the border of the areola, so that it doesn't show later. Once the pus is drained, it's okay—for the time

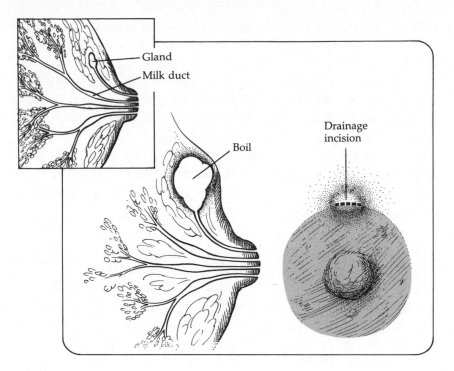

Figure 3.10

being—since this type of infection is apt to recur. The gland is a little blind passage with no internal opening, so it can reinfect itself and drain again at the same point. Eventually this leaves a permanent open tract.

I had some luck reducing these recurrences by removing the entire gland or tract. To get the whole tract, the surgeon must excise a wedge of nipple. The method isn't perfect, but its success rate is a lot better than that of other methods.

We don't yet know the reason for the frequency of recurrence, even in the most skillfully done operations.[23] Perhaps there is disease in more than one duct that makes it susceptible to infection. This has been termed duct ectasia or periductal mastitis. There are multiple descriptions of this condition, and there has been much hypothesizing about what causes it. Perhaps the infection spreads from one gland to another, or perhaps there's still lining left from the old gland that the surgeon isn't aware of. So if you have a chronic subareolar abscess, it's well worth trying to have it taken care of. But understand that you may have to keep dealing with it. About 40 percent of these infections do recur, sometimes as often as every few months, especially if you are a smoker.

As so often happens, many doctors think surgery is called for, no matter how disfiguring it may be. One patient came to me after her doctor said he was fed up with these recurrences and wanted to remove both breasts. Fortunately she had the sense not to listen to him. A well-planned, nonmutilating operation solved her problem. But even if it hadn't, the most drastic procedure that would have made any sense at all would have been to remove the ducts behind her nipple, leaving the breast intact.

INFECTION AND CANCER

To repeat, breast infections do not lead to breast cancer. However, some breast cancers lead to infections or look like infections. As the cancer cells grow, noncancer cells die off for lack of blood supply, and the necrotic (dead) tissue can get infected. So it's possible, though extremely unusual, for a breast cancer to show up first as a breast abscess.

Inflammatory breast cancer can be mistaken for infection (see Chapter 13). This starts with redness of the skin, warmth, and swelling. There usually is no lump. What distinguishes it from infection is that it doesn't get better with antibiotics. Anyone with a breast infection that persists after 10 days to two weeks of antibiotics should see a breast surgeon, who will probably want to do a biopsy.

If you get an infection, don't worry about it—but do see your doctor right away. The infection won't give you cancer, but it should be treated and gotten rid of, and you do want to make sure it is in fact an infection.

NIPPLE PROBLEMS

Cracked or Sore Nipples While Nursing

The nipple is an especially sensitive area and subject to a number of problems, such as the subareolar abscess discussed earlier. A new mother who is nursing sometimes develops a cracked or sore nipple, and it isn't a pleasant experience. The pain can be severe and the guilt from feeling unable to suckle her child adequately is hard to tolerate, especially since her hormones are surging. Such pain occurs in as many as 17 percent of women in the first few weeks postpartum. Typically there is a small erosion or crack on the nipple. Although it usually goes away on its own, if the baby is having trouble sucking or is sucking hard, the nipple may become painfully raw and progress to a cracked nipple in about a week. It is often infected with bacteria. A recent study looked at four different strategies to treat a cracked nipple and found that oral antibiotics provided the best relief and reduced the chance of developing mastitis.[24] This and good nipple hygiene are key to preventing this distressing condition.

Another source of pain in the nipple and/or breast while nursing is infection resulting from candida (a fungus that causes yeast infection). A recent study based on a microbiologic analysis of the mother's nipple, her milk, and the baby's mouth found 19 percent of the women had candida. The involved nipples were mildly inflamed and tender to the touch. It's easy to treat with a topical miconazole (antifungal) oral gel to the nipple and baby's mouth, and oral nystatin can resolve this problem.

Discharge

The most common nipple problem—or rather concern, since it's not always a problem—is discharge. Most women do have some amount of discharge or fluid when their breasts are squeezed, and it's perfectly normal (Figure 3.11). In a study at the old Boston Lying-in Hospital breast clinic women had little suction cups, like breast pumps, put on their nipples and gentle suction applied.[25] Eighty-three percent of these women—old, young, mothers, nonmothers, previously pregnant, never pregnant—had some amount of fluid. As I will explain in Chapter 6, this fluid can be analyzed for precancerous cells.

The ducts of the nipple are pipelines; they're made to carry milk to the nipple, so a little fluid in the pipes shouldn't be surprising. (It can come in a number of colors—gray, green, and brown, as well as white.)

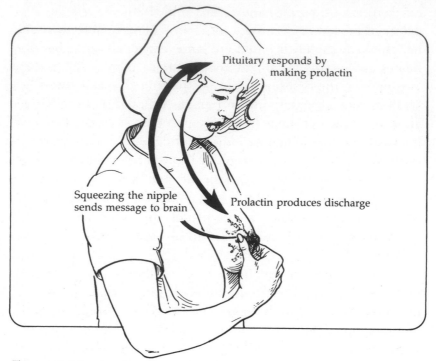

Pituitary responds by
making prolactin

Squeezing the nipple
sends message to brain

Prolactin produces discharge

Figure 3.11

Sometimes people confuse nipple discharge with other problems—weepy sores, infections, abscesses (see above). Inverted nipples (see Chapter 2) can sometimes get dirt and dried-up sweat trapped in them, and this can be confused with discharge.

Some women are more prone to discharge than others: women on birth control pills, antihypertensives, or strong tranquilizers tend to notice more discharge because these medications increase prolactin levels. The discharge may be aesthetically displeasing, but beyond that there's nothing to worry about.

There are also different life periods when you're more likely to get discharge than others: there's more discharge at puberty and at menopause than in the years between. And there's the "witch's milk" discussed earlier in Chapter 1 that newborn babies get. This makes sense, since the discharge is a result of hormonal processes.

When Should You Worry?

The time to worry about nipple discharge is when it's sponta-neous, persistent, and one-sided. It comes out by itself without squeezing, it keeps on happening, and it's only from one nipple and usually one duct. It's either clear and sticky, like an egg white, or bloody. You should go to the doctor for evaluation of the dis-charge. There are several possible causes:

1. Intraductal papilloma. This is a little wart-like growth on the lining of the duct. It gets eroded and bleeds, creating a bloody discharge. It's benign; the surgeon removes it to make sure that's what it is.
2. Intraductal papillomatosis. Instead of one wart, you've got a lot of little warts.
3. Intraductal carcinoma in situ (DCIS). This is a precancer that clogs up the duct like rust; it's discussed in detail in Chapter 13.
4. Cancer. Cancers are rarely the cause of discharge. Less than 10 percent of all spontaneous unilateral bloody dis-charges are cancerous. But it's important to have it checked.

Age is an important factor in predicting whether the discharge is related to cancer. Among patients with nipple discharges, only 3 percent who are younger than 40, and 10 percent who are be-tween 40 and 60, will have cancer, but the number jumps to 32 percent of those over 60.[26]

Your clinician should first test for blood by taking a sample, putting it on a card, and adding a chemical (hemacult test). If it turns blue, there's blood (which may not be visible to the eye be-cause of the color of the discharge). The doctor may do a Pap smear, much like the Pap smear you get to test for cervical cancer. Discharge is put on a glass slide and sent to the lab for the cells to be examined. A recent study from Vermont showed this to be quite accurate when it showed malignant cells but less accurate when it showed only apparently benign cells.[27] Next the doctor will try to locate the "trigger zone" by going around the breast to

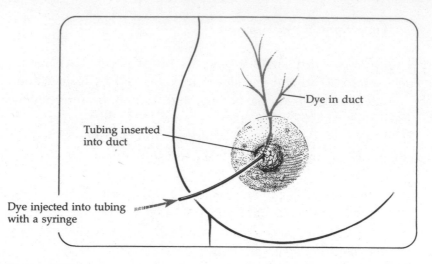

Figure 3.12

find out which duct the discharge is coming from, though often the woman herself can give the doctor this information. An ultrasound evaluation can often identify an intraductal papilloma. If the patient is over 30, she'll be sent for a mammogram to see if there's a tumor underneath the duct. If all these steps are negative for cancer, then surgery is not necessary.[28]

If there is any question or if further investigation is warranted, many doctors will follow this with either ductoscopy or a ductogram. Ductoscopy is exactly what it sounds like: a tiny endoscope (a long, flexible tube used to check out an interior body part) is passed through a numbed-up nipple for the doctor to look around for problems. This has been very useful in finding intraductal papillomas, and a new version of the scope from Germany even has the ability to remove the papilloma through the nipple.[29] Other tools for determining both the cause and location of ductal pathology include ultrasound and ductography in which the radiologist takes a very fine plastic catheter and, with a magnifying glass, threads it into the duct, squirts dye into it, and takes a picture (Figure 3.12). This may sound ghastly, but it really isn't that bad; the duct is an open tube already, and the discharge has dilated it.

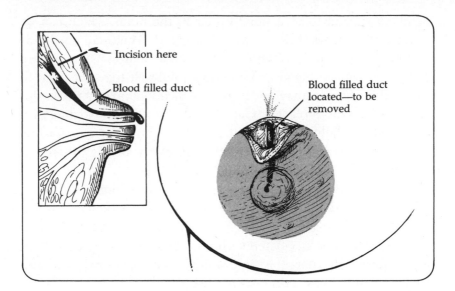

Figure 3.13

Two studies have documented that preoperative ductography increases the chance that if there is any abnormal tissue causing the pathology, it will be found. So if your doctor does not recommend one of these techniques, you may want to look around for someone who does.

You may also have a simple operation under local anesthetic on an outpatient basis. A tiny incision is made at the edge of the areola; the areola is flipped up, and the blood-filled duct located and removed (Figure 3.13). Sometimes the radiologist will cut a fine suture and pass it into the duct to the point to be removed, or blue dye can be injected into the duct to help identify it. Both of these techniques will help pinpoint the right area. Sometimes if the ductogram has shown the lesion to be far from the nipple, the surgeon will localize the area with a wire, as described in Chapter 14.

Another form of problematic discharge is spontaneous, bilateral (on both sides), and milky. If you're not breast-feeding and haven't been in the past year, this is probably a condition called galactorrhea—excessive or spontaneous milk flow. It occurs because something is increasing the prolactin levels. Rarely, the source turns out to be a small tumor in the brain, which can be detected on an MRI of the pituitary gland. This may not be as alarming as it sounds: often it's a tiny tumor that may not require surgery. A neurosurgeon and an endocrinologist together need to check this out. You may be given a medication called bromocriptine to block the prolactin. Galactorrhea is often associated with amenorrhea—failure to get your period. It can also be caused by major tranquilizers, marijuana consumption, or high estrogen doses.

Galactorrhea is diagnosed only when the discharge is bilateral. Many doctors don't understand this, and send patients with any discharge for prolactin level tests. They shouldn't; the unilateral discharges are not associated with hormonal problems. Unilateral spontaneous discharge is anatomical, not hormonal, and the money spent on prolactin tests is wasted.

Other Nipple Problems

There are a few other problems women can have with their nipples. Some patients complain of itchy nipples. Usually this doesn't indicate anything dangerous, especially if both nipples itch. You can get dry skin on your nipples as elsewhere. You may be allergic to your bra or to the detergent it's washed in. Pubescent girls with growing breasts often experience itching as the skin stretches. Otherwise, we don't know what causes itchy nipples. If they bother you, you can use calamine lotion or another anti-itch medication.

There is a form of cancer known as Paget's disease that doctors and patients often confuse with eczema of the nipple. It looks like an open sore area and it itches. If it's on only one nipple and doesn't go away with standard eczema treatments, check it out. A biopsy can be performed on a small section of the nipple. (Paget's disease is discussed at length in Chapter 13.) If the rash is on both nipples and you tend to get eczema anyway, don't worry. The eczema has just decided to try a new place to show up.

Most of these infections and irritations are benign—they're more of a nuisance than anything else. If they appear, get them checked out, just to make sure they're what they seem to be and to get the relief available.

Finally, I should mention currently fashionable nipple piercings. In general they are not harmful, although, like any piercing, they can get infected. What is really worrisome is that such piercings can interfere with, and even scar, the openings of the milk ducts, affecting both later breast feeding and potential new avenues of treatment and prevention of breast cancer (see Chapter 7). For this reason I think it's wise to discourage it.

Part Two

WHAT CAUSES BREAST CANCER AND HOW DO WE PREVENT IT?

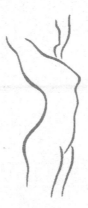

Chapter 4

UNDERSTANDING
BIOLOGY AND RISK

In Chapter 1, I compared the breast to an interactive community in which the cells of the ducts and lobules interact and influence the surrounding fibrous tissue, blood vessels, immune cells, and even fat. The cross talk and elegant dance that results have begun to be studied in recent years, and already what we have learned is pushing us to change how we think about what causes breast cancer.

It appears that at least two critical elements are necessary for any cancer to develop and flourish. The first is a cell that for some reason, either hereditary or carcinogenic, has developed a mutation in a critical part of its DNA, and the mutation changes the cell's potential behavior. Figuring out all of these many mutations and what part of the cell's activity they control is a huge part of current cancer research.[1] An example (which I discuss at length in Chapter 6) is the gene known as BRCA, which is found in all the cells of the body.[2] BRCA is an important gene because it can repair DNA that has been damaged by a carcinogen. When one copy of BRCA has a hereditary mutation, the backup second copy

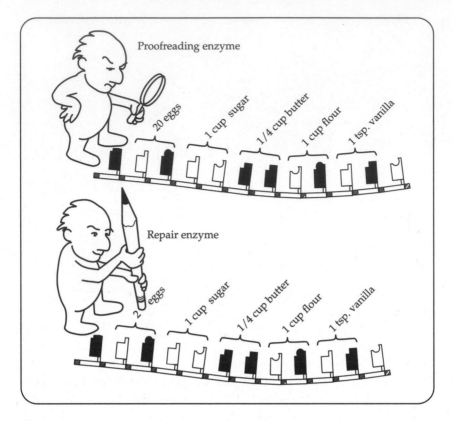

Figure 4.1

from the other parent can still function. It's like being born with one blind eye but still being able to see through the other. This is what occurs in women who inherit the gene.

However, if something happens in the breast to cause a mutation in the second copy (like losing the second eye), then her body can no longer repair damaged DNA, allowing it to propagate with errors and leaving patches of mutated cells in the breast (Figure 4.1).

This by itself is not enough to create cancer, and here's where the second element comes in. The mutated cells are in a neighborhood of other cells—fat cells, immune cells, blood cells, and so on—known collectively as the *stroma*. If these cells are all well behaved, they will have a good influence on the mutated cell,

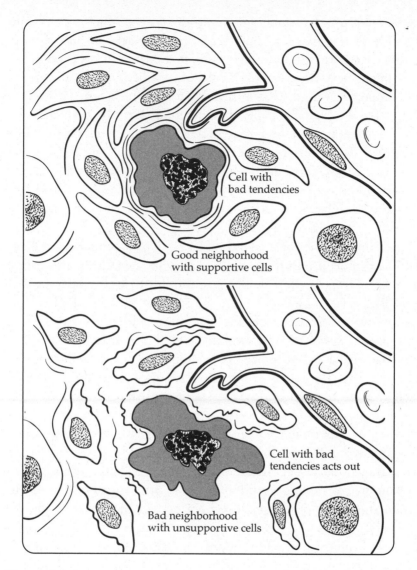

Cell with
bad tendencies

Good neighborhood
with supportive cells

Cell with
bad tendencies acts out

Bad neighborhood
with unsupportive cells

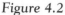

Figure 4.2

which will coexist peacefully with them, and no disease will occur. But if the neighborhood is not so "law-abiding" and stimulates or even tolerates bad behavior, there may be trouble. The
combination of the mutated cells and the stimulating, or tolerant,
neighborhood will create breast cancer (Figure 4.2). Think of this

as the plot of a *Law and Order* episode. As the officers delve into the life of the suspect, they learn that she grew up in a strong, supportive community, and seemed at the time like a good kid— she might have irrational outbreaks of hostility, but there were always people around to calm her down and she'd settle back into her usual affable personality. The neighbors tell the cops that she was a nice person and they don't see how she could have changed. But then our investigators learn that she fell for the wrong guy and moved into his crime-filled neighborhood. Her boyfriend abused drugs, and soon she was joining him. Now her hidden hostility was nourished and encouraged, and she began to fall into a pattern of crime.

Meanwhile, her best friend had a similar upbringing and early life, and moved into the same bad neighborhood; but the friend remained uncorrupted by her surroundings. As the lawyers discuss the case, they decide that the suspect probably had an impulse toward violence from the beginning, which burst out when she was in a violent neighborhood, while her friend lacked this original impulse. Our plot is very simplistic, but it demonstrates the fact that for cancer to occur, it requires both the abnormal cell and the bad neighborhood. The actual story is more complicated than that, and we'd need an entire season of *Law and Order* to keep our metaphor going. For one thing, we don't even know how many kinds of mutated cells may exist. We have discovered two, those that affect BRCA 1 and BRCA 2. There probably are others, which mutate in different ways. Still, it gives us a way to understand the processes of breast cancer and, eventually, all cancers.

I find this new way of thinking about cancer very exciting because it explains a lot and gives me a new way to think about the disease, its cause and risk factors. We can figure out what causes mutations and how to detect them. Maybe all the "children" in the neighborhood are not quite the same, and differing negative personalities create different pathologies—maybe some will turn into killers and others bank robbers and others arsonists (all representing different kinds of cancer) (see Chapter 11). We can also figure out what affects the community (stroma) around the mutated cell. Since the community is also composed of cells, they

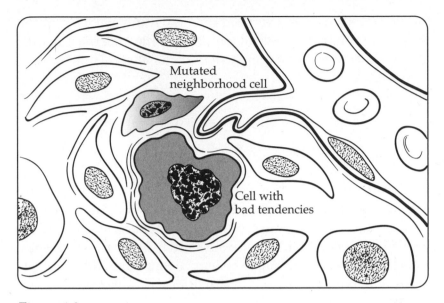

Figure 4.3

too can undergo mutations and alter their behavior (Figure 4.3). Say the original nice neighborhood gets run-down and criminals begin to move in, or a factory gets built and pollutes the water, or a huge department store chain drives out all the small businesses. Each change in any part of the community can affect all of its inhabitants, including our budding young criminal.

So in this chapter we will first explore the basic molecular biology needed to understand cancer and then describe the epithelial (ductal) cells and surrounding tissue. In the next chapter we will make things more specific by looking at the known and suspected risk factors for breast cancer, using this framework.

To me, all of this is both useful and immensely fascinating. It may be less so for some readers. Some of you are probably like my coauthor: she got Ds in college biology and always hated it. She moaned and groaned all the time we worked on this chapter, threatening to resign if it got any worse. She, of course, was being paid to work with it. But you, the reader, are not. Indeed, if you bought the book *you've* done the paying. So if the thought of reading about biology makes you unhappy, feel free to skip on to the section on how to understand studies of risk at the end of this chapter and beginning of the next. You now have my version of the CliffsNotes. All you need to know is the metaphor of the cell in its community. But if you are like me and enjoy delving deeper into the why of things, then come along. I'll make it as easy as I can!

Background

DNA

Life works through a magnificently elegant system. Every bacterium, every tree, every dog, every human being has its vital information coded into the DNA (deoxyribonucleic acid) in the nucleus of its cells. This is responsible for transferring genetic characteristics. With a single system of four bases (like four letters), everything that's alive is programmed. It's like realizing that with a single alphabet of 26 letters we have Shakespeare, *Mein Kampf,* and the Julia Child cookbooks.

These "letters" are called nucleotides, and they are the smallest unit of information in the body. How they combine to form DNA is crucial, because DNA codes all the information that your body contains. It determines the color of your eyes and your hair; it tells your lungs how to take in oxygen from the air and use it for energy. It's also complicated, so I'm going to use another metaphor for a while. I'm borrowing this metaphor from Mahlon Hoagland and Bert Dodson's superb book, *The Way Life Works.*[3] They call DNA a recipe. This recipe uses a definite code—four different "base pairs," to which we have assigned letters (Figure 4.4). Each letter represents a nucleotide. In itself a nucleotide doesn't convey a message; rather, it contributes to the message's creation. The four nucleotides are adenosine (represented by the letter A), thymine (T), cytosine (C), and guanine (G). Each nucleotide is a specific arrangement of carbon, nitrogen, oxygen, and hydrogen atoms. Each nucleotide is also bonded to a sugar called deoxyribose as well as to a phosphate. The nucleotides combine in pairs, and the pairs become the basis of whatever comes next; that is why they are known as base pairs. This pairing is very precise, like a tiny jigsaw puzzle. A and T fit together, as do G and C, and that can never vary.

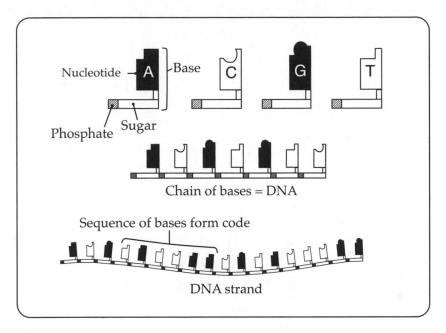

Figure 4.4

Hoagland and Dodson use the analogy of the letters of the alphabet and the paragraphs the letters make, which as you can see I've borrowed, but I'm changing it slightly for my own use. These letters and paragraphs will all combine to create a "cookbook." The base pairs can be seen as two-letter combinations, and they come together in a chain to form a gene, which can thus be seen as a recipe made with those letters. The genes are arranged in a long row, side by side, to form a chromosome (a volume of the book). All the chromosomes together form the genome (or a set of volumes that contains all the recipes needed to make a full-scale banquet—a human being) (Figure 4.5). Here's a multivolume creation indeed!

There are about 3 billion base pairs in the human genome. There are tens of thousands of genes as well—about 5,000 base pairs per chromosome represent a gene. There are punctuation marks and spaces in between genes that affect how the gene is expressed. Thus some series of these bases are important, telling you something crucial, while others represent a dash or a semicolon.

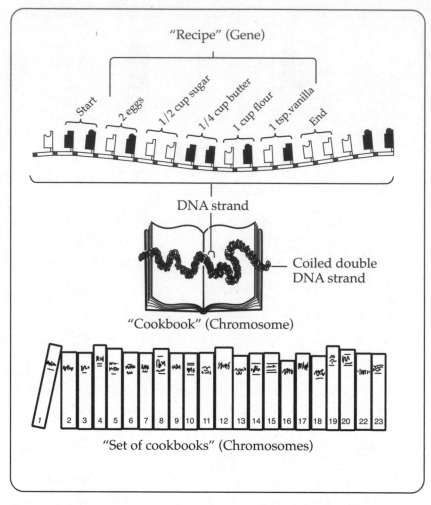

Figure 4.5

But the punctuation and spaces in between genes are just as important in one's chromosomal makeup as the actual genes that are expressed.

Why do the bases have to come in pairs? Each message is encoded in only one chromosome strand. But genes need to be able to replicate themselves or no growth takes place. So the strands come in pairs that are actually mirror images of one another. This is the famous double helix. When a cell needs to divide—as it will for any number of reasons, from healing a scratch on the body to

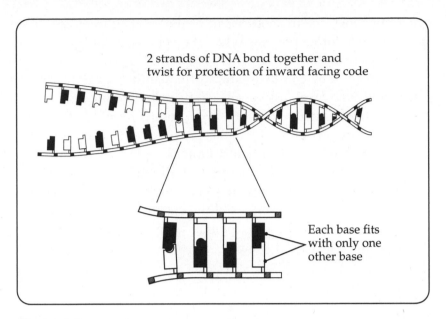

2 strands of DNA bond together and twist for protection of inward facing code

Each base fits with only one other base

Figure 4.6

creating a pregnancy—it can do so because there is a mirror image attached to the original strand. In order to replicate, the helix separates, and mirror images are made of each strand from other bases that are floating around in the cell (see Figure 4.6). The two mirror images then reconnect as a new double helix—a nifty way to make sure the code is unaltered.

RNA

In case DNA hasn't confused you enough, you need to know that it doesn't work alone. It's got a temporary partner, called RNA (ribonucleic acid). DNA, remember, is just a code—a code for creating proteins. By itself, it doesn't do anything. Let's use our recipe image again. You've got a wonderful recipe book in your kitchen, but it's a very rare, expensive old book and you don't want to splatter stuff on it while you're cooking. What you'd like to do is have a copy of one page, which you can bring to the counter and use to make your soufflé. Well, the RNA provides that copy. It duplicates the gene that it needs at the moment. Then it takes the coding message to another part of the cell and translates that piece of code into a protein. When the copy is no longer used, it disappears (you throw it into the trash bin).

The RNA copy can be produced frequently for certain genes (like your daily breakfast cereal) or it can be produced less frequently (like a holiday dinner). The production of RNA determines how much protein will be produced and therefore the levels of expression of a particular protein.

So the gene is like one recipe: it will make one thing. The DNA is the information that has gone into writing that recipe. The chromosome is one volume of the cookbook. And the RNA is the disposable copy of the recipe that keeps the whole cookbook from having to be carted around.

Proteins

Proteins are the body's building blocks, which are needed throughout our lives—making this recipe system vital. As Hoagland and Dodson write, proteins "do the daily business of living, giving cells their shapes and unique abilities." There are many kinds of proteins (just as there are many dishes)—enzymes, transporters, movers, and so on. There are 21 amino acids (ingredients) that are hooked together as proteins, and the RNA is what directs how they're strung together. Proteins are the end product of a recipe—your delicious soufflé (Figure 4.7).

GENES AND BREAST CANCER

When you understand DNA, RNA, and protein, you can begin to comprehend what may happen with cancer. The process can break down at any of these levels. The first level is at DNA. When your eggs are made, the cells divide and put only one DNA strand into each egg. So you give your child half of your DNA, the child's father gives half of his, and the combination makes a unique whole.

A mutation occurs when the wrong nucleotide gets inserted into the new strand as it's being made. Going back to our analogy, let's say there's a typo in the recipe (Figure 4.8). Another impor-

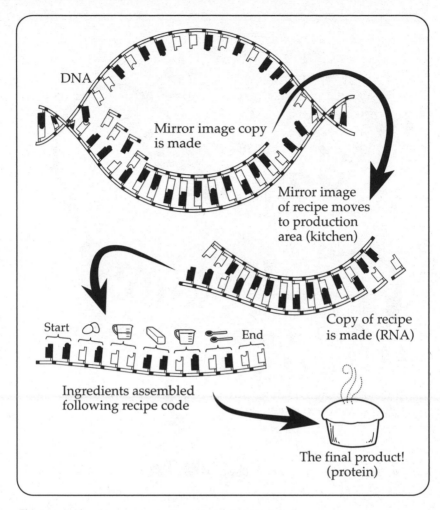

DNA

Mirror image copy
is made

Mirror image
of recipe moves
to production
area (kitchen)

Copy of recipe
is made (RNA)

Start   End

Ingredients assembled
following recipe code

The final product!
(protein)

Figure 4.7

tant way to look at it is that mutations can occur in somatic cells
(the ones that form the tissues of the body) or in germ cells
(sperm and egg) that are passed on to your offspring. Both types
of mutations are important: the first to the given individual and
the second to the next generation.

Examples of germ cell mutations are represented by BRCA 1
or BRCA 2, which are mutated in some hereditary breast cancer.
If your mother or father carries a mutation for BRCA 1 in one
strand of DNA, there is a fifty-fifty chance that you have inherited

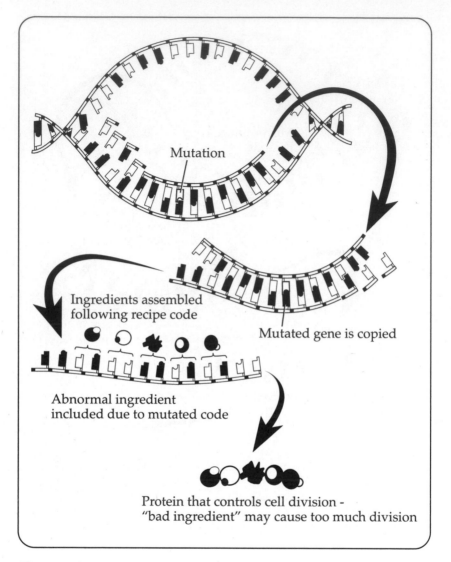

Figure 4.8

it. Remember you only get half a DNA strand from each parent, so you could get the mutated one or the good one. If you inherit the mutation it will be matched with a good strand from the other parent in every cell in your body. This puts you closer to getting cancer because you need only to develop another mutation in your good strand of DNA in the breast or ovary to develop cancer.

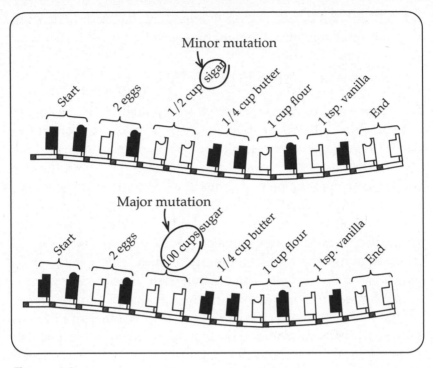

Figure 4.9

This is one reason that women who carry the mutation often get breast cancer at a young age: they start out halfway there. Luckily this situation is not too common—only 5–10 percent of women who develop breast cancer carry a mutation in one of the BRCA genes. (See Chapter 6 for a full discussion of this topic.)

Somatic mutations are more common. They happen with frequency over a person's lifetime because of exposure to carcinogens: radiation, electricity, infrared light, and dozens of other things can create a mutation. But most are no problem. If you have a typo in a recipe no one ever uses and it never gets retyped, it doesn't matter. There are other mutations that don't matter either, because the "typo" doesn't obscure the meaning (Figure 4.9). If your recipe says, "Add one cup of sigar," you may smile at it, but you know you need to add a cup of sugar. Once in a great while a mutation even creates an improvement. (If the recipe says to add a half cup of sugar, it may end up tasting just as good and being healthier.) In fact, there's an argument that civilization itself depends on mutations—the mutations involved in evolution.

Oncogenes and Tumor Repressor Genes

Oncogenes and tumor repressor genes normally function in cell growth. But if altered by mutation, they can lead to cancer because they change DNA quality control, repair, or growth. Like BRCA, these genes in themselves are harmless, even useful. But then again comes the nemesis, mutation. Mutations in these cancer genes are usually caused by outside forces such as radiation, toxins in food, or environmental pollutants. It usually takes more than one of these mutations for a cancer to develop, and of course it also requires the right community of surrounding cells, all of which can also develop a somatic mutation. In other words, cancers are due to multiple alterations in a number of genes.

It's as though the recipe gets typed by a number of different typists at different stages. The first typist makes the mistake, which then gets built into the manuscript, and it's always typed that way from then on. Then somewhere down the line another typist makes another error, and it too gets replicated. So now there are two mutations. And so on down the line. At some point the errors corrupt the document's original meaning.

Luckily the body has a technique for DNA repair—its own internal proofreader, enzymes I call the repair endonucleases (Figure 4.10). These enzymes cut through the strands of DNA, creating fragments. The proofreader reads through the recipe periodically, searching for mistakes and then fixing them. These enzymes are responsible for quality control: they check every cell before allowing it to divide. So if, for example, you've been out too long in the sun and the ultraviolet rays cause a mutation, repair endonucleases will catch it. Then the repair endonucleases have to decide what to do. How badly damaged is this cell? If it's in decent enough shape, then it's fixed. If the damage is so great that the repair nuclease can't repair the damage in time, the cell senses this and self-destructs. It is estimated that our normal cells in the course of cell division contain thousands of DNA errors, which are fortunately detected and repaired. The repair nucleases

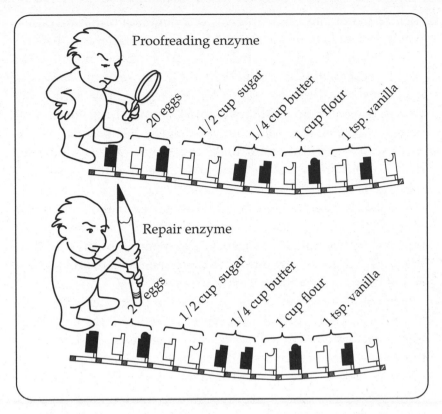

Figure 4.10

are usually pretty good workers, but once in a great while they fall asleep on the job, and the cell doesn't self-destruct (Figure 4.10 and 4.13). Like the proofreader who's daydreaming and misses a serious error in the text, the repair nuclease can sometimes let a mutated cell remain, and then divide. Now there are two mutated cells. Whether or not this will cause major problems depends on how important the mutation is. The fact that this doesn't happen more often than it does is testimony to the body's complex network of protection. There's a lot of redundancy built into the system. There's not just one pathway for repair; there are two or three (we've got several proofreaders and a copy editor at work here).

BRCA 1 and 2 are genes involved in double-strand DNA repair. When women who carry a mutation in one of these get a second mutation in a breast cell, they can develop cancer because their bodies are less able to repair other mutations that may arise (caused by radiation, for example). There is, however, a backup DNA repair system, based on poly (ADP-ribose) polymerase, which we call PARP, since poly (ADP-ribose) polymerase is ridiculously hard to say (Figure 4.11). Targeting this pathway is the basis of new drugs that we have been studying for several years and have now moved up to the stage of being tested on humans with breast cancer.[4] If those tests go as well as we expect them to, the drugs will be available in the next few years (see Chapter 13).

Another kind of cancer gene involves making cells divide. When they're normal, these are called proto-oncogenes; when they're mutated they're called oncogenes. Proto-oncogenes involved in breast cancer are mostly ones that cause more cell division—they contribute to making the cell cycle speed up.

One of the proto-oncogenes is related to the epidermal growth factor receptor (EGFR). This receptor is on a cell; the epidermal growth factor comes in and attaches to the receptor and directs it to divide—so until the factor comes along, it's just a passive receptor (a lock without a key). These growth factors and receptors are necessary at certain times of your life, such as puberty when big changes are going on in your growth and you need growth factors egging on the cells yelling "Grow! Grow! Grow!" The epidermal growth factor finds a receptor, attaches to it, and signals the cell to replicate (grow). There are different types of epidermal growth factor. An important one is epidermal growth factor 2. In the United States this is commonly known as Her-2/neu and in Europe as erb-B2. The type of genetic alteration in Her-2/neu is called amplification. Instead of having only one copy, the cell makes many (10–60) copies of this gene. When this happens the cell has more Her-2/neu receptors than normal, which helps to create more protein and a louder message—like more speakers on your stereo, if you still have a stereo. This accelerates the growth of any cancer cells that may be in the neighborhood (Figure 4.12). Either the gene overexpression or the extra protein can be measured in a woman's tumor by studying the tissue that has been removed.

Tempering the oncogenes and proto-oncogenes are the tumor suppression genes. These are the brakes in the cell system—so

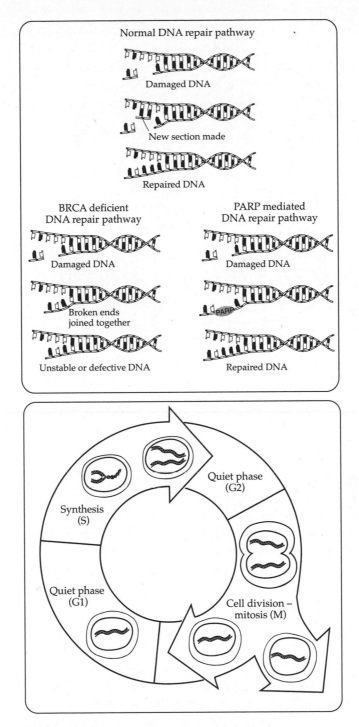

Figure 4.11

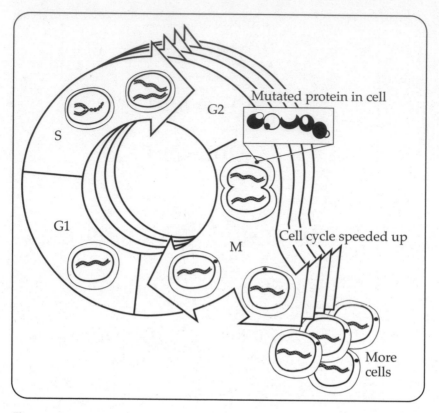

Figure 4.12

that while you have some genes that push the cells to grow and divide, you have others there to say, "Well, no, growing and dividing really isn't such a good idea."

For example, one suppressor gene, p53, keeps cells with mutated DNA from dividing (Figure 4.13). If the p53 itself becomes compromised, nothing remains to slow down that mutated DNA.

Tumor Stem Cells

One of the most exciting concepts in figuring out the biology of breast cancer has been that of *tumor stem cells*. You hear a lot about stem cells in the news, usually in relation to using healthy embryonic stem cells to grow new organs or treat diseases. From the point of view of cancer, our interest lies in what we might call "stem cells gone bad."

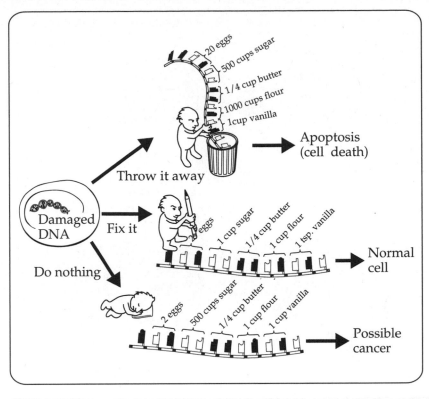

Figure 4.13

It all started when a group at the University of Michigan tried to transplant tumors into mice. Doing that requires a lot of tumor cells, and even then the process doesn't always work. At first, researchers thought that it was just inefficient. But Michael Clarke and his team found that when they separated the cells into groups based on surface markers (like dividing up a group of people by what clothes they're wearing), one group was always very efficient (needing only 20 cells for the transplant), while another could not get the transplant to take even with 20,000 cells.[5] It seemed that not every cell in the cancer was able to generate a new tumor when transplanted. This was counter to the prevailing view that any cancer cell can spread to other areas of the body and grow new tumors there. But if not all tumor cells could generate a cancer, which ones could? When researchers studied the new cancers, they found something interesting. The transplanted tumor

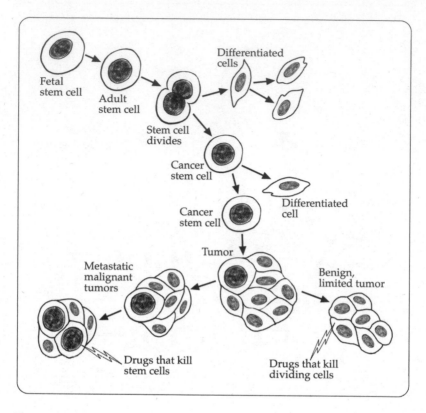

Figure 4.14

cells were all the same, based on their surface markers, but the tumors that grew from them contained a variety of different kinds of specialized cells. This suggested that the original cells were able to self-renew (clone themselves) and also differentiate into less primitive cells. These characteristics are the fundamental properties of stem cells. When stem cells divide, the division can give rise to new stem cells as well as differentiated cells of the organ or tumor (daughter cells) (Figure 4.14). Usually the number of normal stem cells present in an organ is tightly regulated, but cancer stem cells lose this regulation, giving them the ability to self-renew and constantly expand. These cells are like the queen bee. They can make a new queen or they can make lots of worker bees that are not able to become a queen. And only a queen can set up a new hive.

Normal breast stem cells live in the milk ducts and are important in maintaining the ductal lining. Exactly where they are located in the ductal system and what they look like is not yet known. If the setup is like that of white blood stem cells versus leukemia stem cells, then the differences may be subtle. Both normal stem cells and tumor stem cells are tough: they are made to survive. After all, the organ depends on them to maintain itself as cells die naturally. So the stem cells have the ability to pump out toxic drugs like those used in chemotherapy to prevent them from causing harm, making them harder to kill with our normal cancer treatment regimens. They also divide slowly and methodically to avoid errors. This would make them more resistant to irradiation and other DNA-damaging agents.

This new paradigm suggests what may be an important flaw in our approach to cancer treatment. We give drugs that are based on the idea that cells are dividing. But the stem cell actually doesn't divide very much. That means that we may see a tumor shrink but not be cured, which is exactly what happens in metastatic breast cancer. It's a bit like capturing a lot of drug dealers but not the leaders of the drug cartel. In addition, when we carefully study tumor cells and compare them to normal cells in order to find ways to target them, we may be finding targets on the daughter cells and not the stem cells. Finally, when we find cancer cells in the bone marrow of women with breast cancer, they do not reliably predict who will develop metastatic disease. This may be because some of the cells in the circulation are daughter cells that are not capable of setting up a new tumor.

Needless to say, researchers are feverishly trying to learn more about these stem cells, how to find them and eventually how to destroy them. It may be difficult to differentiate between the bad guys and the good guys, at least at first. It won't be tomorrow, but I am sure this new hypothesis will become more and more important in the future.

THE ENVIRONMENT OF THE CELL

We have considered the fact that a cell carrying a mutation requires the appropriate community in order for a cancer to develop. But can you really have mutated cells and no cancer? The answer, surprisingly, is yes. As we get older, we probably all walk around with mutated cells in our bodies. One study examined breasts that were removed at autopsy from women age 40 to 50 who had died of other causes. The researchers did not expect what they discovered—39 percent of the breasts had nests of cancer cells lying dormant inside them. Thea Tlsty of UCSF has been studying early mutations in breast cancer. At one point she was looking at tissue from reduction mammoplasties (when breasts are made smaller because they are too big; see Chapter 2). To her surprise she found cells with the same early cancer markers just sitting around doing nothing.[6] Mutated cells in a good neighborhood!

The proof comes from studies by my friend Mina Bissel, a researcher in Berkeley, California, who has spent her career studying the environment of breast cancer cells in a breast tissue environment. She has taken cells that have the mutations of breast cancer and grown them in a culture of normal breast stroma. In that environment, the cancer cells behaved like normal cells—they made ducts and did the other things that normal breast cells do.[7] The healthy influence of the surrounding cells caused the cancer cells, even though they were genetically altered, to behave well. When Dr. Bissel and her associates put the same cells in a malignant environment, the cells went back to behaving like cancer (see Figure 4.15). Recently Charlotte Kuperwasser and her team did an elegant experiment demonstrating that breast cancer cells can be influenced in women as well.[8] They developed a mouse model that used human mammary cells from reduction mammoplasties and human stroma with added growth factors. When they grew the "normal" epithelial cells in this "activated" stroma, it gave rise to hyperplasia and in one case DCIS. The researchers concluded that these human epithelial cells had undergone one or several premalignant changes before they were put in the mice even though they looked perfectly normal under the microscope. They showed up only when placed in an environment that encouraged cancer. This means that if we knew the right environment, the reverse would be possible as well: we might be able to keep the cancer stem cells from misbehaving. The ability to control or reverse cancer may also explain a phenomenon known as *tumor dormancy* (Figure 4.16). This is thought to happen in women who appear to

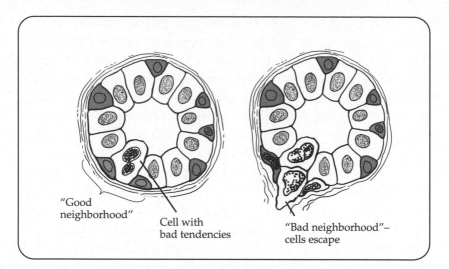

Figure 4.15

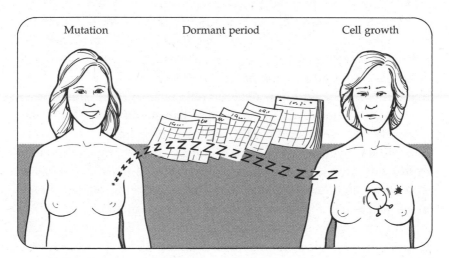

Figure 4.16

be cured at the end of treatment but have a recurrence 10 years later. What were the cells doing for 10 years? They were asleep. What put them to sleep? What woke them up?

In summary, all cancer is probably caused by a combination of genes that are altered by carcinogens and stimulated by an environment conducive to growth and spread.

One question is whether it is the local community of cells that causes the effects or the larger environment of the whole body. My guess is that it can be either or both. For example, we all know of people who go through a lot of acute stress in their lives and then get cancer? Did the stress cause the cancer? Probably not. But it certainly might have changed the body's hormones, as well as the immune system—thus leading to an environment that might make some dormant cells grow.

How does this work? How do the cells talk to each other? As the cells grow they make certain proteins—growth factors, cytokines, enzymes—that are messengers telling the surrounding cells what to do. The surrounding cells then respond to these messages with messages of their own. One aspect of this cross talk is called *epigenetic modification*. Most commonly this is known as *methylation*. A methyl group (carbon with three hydrogens) is attached to a cysteine base (one of the four base pairs in DNA), and functions almost like someone covering a switch with duct tape so that no one can turn it off (see Figure 4.17). An epigenetic change is temporary change because it has the potential to be reversed, as opposed to a permanent mutation, which is, well, permanent. The switch is deactivated rather than destroyed. Interestingly, some epigenetic changes can be inherited from one generation to the next, but with the right drug the change, in this case the methyl group, could be removed, thus changing the gene expression. This is an area of extensive research both in diagnosis, where specific genes are examined for methylation, and in treatment, where demethylating drugs are being explored.

As I was writing this chapter, the *New York Times* ran an article focusing on this new approach to thinking about cancer, a sure sign that it is becoming more mainstream.[9]

Imagine a drug that kills stem cells and can be used as treatment or even prevention. Or if we can find the right tools to change the neighborhood, cancer may be reversible or at least controllable, and we wouldn't have to try to kill every last cancer cell. Or we can destroy only the nests of cells, or prevent them from developing in the first place. This is much more complicated than the standard message of "early detection is the best prevention," but in my mind it is much more promising because it tells us there are many routes to eradicating this disease. Stay tuned!

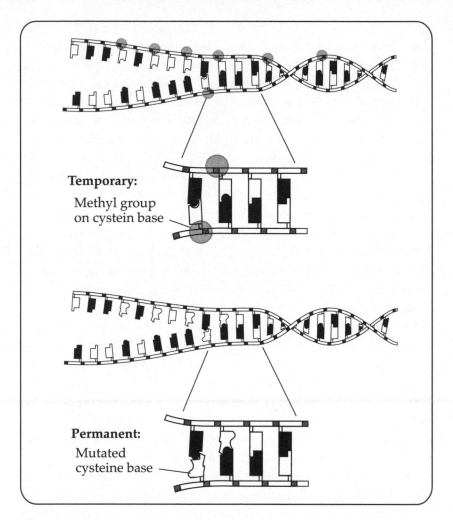

Figure 4.17

RESEARCH ON THE CAUSE AND PREVENTION OF BREAST CANCER

Molecular biology has given us an important understanding of how abnormal cells develop. However, molecular biology is slow when it comes to finding the cause or prevention methods. Here we may have to move to a bigger picture: what causes the cell to mutate in the first place, and what influences the neighborhood? To learn this, we need to look at big groups of women in whom we can find the commonalities as well as differences. This is where *epidemiology* comes in. Many of the studies you hear about when you turn on the television or open a newspaper suggest that food X increases the risk of getting breast cancer or activity Y prevents the disease. Typically, these are big studies that compare groups of women. The problem is that while this type of study can give us clues, it cannot prove cause and effect. It provides, at most, circumstantial evidence. For example, if you studied drug addicts' lives, you would probably find that most of them drank milk as children. But you wouldn't conclude that drinking milk causes drug addiction. To find a connection, you'd need to study both addicts and nonaddicts, calling for a much larger, more complicated study.

The problem is that the media rarely distinguish between kinds of studies—and thus most of us don't learn the importance of this. Different studies have different degrees of significance, and to understand what a particular study means, you need information about the study itself.

There are many ways to conduct studies of diseases and possible ways to control, treat, or prevent them. Unfortunately a completely accurate, comprehensive study is impossible to achieve. There are too many variables in even the simplest area of research. But some studies are better than others. To understand how accurate a study is, you need to look at how it was designed. It may be weak in one area, strong in another, and excellent in a third. Different aspects of a study will make it more or less believable.

Few people understand study design. Doctors are as predisposed to self-deception as anyone else: we all tend to believe the studies that feed our biases rather than the ones that don't. This same tendency is reflected by the media. Reporters often don't understand the nuances of a study, and their sound-bite reports usually fail to address limitations in the study's design. In addition, they often exaggerate the study's implications. Data that form only one brick in the complex design of a wall are presented as if they were the cornerstone. It's no wonder nonscientists are confused about what a study's results mean in real life.

Observational Studies

There are two basic categories of study, each with its own values and limitations. The *observational study* observes, without intervention, people doing what they would normally do. The *clinical trial,* or *intervention study,* tests a certain treatment on a group of people who are assigned to use it in certain ways over a certain period of time. We will examine this category later. Here we will review the observational studies, which are more relevant to risk and prevention.

Observational studies are great for generating a hypothesis. The researchers observe a phenomenon and then try to think of an explanation. They do not, however, prove cause and effect. For example, a study done in Boston observed that women with breast cancer were more likely to get their clothing dry-cleaned, have exterminators come to their homes, and use lawn treatments. The hypothesis was that these poisons might lead to breast cancer. This is an interesting idea, but a connection is far from proven. The next step might be to do an animal study and see if dry cleaning fluid increases cancers. We could also study women who work at dry cleaners to see if they had more cancer. If these studies still seemed to show a relationship, we could then go on to a controlled study in which women were randomized to use dry cleaners or not and then see how many developed breast cancer. This last study, of course, would be difficult to do, but it would be essential to give us the final proof. Many of the studies we hear about in the news are observational, but they are presented as if they demonstrate cause and effect.

These limitations do not mean such studies are useless. They are great at telling us what to study in greater depth. They may even function as a warning sign against possible temporary actions: you may decide to wait and see about making a change until the definitive study is done.

Observational studies take the form of cross-sectional studies, case control studies, and cohort studies. In a cross-sectional study a large number of people are asked questions—about diagnosis, symptoms, habits, and so on—at a specific time. It may study all women diagnosed with breast cancer in a particular year and look at how many of the women with hormone positive tumors (see Chapter 5) were taking hormone replacement therapy (HRT). If this was a high number you would be suspicious, but it would not prove that the HRT was the culprit. The next step is often a case control study because it is easy and cheap to do. A case control study looks at a group of people with a certain condition, comparing them to another group without that condition but with other similarities to the first group. For example, we could take 100 women who had taken HRT for 10 years and match them as carefully as possible with 100 women in the same age-group with the same socioeconomic environment who had not. Then we could see how many breast cancers occurred in each group. This is a cheap and relatively easy way to test the hypothesis generated by an observational study. If the difference between the two groups is statistically significant (it couldn't happen by chance alone), we conclude that there is an association between HRT and breast cancer. This does not prove, however, that one caused the other, a fact often missed by the media.

If many case control studies support the hypothesis and findings, then it may be worth doing a cohort (follow-up) study. In a cohort study a particular group of people are followed over time. Cohort studies have subcategories of their own. Retrospective cohort studies, using information gathered years before, examine subjects at a defined time, usually years later, to see the relationship between the factor being studied and the outcome. For example, they may look at how many of the subjects had a high-fat diet as children. This is not as expensive and time-consuming as a *prospective* cohort study, which starts at the opposite end. These are done only if many case control studies are positive and the question is of considerable clinical or social importance. A group of subjects is followed forward over a period of years. (See the Epilogue to read about the HOW study in the Army of Women, which uses all of these types of studies to find the cause of breast cancer.)

UNDERSTANDING RISK

Every woman wants to know what her risk of getting breast cancer is and what she can do about it. Before discussing the figures, however, we need to be clear about where they come from, since they're often used in confusing and misleading ways. For example, an advertisement calling milk "99 percent fat free" may suggest that it has 1 percent of the amount of fat in whole milk.

Actually, it means that 1 percent of the milk is made up of fat. Since only 3.6 percent of whole milk is made up of fat, whole milk could be called "96.4 percent fat free." Thus a more helpful ad would say, "less than one-third the fat of whole milk." Likewise, when media headlines say that three alcoholic drinks a week increase breast cancer risk by 50 percent they don't mean you have a fifty-fifty chance of getting breast cancer, but rather that these drinks increase the relative risk by 50 percent and your lifetime risk is now about 5 percent rather than 3.3 percent. Thus it is important that we examine the common statistics used about breast cancer and review exactly what they mean. There are three kinds of risk commonly referred to in connection with breast cancer: absolute risk, relative risk, and attributable risk (Figure 4.18).

Absolute risk is the rate at which cancer or mortality from cancer occurs in a general population. It can be expressed either as the number of cases per a specified population (e.g., 50 cases per 100,000 annually) or as a cumulative risk up to a particular age. This cumulative risk is the source of the familiar 1 in 8 for non-Hispanic white women. (Other racial and ethnic groups may actually have a lower risk; see Table 4.1.)

Future risk at any one time also depends to a great extent on your age. At age 20 the risk over the next 10 years is 1 in 2,152 (0.05 percent), while the risk over the next 10 years for a fifty-year-old is 1 in 36 (2.78 percent) (see Table 4.2).

The second kind of risk we talk about determining is *relative risk*. This is the comparison of the incidence of breast cancer or deaths from breast cancer among people with a particular risk factor to that of people without that factor, or a "reference population." This type of measurement is more useful to an individual woman because she can determine her risk factors and thus calculate how they will affect her chances of getting the disease. Even here you have to be very careful. For comparison, you can't use the 1 in 8, or 12 percent, generated in the absolute risk equation (discussed above) because that is based on all women regardless of risk factors. Rather, you need a number that will reflect a woman's risk without the factors being considered. For a woman with no clear risk factors at all (no previous cancers, no family history, menarche after 11, menopause before 52, first pregnancy

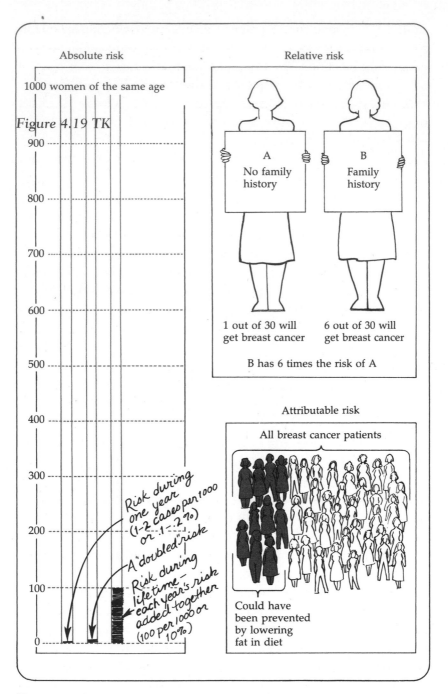

Absolute risk

1000 women of the same age

Figure 4.19 TK

Relative risk

A
No family
history

B
Family
history

1 out of 30 will
get breast cancer

6 out of 30 will
get breast cancer

B has 6 times the risk of A

Attributable risk

All breast cancer patients

Could have
been prevented
by lowering
fat in diet

Risk during
one year
(1-2 cases per 1000
or .1-.2 %)

A "doubled" risk

Risk during
lifetime—
each year's risk
added together
(100 per 1000 or
10%)

Figure 4.18

Table 4-1.   Breast Cancer Incidence in Different Racial/Ethnic Groups

risk	Age-adjusted Cases/ 100,000 women/year	Lifetime risk percent	Lifetime risk
Caucasian	141	14.1%	1 in 7
African American	122	10.2%	1 in 10
Asian/Pacific Islanders	97		
Hispanics	90		
American Indians/ Alaskan Natives	58		

Source: A. Ghafoor, A. Samuels, A. Jemal. *Breast Cancer Facts and Figures 2003–2004.* American Cancer Society, pg 3. Accessed online on 4/17/05 at www.cancer.org

Table 4-2.   Age Specific Probabilities of Developing Breast Cancer

If current age is:	Then probability of developing breast cancer in the next 10 years is:	Or 1 in:
20	0.05%	2,152
30	0.40%	251
40	1.45%	69
50	2.78%	36
60	3.81%	26
70	4.31%	23

Source: American Cancer Society Surveillance Research 2003

before 30) this is 1 in 30, or 3.3 percent, significantly lower than the "average" risk of 12 percent.[10]

If you call the risk of the woman without any particular risk factors 1.0, you can report the risk of those *with* a particular risk factor in relation to this. This is how relative risk is derived. A woman whose mother had breast cancer in both breasts before the age of 40, for example, has a relative risk of 2.7 over her lifetime—that is, 2.7 times that of the woman with no family history, not, as it might appear, 2.7 times the 12 percent mentioned above (see Table 4.3).

Table 4-3.   Factors That Increase the Relative Risk for Breast Cancer in Women

Relative Risk	Factor
Relative Risk >4.0	• Age (65+ vs. <65 years, although risk increases across all ages until age 80) • Certain inherited genetic mutations for breast cancer (BRCA 1 and/or BRCA 2) • Two or more first-degree relatives with breast cancer diagnosed at an early age • Personal history of breast cancer • Postmenopausal breast density
Relative Risk 2.1-4.0	• One first-degree relative with breast cancer • Biopsy-confirmed atypical hyperplasia • High-dose radiation to chest • High bone density (postmenopausal)
Relative Risk 1.1-2.0	
Reproductive factors	• Late age at first full-term pregnancy (>30 years) • Early menarche (<12 years) • Late menopause (>55 years) • No full-term pregnancies • Never breast fed a child
Factors that affect circulating hormones	• Recent oral contraceptive use • Recent and long term use of hormone-replacement therapy • Obesity (postmenopausal)
Other factors	• Personal history of cancer of endometrium, ovary or colon • Alcohol consumption • Tall • High socioeconomic status • Jewish heritage

Source: A. Ghafoor, A. Samuels, A. Jemal. Breast Cancer Facts and Figures 2003-2004. American Cancer Society, pg 3. Accessed online on 4/17/05 at www.cancer.org

How an increase in relative risk affects your absolute risk also depends on your age at the time. For example, a threefold relative risk (compared to that of the general population) at a young age will increase your absolute risk by about 20 percent, while by age 50, the woman with the threefold increased relative risk has a lifetime risk of about 14 percent. One-third of the breast cancers occur before age 50, and so her risk is only two-thirds of that. She has about a 4.5 percent chance of developing breast cancer over the next 10 years and about 10.5 percent in the next 20 years, compared with the average risks of 1.5 and 3.5 percent, respectively.[11]

When you read a study or see one reported in the media, it is important to check the basis for the relative risk numbers. Most authors compare women with a specific risk factor to women without it. They assume that all the other risk factors are equal in both groups, so that only their risk in terms of the risk factor of interest is being compared. It's like the fat in the milk: the numbers can be very misleading if you don't take the time to put them in context.

Finally, we must consider the *attributable risk*. This concept relates more to public policy. It looks at the amount of disease in the population that could be prevented by alteration of risk factors. For example, a risk factor could convey a very large relative risk but be restricted to a few individuals, so changing it would benefit only these individuals. Dr. Anthony B. Miller has hypothesized that if every woman in the world were to have a baby before 25, 17 percent of the world's breast cancer would be eliminated.[12] If you were looking at this from a public health policy perspective, you'd have to weigh the possible advantages of pushing early pregnancy against the problems of young and possibly immature parents, and possible increased population growth.

To understand any of this, we need to go back to the original terminology. What do we mean by risk factors and how are they determined? "Risk factor" is a term referring to identifiable factors that make some people more susceptible than others to a particular disease; for example, smoking is a risk factor in lung cancer, and high cholesterol is a risk factor in heart disease. Medical researchers attempt to define risk factors in order to discover who is most likely to get a particular disease, and also to get clues as to the disease's cause and thus to the possible prevention and/or cure. A risk factor is usually determined by an observational study.

Sometimes, as in the case of lung cancer and smoking, risk factors are dramatic and can make a clear difference in the individual's likelihood of getting the disease. Unfortunately, it usually doesn't work this way. In breast cancer, we have come up with some risk factors—such as family history—which we'll look at in a later chapter. But so far, there is nothing comparable to the connections found between cholesterol and heart disease or between smoking and lung cancer. With breast cancer, the sad reality is that we can't say, as with lung cancer, "You're fairly safe because you're not in this particular population." In fact, 70 percent of breast cancer patients have none of the classical risk factors in their background.[13] It's important to understand this, for two reasons. Overestimating the importance of risk factors can cause needless mental anguish if you have one of them in your background. On the other hand, you may harbor a false sense of security if you don't have them. I can't count the number of times a patient has come to me with a suspicious lump that turns out to be malignant and, stunned, says, "I don't know how this happened! No one in my family ever had breast cancer!" I tell her she's in good company—most breast cancer patients don't have a family history of breast cancer. By virtue of being women, we are at risk for breast cancer.

Risk factors don't necessarily increase in a simple arithmetical fashion. If one risk factor gives you a 20 percent risk of getting breast cancer and another gives you a 10 percent chance, it doesn't always mean that now you're up to 30 percent. The interaction of risk factors is a tricky and complicated process. One interesting example concerns studies on alcohol and breast cancer (which we'll consider later in the book) showing that women with other risk factors who also drank liquor didn't increase their risk very much, while women with no other risk factors who drank raised their risk dramatically.[14]

In the next several chapters we will be exploring the known risk factors and the ways we try to test for risk, but how all this works is still not clear. It reminds me of the old story of the blind men and the elephant. Each man carefully described one section of the elephant's anatomy, but no one got the whole picture. Our descriptions of risk are still fragmentary and there is often the sense that we are missing something big that would tie it all together and enable us to say, "This causes breast cancer so don't do it!" But breast cancer is complex and has many factors that interact with one another in ways we don't understand yet.

So why do we even bother with all these risk factors if they don't really help determine the risk to the individual woman? We do it because it will give us hints as to the cause of the disease— and thus more tools for its prevention and cure. So read on, not to calculate your exact risk or that of your daughter or even to learn how to live your life risk free, but to understand what you read in the media and to explore the mystery that is breast cancer. And if you want to play your own role in sorting it out, join the Love/Avon Army of Women and the Health of Women Study (www.armyofwomen.org) and be part of the research to end breast cancer once and for all.

Chapter 5

Risk Factors

Returning to the metaphor of the mutated cell in a community of supporting cells (Chapter 4), it makes sense to understand the potential causes of breast cancer as those that create mutations and those that affect the community. However, readers who braved the previous chapter will know that nothing is that simple. For one thing, there is some evidence that postmenopausal estrogen can cause mutations in cells,[1] and there is plenty of evidence that it can also quickly change the environment that serves as fertilizer for mutated cells. Further, we now have reason to think that exposures in the womb to various substances can increase breast cancer risk in adult life by modifying the genes epigenetically (mutating temporarily rather than permanently). And we have long known that in a fully formed human we can modify both the potential cancer cell and/or its community.

In addition to the difficulties of trying to figure out a biological cause for breast cancer, we are dealing with the fact that not all breast cancer is the same. As I will explain at length in Chapter 11, there are different kinds of breast cancer that behave differently and respond to different treatments. It is logical to assume that these types of breast cancer may also have different causes and therefore different risk factors. Other than hereditary breast cancer, we have continued to treat them as if they were all one disease. For comparison, it's as if we assumed all lung infections had the same cause by virtue of being in the lung. But tuberculosis differs from strep pneumonia or bronchitis.

Lessons from Breast Cancer Around the World

One clue might be to look at breast cancer as it manifests in different parts of the world. In my work in China over the past five years, I have been struck with the fact that the average age at which breast cancer occurs there is younger than in the United States because older Chinese women are less likely to develop breast cancer than American ones. The average age is 48 in China, as opposed to 68 in the United States.[2] This led me to investigate further. What I found surprised me. The incidence of breast cancer below the age of 50 is about the same in all the countries we have studied (see Figure 5.1).[3] However, after 50 (around the age of menopause) the rates in the nonwesternized countries level off while those in the westernized countries continue to rise.[4,5] There are some hints in these data. African American women have a pattern much like that of women in nonwesternized countries, while the granddaughters of Japanese women who immigrate here have the same pattern as the native-born white residents. Obviously something about the Western lifestyle is at least partially responsible for the increasing growth of postmenopausal breast cancer. This kind of cancer tends to be mostly hormone positive, found on a mammogram, and relatively slow growing. Its increase is probably related to the use of postmenopausal hormones, mammography screening (see Chapter 8), and other factors such as inactivity, age at first childbirth, and perhaps exposure to chemical pollutants.[6] This postmenopausal breast cancer tends to be more common in women of higher socioeconomic status—the ones who had the opportunity to take hormone therapy, get mammograms, postpone childbirth. They often live in major metropolitan areas and may also differ in envi-

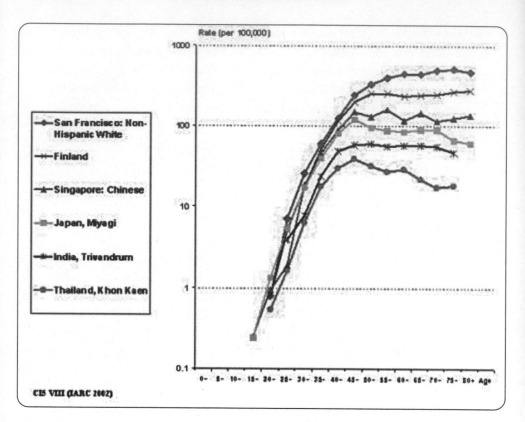

Figure 5.1

ronmental exposures or product use. (Remember these are gener-alizations because I am talking about big groups. There are always exceptions.)

What is more interesting to me, however, is the pre-menopausal breast cancer that has the same pattern around the world. That cancer is aggressive, relatively fast growing, and less often sensitive to hormones. Its causes also seem to differ, though we don't yet know what specifically those causes are. While some of it is related to hereditary mutations, this explains only 5–10 percent around the world.

Premenopausal cancer seems less related to the classic risk factors linked to hormones, like first pregnancy, use of hormone therapy, and menopause. One hypothesis we've been looking at is that it may be related to a viral infection. The limited evidence available on environmental factors also suggest that environment may have more effect on premenopausal cancers.

I am hopeful that the work I'm currently involved in through the Love/Avon Army of Women and the HOW Study (see the Epilogue) will help us learn more about the different causes of breast cancer. With luck, we'll know a lot more by the time this book goes into its next edition. Meanwhile, we do have information about some of the nongenetic causes of breast cancer, if not how they specifically work.

UNDERSTANDING RISK FACTORS

When we talk about the risk of breast cancer, we look at two different types of risk factors: genetic factors and a range of nongenetic factors that include hormones, diet, alcohol consumption, environmental carcinogens, and radiation. I'll explain genetic risk factors in Chapter 6 and address the others here.

As I mentioned earlier, most women who get breast cancer have never had a known risk factor.[7] Often this throws them. As one recent Facebook friend who was diagnosed with DCIS in 2007 writes, "I was only 41 at the time with no family history; a healthy eater with no weight issues; and I had just spent the last two years training for two LA marathons. I was in great shape and on top of the world. I thought breast cancer only 'attacked' women after menopause or those with a family history. My body had let me down. I felt totally betrayed." This anecdote highlights one of the problems when we talk about risk. We have been led to believe that if we do everything right, we will never get breast cancer. As those of you who read the last chapter have learned, breast cancer is a complicated disease. Before enumerating the risk factors we do know, it is worth looking at how we study risk. It's a bit more complicated than most of us have been led to believe.

What do we mean by risk factors and how are they determined? "Risk factor" is a term referring to identifiable factors that make some people more susceptible than others to a particular disease. Smoking is a risk factor in lung cancer, and high cholesterol is a risk factor in heart disease. Medical researchers attempt to define risk factors in order to discover who is most likely to get a particular disease, and also to get clues as to the disease's cause and its possible prevention and/or cure. A risk factor is usually determined by an observational study.

As I noted earlier, the older you are, the higher your chances of getting breast cancer. The publicity about breast cancer, which has increased rapidly in recent years, gives the impression that the disease is hitting younger and younger women. That's partially true. The *percentage* of young women getting breast cancer is the same as it's always been. It's the *number* of younger women in the country that has risen in recent years, because the baby boomers are in their forties and fifties. If you take 10 percent of 40, you get 4; if you take 10 percent of 400, you get 40. There are more forty-something women with breast cancer because there are more forty-something women around. (There's no breast cancer rise among Gen Xers, by the way. There are fewer of them than boomers, and breast cancer in really young women—teens and twenties—has always been unusual.)

Most breast cancer in thte United States still occurs in women over 50—about 80 percent of cases. Your risk at age 30 of getting breast cancer in the next 10 years (see Table 4.1) is 1 in 251. By age 40, it's 1 in 69 in the next 10 years.[8] So the risk of getting breast cancer before you're 50 is very small. The median age for breast cancer diagnosis is 64, which means that half of women who get breast cancer will get it before age 64 and half will get it after.

So whenever you look at risk factors, you need to correct for age. Other risk factors (e.g., family history, hormonal factors) will most likely cause breast cancer only in combination with rising age.

Another factor we need to look at is the variation among ethnic groups. Almost all the data you read are based on non-Hispanic Caucasian women. Table 4.1 demonstrates that the risk for African American and Asian women is lower than for white women. But this is deceptive. At age 30 the 10-year risk for an African American woman is 0.5 percent, while it is 0.4 percent for a Caucasian woman, 0.3 percent for a Hispanic woman, and 0.4 percent for an Asian/Pacific Islander. The disparity between white and black women exists because African American women have rates similar to those of premenopausal white women, but lower than those of postmenopausal white women. That won't necessarily be comforting news to African American women, however. Although it's less common in that group, it's often more deadly (see Chapter 19). When Rowan Chlebowski looked at the postmenopausal women who participated in the large Women's Health Initiative study, he found that most of the differences in incidence attributed to race and ethnicity could be explained by known risk factors except for those in African Americans.[9]

Interestingly, there's also a class variation—white women of higher socioeconomic status get more breast cancer than do poorer white women.[10] Black women of higher socioeconomic status also have a higher risk than poorer black women. Breast cancer seems to "discriminate" opposite to the way our society discriminates.

Radiation

Okay, now you know how we look for risk factors: let's move on the factors themselves. I am starting with radiation because it is a well documented cause of many other kinds of cancer. Radiation is known to cause mutations in the breast cells. In addition, mutations known as *radiosensitizers* intensify the effects of radiation, probably by acting on the surrounding cells.

At least three major studies have confirmed the link between radiation and increased risk of breast cancer. The first study came out of one of the twentieth century's major tragedies—the bombings of Hiroshima and Nagasaki at the end of World War II. The people in the immediate area of the bombings died instantly, or shortly after the bombs were dropped. But it has become evident over time that those within a 10-kilometer radius of the bomb-sites developed far more cancer than others in comparable populations, and scientists began studying these patients to learn more about the dangers of radiation. They measured the amount of radiation the people had been exposed to and then studied them over the years to see what cancers they developed.[11]

The best analysis of this sample reports that women exposed to the bomb had a relative risk of developing breast cancer that was much higher if it happened before they were 20 than when they were older.[12] The effects were greatest among women who had been in their teens and early twenties, and nearly nonexistent in women who had been in their fifties and sixties. Reports have also indicated an increased risk in the women who were less than 10 at the time of the exposure. The effect took longer to be revealed because it didn't appear until the women had reached the age at which breast cancer normally occurs. This supports other findings about the particular vulnerability of the developing breast to carcinogenic agents.

An interesting finding among A-bomb survivors is that those who had early full-term pregnancies were at significantly lower risk than those who hadn't. Remarkably, this protection occurred among women who were exposed as children, as well as among those exposed as adults. Here is confirmation that the maturation of breast tissue occurring during a full-term pregnancy drastically reduces the ability of a cell to progress to cancer, even if it has received earlier damage that would predispose it to the disease.[13] This provides us with even more evidence that it often takes more than one factor to cause a breast cancer.

A second study looked at women who had been treated for tuberculosis with fluoroscopy.[14] This was a common treatment in the 1930s and 1940s, before we knew of the dangers of radiation and instead saw it as a magic cure-all. The typical treatment for TB was to collapse the infected lung to rest it and then check it with X rays every day to see how it was doing. When the women were studied in the 1970s, they were found to have an increased incidence of breast cancer. I came across a similar case in my own practice. A fifty-eight-year-old patient I diagnosed with breast cancer had contracted TB in her early twenties. She lived in France and was treated with intensive radiation in a sanitarium. Her two best friends at the sanitarium, treated with the same radiation therapy she was given, also developed breast cancer.

The third major study examined a group of 606 women in Rochester, New York, who had suffered postpartum mastitis— painfully inflamed breasts (Chapter 2)—and had been given radiation averaging between 50 and 450 rads for both breasts to alleviate their pain.[15] They too had a rate of breast cancer higher than that of the general population. And the risk was dose related. This study is interesting for a second reason. The radiation was given after the first pregnancy, which should have been protective. But it was also given during lactation, a time of high activity in the breast.

There are other studies confirming the existence of radiation-induced breast cancer. One showed an increase in the disease among women with scoliosis who had received a lot of X rays to monitor their backs during puberty.[16] Another showed an increase among a group of women who had had radiation therapy to their chest for acne—also during puberty.[17] Still another study found an increase in women who had had their thymus radiated in infancy or early childhood to shrink it. (The thymus, a normal gland in the middle of the chest, always starts out large, then shrinks with age. But we didn't always know this, and doctors used to "treat" large thymuses with radiation.)[18]

A smaller but still significant study showed that exposure to radiation was linked to an increased risk of breast cancer in a sample of medical diagnostic X ray workers in China, female employees at a nuclear plant, female and male Finnish airline cabin attendants, and radiologic technologists in the United States.[19,20,21,22]

All these studies show that the danger is from exposure to moderate doses of radiation (10–500 rads), and all but the A-bomb and the last study show that the danger is only to the area of the body at which the radiation has been aimed. Thus people exposed to radiation in another area (e.g., for cancer of the cervix) did not show an increased rate of breast cancer.[23] The Nagasaki and Hiroshima survivors had their whole bodies exposed to radiation, and they suffered increased vulnerability to virtually all forms of cancer. Another interesting finding in all these studies is the long latency period. The excess risk does not appear until the age at which breast cancer commonly occurs. This suggests that radiation is only part of the early picture and that other moderating influences come later and affect the development of breast cancer. The duration of the increased risk from radiation is also not known, but in the atomic bomb survivors, fluoroscopy patients, and mastitis patients, it appears to have lasted at least 35 years after the time of exposure.

The exposure in these studies differs in magnitude from the kind you get with diagnostic chest X rays and mammograms. Many people are legitimately concerned about such X rays, but it's a mistake to throw out a highly useful diagnostic tool. Remember that the danger comes with a total cumulative dose of radiation. If you had a chest X ray every week for two years, you probably would increase your risk of getting breast cancer. But the danger of leaving pneumonia undetected, if you have reason to believe it may exist, is far greater than any danger from infrequent chest X rays. Similarly, the level of radiation in up-to-date mammograms (one-fourth of a rad) won't increase your risk of breast cancer very much, unless you start getting the X rays at a young age. As with everything in medicine, you need to balance the risk of having untreated breast cancer against the risk of radiation exposure. As for other diagnostic X rays, I think if a doctor suggests an imaging technique that involves radiation for any condition, you should ask whether the exam is going to change your treatment. For example, will doctors decide you need surgery or a strong drug if the X ray indicates that you have the condition they're looking for? If not, the extra information probably isn't worth the risk the exposure to radiation brings with it. Radiation effects are cumulative, and you want to accumulate only as much as you really need.

But what about radiation used to treat an existing cancer? This radiation falls at the other end of the spectrum: very high levels of radiation are used, on the order of 8,000 rads. In this context, however, the risk from radiation is far outweighed by the risk from the cancer you have. For example, radiation is used to treat Hodgkin's disease, a cancer of the lymph nodes. By itself and in conjunction with chemotherapy it has been responsible for many cures. However, some women who had this treatment years ago are now showing up with breast cancer. We suspect that the chest radiation which saved their lives is responsible for the second cancer.[24] Though this is frightening and disheartening, it's important to remember that the original radiation treatment gave these women those years of life before breast cancer emerged.

ENVIRONMENTAL EXPOSURES

This is an area that has not yet been as well studied as we would like. I used to ask all my patients if they had any environmental or occupational exposures to carcinogens. Almost to a woman,

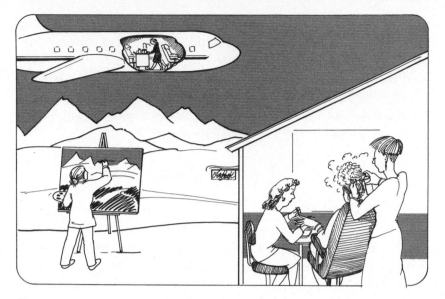

Figure 5.2

they'd say no. Then I'd ask what they did for a living. Very often they did in fact have exposures. For example, one of my patients worked as a manicurist for 15 years, inhaling fumes from nail polish and nail polish remover in a close area. Could that be a carcinogen? Another woman was an artist who used oil paints. She was exposed to the solvents used to clean the oil paint as well as the cadmium in the paint, which some studies suggest may be a strong carcinogen (Figure 5.2).

There are probably a lot of environmental exposures that don't occur to us because we're not used to thinking about life that way. In 1993 the National Cancer Institute held the first conference on occupational risks of cancer in women. (Until then, the assumption seemed to be that women didn't have occupations.) Women who work at home are exposed to many different cleaning solvents and insecticides, which may be among the factors that lead to breast cancer.

If you have questions about chemicals you have been exposed to, the most comprehensive list of chemicals that cause breast

cancer in animal studies is searchable online at www.silent
spring.org/scienceview. Keep in mind, though, that most chemicals in use have never been tested for effects on breast cancer[25]
and that not everything that causes breast cancer in animals will
do so in humans. Joining the HOW study (see the Epilogue) may
be the best way for you to help us figure out any particular links
between breast cancer and the environment.

Electromagnetic Field (EMF) Exposure

Another subject that often comes up is the harm from electromagnetic fields. Electric and magnetic fields arise from the motion of electric charges. They are characterized as *nonionizing
radiation* when they lack sufficient energy to remove electrons
from atoms, as opposed to *ionizing* radiation such as X rays and
gamma rays. EMFs are emitted from devices that produce, transmit, or use electric power such as power lines, transmitters, and
common household items like electric clocks, shavers, and blankets, computers, televisions, heated waterbeds, and microwave
ovens.

Several studies have explored the connection between electric
blankets and breast cancer. A recent large study of breast cancer
in women under 55 found no connection,[26] nor did either retrospective or prospective analyses within the large Nurses' Health
Study cohort[27] or in the large Long Island study based on 1,354
cases.[28] So you can feel free to snuggle up fearlessly in your favorite electric blanket on those cold winter days.

Pesticides and Other Toxic Exposures

Since the 1940s, scientists and engineers have synthesized many
thousands of new chemicals made from petroleum, while other
new compounds have entered the environment as products of
combustion or as industrial byproducts. We have benefited greatly
from plastics, pesticides, inexpensive energy, and other modern
inventions. However, studies in laboratory animals and isolated
cells grown in petri dishes show that some environmental pollutants and consumer product chemicals stimulate biological activ-

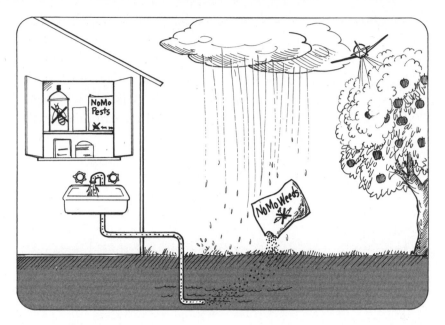

Figure 5.3

ity that raises concerns about breast cancer. Some chemicals can mimic estrogen (a known breast cancer risk factor),[29] damage DNA, and cause breast tumors in animals, or affect the development of the breast in ways that make the tissues more vulnerable in later life (Figure 5.3).

Studying the effects of chemical pollutants in humans is difficult. We use experimental methods called clinical trials to find out whether medicines work or cause harm, but we would never intentionally expose a group of women to chemical pollutants to see if they get sick. Furthermore, breast cancer develops over many years (remember the long lag from the atomic bombs to the cancers women got later on), but we don't want to wait decades to find out if chemicals we use every day cause breast cancer. Some activists believe we should rely on animal or in vitro tests to identify chemicals to avoid in everyday use, while at the same time conducting studies that follow women long-term to learn more. This approach is sometimes called the precautionary principle. While I understand their concern, women are one of the few animals that get breast cancer. And women are complicated. The research has to be done on women if we are going to figure out potential links.

For example, many chemicals in the environment can mimic estrogen in the lab, such as organochlorines (such as DDT and PCBs). These are persistent environmental contaminants that have been identified throughout the global ecosystem in, for example, fish, wildlife, and human tissue, including blood and breast milk. The problem is that, as our studies on the physiology of the nonlactating breast have shown, finding a compound in breast milk does not mean it is found in the breast of a nonlactating woman.

In addition, some of these chemicals and their breakdown products, though not estrogen, have some of the effects of estrogen (in fact, they are often but inaccurately referred to as "weak estrogen"). This has caused many people to think that these substances can stimulate and cause breast cancer just as actual estrogen can. Indeed, they do stimulate human breast cancer cells to grow in laboratory studies.[30]

But not all estrogen-like chemicals have the same effects. For example, tamoxifen acts like estrogen on the uterus but actually *blocks* estrogen in the breast. And soy, which has been called a plant estrogen, has recently been shown to decrease breast cancer recurrences.[31] Finally, recent data suggest that progestin is more carcinogenic than estrogen.[32]

Several observational studies have failed to demonstrate a relationship between occupational exposure to pesticides and breast cancer. For example, neither the Nurses' Health Study nor a European study nor one done in Mexico (where DDT is not banned) has found any relationship between blood levels of DDE, a breakdown product of DDT, and PCBs and breast cancer.[33,34,35] At the same time, observational studies can miss connections. Critics have suggested that these studies used methods that share important limitations. In particular, studies have relied on blood samples taken near the time of a breast cancer diagnosis, long after the cancer began, and the studies typically measure DDE, which is not the same as DDT itself.[36] It could also be that, as with radiation, the age of exposure makes a difference. A 2007 study based on blood samples collected in women who gave birth in California in the 1950s and 1960s found higher breast cancer risk among those who were most likely to have been exposed to DDT as preteen girls.[37]

Breast cancer activists on Cape Cod and Long Island (where there is very high incidence of breast cancer) were responsible for some of the studies done in the early 1990s. They demanded that the government support studies to investigate the high incidence of breast cancer in their areas. Though the studies have not yielded definitive results, they have suggested that there was increased breast cancer risk in women with more DNA damage in their blood from polycyclic aromatic hydocarbons (PAH), which are formed in foods cooked at high temperatures. The women who demanded these studies opened the way to breast cancer activism and raised some questions that remain unanswered.[38] Most importantly, we need to learn why these populations were getting more breast cancer. There must be some cause, even if this study didn't find it. Further studies may help clarify this.

I think that the issue is complex and must take into consideration time of exposure and other associated risk factors. There may be an environmental relationship, but it is probably small. Nonetheless, this lack of definitive answers is no excuse for not evaluating the safety of chemicals in consumer products or cleaning up the environment. There are enough known health problems from environmental pollution to convince us that it needs to be seriously curtailed. This is a fairly new area of scientific study. Who knows what we'll find in the next 5 or 10 years?

Viruses and Bacteria

Many cancers are caused by infections, whether viral (like cancer of the cervix), or bacterial (like cancer of the stomach). Sometimes a virus infects the cell, hijacks its DNA, and inserts some of its own DNA, thus causing a mutation. Other times a virus or bacteria causes a chronic low-grade inflammation, which in turn leads to conditions that promote the development of cancer. Could a bacteria or a virus cause breast cancer? Sure! Mouse mammary tumor virus (MMTV) creates breast cancer in both captured field mice and laboratory-bred mice. MMTV-like viral genetic material has been found in human breast tumors.[39] To date this is only guilt by association: the virus may not be the cause but simply an innocent bystander. Other viruses, such as high-risk human papilloma virus and Epstein Barr virus have also been found in human breast tumors. Again, we don't know what connection there is, if any.[40] In the past decade there has been a resurgence in interest in investigating a possible viral cause of breast cancer. With luck, we'll soon have some answers about this. The study of AIDS has given us knowledge about not only that disease but, as a highly useful by-product, about viruses in general.

HORMONAL RISK FACTORS

How hormones exert their influence on breast cancer is not clear. They may bring epigenetic (see Chapter 4) influences in the womb, and carcinogenic effects; further, they are virtually certain to be a factor that makes the neighborhood more encouraging to cancer cells. They most definitely are a major influence on, if not a cause of, breast cancer.

Our Own Hormones

When you think about hormones and breast cancer, you tend to think in terms of hormone pills. Much attention (and much *needed* attention) has been paid to the relationship between cancer and use of oral contraceptives, menopausal hormone therapy, and fertility drugs. Less consideration has been paid to our body's own hormonal levels. Do women with naturally high levels of estrogen have higher risks of breast cancer? What about testosterone? (As I mentioned in Chapter 1, women have testosterone, though in much smaller amounts than men do.) Multiple studies have shown that circulating levels of estradiol and of testosterone are associated with breast cancer risk in postmenopausal women: women with the highest level of hormones have two to three times the breast cancer risk of those with the lowest level. Cumulatively, epidemiological data suggest that there is a role for prolactin in breast cancer as well.[41] While these results are interesting, they may be deceptive, since the information has been obtained through blood tests. But we now know that in at least some women the breast tissue is capable of making its own estrogen locally through the enzymes *aromatase* and *sulfatase*.[42] We know also that the tissue around a tumor has higher estrogen levels than the tissue far from it.[43] Even though what we measure in the blood may not represent what is going on in the breast, studies do show that blood levels can be highly predictive of breast cancer risk.

Early Influences

Some of the most intriguing data on the influence of hormones suggest that prenatal influences may affect breast cancer risk. In studies, fetal mice were exposed to the estrogen-like bisphenol A (a substance used in making plastics). This resulted in long-lasting effects in the mice's mammary gland that manifested as precancerous changes during puberty.[44] A similar mechanism may work in human females as well. This was tragically demonstrated during the 1950s and 1960s; a synthetic estrogen, diethylstilbestrol (DES), was widely prescribed to pregnant women to prevent miscarriages. Many years later we discovered that DES increased the risk of vaginal and cervical cancer in those women's daughters. A recent follow-up study suggested, but did not prove, an increased risk of breast cancer in daughters under 40 and a definite increase in risk in those over 40.[45] While far from definitive, this leads us to believe that there may be influences in the womb that set the stage for later disease.

Another way of viewing these influences is to look at factors at birth. Data are pretty consistent that high birth weight (which gives us clues about in utero estrogen levels) correlates with later breast cancer risk.[46] On the other hand, preeclampsia, a condition associated with low estrogen levels, decreases the child's subsequent breast cancer risk.[47,48] Other factors indicate that good nutrition during childhood also correlates with breast cancer risk. One hypothesis is that early stimulants for growth (internal and external factors that lend themselves to growth, the way rain, sun, and fertilizer encourage a plant's growth) also increase the number of breast stem cells that are available to undergo mutations later in life.[49] These mutations can be inherited or acquired by exposure to carcinogens. Another theory is that the early hormones cause epigenetic changes of the DNA (changes that have the potential to revert, though such reversion is not inevitable).

Adult Hormones

There is no question that exposure to hormones affects our risk throughout life. For example, the younger a woman is at her first period and the older she is when she goes into menopause, the longer she has reproductive levels of hormones, the more likely she is to get breast cancer than is a woman with a shorter reproductive period (Table 4.3). If she menstruates for more than 40 years, she seems to have a particularly high risk. A woman whose ovaries are removed early and who doesn't take hormone therapy has a greatly reduced risk of breast cancer.[50] Oddly enough, however, one recent study has suggested that ovarian removal increases mortality overall: while protecting you from breast cancer, it increases your vulnerability to other conditions such as heart disease.[51] If you've had a hysterectomy, it may or may not influence your risk of breast cancer, depending on whether your ovaries were removed. If you still have ovaries, your body continues to go through hormonal cycles, even though you have no periods; these cycles continue until the time you would normally go into menopause.

Pregnancy appears to affect breast cancer risk in two ways. During a pregnancy and for the 10 years following it, a woman has a greater risk of developing breast cancer, presumably because the hormones of pregnancy have caused more cell division.[52,53] A recent hypothesis suggests that involution (resetting of the breast after weaning) sets the stage for more cancer.[54] However, women who have never been pregnant seem to be more at risk than women who have a child before 35. The hormones of a pregnancy carried to term will mature the breast tissue, making it less susceptible to carcinogens. Women who have their first pregnancy after 35 have a greater risk than women who have never been pregnant at all. Although it had been hypothesized that therapeutic abortion or miscarriage might increase breast cancer risk, large studies have shown no association.[55,56,57] Breast-feeding is protective against breast cancer, the relative risk decreasing 4.3 percent for every 12 months, in addition to a decrease of 7 percent for each birth. This in part explains some of the discrepancy between more developed and less developed countries, as there tends to be more and longer breast-feeding in poorer countries.[58]

After menopause most estradiol (estrogen) comes from converting androgens—hormones from the adrenal glands—into estradiol. Most of this conversion is done by fat tissue. Thus estradiol levels tend to increase with body weight. In contrast, body weight is not a risk factor for breast cancer before menopause: premenopausal estrogen comes from ovaries (see Chapter 1).

LIFESTYLE FACTORS IN BREAST CANCER

Birth Control Pills

The birth control pill also has a place in this story. Originally seen as the magic solution to unwanted pregnancy, "the pill" was vilified when its negative side effects became apparent. As is often the case, the reality of the pill is more complex. Especially in its early forms, the pill seemed to contribute to a number of illnesses, including stroke (especially in combination with cigarette smoking in women over 30). Later studies, however, have suggested that it may also be useful in protecting against certain diseases, such as ovarian cancer.[59] It stops ovulation, and the more you ovulate the more chance you have of getting ovarian cancer. So if you take the birth control pill and decrease the total number of ovulations, you can decrease your risk of ovarian cancer. And the pill has consistently been shown to reduce endometrial cancer as well. So what, then, is its relation to breast cancer?

Part of the problem in discussing "the pill" as though it were a single entity is that it, like some other inventions, has gone through many permutations. Earlier pills used much more estrogen and progestin than current pills do; we've changed both the amounts and the proportions of those hormones. So early findings aren't necessarily applicable to the pill used today. A study that says it's looking at women who have been on the pill for 10 or 20 years is actually likely to be looking at women who have been on a number of different pills at different times—which explains in part why we seem to get so many contradictory results with studies on the relationship between breast cancer and the pill. A 2002 study looked at 9,257 women between 35 and 64 (old enough to have taken oral contraceptives early in their reproductive years). It found no increased risk of breast cancer in either current or former users of the pill.[60] This may not be true for all women, however; some data suggest that women with a family history of breast cancer who start taking the pill between 18 and 20 and carry the BRCA 1 gene for breast cancer had an greater risk than the gene carriers who did not take the pill.[61] One interesting study suggests that the risk of breast cancer in regard to oral contraceptives may be related to the way they are broken down by the body, and that this may be different in different women.[62]

Postmenopausal Hormone Therapy

Over the past several decades we have shifted from considering menopause a natural part of life to thinking about it as a disease that needs treatment. It is hard sometimes to determine how much of that approach is thinly veiled marketing for the panoply of drugs offered to us as we age. Menopause is as natural a part of life as fertility is. Just as our bodies need high levels of hormones to reproduce, they also need the downshift to a more reasonable level after menopause (see Chapter 1). Those who favor long-term hormone therapy argue that we're not "supposed" to live long enough to go into menopause in the first place; in the old days people died in their thirties and forties. But in fact people didn't all die so soon. True, the "average life expectancy" was low—as low as 32 in 1640. But that average was drawn from all deaths and did not represent a typical age of death. Until modern medicine came along, there were large numbers of deaths at all ages, and especially in childhood. It was no more usual to die at 35 than at 65. Men were considered fit for military service until they were 60, and a fair number of people of both genders lived into their nineties.[63,64,65] So that argument makes no sense.

We once believed that the ovaries stopped functioning at menopause. Recent studies have shown that to be a fallacy—most women's ovaries don't stop functioning. But until recently, there was no test available that could detect lower levels of estrogen, and so it was assumed that there weren't any such levels. Actually most women continue to produce hormones well into their eighties—testosterone, androstenedione (both estrogen precursors), and even some estrogen.[66]

We are also starting to understand the symptoms of menopause. The traditional belief is that the symptoms of perimenopause come from low levels of hormones, but recent studies have shown that what's really at the core of symptoms is the *fluctuation* of hormones as the body rebalances at a new level. The transition typically takes between three and six years, and then the body settles into its new situation.

It's important to remember that there are two very distinct reasons for women to consider hormone therapy: symptom control and disease prevention. (Note that this refers only to estrogen and progestins: we will examine estrogen alone in post-oophorectomy women shortly). Hormone therapy does help reduce hot flashes, vaginal dryness, insomnia, night sweats—the vast range of uncomfortable, usually short-term symptoms many experience during their perimenopausal years. Typically, these symptoms are transient—they last about three to five years. After that, the body readjusts itself and the woman is fine. Although we used to think that the short-term use of hormones (three to five years) for women without breast cancer or clotting disorders was probably safe, a recent study from France has shown that women who start hormone therapy close to menopause have approximately a 50 percent increased breast cancer risk relative to nonusers even when they had used this regimen for two years or less.[67] As my colleague Leslie Bernstein wrote in her editorial regarding this paper, "It would seem that a conservative approach regarding the use of combined HT at menopause is warranted, using hormones briefly and only when menopausal symptoms are so intense that no other approach will work."[68] (For women who have had breast cancer, see Chapter 19.)

In the third edition of this book I discussed my concerns about the widespread use of hormones after menopause; in the fourth edition I told readers about the Women's Health Initiative (WHI), a study that had two components, one considering estrogen alone and the other, estrogen combined with a progestin. It showed that even relatively short-term use of estrogen plus progestin increases the susceptibility to breast cancer. In addition, by keeping breasts in a premenopausal state, the hormones create denser breast tissue, making mammograms less likely to catch cancers.[69] In this edition I can report that my fears and the WHI findings (see Chapter 7) have been confirmed by other studies.

When the results were announced in 2002, many women throughout the world abruptly stopped taking hormone therapy (HT), causing a sudden decrease in sales. In parallel there was a 28 percent decrease in breast cancer diagnosis in the United States, Australia, New Zealand, Canada, Germany, and France.[70] Significantly, the decrease was only in women over 50 and only in estrogen-sensitive tumors. Follow-up showed that within two years of starting HT, women taking both estrogen and progestin have an increased risk of breast cancer and within two years of stopping the risk disappears. Some critics suggested that the effect on cancer was too fast for it to have been caused by the HT. However, it is probable that the hormones were like fertilizer on nests of mutated cells already present (see Chapter 4). Interestingly, a study by Karla Kerlikowske has demonstrated that only the women who showed dense breasts on mammography and took estrogen plus progestin had an increased risk of breast cancer.[71]

Since estrogen has the potential to cause mutations, you would expect that, as with other cancers, breast cancer would take many years to appear. But if in this case estrogen with or without progestin may be simply *promoting* an existing dormant cancer, it "wakes up" the cancer cells. Thus the women who stopped taking the hormones might have, in effect, sent the cells back to sleep.

Because of the dangers of the combined hormones, the studies were stopped when that data emerged. The estrogen-only study was continued for a while, but it too was stopped prematurely, in 2004.[72] Here the findings were even more surprising: there was no increase in breast cancer risk or benefit to heart disease (which early studies had suggested was a good reason to take estrogen). The women had been on estrogen for only 6.8 years. Then in 2009 the American Cancer Society study showed that estrogen alone increases the risk of lobular (as opposed to ductal) breast cancer by 50 percent after 10 years.[73] Again, this was consistent with earlier observational studies, which had shown that the risk of estrogen alone was significantly less than that of estrogen plus progestin.[74] Estrogen alone has less effect on mammographic density than it does when combined with a progestin.[75] In addition, studies that have looked at the *duration* of estrogen use show the biggest risk in the women who take it the longest. Bruce Ettinger of Kaiser Permanente looked at a series of women who had used estrogen for at least 17 years. The study found a doubling of the risk of breast cancer.[76] All of this would suggest that the woman who has had her ovaries removed can safely take estrogen alone for at least seven years.

Criticisms of the Women's Health Initiative include the fact that it studied conjugated estrogen (Premarin) and medroxyprogesterone acetate (Provera), synthetic hormones, rather than the newer "bioidentical" hormones that are closer to what our bodies make (see Chapter 1). The implication is that natural progesterone and estradiol are safer for the breast.

A recent study from Europe, where a wider variety of HT is used, has shed some light on this. The study, called E3N, compared a range of commonly used progestogens. The researchers found that bioidentical forms such as micronized progesterone and dyhdrogesterone combined with estrogen had the lowest risk among the existing formulations of progestins. In addition they found a 1.3 increased risk of breast cancer in those who used estrogen alone, mostly in the form of estradiol cream.[77]

I still worry when I notice television celebrities suggesting that as long as we take postmenopausal hormones that are identical to

the ones our bodies make, we will be okay. Micronized progesterone may be *less* dangerous than other forms; but "less" is a far
cry from "none." Indeed, since high levels of the hormones made
within your own bodies increase your risk of breast cancer, it
would seem that hormones made to mimic your own hormones
would have the same effect.

One crucial question currently being studied is whether cancers caused by postmenopausal hormone therapy are the same as
cancers caused by other factors. At least four recent studies have
shown an increase, predominantly in lobular cancers in women
on HT.[78,79,80,81] This makes some sense, since lobular cancers are
almost always sensitive to estrogen.

In recent years there has been an increased use of testosterone
to treat the diminished libido that often occurs in postmenopausal women. Unfortunately, there are no long-term safety
data on this drug. As we have learned, just because you had more
of a hormone when you were premenopausal doesn't mean it is
safe to take when you are postmenopausal. Women whose bodies
make higher levels of testosterone have higher levels of breast
cancer.[82] A review of HT use in the Nurses' Health Study demonstrated two and a half times increase in breast cancer in users of
estrogen plus testosterone—significantly greater than that of estrogen alone and marginally higher than estrogen plus a progestin.[83] You need to be careful about what you put in your body,
and always demand long-term safety data. At the very least, ask
yourself if the risk is worth what you believe the gain to be, before
you decide to take any medication long-term. (Remember, just
because a substance may be called a "supplement" doesn't mean
it isn't a medication. It is.)

Fertility Drugs

Fertility drugs are being used a lot these days as younger baby
boomers who postponed childbearing are now trying to get pregnant. We don't know how safe these drugs are or how they interact with breast cancer. Some data suggest that use of clomiphene
citrate (Clomid) may increase breast cancer risk.[84,85] By the time

you're taking fertility drugs you're probably over 30 and haven't had a child yet—a combination that already increases your risk of breast cancer. Some of these drugs may add a promoter effect to an already existing cancer. Data regarding the safety of in vitro fertilization are mixed, with some showing no increased risk and others suggesting that women over 40 doing IF may have a higher risk of breast cancer.[86]

Some of the differences in effects between our own levels of hormones and those we take from any of these drugs may be from our ability to metabolize them. Some bodies metabolize at a different rate than others, which may be why the effects are variable. This may explain why postmenopausal hormones don't increase breast cancer risk even more than they do.

Diet

The idea that dietary fat can contribute to breast cancer has been around for a long time. It began with the observation that breast cancer is lower in Japan than in the United States, and that the incidence increases when women move from Japan to the United States. As proponents of this theory note, one of the many cultural differences in the immigrant group is diet. Charts of fat intake in different countries overlaid on charts of breast cancer incidence appear to confirm the association.

But as I've mentioned a number of times, this kind of parallel doesn't necessarily mean cause and effect. Northern European countries tend to have both a high-fat diet and an increase in breast cancer. But they also have a high-calorie diet. Further, they tend to have the same genetic background, which has been passed on to most of us in the New World. These, or other factors, might be equally or even solely significant.

The high-fat breast cancer hypothesis was put to the test in rats, and it was found that the total calorie count seems to be more important than the amount of fat. A retrospective study on Swedish women who had been hospitalized for anorexia nervosa before age 25 showed a significantly lower risk of breast cancer than that of women who were hospitalized after 25 or did not have the disease.[87] Whether this is due to the fact that they are less obese, had later first periods, or overly restricted calorie intake is not yet clear.

Some researchers feel that the type of fat may be important, but a recent analysis of the Nurses' Health Study failed to find an association between any type of fat and breast cancer.[88] Although the large numbers of women in this study increase its power to demonstrate a relationship, it is an observational study and thus not as conclusive as we'd like. The Women's Health Initiative, which is randomized and prospective, also showed that low-fat diets have no effect on breast cancer risk.[89] Finally the Women's Healthy Eating and Living (WHEL) study, which randomized survivors to a diet very high in vegetables, fruit, and fiber and low in fat showed no difference in breast cancer recurrence or survival after seven years.[90]

Weight

Some studies suggest that the amount of fat we eat may have an *indirect* effect on breast cancer. Fat is by definition high in calories, thus creating greater weight. Some data show that the taller and fatter a postmenopausal woman is, the more susceptible she is to breast cancer. Indeed, overall nutrition may play a role in the disease: people who eat more may be more vulnerable to breast cancer. Overeating may also connect to other risk factors: girls with lower food consumption stay thinner and often begin menstruating later than more heavily nourished girls. We need another study, one that starts in adolescence and monitors the young woman's diet throughout her life. Luckily, the National Institutes of Health and the Breast Cancer and the Environment Research Centers, which are following girls from the time they are about six years old, should have some preliminary answers soon about effects of diet on girls' developmental milestones that affect later breast cancer risk.

It's also possible that cancer cells grow better in an environment with a lot of overnourished cells, and the fatter you are the more such cells there are for the cancer cells to grow with.

Overall, the various studies suggest that being overweight or obese and/or gaining weight will increase your risk for post-

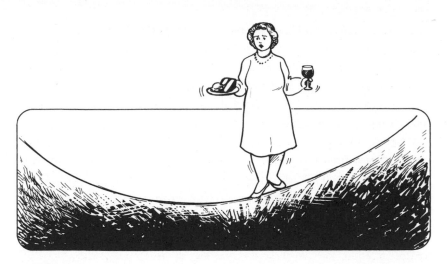

Figure 5.4

menopausal breast cancer.[91] While there isn't nearly the solid proof that there is with smoking and lung cancer, the data are strong enough to make it worthwhile to seriously consider cutting back the calories and definitely start exercising (see Chapter 7).

Alcohol Consumption

Alcohol, the other major dietary substance that has been associated with breast cancer, has received less attention—which is ironic, since the data are more solid. A number of studies suggest that drinking alcoholic beverages, even in moderate amounts, may increase your risk of breast cancer. A combined analysis of observational studies reported that postmenopausal women who drank alcohol had a 22 percent higher relative risk of breast cancer than those who did not. This analysis estimated that for every additional drink per day there was a 10 percent increase in relative risk.[92] Remember this is an increase in *relative* risk. That means if your risk is 10 percent it will go to 11 percent.

Fortunately, good eating habits can help. Several large studies show high intake of folic acid, found in spinach, broccoli, corn, legumes, and multivitamins, appeared to mitigate the excess risk of breast cancer from alcohol.[93,94,95] Since one to two drinks a day have been shown to decrease heart disease, this gives those of you who enjoy your cocktail or glass of wine an out: increase your green leafy vegetables and take a multivitamin. I can just picture it—a spinach martini, with a multivitamin instead of an olive.

Seriously, whether to stop drinking or not is one of the many decisions we all must make on inadequate information. The increase in breast cancer risk from alcohol isn't great, but it definitely exists. You alone know how much pleasure you get from your glass of wine or beer, and how alarmed you are at the thought of breast cancer. If drinking is not all that important to you, you may want to reduce your alcohol consumption to a glass of champagne at major celebrations (Figure 5.4).

Chapter 6

TESTS FOR RISK

IN CHAPTER 5 WE EXAMINED DIFFERENT RISK FACTORS FOR breast cancer. These factors are important to researchers trying to figure out the cause of the disease. But they are less helpful to you individually, with the questions you have at this particular point in your life. That is because the statistics come from comparing women who have had breast cancer to women who haven't had it. So they can tell us, for example, that more women who got their periods before they were 13 will develop breast cancer than will women who got their periods after 13. But it won't tell *you* that you are or aren't going to get it, whenever your period began. Frustrating. In this chapter we are going to consider tests that examine individual women and determine which ones have something in their genes or in their breasts that indicates a higher risk of getting the disease.

I am starting out with the genes, since we know the most about them, and then I'll move to ways doctors can examine the breast itself for prediction. This, of course, won't give you—the reader—any absolute answer. For that, you need a crystal ball.

Because we don't yet know the cause of breast cancer, most of what we measure can give us only clues. For example, before we knew that cancer of the cervix was caused by HPV virus, we knew that having an abnormal Pap smear meant you were at increased risk of developing the disease. But many women with abnormal Pap smears never got cancer of the cervix, and some with normal Pap smears did. Now we test for HPV. It doesn't guarantee that you will or won't develop cancer, but at least it tells you if you have been exposed to something that can cause it. So it's more accurate than the earlier tests, but still not definitive. On the one hand, a negative finding doesn't mean you can breathe a sigh of relief, knowing you'll never have the disease. On the other hand, it may be comforting to those of you who do have the risk factor to learn that you're not facing the certainty of getting the cancer.

Genetic Tests

When we try to determine the cause of a disease, it sometimes helps to look for commonalities among the people who get it and then turn our attention to these groupings for further hints. In the last chapter I divided breast cancers into those that typically occur in young, premenopausal women and those more likely in older, postmenopausal women. But there are numerous other groupings to explore. One important division is between women whose cancer appears to be what we call sporadic—they have no known family history of it, and therefore are unlikely to have inherited their risk (the largest number of women with the disease)—and those whose cancer appears to be hereditary. Within the latter category there are further groupings. One group has a cancer that is clearly genetic—a dominant cancer gene is passed on to succeeding generations from either the father or the mother. Not everyone with the gene will develop breast cancer, but those who inherit it will have a higher risk. Much larger is the group of women whose cancer is polygenic. This means there is a family history of breast cancer that isn't directly passed on through each generation in one dominant gene—some members of the family get it and others don't. In this category we also include the possibility that the cancer actually is genetic—there may be a dominant gene that we haven't discovered and thus don't know how to test for. Women in this category are at greater risk for cancer than the general public, though less so than women with identifiably hereditary cancer.

There are many possible genes that might make someone more prone to breast cancer. She may, for example, inherit a gene that causes her to begin menstruating at an early age—which means other family members, inheriting the same gene, are also more likely to get breast cancer.

Another possibility is exposure to similar external risk factors. I have a friend who is one of five sisters who got breast cancer. The sisters were all tested for BRCA 1 and 2, and were shocked to discover they didn't have it. When all the cancer is in one generation, as in my friend's case, it's possible that they were all exposed to an environmental factor that caused the cancer by creating either a temporary or a permanent genetic mutation.

I often hear from a woman newly diagnosed with breast cancer that she fears her daughter is doomed—and that it is she, the mother, who has doomed her. But it's unlikely that the daughter is fated to replicate her mother's experience, and of course the mother's guilt is wholly irrational. Although having first-degree relatives with a history of breast cancer increases a woman's risk of the disease, most will never develop it. In countries where breast cancer is common, the lifetime increased incidence of breast cancer is 5.5 percent for women with one affected first-degree relative and 13.3 percent for women with two.[1] This should be reassuring for the majority of women.

BRCA 1 AND BRCA 2

Approximately 50 to 90 percent of hereditary breast cancer cases are caused by mutations in the BRCA 1 and BRCA 2 genes; or, more accurately, 90 percent of cases from families with hereditary breast and/or ovarian cancer and 50 percent of cases from families with hereditary breast cancer. (Remember that the actual BRCA genes aren't bad: we all have them. It's the mutations that sometimes happen to them that we need to worry about.) We have learned a lot about these genes since they were discovered in the early 1990s. For one thing, in addition to breast cancer, they also predict higher rates of ovarian and pancreatic cancers (the latter, however, is a much smaller risk). The two genes are equally common, and men can carry both of them.

The risk that women who have mutations in BRCA 1 or BRCA 2 will develop breast cancer is somewhere between 50 and 80 percent. At first researchers believed that anyone with the BRCA 1 gene had an 80 percent lifetime risk of getting breast cancer, based on studies of families with a lot of breast and ovarian cancer.[2] Additional studies were then done on women who, though they had the gene, had only one or two relatives with breast cancer. The studies found, predictably, that the risk was commensurately lower in this group—more like a 37–60 percent chance.[3]

Men who carry mutations in BRCA 1 or BRCA 2 are also susceptible to cancer; however, their risks remain less well understood. In women BRCA 1 mutations carry the greatest risk; in men it is BRCA 2. The relative risk of developing cancer for male BRCA 2 breast cancer mutation carriers is high before age 65, mostly due to breast, prostate, and pancreatic cancer. And of course they can also pass the mutated gene on to their children.[4]

As I have already noted, not all mutation carriers develop breast cancer. The word we use to describe this variability is *penetrance*, which means the lifetime (usually defined as up to age 70) risk of developing breast cancer. Whether or not the mutation in the gene results in cancer depends on whether that mutation has an effect. We don't know what causes this difference in penetrance, but some carriers probably won't get cancer unless there is an additional key genetic alteration. Or they may have inherited other genes that protect them. Several mutations in sequence are probably needed to cause breast cancer (See Figure 4.1). For example, initially you'd be susceptible to a mutation caused by hormones; the second mutation would be caused by diet. The person with genetic breast cancer passes the gene on to her daughter, so the girl is born with her first mutation and needs only to acquire the second to get breast cancer. If the second mutation was for something that could be altered (e.g., exposure to radiation, discussed in Chapter 5), it would hypothetically be possible for her to avoid exposure to that danger and thus escape breast cancer. In fact, studies have shown that the risk of developing cancer has increased in recent generations, implying that nongenetic factors may modify the inherited risk. Not surprisingly, the factors that appear to modify the risk most strongly include reproductive histories and hormones. Oral contraceptives are associated with a profound reduction in the risk of ovarian cancer with little or no increase in the risk of breast cancer. Other factors include how old you are at your first period, whether you have been pregnant, whether you have breast-fed your child, and whether you have had your ovaries removed. Also these factors can have different effects depending on which gene is mutated. Having more than one pregnancy appears to be protective in BRCA 1 carriers but is associated with an increased risk in BRCA 2 carriers.[5]

All that being said, penetrance for breast cancer is about 80 percent for both BRCA 1 and BRCA 2; for ovarian cancer it is about 40 percent for carriers of BRCA 1 and 20 percent for carriers of BRCA 2.[6] The risk of ovarian cancer rises steeply after age 40 in both BRCA 1 and 2 carriers, with an average age of 51.2 years at diagnosis.[7]

Men who carry BRCA 1 mutations have a 1.2 percent lifetime risk of breast cancer; those with BRCA 2 mutations, a 6.8 percent risk.

Founders Mutations

There are over 700 possible mutations in each of the BRCA genes, just as the same word can be mistyped in a number of different ways. Interestingly, three of these mutations were found consistently in women of Ashkenazi (eastern European Jewish) descent, like a word always mistyped in one of the same three ways. The mutations are 185delAG, 5382InsC, and 6174delT. These are often called founder mutations because they're more common in small, tightly knit populations. The founder is the first person who got the mutated gene, inadvertently "founding" it and then passing it down to her or his descendants. Intermarriage perpetuates the gene through many generations. Since one of the three founder mutations is present in 2.5 percent of Ashkenazi Jews, this group has been studied extensively. Much of our knowledge about penetrance and the natural history of hereditary breast cancer has come from this relatively small group.

Of course, such an effect isn't exclusive to Ashkenazi Jews. When researchers started looking at other populations, they found similar situations. In Iceland, where there's a lot of intermarriage, there is also a predominant mutation of BRCA 2. Only 9 percent of people in Iceland with a mutated BRCA gene have a BRCA 1 mutation, while 54 percent have BRCA 2.[8] This is the reverse of the case in most other Western countries, in which BRCA 1 mutations are far more common than BRCA 2. In Norway it's even more specific. Though Norwegians may have either a BRCA 1 or BRCA 2 mutation, which mutation a person gets depends on which fjord she lives on.[9] One fjord has one mutation, while another has one of the others. It is not always so simple, however. In a study of Hispanic women living in Los Angeles, Jeff Weitzel found that six mutations were responsible for 47 percent of the positive genetic tests, with four of the six seeming to be almost exclusively in families with Latin American/Caribbean or Spanish ancestry. Even more interesting was that another of the six mutations was the same as one of the three Ashkenazi Jewish founder mutations, suggesting that it dates back to the Jews who remained in Spain during the Inquisition, assimilated into Spanish culture, and immigrated to the Americas in the late fifteenth century.[10]

Another recent study from California looked at 3,000 women who developed breast cancer before the age of 65. They found that 8.3 percent of women of Ashkenazi heritage and 3.5 percent of Hispanic women were carriers of one of the mutated BRCA genes; while 2.2 percent of non-Hispanic white women and 0.5 percent of Asian women had a BRCA 1 mutation. Although only 1.3 percent of black women overall had a BRCA 1 mutation, 16.7 percent of black women diagnosed with breast cancer before age 35 had the mutation.[11]

Returning to the typo metaphor, there are thousands of possible typos with the BRCA 1 or BRCA 2 genes. It's as though all Ashkenazi Jews used the same typewriter, with an *e* that didn't work. Icelanders used a different typewriter, on which the *t* didn't work. (In the next edition of this book, I'll have to come up with a new metaphor, or any readers born during the computer era won't know what I mean!)

All of this is important when it comes to testing. If you're from an Ashkenazi family and have breast or ovarian cancer, instead of looking for any of the thousands of possible mutations, doctors focus on the three mutations that are most common in this population—and the gene is much easier to test. Investigators have shown that if a Jewish woman does not carry one of those three founder mutations, it is highly unlikely that a different mutation will be found. On the other hand, if testing for a mutation means studying the whole paragraph to find the typo, it's more time-consuming, and thus more expensive, to test.

What do these genes do? Why does a mutation in BRCA 1, which exists in every cell of your body, cause breast and ovarian cancer and not, say, kidney cancer? BRCA 1 and 2 are thought to be involved in checkpoint or quality control of the DNA. Before a cell can divide and replicate, its DNA has to be checked out to make sure there are no mutations. As part of their quality control job, BRCA 1 and 2 are involved in tagging badly damaged DNA for degradation. As mentioned in Chapter 4, both BRCA 1 and 2 are also involved in DNA repair. When a carcinogen like radiation causes a mutation in the DNA, these genes are critical to the machinery that repairs it (See Figure 4.10). When the genes themselves are mutated, they cannot do the repair and the damaged genes accumulate. But this still does not explain why the cancers occur in the breast and ovary specifically. One theory is that absence of functioning BRCA 1 and 2 can exacerbate the action of tissue-specific promoters like estrogen and progestin. As I was researching this chapter, I thought for a minute about this theory and then said, "Hmm. I thought BRCA 1 caused cancers that aren't sensitive to estrogen. So why would it care about estrogen?" This sent me back to the books, only to find a new hypothesis: the breast cancer stem cells that seem to develop into BRCA 1 cancers are indeed estrogen receptor negative—but the cells right next door are not. Could it be that these surrounding cells might respond to estrogen and send pro-survival signals to the estrogen receptor negative cancer stem cells? I'll discuss this later when I review the options for mutation carriers. For now, I simply want to note that most of the treatments that reduce estrogen also reduce the estrogen receptor negative tumors of BRCA 1. Obviously we have a long way to go to understand how these mutations work, but research is moving rapidly and I am sure the answers are not far off.

Genetic Testing

Now that we have a simple blood test that can detect many of the mutations that occur in BRCA 1 or BRCA 2, the questions become, who should undergo it? And what does it mean?

As usual in medicine, we are using the test clinically at the same time we are researching it. If you test positive, we don't know how much of a risk that gives you. If you test negative, it doesn't mean you don't have *any* breast cancer gene, it just means you don't have a mutation in BRCA 1 or BRCA 2. You could have an as yet undiscovered BRCA 3 or BRCA 4. All we can do is look for "typos" in these two different paragraphs we already know about. If you happen to have a typo in another paragraph and that mutation causes breast cancer, we won't know it. Or if you have a typo that doesn't change the meaning of the sentence, you might test positive and not get breast cancer. With each new bit of discovery, the answers to those questions can change.

In an interesting article for the *Annals of Surgery*, J. D. Igelhart looked into the responses of women who were considering getting tested for BRCA genes and sought counseling at the testing center.[12] Even after they had talked it over with counselors who explained the test's limitations, most women still believed that if they tested negative they wouldn't ever get breast cancer. When you desperately want something to be true, you often mentally edit what you hear to transform it into what you want it to be.

Whatever the limits of counseling, however, it's far more frightening when women go into testing without it. And for the most part, they do. Says Dr. Iglehart, "Physicians without genetic training are more likely to provide testing and least likely to provide counseling." And in fact few doctors have genetic training.

In the Iglehart study, high-risk women were asked before testing to estimate their risk of having the gene. The patients far overestimated their risk, thinking they had a 100 percent risk. The doctors not specializing in inherited risk thought most patients had zero risk. They thought a few had a 10 percent risk, and a few had a 20 percent risk.

Interestingly, women with doctors who do have expertise—the ones who work in clinics where counseling is part of the process—

are much less likely after the counseling to get tested. When they recognize the limits of what the test can do, they reconsider. Those who go to their local doctors and receive no counseling are more likely to have it done. A recent study by Della White and her colleagues surveyed family physicians regarding their likelihood of referring a low-risk woman for genetic services if she had asked for testing. Family physicians regarded it unlikely that the patient carried a mutation, but 65 percent believed if they refused to refer her for genetic services it would harm their relationship with the patient![13] At $3,000 a test, that is an awfully expensive way to keep the patient happy.

Some people have asked why the test for the breast cancer gene is being offered only to women at high risk for the disease. Why isn't it being suggested for all women with breast cancer, or even all women in the country? Part of the reason is that the chance of having the gene is so low for most people that testing wouldn't be worthwhile. A study by Beth Newman, reported in the *Journal of the American Medical Association,* looked at a general group of women between 20 and 74 with breast cancer to see how many had the mutation.[14] Only 3 percent had the BRCA 1 gene.

J. Peto and his colleagues did a study in the United Kingdom in the summer of 1999, looking at women with hereditary breast cancer.[15] They divided them into age-groups and looked at the correlation between hereditary cancer and the BRCA genes. They estimated the incidence to be 3.1 percent BRCA 1 and 3.0 percent BRCA 2 in women with breast cancer under 50; 0.49 percent (BRCA 1) 0.84 percent (BRCA 2) in women over 50; and 0.11 percent (BRCA 1) and 0.12 percent (BRCA 2) in all women. So it's a very small percentage, even among young women.

Results of Genetic Testing

If you want to be tested, it makes sense to find out if there is a breast cancer gene in your family by having a relative who has had either breast or ovarian cancer tested first. If your mother has had breast cancer, is tested, and discovers that she doesn't have a genetic alteration, there's no need for you to get tested. If we find that she has a mutation in the BRCA 1 gene and you don't, then we know you didn't inherit that gene. This is called a true negative. Again, it's no guarantee that you won't get breast cancer, but the risk is much reduced and is the same as that of anyone whose parents don't carry the genetic mutation. My friend, Mary, of Ashkenazi Jewish descent was diagnosed with breast cancer and was found to carry a mutation in the BRCA 1 gene. This led her sister and brother to be tested. Both her siblings were found to be carriers. Within a few months, her sister was diagnosed with breast cancer. The good news came when her twenty-five-year-old daughter decided to be tested after reviewing her options with a hereditary breast cancer specialist in Washington. Everyone breathed a sigh of relief when she was found to be negative for the mutation carried by her mother, her aunt, and her uncle.

Less clear are the families with a lot of breast cancer (two or more breast cancers in relatives under the age of 50 or three or more breast cancers in relatives of any age) who test negative. This is called a noninformative test because it tells you that though we can't detect anything amiss with our current testing, this does not guarantee that there is no increased risk. Since only 25 percent of families in which there is breast cancer and no ovarian cancer will carry a mutation, this population with lots of breast cancer but no identifiable mutations is a large group. One analysis by Steven Narod's team in Canada calculated that they still had approximately a fourfold increased risk of breast cancer compared to the normal population and still warranted screening and maybe even chemoprevention (see Chapter 7).[16] A Facebook friend of mine was the ninth person in her family to get breast cancer. All the computer modeling and genetic consultations predicted a 98 percent chance that she would be a carrier of BRCA 1 or 2, and yet she tested negative. Obviously she was at increased risk. She probably has a gene/mutation/condition/exposure we just don't know how to test for yet.

Current testing looks for mutations, deletions (areas where something is missing), and sequence change. The sequence may be only one nucleotide off (see Chapter 4), and it may or may not be important. Often we don't know whether this variant is significant or not and therefore call it a variant of uncertain significance

(VUS). This can be very frustrating for the doctor and the family. Between 10 and 15 percent of people undergoing genetic testing for BRCA 1 and BRCA 2 mutations will be found to have a VUS.[17] They are even more common in nonwhite populations, with frequencies as high as 46 percent among African Americans[18] and 22 percent among Hispanics of all racial categories.[19] Sometimes genetic detective work can help sort them out, but frequently a woman is left not knowing whether to consider herself at risk.[20] In these situations it is important to be followed in a high-risk setting (clinic or university medical center) where research is going on all the time. Ask about registries of these variants, so that you will become aware of any new information as soon as it becomes available. Again, as research continues, we'll learn more and more about this, but we don't have all the answers now.

The Risks and Benefits of Getting Tested

What precisely are the risks? As I noted, one is financial. The testing can be expensive. And insurance companies don't always pay for it. If a particular mutation is identified, then other family members can get tested for much less money—around $400. That's because the really hard work is searching for the specific mutation. It's like proofreading an entire manuscript to find the typo; once you know where it is, finding it in other copies is fairly easy.

Initially there was fear that insurance companies would discriminate against women who had been tested. So far this has not been the case. Still, it would be smart to check the laws in your state and the policy of your insurance company before proceeding.

Keep in mind that it isn't only you who will need to deal with the consequences of your decision. It becomes a family issue. If I get tested and I'm positive, this will have implications for my sisters—who may or may not want to get tested. It also has implications for my daughter. If you choose to be tested and learn you have a mutated gene, you will then need to decide what to do with the information.

When you already have breast cancer, the emotional conflict over gene testing intensifies. You tend to think that you're unlucky and you must have the bad gene. Further, your own psychological issues almost inevitably get mixed into your perceptions. Were you mean to your mother when she had breast cancer, so now you're being punished by inheriting a killer gene? Even highly sophisticated people are to some extent trapped by unconscious expectations.

One benefit of being tested is the reduction in uncertainty. If the result is positive, the knowledge can allow you to make a plan for risk reduction (see Chapter 7). My Ashkenazi Jewish friend mentioned above told me that she highly recommended the daughters of BRCA 1 women be tested. It was an enormous relief for her and her daughter that she was negative, and she suspects that it would also be helpful to know if her daughter is a carrier. Not knowing was too anxiety-causing for that family.

A Facebook friend wrote that she had herself tested because there was ovarian and breast cancer on her father's side of the family, and her oldest sister had ovarian cancer. Ideally her sister would have been tested, but she refused because she did not want to know. However, my friend wanted to know for her own sake and her daughter's.

Testing for Women Without Breast Cancer

If you don't have breast cancer, should you get tested? The general recommendation is that someone with a 10 percent or greater risk of getting breast cancer should be seen by a genetic counselor and consider testing.[21] This would include:

1. Family history of relatives with a BRCA 1 or 2 mutation
2. Close family member with breast cancer diagnosed before 40
3. Close family member with ovarian, fallopian tube, or primary peritoneal cancer
4. Personal history of ovarian cancer at any age, particularly for those of Ashkenazi Jewish heritage
5. Family history of male breast cancer, particularly if at least one first- or second-degree relative has had breast cancer and/or ovarian cancer

If you decide to be tested, there are several possible results. Most satisfying are the true positives and true negatives. In a true positive, the test finds a clear mutation. In a true negative, the patient tests negative but another family member has an identified mutation. In this case you know you did not inherit the family gene. More complex is the situation in which the test identifies no known mutation, and no one else in the family has a specific mutation. Then you do not know whether there is a mutated gene that is not one of the ones we know how to look for, or if there is no genetic alteration. Also, abnormal genetic alterations of unknown clinical significance can be found that have not been linked to breast cancer. In both of these situations you are left with as many questions as answers.

If you are going to be tested, do it through a genetic counselor. You can get a referral from your gynecologist or primary care doctor, bypassing a genetic counselor, but I do not recommend this approach. First of all, it may not be appropriate for you to be tested, and given the tendency for family physicians to inappropriately refer patients for testing, you need to be doubly careful. In the United States one company, Myriad Genetics, has patented the genes and their mutations. This makes Myriad the only company that can perform the test legally. The ACLU has won a lawsuit to challenge the concept that genes and mutations can be patented. It will now work its way through the courts. This is important to women not only because the monopoly blocks competition and therefore keeps costs high but also because it blocks the ability to have a second test done elsewhere to confirm the results. Recently Myriad Genetics started direct-to-consumer advertising, leading many women with no particular risk to demand the test. Not only is this a waste of resources, but it can also give many women a false sense of security about their real risk of breast cancer. A genetic counselor can help you determine whether the test should be done, and if it is done, can help you interpret the results. To find such a counselor, you can check with a nearby medical school. You can also call 1-800-FOR CANCER. There is a website that lists genetic counselors for cancer geographically throughout the United States: http://cancer.gov/search/geneticsservices.

Testing for Women Who Have Been Diagnosed with Breast Cancer

There are good reasons for women with breast cancer to consider getting tested. They may want to know if others in their family are likely to get cancer. Or they may be thinking about having children, and the possibility of passing on a breast cancer gene could play a role in their decision making. Women with cancer in one breast are more likely to get it in the other, and they may want to consider having a double mastectomy if they know they have the gene. In women without the mutated gene, the risk of a second primary is between 0.5 and 1 percent a year, and 15–25 percent over their lifetime. For someone with the gene, it's probably between 1 and 2 percent a year, 30–50 percent over their lifetime. A woman with BRCA 1 or BRCA 2 may want to have her ovaries removed, which reduces breast cancer risk by 53 percent.

It doesn't make sense for every woman with breast cancer to be tested, since hereditary breast cancer is so rare. Still, there are some profiles showing your likelihood of carrying a genetic alteration. If you are an Ashkenazi Jewish woman younger than 40 with breast cancer, there is about a 33 percent chance that you are a carrier. If you are not Ashkenazi Jewish and have breast cancer before 30, you have a 12 percent chance of having a mutation. If you develop bilateral breast cancer between age 40 and 50 and have a first-or second-degree relative with breast or ovarian cancer before 50, there is a 42 percent chance that you carry a mutation. If you got breast cancer after 50, there is a lower risk that it is hereditary; in fact, having more than two breast cancers in first-or second-degree relatives after 50 gives you a risk of only about 2 percent of having a mutation.[22,23]

Hereditary Breast and/or Ovarian Cancer Syndrome Testing Criteria (NCCN Practice Guidelines 2009)

- Individual from a family with a known BRCA 1/BRCA 2 mutation
- Personal history of breast cancer with one or more of the following:
  - » Diagnosed before age 45
  - » Diagnosed before age 50 with more than one close

blood relative with breast cancer before 50
  » Two different breast cancers with the first diag-
     nosed before 50
  » Diagnosed at any age with more than 2 close blood
     relatives with breast and/or ovarian. Fallopian tube
     or primary peritoneal cancer at any age
  » Close male blood relative with breast cancer
- Personal history of ovarian/fallopian tube or primary
  peritoneal cancer
- Personal history of male breast cancer
- Family history only but a close family member with any
  of the above criteria

CHOICES AFTER A POSITIVE TEST

If you test positive for the BRCA 1 or BRCA 2 gene, what next? First, getting a positive test result is not an emergency. It just confirms what you undoubtedly suspected: that you are at high risk for breast cancer. The question is, what are you comfortable doing about it? The choices range from ignoring it (probably not too wise) to close monitoring through chemoprevention or surgical prevention (examined in Chapter 7).

Again, you want to be seen by a clinic that specializes in high-risk women or women with genetic risk. They will review your options with you and consider your particular situation. Many factors have to be taken into consideration, from whether you still want to conceive children (which would preclude having your ovaries removed immediately) to whether you are claustrophobic and cannot tolerate an MRI. You need to discuss and digest all of these matters before you launch into a plan that will work for you and your life.

Surveillance

Monitoring for mutation carriers has been evolving. Usually it involves having an exam every six months beginning around age 25–35, as well as a yearly mammography. The latter is controversial because, as we will see in Chapter 8, mammography doesn't work as well in young women with dense breasts. In fact it detects less than half of the breast cancers in mutation carriers.[24,25,26] Still, that's better than nothing, and it can find microcalcifications. Ultrasound is often added to the mammography, especially if there are palpable lumps. Since the last edition, there have been six studies regarding the use of MRI for screening in this setting, and they indicate that it has a higher sensitivity than mammography. MRI is far from perfect, however. Most of the studies include a few cancers found by the woman herself in between scans. This is probably because women who carry the BRCA gene often get aggressive cancers that grow faster between screenings or metastasize sooner or are just harder to see than the sporadic ones. Another problem with MRI is that it is also sensitive to lots of things that are not cancer. But if you are at high risk, you want a very sensitive test and are probably willing to trade off unnecessary biopsies for the chance of finding a tumor early. At the current time, MRI with mammography and ultrasound starting when you're around 25 or 30 seem to be the best approach to surveillance. But you must make sure you are getting the best breast MRI available, in a high-risk or genetic clinic. Images are only as good as the people who take them and those who read the pictures.

Of course, the cancer risk of having one of the BRCA mutations is not limited to the breast. You also need to monitor for ovarian cancer. In many ways, as I noted earlier, ovarian cancer is more deadly than breast cancer, although it's also much less common. Breast cancer is often more treatable when found on screening, while ovarian cancer is less often found at an early stage. It is a very sneaky cancer: there are no symptoms until it's far developed. Pelvic exams rarely show signs of ovarian cancer. A blood test called CA125 is good for monitoring metastatic ovarian cancer, but it works only about 50 percent of the time when the cancer is in an early stage. It's particularly tricky in premenopausal women. There are a lot of false positives, leaving the patient terrified that she has an incurable disease and leading to unnecessary surgery. Transvaginal ultrasound is a more recent technique. An ultrasound tool is placed in the vagina and the technician can look around the ovarian area. The process has a very high resolution, but most of what it finds is benign. It may be a good idea for very high risk women, but if used for screening, suspicious signs would be found in about 50 out of 1,000 women, all of whom would undergo major surgery and only one of whom would turn out to have cancer.

Other Genes and Tests

BRCA 1 and 2 are by far the most common culprits in hereditary breast cancer, but there are others—less common inherited mutations that also influence the risk of breast cancer.[27] CHEK 2 is associated with DNA repair and is most common in women of northern and eastern European descent. It doubles breast cancer risk. Most cancers resulting from this mutation are estrogen positive and so a chemoprevention program with raloxifene or tamoxifen can be considered (see Chapter 7).

Li Fraumeni syndrome is a rare hereditary condition characterized by multiple types of cancer, including soft tissue sarcomas, osteosarcomas, leukemias, brain tumors, adrenocortical malignancies, and early onset breast cancer. It results from a mutation in the tumor suppressor gene p53. It has been estimated that 50 percent of carriers will develop some kind of cancer by age 50 and 90 percent by age 70. Recommendations are for MRI screening starting at age 20 to 25 and consideration of prophylactic mastectomy.

PTEN is a mutation associated with a disease called Cowden's syndrome. It is a rare hereditary syndrome characterized by multiple characteristic skin lesions and an increased risk of early onset breast cancer and thyroid cancer.

When BRCA 1 and 2 were identified, we thought that in a year or two we would find BRCA 3 and 4. But that has not happened. There are families with a lot of breast cancer who do not have the mutations that we know how to test for. Do they carry another mutated gene? Possibly, but it is beginning to seem like the genes that explain most hereditary breast cancers have been found. The next discovery may be many mutations that are found in only a few people. Or maybe we'll find common mutations that actually lead to breast cancer in a few people. These, of course, are more difficult to detect. In search for these low frequency, low penetrance genes, researchers have been taking another tack. They look at the DNA of many people with a disease and compare it to the DNA of people without the disease. These studies are called genome-wide association studies (GWAS). By doing such comparisons they can identify single nucleotide polymorphisms (SNPs, pronounced "snips")—single changes in the DNA of chromosomes that seem to be found more commonly in women with breast cancer. It all ends up being a statistical exercise, but the hope is that they can predict who is at increased risk. As I write this in 2010, at least 14 SNPs have been identified with breast cancer risk.[28] None by itself creates even a doubling of breast cancer risk. In other words, the risks they entail are about the same as the risks of delaying your first pregnancy or getting your first period at a young age. Certainly they are not strong enough to cause you to consider preventative surgery. On the other hand it is possible to have multiple SNPs, and perhaps such combinations could be more accurate at predicting risk. There are commercial companies marketing tests based on SNPs directly to the public (DeCode and 23 and Me). While I generally think that more knowledge is better, we don't yet know what to do with the information. Should you start screening earlier? Have routine MRIs with the attendant increase in biopsies? If you test negative for the SNPs, does that mean that you have no risk of breast cancer? It's a lovely thought, but I doubt it will prove true. At this point I would caution anyone interested in pursuing this route to think first about what she would do with the information if she got it.

PRECANCER FOUND ON BIOPSY

The presence of a BRCA mutation covers only a small number of women who are going to get breast cancer. There are other, more specific indications of the likelihood of the disease. One of these is the presence of cells that look like they are on the way to becoming cancer. These are far more common, and far more conclusive.

To understand the conditions we call precancer, we need to back up a minute and return to the breast's biology. As noted in Chapter 1, the breast is a kind of milk factory. It has two parts—

lobules that make the milk and ducts like hollow branches that carry it to the nipples (See Figure 1.10).

Over the years, you can get a few extra cells lining the duct—sort of like a fungus on the branch. This is called *intraductal hyperplasia,* which simply translates to "too many cells in the duct." We call these *proliferative cells.* In themselves they aren't a problem. Sometimes the cells become a bit strange looking, and this condition is called *intraductal hyperplasia with atypia* (also known as atypical hyperplasia, or ADH). If they keep on looking odd and multiply within the duct, clogging it, they get another name—*ductal carcinoma in situ* (meaning "in place") or *intraductal carcinoma* or *DCIS* (Figure 6.1). You might imagine that this means there is a big difference between these two steps. After all, that deadly word "carcinoma" has been inserted into the phrase. But in fact, the only difference between ADH and low-grade DCIS is that DCIS requires two adjacent ductal structures to be filled with cells and ADH does not—a fairly arbitrary definition. We think that these DCIS cells represent the "seeds" of a potential cancer and can reverse themselves if the neighborhood changes. It isn't until the cells are let out of the ducts and into the surrounding fibrous tissue or fat that they are called *invasive or infiltrating ductal cancer.*

You can tell the same story about the lobules with lobular hyperplasia, atypical lobular hyperplasia (ALH), and lobular carcinoma in situ (LCIS). And sometimes you see a mixture of ductal and lobular cells (Figure 6.2). This is not surprising, since the very first changes that lead to cancer are thought to start at the junction of the duct and the lobule.

Of course, we are making these distinctions based on how the cells look under the microscope. We need to analyze further with genetic tests. It would not be surprising if they represented different types of DNA damage or mutations. Studies are now being done to try to figure this out.

The proliferation (hyperplasia and atypia) takes place inside the duct or lobule, so you can't feel it by examining your breast. In the past it was found only incidentally (2–4 percent of the time) during a surgical biopsy, not in the lump itself but next to the lump in the rim of apparently "normal" tissue, and the pathologist

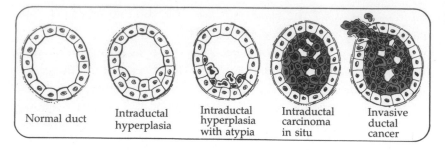

| Normal duct | Intraductal hyperplasia | Intraductal hyperplasia with atypia | Intraductal carcinoma in situ | Invasive ductal cancer |

Figure 6.1

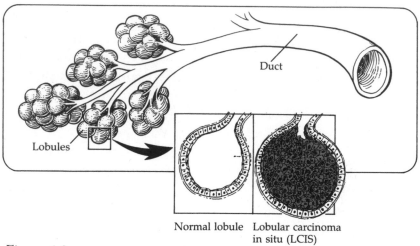

Normal lobule   Lobular carcinoma in situ (LCIS)

Figure 6.2

came across it by accident.[29] A recent review by the Mayo Clinic followed all women who had benign biopsy findings between 1967 and 1991. They found that 67 percent of biopsies showed tissues that were nonproliferative, meaning they represented some of the common conditions discussed in Chapter 3. Thirty percent of the biopsies showed proliferation but no atypia (hyperplasia), and only 4 percent revealed proliferation with atypia (atypical hyperplasia). Now with mammographic screening we are finding that some (12–17 percent) of the microcalcifications biopsied are associated with ALH or ADH.[30] In addition to increased detection by mammography, a French study showed that women who were on postmenopausal hormones had twice the risk of ADH as women who were not. It will be interesting to see if the recent decrease in postmenopausal hormone use will result in less apparent ADH. I say "apparent" because autopsy findings on women who have died of causes other than breast cancer reveal that 30 percent or so had some degree of either hyperplasia or atypical hyperplasia.[31] So probably a lot of us are walking around with these conditions and don't know it because we have no reason to have biopsies, they don't show on mammograms, and the cells are dormant.

Risk of ADH and ALH

The fact that we are finding more atypical ductal hyperplasia has led to several studies about what it means.[32,33,34] In general we believe that there is a progression of increased risk with each of these entities.[35] Four large studies with follow-up show an increased risk of 1.5, or half again as many cancers as in women who do not have proliferative changes without atypia. Women with proliferative disease with atypia (atypical hyperplasia) have four times the risk of those without these changes.[36] Premenopausal women with hyperplasia have a higher risk than postmenopausal women with the condition.

This may connect with another factor that seems to affect risk—the woman's age. Premenopausal women have a higher risk of getting cancer over their remaining lifetime than postmenopausal women. Until recently no one had reported specifically on the significance of atypical lobular hyperplasia in terms of this age factor. Dr. David Page remedied the situation with a study of the 252 women in his records in whom a surgical biopsy showed atypical lobular hyperplasia.[37] He found that 50 of them went on to develop invasive cancers, giving them a relative risk of 3.1. The cancers were on the same side as the ALH 75 percent of the time and took, on average, 14.8 years to show up. Obviously these lesions don't progress rapidly and often don't progress at all.

There are still many questions. For the woman diagnosed with atypical ductal or lobular hyperplasia, the most vital question is, what does it mean? The first step is to look at how it was diagnosed. If atypical hyperplasia shows up on a core biopsy, there is a consensus that an open surgical biopsy is indicated. This is because of a 20–25 percent risk that the hyperplasia is the tip of the iceberg—that next to it there may be an in situ or invasive cancer.[38]

On the other hand, if it was found during a larger surgical biopsy and it is not at the margins we can be more confident that the whole area has been removed. Most surgeons would agree that the best program is close follow-up, so that any in situ carcinoma or invasive cancer is found. This would include a physical exam by a doctor every six months and yearly mammograms.

For women who want a treatment, studies using tamoxifen for prevention have given us another option. The women with ADH who took tamoxifen for five years had 86 percent fewer subsequent breast cancers over the period of the study than those who had no treatment.[39] It is certainly worth considering the risks and benefits of this approach (see Chapter 7). As shown in Chapter 17, the benefits persist long after the five-year course is over. Some women may even consider a more drastic approach and have preventive mastectomies.

Lobular Involution

Another recent finding on biopsy that may give information about breast cancer risk is whether there is *lobular involution*. (Involution refers to what happens when the tissue regresses or retires.) You will remember from Chapter 1 that the breast develops lobules at puberty, and it develops even more with pregnancy, when they're needed to produce milk. After you've finished breast-feeding your child, the lobules all undergo cell suicide. But don't be sad for the poor lobules; they've lived a good life—and new ones form to replace them and prepare your body for its next pregnancy. This is one form of involution.

As we age, and especially after menopause, our lobules are no longer stimulated by hormones and become permanently involuted. These changes can be seen on a breast biopsy. Lynn Hartmann at the Mayo Clinic looked at a large series of benign breast biopsies from the past in women who had later developed cancer. She found that women who experienced lobular involution had a significantly reduced risk of breast cancer. For example, women over 55 who didn't appear to have involution had a threefold increase in breast cancer risk. This permanent involution occurs around menopause, with only 5 percent of women under 50 showing it but 20 percent of women between 50 and 59.[40] Much additional work is required to understand how lobular involution is induced, why some women demonstrate it before menopause while others never show any involution, even after menopause, and how lobular involution protects from breast cancer. Nonetheless these observations seem likely to give us further insight into how the interactive community of cells in the breast can work for good as well as harm.

RESEARCH TOOLS FOR FINDING THE ABNORMAL CELLS

It is all well and good to find precancerous changes on a biopsy, but it would be much more helpful if there were an easy way to identify abnormal or precancerous cells. There are three current approaches to sampling cells: collection of nipple aspirate fluid (NAF), ductal lavage, and random periareolar fine needle aspiration (RPFNA). They all depend on cytology (the study of cells), which involves looking at isolated cells under the microscope and determining by their appearance whether or not they are precancerous. Although they are considered research tools, they are teaching us a lot about who is at risk.

Nipple Aspirate Fluid (NAF) Collection

As noted in Chapter 4, all breast cancer starts in the milk ducts. The idea of studying the ducts and their fluid was first mentioned in 1946 when a Uruguayan doctor, Raul Leborgne, described a way to pass a small catheter into a breast duct and squirt saline in, take the catheter out, and collect the fluid as it dripped out.[41] He termed his procedure a "ductal rinse." Then in 1958 American George Papanicolaou, the inventor of the cervical Pap smear, described applying suction to the nipple to obtain small drops of fluid from the milk ducts. He termed it a "breast Pap smear."[42] (As

I explained in Chapter 3, it's not unusual to be able to obtain fluid from a woman's breast.) The timing was not right, however, and the technique languished for years. This was probably because no one knew at the time how the information could be used to help women. But curiosity remained, and in the 1970s, several researchers reevaluated Papanicolaou's approach. Three major series of studies took place, each advancing our understanding in a slightly different way: one by Gertrude Buehring, another by Otto Sartorius, and the third by Eileen King and Nicholas Petrakis.[43,44,45] In all of them researchers were able to obtain breast fluid from about 80 percent of premenopausal women and 50 percent of postmenopausal women by using a suction cup on the nipple.

King and Petrakis took the long view. Between 1973 and 1980 they collected fluid and then analyzed it. After 21 years of follow-up, 285 of 3,633 women developed breast cancer. The researchers compared the outcome with their initial evaluation of the fluid they'd taken 21 years earlier. Not surprisingly, they discovered that the women who'd had no fluid had the lowest incidence of breast cancer (4.7 percent). Those with fluid but with normal cells had a slightly higher incidence (8.2 percent) than those without fluid. Those with hyperplasia showed a bit higher (10.8 percent) incidence, and those with atypical cells the highest (13.8 percent). The researchers took into account differences in the women's ages and the years they entered the study. The women with atypical cells had nearly three times the amount of breast cancer of the women with no fluid at all.

They also concluded from this study that women with atypical cells and a first-degree relative with breast cancer were nearly twice as likely to develop the disease as were women who had atypical cells but no first-degree relatives with breast cancer. This suggests that if you have both atypical cells and a family history of breast cancer, you have a fairly high risk of getting the disease. Gertrude Buehring recently completed a 25-year follow-up of her series of NAF volunteers and confirmed a higher risk of cancer in those who had both NAF and abnormal cells.[46] Kim Baltzel has now completed the follow-up of the Sartorius series of 946 women and found that women with abnormal epithelial cells in

NAF have a greater risk of breast cancer than those without fluid. Even women with normal cells had a higher risk than women without cells or without fluid.[47] So we now know how most of the 6,000 or so women who underwent the procedure more than 20 years ago have fared.

In addition to cells, there are also proteins, hormones, and even carcinogens in the fluid. Since cells require a cytologist to look at them, it would be better if there were something that could serve as a *marker* of what was going on biologically in the duct—a protein secreted by precancerous cells, for example. Ed Sauter, a surgeon from Fox Chase Hospital in Philadelphia, improved the suction technique of obtaining nipple aspirate fluid so that he was able to retrieve fluid from close to 100 percent of women.[48] He then looked for PSA (the same marker that is used for prostate cancer) and other markers. As yet the perfect marker—one that can predict who is at risk for breast cancer—has eluded us.

We have been doing research on this approach at the Dr. Susan Love Research Foundation and are working on an easy, inexpensive home test based on finding markers in nipple aspirate fluid to help young women determine whether they are at risk. We're also looking at the immune cells in the fluid. Could they be a hint about to the cause of breast cancer? Does the fluid represent a low-grade inflammation, and if so, does that inflammation set the stage for breast cancer? I hope by the next edition of this book there will be lots to report on this front.

Ductal Lavage

The problem we came up against with nipple aspirate fluid was that not all ducts had it. I found this surprising; the common belief among doctors, when they gave it any thought at all, was that it was always there. So I thought it would be important to look at cells and fluid from every duct. I developed a tiny catheter that could be used to thread through the nipple into a milk duct for a distance of about 0.5 inch (1 cm) (Figure 6.3). Using this catheter, we washed each duct with saltwater and then retrieved cells from deep in each ductal tree. The fluid was then sent to be examined

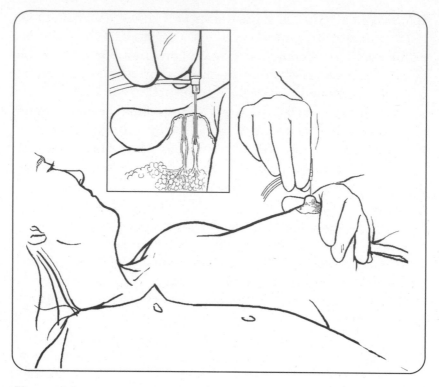

Figure 6.3

for cells, as we had done with NAF. In an early study we compared these cells to those in the fluid obtained by suction alone. We found that lavage, as we called the process, collected more cells than NAF and was better able to detect abnormal cells.[49] Although the procedure was approved for high-risk women, the question remained, How do we know that these cells are precancerous? We found that there were limits to our procedure. First of all, not all ducts with cancer gave fluid that contained any cells, let alone cancer cells. In addition when we repeated lavage in the same duct six months later, we found that most of the time the atypical cells had gone away on their own, much as they do when the doctor repeats a Pap smear. One of my colleagues, Dr. Bonnie King, looked at not just the cells themselves but the DNA inside them. This turned out to be more accurate.[50] The research is continuing and expanding. Some researchers are looking for substances in the fluid that can identify who has cancer or is at risk: patterns of proteins, for example, or hormone levels. Although this is still a research tool, I am confident that we will find a good marker of risk in the fluid, and when this happens lavage will become a useful test on a wider level. Another aspect of this approach is ductoscopy. This involves threading a very small scope through the nipple and down a milk duct and biopsying the lining. Although many surgeons have identified known cancers through this technique, it is not clear whether it will be a good diagnostic test for precancerous lesions.[51]

Random Periareolar Fine Needle Aspirate (RPFNA)

In a different approach to the problem of identifying the woman with high-risk changes in the breast, Carol Fabian in Kansas explored the use of fine-needle aspirates (see Chapter 8)—sticking small needles into both breasts on both sides of the nipple and then suctioning out some cells (Figure 6.4).[52] Although this technique has found more atypical changes in the tissue of high-risk women than in those of normal risk, it also has its limitations. Since the needles are placed blindly, they will detect the changes that are going on throughout the breast. If atypical cells are identified by random needle sticks, it is more difficult to ascertain which duct they are in and get back to the precise spot six months later. Nonetheless, this approach has proved useful in testing new drugs to see if they have any effect on the breasts of high-risk women. First RPFNA is done and then the women take a new drug for six months, at which time the needle biopsies are repeated looking for changes in markers of hyperplasia and atypia.

BREAST DENSITY

As you will see in Chapter 8 breast tissue, which is dense, shows up white on the mammogram, while the more transparent fat tissue shows up gray. Women whose mammograms show very dense tissue are at significantly higher risk of breast cancer than those whose mammograms are less dense, and this applies to women of any age. Although some researchers have attributed this to an

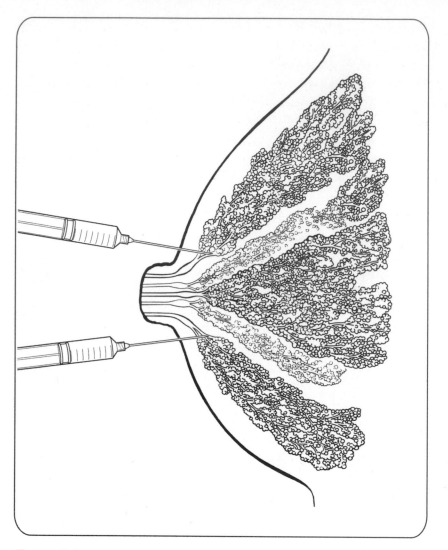

Figure 6.4

increase in breast cells, the evidence suggests it is the stroma, or local neighborhood, that is responsible. Some epidemiological data suggest that breast density may have two different effects. One is that dense tissue makes it more difficult to see lumps on the mammogram. The other is that the stroma in the breast tissue is being stimulated. When I was first told this, I thought it was foolish—the dense breast tissue that shows on the mammogram isn't what gets cancer; the cells within the ducts get cancer. But now we're learning that there is constant "cross talk" between cells and their neighbors, and it isn't quite so easy to dismiss.

For example, one of the dangers of hormone therapy, as noted in the last chapter, is that a third of women taking it show increased breast density on mammogram, which starts as soon as the woman begins taking the medication. Further, observational studies have suggested that progestin added to estrogen increases the density, resulting in more risk than estrogen alone causes.

There are increasing data to support this theory. The studies regarding HRT have suggested that it is the women whose breasts become denser who have the increased risk. We have also seen that tamoxifen reduces breast density almost immediately.

This is getting more and more attention. As I was writing this chapter, Connecticut passed legislation requiring that women be given information about their breast density when they get mammograms. I find this a bit premature. While exploring breast density is a very exciting research tool, there are many problems with it in a clinical setting. First, there is no universal scale for measuring it. Karla Kerlikowske, a researcher who has been very enthusiastic about these studies, has suggested that simply giving the women information about the density of their breasts is likely to create useless stress. It may well become useful in the next few years to determine who needs more screening or even chemoprevention. But we're not there yet. For the moment, it remains simply another interesting research tool.

STATISTICAL RISK

In this chapter we have focused on concrete ways to determine your risk based on either your genes or changes in your tissue. Sometimes we resort to calculating a statistical risk based on some of the family history and lifestyle risk factors. In an attempt to do this several statistical models have been developed based on population risks, and then applied to individual women. These are usually based on various combinations of family history, age, reproductive history, race/ethnicity, hormonal factors, and benign breast disease. The one most commonly used in the United

States is the NCI breast cancer risk assessment model based on the Gail model (www.cancer.gov/bcrisktool). It has been validated for use in most women age 35 years or older and provides an individual's five-year and lifetime risk estimates for developing breast cancer on the basis of five to six questions. The women's contraceptive and reproductive experience (CARE) model has allowed them to update it for African American women.[53] A new model from Tice incorporates breast density into its calculations and has been shown to be a good tool in a multiethnic population.[54]

Another model based on the Women's Health Initiative Study predicts the risk of ER positive cancers in postmenopausal women. None of these models work well in women with a strong family history, however, and so the Claus or the Tyrer-Cuzick[55] models, which include detailed family history, are often used in these situations. Finally, a model known as BRCAPRO is frequently used to estimate how likely a woman is to carry a mutation in BRCA 1 or 2 and whether testing is worthwhile. These last three are most often used in high-risk or genetic clinics.

Risk models that do well in predicting the proportion of women in a population who develop cancer have only a modest ability to discriminate whether an individual woman would or would not develop breast cancer. It is like predicting that women who graduate from college and live on the East Coast are more likely to go to Europe at some point in their lives versus predicting that *you*, who live on the East Coast, will go to Europe. Most women who are identified as being at increased risk for breast cancer will never develop the disease, and most women who develop breast cancer have no known risk factors and would not be identified ahead of time using any of these models. But if these models are so limited, why do we even use them? We use them to figure out whom to include in studies of chemoprevention so that we know we are comparing similar women. That way we can say if you have this risk, and based on this model, you may be a candidate for this type of prevention. As of yet we do not have the perfect test, statistical or otherwise, to identify the woman most strongly at risk.

Chapter 7

PREVENTION AND RISK REDUCTION

THIS FIFTH EDITION OF THE BOOK HAS LOTS OF NEW INFORMATION about the biology of breast cancer. I wish I could say that it had a corresponding amount of information about preventing the disease. Research has not yet been able to take that next step—using its findings to stop the cancer before it starts. We'll get there; we're just not there yet. Our current approaches to breast cancer prevention are the ones we've used for years—lifestyle changes, drugs, and surgery. Once our current research into the biology takes us to the realm in which we learn what causes breast cancer, we will have the tools to help us find more specific ways to prevent it.

Meanwhile I'll talk about the measures we do have. There are a few of them; what you decide to do will probably depend at least partly on your level of risk. A woman with average risk will likely stick with lifestyle changes; someone whose mother has had breast cancer may want to consider chemoprevention as well. Finally, a carrier of the BRCA 1 or 2 mutations may want to look into preventive surgery. In this chapter I'll review all these options and the data supporting them.

LIFESTYLE

As I was writing this chapter, the American Institute of Cancer Research released a new review of all the studies examining lifestyle changes that could prevent breast cancer. Their conclusion was that more than 70,000 breast cancer cases a year, or 40 percent of all cases, could be prevented with lifestyle measures such as maintaining a healthy weight, breast-feeding, eating well, exercising, and limiting alcohol consumption (see Chapter 5). Of these measures, the biggest single thing a woman can do to lower her risk, especially after menopause, is maintain a healthy weight. There is a growing body of evidence indicating that being overweight as we get older increases estrogen and also affects insulin and other growth factors in ways that give cancers a more stimulating neighborhood in which to grow, at the same time making it more difficult for the body to eliminate emerging abnormal cells.

A lifestyle issue that is not discussed much is age at first pregnancy. The data are clear that early first pregnancy is protective and that getting pregnant for the first time after 35 increases the risk more than never being pregnant at all. The full explanation for this finding is not clear, but it suggests that you might choose to have your family first and then focus on career—or combine child rearing and a career with an equal opportunity husband or partner. Breast-feeding also has been shown to decrease breast cancer risk, especially in women with a family history of the disease. The greater the total number of months of breast-feeding, the greater the risk reduction.[1]

Diet

Since the fourth edition we have more data about the connection between diet and breast cancer. The role of dietary fruits and vegetables as a means of preventing breast cancer was given a blow when the report came out in 2005 from the European Prospective Investigation into Cancer and Nutrition (EPIC). An amazing 285,526 women between the ages of 25 and 70 completed a dietary questionnaire and then were followed prospectively for a median of 5.4 years. Although 3,659 breast cancers were reported, the study found no association between consumption of fruits and vegetables and the risk of developing breast cancer.[2] However, this didn't tell us whether certain fruits or vegetables, consumed at certain times in a woman's life, may have an effect. Then in 2006 the Women's Health Initiative reported on its randomized controlled study of low-fat diet. This study began in 1992 and randomized women between 50 and 79 to a diet with less than 20 percent of calories from fat, at least five daily servings of vegetables and fruit, and at least six of grain. Between 1993 and 1998, 48,835 women were studied. After approximately eight years of follow-up, breast cancer incidence was 9 percent lower for women in the dietary intervention group than for those in the comparison group. While this sounds great, the statistical calculations showed that it could have happened by chance. Add that to the fact that sticking to a restrictive diet that might not be to your taste is a lot to do for a measly 9 percent reduction in relative risk.[3]

Further, the question is complicated by the fact that weight gain is a risk factor for breast cancer, as noted in Chapter 5. Since a diet high in fruits and vegetables is usually lower in calories, any apparent connection may be incidental. It's not the apples and carrots you are eating but the hamburgers and cheesecake you *aren't* eating that probably make the difference. The overweight women who manage to lose weight in all of these studies reduce their risk more than the women who were thin and therefore at lower risk to start with. At this point I think it is wise, for many reasons, for all of us to eat a diet low in animal fat and high in fruits and vegetables, but I wouldn't count on it to save us all from breast cancer.

Soy, Flaxseed, and Green Tea

Soy as food has had a mixed reputation regarding breast cancer prevention. It has often mistakenly been termed a phytoestrogen (literally plant estrogen) when in fact it has a much more complex hormonal composition. Studies in Western populations have shown no association between high soy intake and breast cancer prevention.[4] However, a large study from Shanghai found that adult soy food consumption was associated with a lowered risk of premenopausal breast cancer.[5] It appears that most important is a high intake of soy foods during adolescence. Soy contains some weak plant estrogens that may enhance early differentiation and maturation of the breast tissue, which in turn may protect a woman from developing breast cancer.[6] A U.S. study of Asian American women confirmed that soy intake during childhood, adolescence, and adult life was associated with decreased breast cancer risk, with the strongest and most consistent effect from childhood intake.[7] This is encouraging and you may want to try and coax your adolescent into eating more tofu. But we can't be totally certain it will help: there remains the possibility that these children and adults had other elements in their lifestyle that were also, or even exclusively, protective. We get a hint of this in the study: when adjustments were made for measures of westernization, they found reduced benefits of soy intake among adolescents and adults, but not among younger children.

Regarding soy supplements, it's probably a good idea to play it safe and stay away from them, as they may not have the same effects as soy in real foods. Although you would think the label would tell you the dose, supplements do not need to either control or report this information the way drugs do. They could have no soy in them at all or a lot, since supplements are not regulated.

Flaxseed, sesame, and several other oily seeds and edible fibrous plants contain high amounts of lignans (complex elements in a plant cell's walls that give the plant rigidity and strength), which have some weak estrogenic and antiestrogenic properties distinct from those of soy. Flaxseed is currently advocated by professional gynecologic associations in Canada as a treatment for cyclic breast pain,[8,9] and a small placebo controlled trial in early breast cancer has also shown that it can reduce growth of cancer cells.[10] It currently is being studied in clinical trials to determine if it might be helpful in preventing breast cancer.[11]

Another substance being studied is green tea, which, like soy, is often part of an Asian diet. A study of Chinese women in Singapore found that daily intake of green tea had a strong effect on decreasing mammographic density. Black tea, much more common in the West, had no effect.[12] I must say this finding brought a smile to my face as I sipped my evening cup of green tea!

Vitamins and Minerals

Changing one's diet is never easy, and researchers have tried to figure out the key ingredients in vegetables, fruits, and fats so they can put them in a pill. This can be a tricky business. I am always reminded of the study done to prevent lung cancer. Initial work had shown that people who ate a lot of carrots had less lung cancer. Researchers postulated that it was the beta-carotene and decided to test it. They gave smokers beta-carotene capsules and were shocked when they found more cancers in the smokers taking the pills than those in the control group.[13] The answer is probably that vitamins and minerals are meant to be eaten together in a healthy diet. Beta-carotene needs to be eaten with all the other vitamins and minerals in the carrot, not in isolation.

Still a lot of research continues to focus on specific vitamins, hoping that one will be the holy grail. At the time of this writing it is Vitamin D, which also is thought to help maintain healthy bone, muscle, immune system, and probably other tissues as well. We make most of our vitamin D in the skin as a result of sun exposure. Our current indoor lifestyles and increased use of sun screen limit this route for many women. As a result there are a lot of women, including some with breast cancer, who have low blood levels of vitamin D. This has led some researchers to question whether vitamin D can prevent breast cancer. Epidemiologic studies comparing women in areas of high versus low sun exposure, animal studies, and some case control studies, particularly in young women, suggest that it can, especially if higher blood levels are achieved than we usually see with conventional doses of supplements. However, these investigations are only first steps. Women who have lower body fat from diet and exercise are also likely to have higher levels of vitamin D. We are not sure of the target blood level of vitamin D or the age at which vitamin D supplementation would need to start to prevent breast cancer. Further, overly high levels of vitamin D can result in side effects such as kidney stones.

Only two studies have evaluated cancer incidence in women randomized to placebo or calcium plus vitamin D. A small study in postmenopausal women in which the vitamin D dose was 1100

IU suggested a benefit in reducing all types of cancers, including breast cancer, but the numbers of developed cancers were too small to single out reduction of a specific cancer.[14] The Women's Health Initiative (WHI) randomized postmenopausal women to take calcium and 400 IU of a specific form of vitamin D or placebo. Women in both the placebo and treatment arms were allowed to take up to 1000 IU of nonstudy vitamin D since they were actually focused on calcium preventing fractures in this study. No reduction in risk of breast cancer comparing the treatment arm to placebo was observed in the WHI, nor were baseline blood levels of vitamin D correlated with breast cancer risk,[15] although these baseline levels were rarely in the range associated with substantial risk reduction in other studies.[16] They did find that baseline levels correlated with weight and exercise.[17] So one possible explanation of the previous studies may be that the women with higher vitamin D levels were also more likely to be thinner and also to exercise. Since these factors can also reduce breast cancer risk, it is hard to know which is more relevant. While we are waiting for further information about vitamin D, particularly for younger women, taking a supplement or spending 15 minutes a day in the sun without sun block will probably not harm you unless you are very fair or have a personal or family history of skin cancer. Many vitamin D experts recommend taking a supplement of 1000 IU daily for general health.[18]

Vitamin A studies have also been equivocal, with some suggesting a benefit and some not.[19] However, in studies that measure vitamin A compounds in the blood, low levels of the vitamin correlated with an increased risk of breast cancer.[20,21] Recent reviews of epidemiological data suggest that vitamin E in foods may provide some protection against breast cancer while vitamin E supplements appear not to.[22]

Finally the Women's Health Initiative looked at whether taking a multivitamin would reduce the risk of getting cancer. The WHI observational study[23] found that taking a multivitamin had little or no influence on the risk of common cancers, cardiovascular disease, or total mortality in postmenopausal women.

Overall the data are not strong enough to talk about a "breast cancer prevention diet," but in general a diet low in animal fat and high in whole grains, fruits, and vegetables is most likely to keep you healthy and help you maintain a good weight. It also makes sense to drink alcohol only in moderation, since, as discussed in Chapter 5, regular consumption of alcohol may affect your vulnerability to breast cancer.

Exercise

Exercise is important for cardiovascular health and for preventing osteoporosis, heart disease, and breast cancer. A 1994 study by my friend and colleague Leslie Bernstein at the City of Hope Medical Center demonstrated that women who participated in four or more hours of exercise a week during their reproductive years have a 58 percent decrease in breast cancer risk.[24] This was very exciting because it is one of the first lifestyle changes shown to decrease risk. Bernstein has recently updated this finding in a prospective study of retired and active California teachers and other public school professionals followed for 10 years.[25] She found that strenuous long-term exercise can indeed protect against invasive and in situ breast cancer, with a 20 percent greater risk reduction in women who exercised more than five hours a week than those who exercised minimally or not at all. Interestingly, participation in moderate to strenuous activity also reduced by about half the risk of estrogen receptor negative breast cancer. More than 50 studies have shown that women who are physically active have a lower risk of invasive breast cancer. Several have shown the same is true for in situ breast cancer. This suggests that physical activity affects early phases of breast cancer development. What causes this to happen is not clear, and the benefits may differ at different times of life. In young women the mechanism is thought to be hormonal, since exercise results in alterations in menstrual cycle patterns and ovulatory frequency, both of which are correlated with lower risk[26] (Figure 7.1). Even though affecting the menstrual cycle may seem like it should prevent hormonal tumors, it is also possible that the effect is on the interactive community of cells in the stroma that support estrogen negative tumors. Other possibilities are that exercise has an anti-inflammatory effect, which reduces the incidence of cancers.

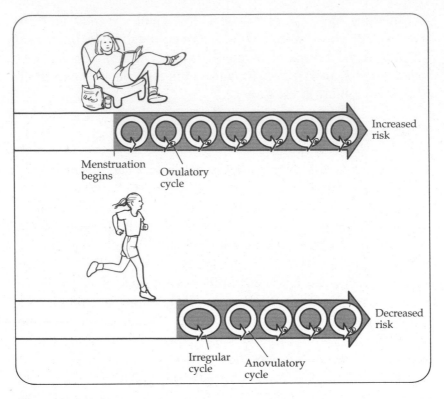

Figure 7.1

Finally there is the fact that it helps maintain a healthy weight, which is important in postmenopausal women.

A long-term prevention approach would be to get girls into the habit of exercising. Rose Frisch of Harvard Medical School and Harvard School of Public Health has shown that women who were involved in athletics during high school and college have a decreased risk of breast cancer.[27]

A delightful proposal has been put forth: increase funding to high school athletics for girls. Expanded participation in athletics would likely decrease breast cancer, strengthen bones, and prevent future osteoporosis; it would also help prevent heart disease. But physical activity doesn't have to be athletics. My daughter joined the folk dancing club in college and gets a great workout that way. And it is never too late to start! I am a born-again exerciser, having started running at age 50. I have learned to enjoy the stress reduction from my regular slow run, as well as the sense of moral superiority I feel for the rest of the day.

Lifestyle changes are interesting from a public health standpoint, and probably are worthwhile to consider on an individual basis, but they may or may not be applicable to any particular woman, and I don't advise using them as the sole influence in decision making. For example, I had my first child at 40 and do not regret it. The advantages to me far outweighed the slight potentially increased risk for breast cancer. Would I have been wiser to have had a child in my twenties, when I wasn't ready for it? Or, since having no children is actually less of a risk than having a first child later in life, should I have deprived myself of the joy Katie has brought me? For me, there was no question. On the other hand, I do eat a good diet high in fruits and vegetables and low in animal fat. The occasional twinge I feel at the sight of a juicy hamburger or wedge of Brie is a reasonable price to pay for the possibility that I may be decreasing my breast cancer risk and improving my overall health. Another woman in my position might decide to adopt rather become pregnant, or she might decide that the pleasure she gets from some of her fatty foods isn't worth abandoning. These are very personal decisions.

CHEMOPREVENTION

Hormones

Since hormones are heavily implicated in the development of breast cancer, and the more menstruating years you experience the higher your risk of breast cancer, one proposed approach has been to put women into temporary menopause.[28] This approach, which could combine birth control and breast cancer prevention, has been shown to reduce mammographic density,[29] but so far no long-term studies have been done to demonstrate its safety and effectiveness for breast cancer prevention.

Another approach is based on the recognition that the younger you are when you have your first child, the lower your risk. There has been some thought that we might have an effect on breast cancer risk by coming up with a way to induce a hormonal "pregnancy," in which a teenager would be given pregnancy hormones for nine months to mature the breast tissue. To my knowledge, this has been tried only in rats, but it's an interesting possibility. One ingenious study took advantage of the fact that HCG (a hormone of pregnancy) was once used in weight loss clinics allegedly to help women lose weight (it has no such effect, but many women took these shots). Leslie Bernstein was the only one ever to collect such data, and she showed that it does reduce breast cancer risk in premenopausal women, just as the animal studies would have predicted, with the strongest effect seen in women who had never been pregnant and therefore had not had a chance to be exposed to their own pregnancy-induced HCG.[30] There are several small studies looking at whether HCG could be used for prevention.

Tamoxifen and Raloxifene

Another use of drugs to prevent breast cancer is based on the idea of blocking the estrogen receptor to keep estrogen from having its usual effect. This is the theory behind efforts to avert the disease by giving women tamoxifen or raloxifene.

These drugs are actually not estrogen blockers but selective estrogen receptor modulators, or SERMs. Tamoxifen as a breast cancer prevention tool was discovered from an observation in breast cancer treatment studies. Researchers who had used it to treat existing cancers had realized something: when women with breast cancer took tamoxifen, not only did they have fewer recurrences of the original cancer, but they also had 30–50 percent fewer cancers in the opposite breast. A woman who usually had a 10 percent risk of cancer in the other breast now had a 5–7 percent risk. If the drug could prevent new cancers in women who already had the disease, thought the researchers, perhaps it could further reduce the susceptibility of women who were at high risk. A study, the National Surgical Adjuvant Breast and Bowel Project (NSABP), was devised to examine that possibility.[31] It was a huge study—13,388 women. First researchers used the Gail model, a statistical combination of risk factors, to calculate who was at increased risk (see Chapter 6).[32]

Having picked the subjects for their study group, they then randomized them, giving half the group tamoxifen and half a placebo. Among these women, some had already been diagnosed with lobular carcinoma in situ or atypical ductal hyperplasia and others were calculated by the Gail index to be at high risk. Although the study included women with a five-year risk of 1.6 percent or more, most people in the study had a higher risk—and half of them had more than a 3 percent risk.

Overall, the study showed that taking tamoxifen decreased by 49 percent the danger of getting invasive cancer. Fewer cases of breast cancer were found among the women who took tamoxifen than among those who didn't. The benefit persisted in all age-groups, though the numbers were small. In certain groups the difference was more dramatic. For example, women with previously diagnosed atypical hyperplasia had an 86 percent decreased risk.

Tamoxifen prevented tumors that were estrogen receptor positive (sensitive to estrogen) for pre-and postmenopausal women, including both invasive cancer and DCIS. This study lasted only four years, and it couldn't look at death from breast cancer because cancer takes time to develop, be detected, and induce fatality. So there's no way of knowing if the tamoxifen prevented cancer deaths or prevented only the appearance of cancers that wouldn't have been fatal anyway. Since the first report, three other randomized controlled studies have confirmed this effect.[33,34,35] Interestingly, a lot of the prevention happened within the first year or two. This is reminiscent of the rapid effect from HT (see Chapter 5), suggesting that it may be affecting the stroma around the cells and suppressing dormant cancer cells in the breast. Even more interesting is the fact that the risk reduction from tamoxifen appears to last for at least five years after the drug has been stopped.[36]

The big question remains whether the cancers we are preventing are also the ones we are most successful at treating anyway and therefore will not impact the numbers of deaths from breast cancer.

Risks and Benefits of Tamoxifen for Prevention
Like all drugs, tamoxifen has some risks.[37] Most worrisome are clotting problems leading to deep vein thrombosis, pulmonary

embolism, and strokes, as well as the uterine cancers that have been found with tamoxifen use.

The good news is that the greatest risk of uterine cancer appears to occur in women who previously took estrogen therapy (without Provera) for menopause or were extremely overweight.[38] For women who have not been on ERT and for normal-weight women the risks may be lower (see Chapter 9). In these women there were also fewer severe problems—hot flashes and vaginal dryness.

Overall, the best use of tamoxifen is in women for whom it has been shown to have the biggest benefit—those with atypical hyperplasia or lobular carcinoma in situ (see Chapter 13).

Raloxifene

The accidental discovery of tamoxifen's potential effect on breast cancer was followed by a furious search for drugs with similar capabilities. Raloxifene (Evista) was the first such drug—the first true designer SERM. Marketed in 1999, it was created to have the positive effect of estrogen on the body with none of its negative effects—particularly uterine cancer. Preliminary data from studies designed to look at raloxifene as a drug to treat low bone density suggested that it might also be able to prevent breast cancer.

The Study of Tamoxifen and Raloxifine (STAR) trial, sponsored by the National Cancer Institute, compared tamoxifen and raloxifene head to head in 20,000 postmenopausal high-risk women, average age 58. There was no placebo group. The results of this study suggested that tamoxifen and raloxifene were equivalent in reducing the risk of invasive breast cancer. As this edition went to press, the eight-year follow-up of this study was reported. While both drugs continued to reduce risk, raloxifene was less helpful than tamoxifen (38 percent decrease versus 50 percent) in reducing the risk of noninvasive or invasive cancer, but it had fewer objective side effects than tamoxifen—including fewer total uterine events (hyperplasia, biopsies, hysterectomy, cancer) and cataracts. The incidence of subjective side effects and quality of life were about the same, although individual side effects differed slightly between the two. For example, the incidence of vaginal dryness and sexual side effects was greater in the raloxifene arm but hot flashes somewhat higher in the tamoxifen arm.[39]

The good news is that now we have solid data to recommend chemoprevention in high-risk women: tamoxifen for premenopausal women and raloxifene for postmenopausal women. No drug is risk free, of course, but the risks last only for the first five years, while it appears, at least for tamoxifen and probably for raloxifene, that the benefit lasts a lot longer.

PREVENTIVE SURGERY

Most people assume that the foolproof way to prevent breast cancer is to remove the breasts. If you don't have breasts, the reasoning goes, you won't get breast cancer. There are two problems here. For one thing, it's a drastic solution. Most women like their breasts for esthetic and erotic reasons, even if they're not planning to use them for breast-feeding. Yet some are so terrified of the possibility of breast cancer that preventive mastectomy seems to be a good idea.

Most of the studies have followed women who are at high genetic risk because of mutations in BRCA 1 or 2, and they show that preventive mastectomy reduces the risk of subsequent breast cancer by 90 percent. That's the other problem. It's a large reduction, but not a total one. No mastectomy can be guaranteed to remove all the breast tissue, which extends from the collarbone to below the rib cage, from the breastbone around to the back. Further, it doesn't separate itself out from the surrounding tissue in any obvious way (Figure 7.2). The most brilliant surgeon in the world couldn't be certain of digging all the breast tissue out of your body. When we do a mastectomy we do our best to get out as much as possible.[40]

This drastic approach may well make sense for some women who are carriers of the BRCA 1 or 2 mutations, as we will see below, and maybe even women who have had breast biopsies showing precancerous changes such as lobular carcinoma in situ or atypical hyperplasia. Recently, however, its use in nonmutation carriers has risen, particularly in those who have been diagnosed with breast cancer in one breast and decide to have the other one removed "just in case." Without discounting anyone's right to make such a choice, I have to say that this trend makes me a bit uneasy.

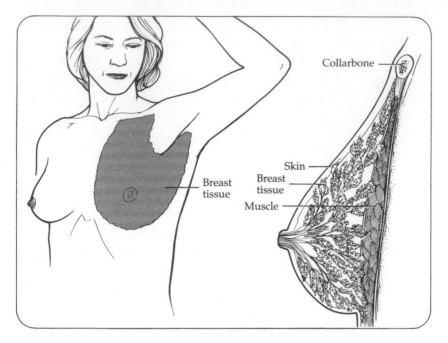

Figure 7.2

Interestingly, part of the growing popularity of preventive (often called prophylactic) mastectomies seems to be driven by the use of preoperative MRIs. As this test (see Chapter 8) finds lots of "things" that may not be cancer but need to be investigated, it often scares women so much that they want just to get rid of both breasts once and for all.[41] In fact the risk of cancer developing in the second breast is not high, about 10 percent over a lifetime, and most women will not have further problems, particularly if they are taking or have taken a hormonal treatment that has been shown to decrease the risk of contralateral breast cancer. Often the risk of recurrence of the first cancer is higher than the risk of a new cancer in the other breast. This is relevant because having a bilateral mastectomy with immediate reconstruction and the subsequent recovery time often leads to a delay in starting chemotherapy or other systemic treatment (see Chapter 17) for the first cancer.

I think part of the problem is that surgeons are rushed and often don't take the time to explain to women the risks and benefits.

But then I may be a bit biased. We fought so hard in the 1980s to give women the option of lumpectomy, which conserved the breast and equaled the effectiveness of mastectomy, that I find it hard to see public opinion shifting the other way without data to suggest its usefulness.

Some women who are newly diagnosed or consider themselves high risk wonder about having their ovaries removed. Although this will reduce the risk of breast cancer and ovarian cancer, there is a significant downside. Recent studies have shown that preventive removal of the ovaries increases the risk of early death from other diseases, including lung cancer, which overrides any benefit from decreasing breast or ovarian cancer.[42] And removing the ovaries after menopause has no effect on breast cancer risk. Further, because ovarian tissue, like breast tissue, still remains in the area surrounding the organs, removal of the ovaries isn't a guarantee against getting the disease (see below).

Prevention in BRCA 1 and 2 Mutation Carriers

In women who are carriers of a genetic mutation in BRCA 1 or 2, the situation is a bit different. Their risk of developing cancer is 65–80 percent over their lifetime, and in the absence of other alternatives, they may well decide that it makes sense to choose preventive surgery. In a multicenter study of 483 mutation carriers from the Prevention and Observation of Surgical End Points study group (PROSE), the women were monitored for an average of 6.4 years. Two of 105 carriers (1.9 percent) who had preventive mastectomy developed breast cancer, as opposed to 184 out of 378 (48.7 percent) matched controls. When they looked only at the women who still had their ovaries, prophylactic mastectomies led to a 90 percent reduction in risk.[43] The Rotterdam Family Cancer Clinic updated its experience with risk-reducing mastectomies in 358 women with known mutations. The women underwent skin-sparing mastectomies (see Chapter 14), often followed by immediate reconstruction. In 4.5 years there was only one case of metastatic breast cancer in a previously unaffected woman. The mastectomy specimens were carefully examined for the presence of cancers, which were found in 10 out of 358 women, or 2.8 percent.[44]

If you are a mutation carrier, having your ovaries removed before age 50 reduces the risk of ovarian cancer by 96 percent and decreases the risk of breast cancer by 47–61 percent.[45] It doesn't reduce the risk of ovarian cancer 100 percent, since there can be specks of ovarian tissue in the peritoneal lining of the abdomen (this is the smooth, glistening lining of the inside of your belly, something like the inside of your mouth) that can still become cancerous. In a large follow-up study of women at high risk for ovarian cancer at the Gilda Radner Familial Ovarian Cancer Registry, 6 of the 324 women (2 percent) who underwent prophylactic oophorectomy developed peritoneal carcinomas.[46] And finally, in women over 50 the risk reduction was 89 percent for ovarian cancer and 48 percent for breast cancer.[47] Interestingly, in at least one study, taking estrogen after oophorectomy did not seem to affect this lowered risk, probably because the hormones are given at a lower dose than premenopausal women are likely to have naturally.

And what if you do both? Have your ovaries and breasts removed? We are unlikely to get this information because the number of mutation carriers who have had this surgery is not large enough to do the kind of randomized controlled study that would be needed.

If all this seems overwhelming, remember that you don't have to do everything at once. One of my Facebook friends had a strong paternal history of breast cancer (great-grandmother, grandmother, father, two cousins, and three aunts), and they all tested positive for BRCA 2. Initially she opted for close surveillance and then after many years had bilateral oophorectomy. Five years later she decided to reduce her risk further with bilateral preventive mastectomy. Now two years later she is very happy with her decision: "My husband and I talk about it every once in while, satisfied with the knowledge that we can grow old together without the huge threat of cancer for me."

Having a genetic risk of breast cancer is not an emergency, and you do not have to rush. Take your time to decide what is appropriate for you, and don't be afraid to change your mind over time.

Not all women who are carriers of the BRCA genes and thus face a very high risk of breast cancer choose to undergo preventive surgery. They still have options. One choice, as mentioned in the last chapter, is close monitoring, which, though not prevention, aims to find a cancer as soon as it becomes detectable. This approach has not yet shown a reduction in breast cancer mortality. The current guidelines for a BRCA carrier are to start screening with mammography and MRI at age 25, but many imagers and oncologists feel more comfortable with utilizing only MRI (sometimes combined with ultrasound) until the carrier is 30 or has had her first child. One interesting analysis modeled the benefits of screening versus preventative surgery for a twenty-five-year-old BRCA 1/2 carrier. The researchers found that preventive mastectomy at age 25 plus preventative oophorectomy at 40 maximizes the probability of survival. However, mammography plus MRI screening starting at 25 with preventative oophorectomy at 40 is about the same.[48] Note that there are also downsides to oophorectomy prior to 40, such as increased heart disease.

Beyond surveillance, there are lifestyle changes that may have some impact. As noted in the last chapter, modulating estrogen appears to be relevant; for example, oral contraceptives decrease ovarian cancer. So too does breast-feeding.[49]

There are several interesting new approaches on the horizon. An animal study at Johns Hopkins found that giving low-dose chemotherapy into the ducts results in the equivalent of a chemical mastectomy.[50] It removes the ductal cells but not the others. My research has involved safety studies in which we put chemotherapy into the ducts of women scheduled for mastectomies to see if it has any side effects. The original studies have gone well and we are now looking at the effects of this approach in women with DCIS. My hope is that one day it will allow women to prevent breast cancer without removing the breast.

Another possibility would be a drug specific to the BRCA defect that could prevent cancer from developing. This class of drugs (PARP 2 inhibitors, which we considered in Chapter 4 and will examine at length in Chapter 21) has been developed and tested in women with metastatic disease and has had very promising results. Whether these drugs will be useful for prevention has yet to be determined, but it is certainly a possibility. Because so much research is going on, mutation carriers who want to take measures to prevent the disease should go to a high-risk center that specializes in women with genetic breast cancer, where they will get the very latest and best advice available.

As this book was being written a promising announcement regarding some mouse experiments with a breast cancer vaccine against lactalbumin, a protein found in breast feeding women and breast cancers, made headlines. While preliminary this type of approach holds promise for real prevention.[51]

Putting It Together

So, once again, what can most women do? There are some steps that the average woman can take to reduce her risk.

1. Exercise for at least 30 minutes a day, preferably 4–5 hours a week (enough to break a sweat).
2. Maintain a normal weight, especially if you are post-menopausal.
3. Have your children before 35 if you can.
4. Breast-feed your children.
5. Avoid unnecessary X rays.
6. Drink alcohol only in moderation and make sure you take folic acid when you do drink (see Chapter 5).
7. Avoid taking hormones (HT, fertility drugs) unless necessary.
8. Have a doctor evaluate any breast symptoms or changes that develop.
9. Have a mammogram when appropriate (see Chapter 8 on screening).
10. Join the Love/Avon Army of Women (online at www.army ofwomen.org) to participate in studies to find the cause and prevention of breast cancer.

If you have a family history of breast cancer or think you are at risk, you can be evaluated at a high-risk center to see where you stand. Those who are at increased risk may consider taking raloxifene or tamoxifen for five years. If you fit the criteria for genetic testing (see Chapter 6), you should see a genetic counselor to consider your options.

Part Three

DIAGNOSIS AND SCREENING

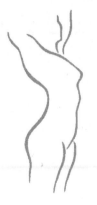

Chapter 8

Diagnosis: Mammography, Ultrasound, MRI, and Biopsies

Imaging has become more and more important in the diagnosis of all breast problems, and even biopsies are now often image directed. "Imaging" means ways of seeing body tissue.

In this chapter we'll look at diagnostic mammography and other commonly used diagnostic tools (the same equipment is used for screening and diagnostic mammography, but different types of pictures may be taken) and finish with a description of biopsy techniques.

Mammograms

A mammogram is an X ray of the breast—"mammo" means breast and "gram" means picture. It isn't the same as a chest X ray, which looks through the breast and photographs the lungs. Mammograms look at the breast itself and take pictures of the soft tissue, allowing the radiologist to see anything unusual or suspicious. Mammography can pick up very small lesions—about 0.5 centimeter (or 0.2 inch), whereas you usually can't feel a lump until

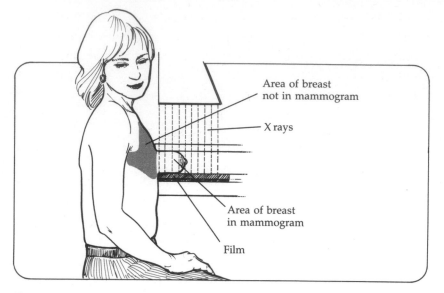

Figure 8.1

it's at least a centimeter (0.4 inch). These lesions can be benign or malignant. In addition, mammograms can sometimes pick up noninvasive cancers (see Chapter 13).

Mammography has its limits, though. The mammogram can photograph only the part of the breast that sticks out—the plates are put underneath the breast or on the sides of the breast—so it's easier to get an accurate picture of a large breast than of a small one. The periphery of the breast does not get into the picture at all (Figure 8.1). In addition, if your breasts are dense, the lump may not be visible through the tissue. So a mammogram isn't perfect. Physical exams and mammograms complement each other. You can see some lumps on a mammogram that you can't feel, and you can feel some lumps (palpation) that you can't see on an X ray.

You get a diagnostic mammogram (as opposed to a screening mammogram) when you find a lump or have another breast complaint and your doctor wants to get a better sense of what the problem is or look more closely at an area that may have changed from a previous mammogram. If, for example, you have lumpy breasts and there's one area that may be a dominant lump, your doctor may send you for a mammogram. If a lump looks jagged, rather than smooth on the mammogram, it's a sign that further investigation may be called for. If you've got a lump your doctor thinks may be cancerous, a mammogram can help determine if there are other lumps that should be biopsied at the same time; it can also document the location of the lump.

What Mammograms Show

A mammogram, like any other X ray, presents a two-dimensional view of a three-dimensional structure. Denser areas appear brighter. Breast tissue, for example, is very dense, and shows up white on the mammogram. Fat, which is not very dense at all, shows up gray (see photographs on pages 216–217).

As you'll recall from Chapter 1, when you're young—in your teens and early twenties—your breasts are made up mostly of breast tissue and are very dense. As you grow older, the breast ages, much as your skin does, and there's less breast tissue and more fat. However, women vary in the proportion of breast tissue remaining after menopause.

Beyond assessing breast density, mammography is looking for lesions or abnormalities. If you have felt a lump, the imaging will look particularly in that area to decide how suspicious it may be. Generally, when noncancerous lesions expand, they push the normal breast tissue away and create smooth edges (like blowing up a balloon), whereas cancers expand by growing between the normal cells—"infiltrating"—and this leads to indistinct or jagged irregular edges (like a mold expanding into a cheese). Thus when mammograms show something round and smooth, it's likely to be a cyst or a fibroadenoma (see Chapter 3). The mammogram can't distinguish between them; you follow up with an ultrasound (discussed later in this chapter) to see if it's a cyst. If a mammogram shows jagged, distinct, radiating strands pulling inward, it's more likely to be cancer. But until it is biopsied, we can't tell for sure. Several benign conditions can mimic cancer on a mammogram. Scarring or fat necrosis (dead fat) will look very suspicious. A noncancerous entity—a radial scar—is caused by an increase in local fibrous tissue (see Chapter 1) trapping some of the glands in a way that can look suspicious. It can be confusing even under the

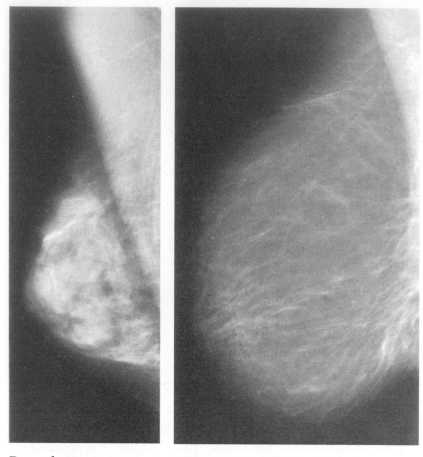

Dense breast in young woman   *Fatty breast in older woman*

microscope and often requires an expert breast pathologist to rule out cancer.

A mammogram may also show intramammary (in the breast) lymph nodes. In fact, until the mammogram came along, we didn't even know there were lymph nodes in the breast. We now know that 5.4 percent of women have them.

Sometimes you'll hear about a "normal" mammogram. But there's really no one normal pattern, since there's no "normal" breast: there is only normal for you. There is a standardized reporting system for mammography that was developed to indicate how suspicious a particular finding may be. It is now used by most radiologists who interpret mammograms. This is called the

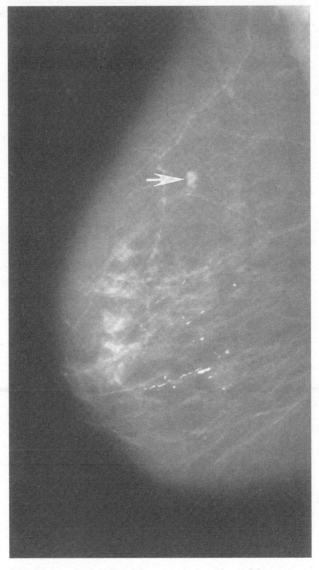

Small cancer in fatty breast (arrow) and benign calcifications

Breast Imaging Reporting and Data System (BI-RADS; see Table 8.1). It is important that the radiologist who interprets your mammogram uses BI-RADS for the report so your doctor won't be confused by the report findings.

Mammogram reports sometimes mention the amount of breast density. In fact the state of Connecticut is looking at

Table 8.1   American College of Radiology Breast Imaging Reporting
and Data System (BI-RADS) Assessment Categories: Mammography

Category 1	Negative	The breasts appear normal
Category 2	Benign finding	This is also normal; the reader is pointing out a non suspicious benign finding
Category 3	Probably benign	Less than a 2% chance of being cancer; repeat test in 6 weeks will confirm it is stable
Category 4	Suspicious abnormality	Biopsy should be considered. Does not have classical appearance of cancer but a chance of 2-7.95%. Actual probability in report will help doctor and patient decide whether a biopsy is indicated
Category 5	Highly suggestive of malignancy	These lesions have a high probability (95%) chance of being cancer; A biopsy is recommended
Category 6	Biopsy proven malignancy	This is for lesions that have already been biopsied
Category 0	Incomplete	Need additional imaging evaluation and/or prior mammograms for comparison

BI-RADS Breast Density Classification

Category 1	Entirely fat	Lowest risk
Category 2	Scattered fibroglandular densities	
Category 3	Moderately dense	
Category 4	Extremely dense	Highest risk

requiring mammographers to quantify the amount of density in
their reports, and there are BI-RADS categories for density. On
the surface this sounds like a good idea. After all, in Chapter 6 I
mentioned that having density on a mammogram increases your
risk of getting cancer. In general, half of screened women have
fatty or scattered density, which is considered lower risk. The
problem is the lack of a standardized measurement of density.
One doctor may call your breasts dense while another may say
they are fairly transparent. So while it is worth knowing whether

your breasts are more dense than those of most women your age, we cannot use it as a measure of risk. The main reason to know how dense your breasts are is that you will have a sense of how accurate the mammogram may be. If your breasts are extremely dense, the accuracy is only about 69 percent.[1] This is because dense breast tissue can hide a cancer, so it's sort of like looking for a polar bear in the snow. If your breasts are mostly fatty, you can be more assured that when a mammogram shows that there is nothing suspicious in your breast, there probably isn't.

Types of Mammograms

Though early mammography in the 1950s produced a fair amount of radiation, over the years X ray techniques have been refined so that very little radiation is actually used. It's commonly said that a mammogram exposes you to the same amount of radiation you'd get in a plane flying over Denver. One radiologist I used to work with in Boston explained it in more colorful terms: the amount of radiation of one mammogram is equal to the amount you would get by walking on the beach nude for 10 minutes or until you got caught.[2] While one mammogram gives a pretty low dose of radiation, having mammograms every year from an early age can add up, as I explain in Chapter 9. Film-screen mammography, the conventional type, gives a precise definition of what the tissue looks like. It can be a bit uncomfortable because the breasts have to be squeezed between the plates to get an accurate picture. The slight discomfort is well worth the increased accuracy and low radiation. A 1993 study tried letting women control the compression themselves. Not surprisingly, they ended up with the same amount of compression, equally good quality films, and fewer complaints.[3]

A newer technique is the digital mammogram. Like a digital camera, digital mammography is a way of computerizing the image so it can be viewed on a computer monitor screen and printed out like conventional mammograms. Because it's a computerized rather than a photographic technique, the radiologist can magnify different areas to focus on what she or he wants to see. Just as you can play with digital photos on your computer and remove Uncle Jack, on a digital mammogram all the fat can be blocked out so only breast tissue shows up, or all the breast tissue can be erased so that only fat shows up. A recent study has shown that it does this successfully. In a paired comparison of digital and regular screen-film mammograms the same number of cancers were found. But with the digital technique, fewer additional images were needed to sort out an abnormal shadow before a biopsy was recommended. The technique allowed the radiologists to manipulate the images and figure out if what they were seeing was real, whereas the screen-film had to be repeated in a different view to accomplish the same thing.[4,5] Finally, the technique allowed the image to be stored more efficiently and transmitted more easily, as with the photos taken with a digital camera. Though this technique was hoped to be more sensitive and accurate than film-screen mammogram, that has not proven to be the case. A very large multicenter prospective study comparing the two techniques showed no difference in sensitivity (ability to find suspicious lesions), recall (being called back for another picture), or biopsy rates between the two techniques. The only slight advantage was found in regard to pre-and perimenopausal women with very dense breasts. Although digital mammography is easier to perform, the older mammography still works very well. If your mammography center is still doing film-screen, don't panic.

For a time digital mammography in another form promised to be even better. This was computerized *reading* of mammograms (computer-aided detection, or CAD). A computer prescreens mammograms and points out the worrisome areas so that the mammographers can examine them more carefully. It was hoped that this would make reading more accurate, as computers don't get distracted or blink at the wrong moment. In one study it did help find more cancers; unfortunately, this benefit did not seem to translate to the real world when tested in a large clinical practice.[6,7]

At this point, we've gotten almost as far as we can with mammography. Each advance is only slightly incremental. We can hope for other and better imaging techniques to be developed in the future. Some exist already, and we'll discuss them later in this chapter, but so far they work better as adjuncts to mammography than replacement of it.

Calcifications

One of the more important discoveries that has come about from the study of mammograms is that breast cancer is often associated with some very fine specks of calcium that appear on the picture—they look a bit like tiny dust particles on a film.

We discovered that these microcalcifications, as we called them, were sometimes an indication of invasive or noninvasive cancer (see Chapter 13). So the radiologist will always mention in a report any microcalcifications that show up. But it's nothing to panic about—80 percent of microcalcifications have nothing to do with cancer; they're probably just the result of normal wear and tear on your breast.[8] Ironically, when you age, calcium leaves your bones, where it's needed, and shows up in other places, where it's not. It can appear in arteries, causing them to harden, and in joints, causing arthritis. The microcalcifications in your breast won't cause any problems if they're not indications of invasive or noninvasive cancer. (The appearance of this calcium in your body has no relation to how much calcium you eat or drink, by the way.)

How do we distinguish between the ominous calcifications and the harmless kinds? We look at the shape, the size, and how many there are. If they're tiny and tightly clustered, and there aren't a whole lot of them, they're more likely to indicate noninvasive cancer. If they're all over the place they're more likely to be benign.

Noninvasive cancer occurs in the duct or lobule, which is very small. For the calcifications to fit in a duct, they too have to be very small, and tightly clustered. The big chunks of calcium we see on the mammogram couldn't possibly fit in the ductal system, so we know they're benign. They're usually old fibroadenomas that you had as a teenager, which, having faded and become soft and less dense, are now calcifying. Sometimes they're calcifications in a blood vessel that's getting older and harder.

There's a middle group of calcifications that are less easy to characterize. They may be new, but there are just one or two of them. In that situation, we'll usually repeat the mammogram in six months.[9] If it's noninvasive cancer, we may see more calcifications, or a change in the shape or size, whereas if there's no change, it's more likely to be benign. Patients get nervous about that; if it's cancer and we wait six months, won't it grow and kill you? But in fact, if we wait six months it's probably because we don't think it's cancer. And even in the worst-case scenario, it's noninvasive cancer and noninvasive cancer takes 10 years to develop into cancer. So six months won't make any difference, and the wait prevents needless biopsies.

Some noninvasive cancerous calcifications don't grow or change, so they don't get picked up on the second mammogram. But that's because they aren't growing and thus aren't becoming cancer.

Anytime doctors are worried about calcifications, they can proceed to a biopsy. This is usually done as a core biopsy (described at the end of the chapter). If we want to prove an area benign by imaging, usually we need to do a mammogram every six months for between two and three years. In the days of wire-loc excisional biopsies (see Chapter 14) this was acceptable and proven safe. But the more modern invention of the core biopsy has proven even less invasive and can resolve the issue sooner.

Mammographic Workup

Screening is for asymptomatic women (see Chapter 9). In contrast, diagnostic mammography involves working up a lump felt by a woman or her doctor or an abnormal finding on a screening mammogram.

One way to do this workup is to use a spot compression view. We do this when there is a dense area on a film-screen mammogram that we're unsure of. It's an extra magnified view on the mammogram; the radiologic technologist uses a small plate to press right over the abnormal area and takes a picture of that area. Since a mammogram is a two-dimensional picture of a three-dimensional structure, we see overlapping shapes. (It's as if you had a transparent balloon with different pictures on each side. If you took a photo from the front, it would look like one complex image. If you looked at each picture on the balloon from a different direction, you'd see them as separate.) The technologist may

also press on your breast at an angle and change it so that things aren't perfectly juxtaposed. If there is an abnormal density on mammogram or a lump that can be felt but isn't visible on a mammogram, you may be sent to get an ultrasound.

If you have a palpable lump, the technologist should tape a metal BB on your breast as a marker to be sure that the lump is on the film. If it is at the periphery of the breast, special mammographic views may be needed to get it in the picture—like changing the angle of your camera to make sure Aunt Mabel's head doesn't get cut off in the photo. This is especially important for lumps that are near the armpit or in the lower fold of the breast. Markers are also frequently put on moles or other skin lesions and on the tip of the nipple to help with orientation.

If calcifications are present, we often do a magnification view, which is a mammogram that magnifies the area of the breast with the calcifications, so we can see them and characterize them better. So, for the most part, if you're told that the calcifications on your mammogram are worrisome, you should make sure they do a magnified view to see if the calcifications still look bad and how many there are. This is sometimes not necessary with digital mammogram.

A mammogram can't tell for certain what you have. But in some situations the view from the mammogram shows signs that clearly suggest a diagnosis. It's a bit like seeing someone from the back. You don't know for sure that it's your friend Mary until she turns around and faces you. But if it's Mary's shade of red hair, arranged in the kind of ponytail Mary always wears, and she walks like Mary does and carries the kind of large briefcase Mary likes to carry, you can make a pretty good guess that it's Mary. How often you are right, of course, depends on how well you know Mary. An experienced mammographer is better able to diagnose breast problems than an inexperienced one.

When I was in practice, I'd often have a patient tell me something strange had appeared on her mammogram. I would look at the X rays and see a small, smooth lump, like a fibroadenoma, but it would be new. The radiologist had written, "possible fibroadenoma; cancer can't be ruled out." I could have done one of two things. I could have waited six months and checked it out again; if it were cancer, it probably would have grown. If she was really anxious, I could have done a core biopsy under X ray or ultrasound guidance. If it wasn't cancer, that was fine; if it was, we could plan for the cancer surgery.

Quality of Mammograms

Today all mammography units must be accredited by an FDA-approved body (certified by the FDA as meeting its standards) and must prominently display the certificate issued by the agency. The initial quality standards for mammography facilities to meet FDA certification went into effect in December 1994. They include the following: radiologic technologists who perform mammography, physicians who interpret mammograms, and medical physicists who survey equipment must all have adequate training and experience; each facility must have a system for following up on mammograms that reveal problems and for obtaining biopsy results. In 1996 the FDA along with the National Mammography Quality Assurance Advisory Committee developed additional and more comprehensive final standards, including (1) a consumer complaint mechanism to provide women with a process for addressing their concerns about mammography facilities; (2) special techniques and personnel qualifications related to mammography of women with breast implants; (3) communication of mammography results to referring physicians and *all examinees* (*that means you*) in writing; and (4) additional clinical image review and examinee notification requirements when a facility's images are determined to be substandard. In addition, the BI-RADS system provides a standardized reading of mammograms whereby all of them are classified according to six categories (see Table 8.1) and must be used.

Mammography is the one area where we really do have quality control—something we have little of in the rest of breast care, and indeed in much of medicine.

Procedure

What actually happens on the day you have a mammogram? Preparations start before you leave the house. Don't use talcum powder or deodorant (except for those without aluminum, such as Tom's) the day you're scheduled for a mammogram—flecks of talcum can show up as calcifications on the mammogram. Avoid lotions that can make the breast slippery. Some instructions will tell you not to consume caffeine for two weeks before the X ray; unless you have experienced some problem with caffeine, these are instructions you can ignore.

The atmosphere you face when you get there will vary from one mammography facility to another. Some are cold and clinical; others provide a warm ambience and reassuring, friendly personnel. But the actual procedure is pretty standard. You have to undress from the waist up, and you're usually given some kind of hospital gown. You'll probably be x-rayed standing up. The technologist—usually, but not always, a woman—will have you lean over a plastic plate and help you place your breast on the plate. This can feel a bit uncomfortable, especially when the plates press your breast together. Two pictures of each breast are usually taken, one from the side, the other vertical. In addition, the way the technologist takes the X rays is important. The tighter your breasts are squeezed, the more accurate the picture is and the less radiation is necessary to penetrate the tissue.

The process really isn't all that painful. One researcher did a multicenter study interviewing women right after their mammograms, asking how painful the process was and what point they were at in their menstrual cycle.[10] He was pleased that 88 percent of the women reported no pain or discomfort, and was surprised to learn that their cycle didn't seem to have any effect on their comfort level.

For the small percentage of women with unusually sensitive breasts, a mammogram can indeed be painful. In this study none of the women who reported that the procedure was painful felt that the pain would stop them from having another mammogram exam. It's unfortunate that it's not painless, but I think it's well worth the slight—and brief—discomfort. At UCLA we actually timed the technologists, and we found that compression lasted at most 10 seconds. It doesn't leave bruises or tender spots when it's over.

Women with disabilities may have difficulty getting a clear mammogram, particularly if they're unable to stand up. Fortunately a good technologist can do a mammogram while a woman sits for the procedure. If you're told this can't be done, you should insist on it or go to another facility.

The whole process lasts only a few minutes; when it's done, you have to wait while the pictures are developed, so you may want to bring along a book or an iPod. A digital mammogram is faster, since films do not have to be developed and the technologist can check the mammograms on a computer screen a few seconds after they are taken. The radiologist (a physician, not the technologist) who looks at the pictures will sometimes see something on the periphery that isn't completely clear and will want to take another picture, focusing on that area, or possibly a magnification view. If you are having a diagnostic mammogram, the radiologist will usually discuss the results with you immediately following the examination. In some places, the radiologist will also come out and tell you what the screening mammogram shows. In other high-volume settings the radiologists will read the screening mammograms later in the day when they can focus and not be interrupted. Then the results are sent by mail and you have to wait several days to a week to get them. Studies have shown that centers that do a high volume of mammograms and read them later often have more accurate interpretations, so this is not unreasonable.

Please don't ask your technologist to interpret the mammogram for you. Technologists aren't doctors; their job is taking the pictures, not reading them.

Although, as I have often been quoted as saying, mammography must have been invented by a man (and there should be an equally fun test for men), it is the best tool we currently have. We have to be careful, regarding the risks and benefits of screening (see Chapter 9), not to throw the baby out with the bath water. It's an imperfect tool but, particularly for women with confusing breast problems, an important one.

Limitations of Mammography

Frustration with the limitations of mammography has led to a search for other ways of looking at the breast. Mammography uses radiation, which is potentially dangerous, and it is limited in its ability to see through dense breast tissue and determine clearly whether a lump is benign or malignant. These issues are especially important for young, high-risk women. Ultrasound and MRI are used more commonly in these cases. Some other techniques are old, and some are new. The amount of promise varies significantly with each technique.[11] So far none of these techniques promises to do away with mammography. Most are used as adjuncts to mammography, to help figure out which suspicious lesions on a mammogram are really worrisome, to image dense breasts, or to determine which young woman may benefit from a mammogram.

ULTRASOUND

In the ultrasound method, high-frequency sound waves are sent off in little pulses, like radar, toward the breast. A gel is put on the breast to make it slippery, and a small transducer (a device that picks up sound waves) is slid along the skin, sending waves through it. If something gets in the way of the waves, they bounce back again, and if nothing gets in the way, they pass through the breast. Unlike a mammogram, it never picks out small details or microcalcifications, but it can show other characteristics of a lump. Ultrasound is appealing because it doesn't use radiation. It is most effective in the dense breast, where mammography is limited. But it is much less useful in the fatty breast, where mammography is very effective.

We use ultrasound mostly to look at a specific area. If we know a lump is there, we can get more information about it. It can help determine whether a lump is fluid-filled or solid—if it's fluid-filled, like a cyst, the sound waves go through it, and if it's solid, like a fibroadenoma, they do not. If a lump shows up on a mammogram that we can't feel in a physical examination, and we want to determine whether it's a cyst or a solid lump, ultrasound can give us the answer.

Ultrasound can also help us interpret a mammogram. If the doctor feels a lump and the mammogram shows just dense breast tissue, the ultrasound can sometimes see if there's a lump within that tissue.[12] Mammography will show only overlapping areas of brightness, but ultrasound can sometimes distinguish differences in the density of the tissues that cause the shadows. Imagine a balloon with a few colored balls inside it. Where a mammogram would be able to see only the balloon, an ultrasound could distinguish the balls inside, which are different from the balloon itself. Ultrasound adds another dimension to the imaging possible with mammography. Therefore, if there is a suspicious area on a mammogram, most breast imaging centers will also do an ultrasound. Many breast surgeons have an ultrasound machine in their office so that they can immediately check on a lump that you or they may have felt.

Since, as far as we know, sound waves are harmless, ultrasound is often the best tool for studying benign problems at length, particularly in women under 35. So if a doctor has a younger patient with a lump and wants to determine whether it's likely to be a fibroadenoma or a possible cancer, ultrasound in that area can differentiate between a distinct lesion with edges or an irregular area with or without infiltrating borders.

A limitation of ultrasound is that it depends, more than mammography does, on the experience of the person operating the equipment. Unlike mammography, which shows the whole breast on each picture, each ultrasound picture shows only a small section of the breast—so it can be harder to figure out where it is in the breast as a whole. Therefore the technologist or physician who operates the ultrasound equipment must be able to first find the abnormality and then demonstrate it well on the pictures. The technologist or physician holds the transducer directly over the suspicious area, and the angle at which it is held changes the image. Looking at the photograph of the image at another time can be difficult. The ultrasonographer needs to be standing at the patient's side looking at the screen while performing the examination and taking the pictures. It may be hard for the physician to pick up an ultrasound picture after the fact and then interpret it accurately.

We can also use ultrasound in much the same way we use mammograms to guide core biopsies (see Chapter 9).[13] Sometimes ultrasound guides us into the lump more effectively than mammography does. Physicians experienced in breast ultrasound can approach the lump from different directions, which might make it easier to biopsy hard-to-reach areas in the breast, and many find the ultrasound method faster and more comfortable for the patient. It is the way most surgeons prefer to do an image-guided core biopsy, since it is the most comfortable for the patient, who is lying in a supine position. For the same reason, surgeons find it easier to use in surgical planning, since the patient is in the same supine position that she will assume in the OR.

MRI

Magnetic resonance imaging (MRI) takes advantage of the electromagnetic qualities of the hydrogen nucleus. Hydrogen is part of water, and water is part of our bodies. MRI is a huge magnet. You are put in the middle of the magnet, and the hydrogen nucleus lines up with the magnetic field. Then the MRI technologist turns on a radio frequency wave to tip the hydrogen nucleus off the new magnetic axis. When the radio frequency wave is turned off, the hydrogen realigns with the strong magnetic field. The way the hydrogen realigns with the field allows the MRI machine to make an image of the tissues.

This test was initially used in the brain, and has been very accurate in diagnosing brain tumors. It's finally taking its place in breast diagnosis. It is now recognized as the most sensitive and specific way to evaluate whether a silicone breast implant has leaked. A silicone-specific technique has been developed to differentiate rupture of the capsule from other benign breast problems.

MRIs are significantly more complicated than mammography or ultrasound. For one thing, if you are premenopausal you need to schedule your MRI during the first half of the menstrual cycle (days 3–14) to avoid the normal hormonal changes that can affect the interpretation.[14] On the day of your exam, leave metal items (pins, hairpins, removable dental work, pens, eyeglasses, regular and body piercing jewelry) at home or in the locker provided since they can distort the images. Watches, credit cards, cell phones, and hearing aids can also be damaged by the machine. Let your MRI technician know if you have a pacemaker, cochlear (ear) implant, or clips used on brain aneurysms, as well as metal pins, screws, plates, stents. Most joint replacements are okay but it is always good to let the technician and radiologist know in advance. People who weigh over 300 pounds won't fit in the machine.

Traditional breast MRI currently involves a movable examination table that slides into a circular magnet. Some newer machines are open at the sides but may not be appropriate for your exam. If you are worried about feeling claustrophobic, ask which machine will be used. About 1 in 20 women will need sedation prior to the exam, so don't be afraid to ask for it if you want. If contrast material is going to be used in the exam to highlight abnormalities, a nurse or technologist will insert an intravenous (IV) line into a vein in your hand or arm. A saline solution will be dripped through it to keep the vein open during the procedure.

The MRI exam is done with you lying face down on a table with your breasts hanging into cushioned coils and your arms over your head (see Figure 8.2). Once you are positioned on the table, the radiologist and technician will leave the room. They can see and hear you, however, so speak up if you need to. First an exam is done without contrast material to get a baseline. You will be told what to expect but it is good to anticipate that there will be a lot of humming and tapping noises like those of a low-level jackhammer. You can request earplugs if you want. Once the first images have been obtained, the contrast is injected into the intravenous line. This usually causes no side effects, although occasionally it produces a warm feeling. To get good results, you will be asked to stay still during the exam. It can be helpful to try relaxation techniques (see Chapter 18) or imagine yourself somewhere else that you find comforting. The exam itself takes between 30 and 60 minutes; the whole procedure is usually over in an hour and a half. Although the procedure may seem scary, there are no known risks from the magnet and the only side effect is a potential allergy to the contrast material.

The downside of MRI is the fact that it finds all kinds of abnormalities, most of them benign. At first you may think this is a good thing. But actually it means lots of women are getting unnecessary biopsies in an effort to track down every finding on the MRI. If an MRI finds a lesion that cannot be seen on mammography or ultrasound, it then needs to be biopsied with special nonmagnetic equipment, adding yet another level of difficulty.

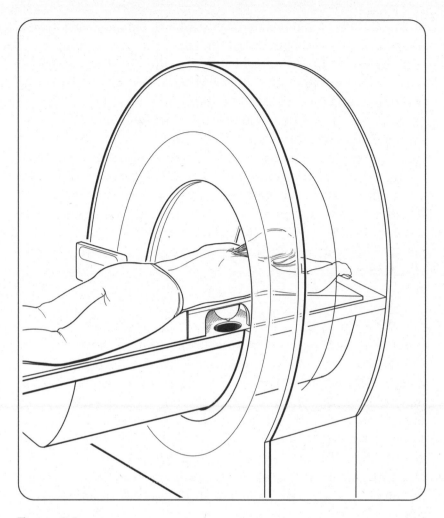

Figure 8.2

Diagnostic MRIs are best done by a dedicated team that does breast MRI full-time using a dedicated machine. To determine how experienced the team is, ask if they are able to do MRI-guided biopsies. Good diagnostic centers should be able to do the whole workup.

MRI, like ultrasound, is useful in conjunction with mammography, not as a replacement for it. Sometimes it is used to further distinguish an abnormality found on mammography and ultrasound. It can also be used to follow the results of chemotherapy in large cancers treated systemically prior to surgery (see Chapter 17) or instances in which there is cancer in a lymph node but none in the breast (see Chapter 13). Finally, as noted in Chapter 7, it is used to follow very high risk women such as those who carry the mutation for breast cancer.[15]

A common practice is to do an MRI preoperatively for a woman diagnosed with breast cancer to make sure that she is a candidate for breast conservation. This has not been shown to be worthwhile in the majority of cases and has the potential to increase the cost of care and delay treatment of the cancer (see Chapter 14). MRI should *not* be used to characterize suspicious lesions (BI-RADS 3 or 4) that need to be biopsied. It is better to just have the core biopsy, since it is more accurate, definitive, and cheaper than an MRI.

PET SCANNING

No, this doesn't mean we scan your little kitten. Positron emission tomography (PET) is another detection technique that has received a lot of press. PET is a completely different way of imaging breast tissue. We don't look at the structure itself, but at the activity going on in it. All tissues need glucose as fuel to survive. Cancers are rapidly growing and turning over, so they use more glucose than normal tissue. PET scanning looks at how much and how fast glucose is being used by a tissue. Like MRI, PET was first developed to study the brain, and it has been very useful for that.

To do this scan we inject the patient with a radioactively labeled glucose molecule, which is taken up and metabolized by the tissue. The scanner can demonstrate how much glucose is taken up by the tissues and how fast. When imaging the brain with the PET scan, we can have the patient do a number of things that use different parts of the brain. If the patient talks, the scan lights up in the area of the brain that connects for talking; if the patient reads, it lights up another area. So it's very useful in mapping the brain and seeing where different problems lie.

Potentially PET scanning could be the answer to detecting virtually any cancer, since it can examine the whole body. PET scans have been able to demonstrate areas of metastatic disease that cannot be seen by other imaging techniques.

Specific PET scanners for the breast have been developed and have demonstrated some promise. The question of how they fit into the detection and treatment of breast cancer remains. Studies are exploring a role for preoperative planning as well as following neoadjuvant therapy (see Chapter 17), but as of yet it is not clear what value they bring.[16] The major question is how small a cancer they can pick up—how sensitive they really are. As with MRI, we are still in the process of determining PET's usefulness. It may have a role in distinguishing benign lumps from malignant ones based on how much glucose they use.

BIOPSY

When the doctor says you need a biopsy, it usually means a needle or core biopsy. A fine-needle (like the kind used to draw blood) biopsy takes only a few cells out of the lump; a larger-needle biopsy, called a core, cuts a small piece out of the lump. In the United States core biopsies are the procedure of choice because they obtain more tissue and are easier for pathologists to read (Figure 8.3). My colleague Ellen Mahoney describes it through a domestic analogy: MRI shows you a house, she says, but a core biopsy shows the house and also tells you what the neighborhood looks like. These are usually done in a doctor's office or mammography suite. Needle and core biopsies can be done on lumps that are palpable or on lesions identified only on imaging. They can be done with ultrasound or mammography guidance if a lump cannot be felt. It is very unusual these days for a surgeon to do an operation to make a diagnosis on a breast lump or abnormal mammogram. If that is being suggested for you, it is important that you find out why and then consider getting a second opinion.

The term biopsy, by the way, refers to the procedure itself, not the process of studying the lump in the laboratory, which the pathologist or cytologist does later. Anything that we cut out of the body is always sent for analysis, and the connection between the two procedures causes people to confuse them with each other. If you're having a biopsy performed, it's useful for you to know the

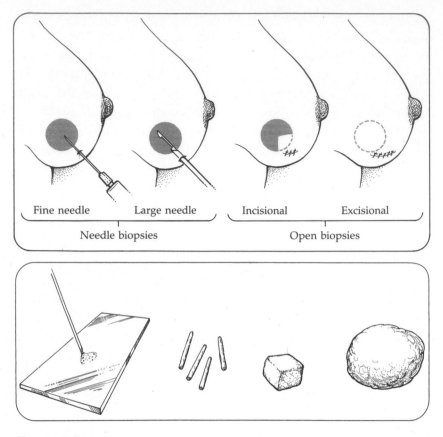

Figure 8.3

precise meaning of the term. The rule of thumb with any biopsy is
that three elements should be consistent to determine that the lesion is benign or malignant.[17] If I think on examination that it's a fibroadenoma, if it looks like one on the ultrasound, and if it also
looks like one under the microscope after a needle aspiration, then
I feel certain that's what it is. But if one of those elements is different—if it seems like a cancer to me, even though the mammogram
and core biopsy suggest it is benign, another biopsy may be
needed.

Core Biopsy

Core biopsies should be the first choice when a woman presents
with a palpable lesion or one that is judged to be BI-RADS 4 or 5

on imaging (see Table 8.1). They can be done by a surgeon or radiologist. Your doctor will get the results and refer you for further treatments if indicated. If the core biopsy shows cancer, you can then have the surgery you need, and you've had only one surgical procedure. If the core biopsy report is benign, you are done. Core biopsy is ideal if you're likely to want a mastectomy, since it entails only one surgery. People with multiple lesions do better with core biopsies because multiple surgical biopsies can leave your breast looking like Swiss cheese, and multiple core biopsies are far less disfiguring. If it's very likely that the lesion is a fibroadenoma (see Chapter 3), a core is also ideal because it will assure you and your surgeon that it is indeed a harmless lump. In the case of a palpable lesion it is better to do a diagnostic mammogram first followed by a diagnostic ultrasound to determine if the lesion is cystic or solid. If it is seen to be a cyst on ultrasound, an aspiration can be done at that time or later (see Chapter 3).

If the lesion can be felt, a core biopsy can be done without imaging, although an improved diagnosis results when ultrasound is used to direct the core into the lesion. This is by far the most comfortable for the patient, who lies on her back while the procedure takes place under local anesthesia. The ultrasound approach is most popular because it does not require equipment such as X ray machines and does not expose the woman to radiation. Surgeons may have an ultrasound machine in their offices but will rarely have X ray equipment. If the lesion is seen only on mammogram, then a stereotactic core biopsy is done under X ray guidance. This is less optimal since it requires a woman to lie still on her stomach for 45 minutes. In lesions seen only on MRI, a core can also be done in the MRI machine. This is the most complicated, since it involves contrast material as well as special nonmagnetic needles and has you lying on your stomach for 45 minutes. This eliminates anyone with significant anxiety (unless the anxiety is controlled with medication), with arthritis in the neck or back, with chronic cough, with severe kyphosis (a condition that causes the person to hunch over), or anything else that prevents absolute immobility for 45 minutes.

Medical device manufacturers have been mobilized by the success of core biopsies and are coming up with machines that will allow a surgeon to do an entire lumpectomy this way. Surgery could be avoided altogether if there were a needle bigger than that used for core—enlarged a centimeter or two—that could take out an entire lesion. There are several devices out there and all have their pros and cons. What is important is that the surgeon or radiologist using the biopsy device is experienced with it and comfortable with the results. Doing a lumpectomy with a device rather than doing an open, surgical one always entails the difficulty of ensuring that the doctor gets clean margins. When there's a small lesion that the doctor feels is probably benign but the patient wants removed, margins are less crucial. In the rare case where the lesion turns out to be cancerous, a surgical reexcision can be done. This kind of lumpectomy also works well for patients sixty or older, those with fairly fatty breasts, and those with small, well-circumscribed cancerous lesions. In this case the doctor should be able to remove the lesion and still get good margins.

The Procedure

When the procedure is done by ultrasound, the woman lies on her back on a table and the radiologist or surgeon identifies the lesion using a handheld ultrasound device. The patient is given local anesthesia and then the doctor makes nick over the site where the biopsy needle will go in. The doctor passes a device through the incision and positions it for the biopsy (Figure 8.4). (This device was first called a "biopsy gun." I assume the inventor was a man—who else would think of aiming a gun at women's breasts? In the UCLA breast center, I persuaded doctors to use the less lethal-sounding "biopsy device.") When the biopsy device is used, the needle enters the lesion rapidly and drills a core of tissue. Although this sounds scary, the experience is similar to having your ears pierced with the tool used in jewelry outlets. Some devices use a vacuum or suction to pull the tissue into the needle rather than drilling out a core. Others use a quick freeze to make the tissue more solid and therefore easier to cut. Which device is optimal depends on the situation and the experience of the doctor. Usually several passes are taken to make sure the lesion is well sampled. The size of the nick depends on how big the core biopsy needle is; generally a little, bandage-like covering called a steri

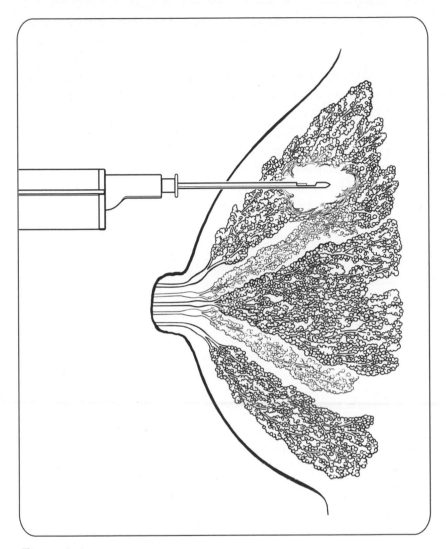

Figure 8.4

strip is enough to close it. Usually five cores are taken out for lumps; for microcalcifications it may be ten or more. Afterward a metal clip is used to permanently mark the site of the biopsy and then pressure is applied to the breast for a few minutes until it stops bleeding. If swelling is a concern, the breast may be covered with an ice pack.

Stereotactic core biopsy differs mainly in that it is done under X ray guidance. The patient lies down on the table with her breast suspended below her between two X ray plates (Figure 8.5). After the area is precisely localized with mammograms and a computer, the biopsy is obtained as above. After the biopsy the breast is x-rayed to confirm the line of air in the middle of the lump, which proves that the doctor actually took out what she was going after.

There are few complications, whether done under X ray or ultrasound. Rarely the doctor might miss the lesion. In 1 percent of patients there may be infection or hematoma (blood collection). You may have some minor bruising.

Fine-Needle Biopsy

If you have a palpable lump, the surgeon will anesthetize your breast with a small amount of lidocaine and then use a needle and syringe to try to get a few cells. The material is squirted onto a slide, which is examined under a microscope. This can often show whether it is benign or cancerous. However, since there's no tissue to look at, just individual cells, the procedure requires a good cytologist (a specialist in the field of looking at cells rather than tissue) who can identify cells out of context.

Fine-needle biopsies can also be done on lesions that can be seen only on mammogram, although generally we use a core biopsy in that setting.

How to Read Your Biopsy Report

There are three possible biopsy findings—benign, cancerous, or not certain. The latter happens when the doctor gets only a piece of the lesion. It's possible that the pathologist will find atypical hyperplasia, which often exists with cancer (see Chapter 5). If that's the case, the doctor is obligated to go back in and take more tissue out, to be certain that there are no cancer cells as well. According to a research article by Dr. Helen Pass, about 50 percent of atypical hyperplasia diagnosed from a core biopsy on a lesion seen on a mammogram turn out to be accompanied by cancer.[18] As with needle aspirations, three elements should be consistent

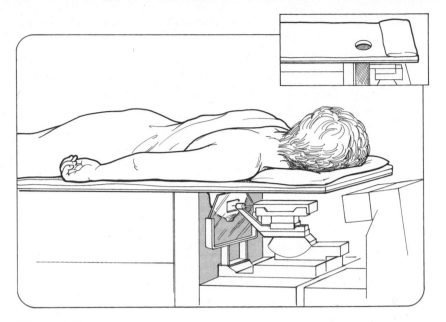

Figure 8.5

to determine that it is benign.[19] The physical exam, mammogram, and pathology have to match. But if one of those elements is different—if it seems to the doctor that it's not a fibroadenoma, even though the mammogram and needle aspiration suggest it is; or if the doctor thinks it is but either the mammogram or biopsy suggests something different—then it's important to go on to a larger biopsy.

Even when the doctor tells you that the lump was benign, it's important to find out exactly what it was. "Benign" isn't enough. You should ask to see a copy of your pathology report.

The report will have two parts. The first is the "gross description." It describes what the surgeon gave the pathologist—a slide with some cells on it, or a core, or a piece of tissue measuring 3 by 5 centimeters. If it's microcalcifications, the pathologist won't see these with the naked eye, and so they won't be described.

The second part describes what the tissue looks like under the microscope. Some reports will give you a detailed description— what the cells look like, what the surrounding tissue is like, and so on. Others cut to the chase and give just the final diagnosis. So it may read, "1. fibroadenoma." It almost always adds, "2. fibrocystic disease" or "fibrocystic change." That's because, as I said in Chapter 3, the "fibrocystic change" is the background that we see normally in breast tissue, so it's always there. The report may say "fibrocystic change" alone if it's just breast tissue. That's not an adequate diagnosis. So it is important to make sure that the correct tissue was biopsied.

In addition, if your biopsy was done for calcifications, you want to be sure that the pathologist saw calcifications under the microscope, so you can be sure that he's looking at the right tissue.

Then you should get a copy of the report and save it. It may become relevant at some later time and it's important for you to have it in your records. We're starting to realize that some of the changes in the basic molecular biology of the breast tissue (see Chapter 10) can be identified in earlier biopsy tissue. It is important for you to be able to have the pathologist go back and look at the slides and determine what kind of fibroadenoma you actually had. Probably they won't keep the tissue, but if you at least keep a record of your biopsy, with the date and the hospital, you can go back and find the slides. That can be very important.

It's really essential, if you've had your biopsy because of a lesion seen on mammogram, to have a new baseline mammogram a month or two after the procedure. If the doctor doesn't suggest it, you should. Sometimes when we take out calcifications, we do not get all of them. If it's benign, that doesn't matter. But it's good to have it documented so that a year from now if you have a mammogram, it won't seem like there are new calcifications.

Similarly, if you have something taken out, your breast is going to look different: there will be scarring. A year later that might look like something new and alarming, unless there's a baseline fairly soon after the surgery for comparison.

With all of the minimally invasive ways to biopsy tissue, it is now much easier to find out what a lump or mammographic lesion is, which leads to many fewer sleepless nights for women and their doctors.

Chapter 9

SCREENING

EARLY DETECTION

One of the most consistent messages in breast cancer discussions has been that early detection is valuable and doable. Most of us in the field have believed that cancers grow at a certain steady rate and at a certain point "get out" into the rest of the body. Thus, we concluded, if we could just find the cancers before this happened we could prevent people dying from breast cancer. In fact the somewhat contradictory message has been that "early detection is the best prevention." While this is good as a sound bite, it is bad as science. For one thing, early detection by definition means finding cancers that are already present. That's hardly prevention. Prevention means stopping them from happening in the first place. Further, in many cancers, including breast cancer, "early detection" doesn't always work. This becomes obvious when we think about the biology of breast cancer and the fact that it takes both a mutated cell and a promoting local neighborhood for a detectable cancer to arise (see Chapter 4). Focusing on finding the mutated cells is one approach, but as I've pointed out earlier, this ignores the fact that the neighboring cells, the cells in the stroma, have a large role to play in the process of the cancer. So rather than putting all our efforts into the search for early detection of the disease itself, we may need to shift our primary focus to early detection of the conditions that prompt cancers—to study the whole "neighborhood" of various cells in the breast.

Is the concept of early detection totally fanciful? Not really. There are some cancers that we *can* detect early. What's misleading is the idea that *every* cancer has the potential to be found early with the techniques we have available at present. Screening is still our current best tool for changing the breast cancer mortality rate. We need to take full advantage of it while working hard to find something better. As we learn more and more about what creates breast cancer, we come closer to finding methods of both prevention and genuinely early intervention.

Evaluating Screening Tests

Amid the fallout over revised mammographic guidelines released in fall 2009, some women remained convinced that screening by mammography is more accurate and reliable than it actually is. The truth is that we have oversold early detection and we need to review what screening mammography can and can't do. What it can do is important—detect some cancers earlier than they would be otherwise—but this isn't really very early. For now, it's what we have, and it makes sense to use it.

Let me start with a definition. Screening is the process by which doctors look at healthy people with no symptoms in order to pick up early signs of disease. The Pap smear for cervical cancer is a perfect example. With it, we can diagnose cancers in women before any symptoms have manifested. We need something similar for breast cancer—a test that's easy to do, widely acceptable to patients (i.e., cheap and painless), sensitive enough to catch signs of the disease or the conditions that lead to it, and specific enough not to miss something dangerous or misread something harmless. (This is what doctors mean when we talk about "false negatives" and "false positives.") False positives can encourage invasive procedures to remove something that isn't

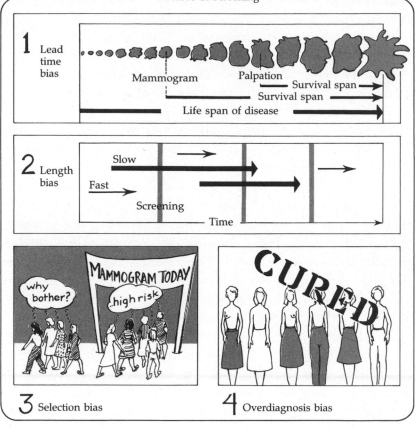

Figure 9.1

even there; false negatives can hide the reality of a present but invisible danger. Meanwhile, most breast cancer screening is done through one of three tests that vary in effectiveness—breast self-exam (BSE), breast exam by a doctor, and mammography.

Several studies have examined these three tests. Accepting that not all cancers will be found early, what evidence is there that the current tools are making a difference? Before we get into the studies, let's look at a few common biases that complicate early detection (Figure 9.1).

One widely held assumption is that detecting a disease early will always affect its rate of progress. This is sometimes true and sometimes not. Let's assume you have a disease that usually kills eight years after it starts (this is not the case with breast cancer). If we diagnose the disease in the fifth year, you'll live three years after the diagnosis. If we diagnose it in the third year, you'll live five years—and we gleefully proclaim that our early diagnosis has given you a longer survival span. Actually, it hasn't—it's just given you a longer time to know you've got the disease, which may or may not be a benefit. So just looking at years of survival after diagnosis isn't enough; we need to know how many people actually die of the disease with and without early detection. Simply finding a tumor does not mean we can change the outcome.

The second assumption is that all tumors are equally dangerous. Screening tests are more likely to catch slow-growing tumors, which have a better prognosis. It's like a nighttime security guard patrolling the bank every hour. The guard will catch a slow robber who takes three hours to get the job done, but the savvy robber, who can do the job in 20 minutes, will probably be in and out before the guard shows up. Since the fast robber is also the most efficient one, the guard will get only the slower, less competent criminal.

The third assumption is that women who get regular screening are representative of the population as a whole. This is probably not true since even if we make mammograms available to all women over 50 while offering no extra incentives to take the test, who's likely to take us up on the offer? For the most part, it'll be the people who perceive themselves as being at high risk—those who have already had breast cancer or whose mother had breast cancer. Women who worry less about getting the disease are less likely to bother getting the test. So the studies represent the benefit of screening a select group of women and can't be extrapolated to all women.

Finally, there is the fact that screening leads to overdiagnosis. A mammogram detects all kinds of breast cancers. Some, as explained in Chapter 4, may be dormant and therefore not in need of treatment and some may be actively growing and thus potentially life threatening. At the moment we do not know how to figure out which ones are which (see Chapter 11). So we treat them all. Then we congratulate ourselves at how well all the patients have done—when many of them would have done just as well if we had done nothing.

We must examine the data supporting each type of screening against these assumptions if we are truly to understand its worth.

BREAST SELF-EXAM

Breast self-exam has always seemed to be the easiest and most obvious way to find breast cancers. But just finding cancers does not mean that you are making a difference in their outcome. Before I start explaining about the data, I want to be clear about my definitions. Those health care professionals or researchers who talk about "breast self-exam" usually mean a formal procedure you do in four positions, covering the whole breast in a certain pattern and taking a half hour to perform. These are the ones you see on the shower card or video version. When a woman talks about breast self-exam she is often talking about poking around either because it is "that time in the month" or because a pain or twinge has brought her attention to her breast. The question is not whether women can find their own cancers. They can. But do they find them while doing a formal regimen every month, like a religious ritual, or simply in the normal poking around that we all do?

To answer that question, a randomized controlled study of formal breast self-exam was done in Shanghai and reported in 1997.[1] In the study 267,040 women from 520 factories were randomly divided between a self-exam instruction group and a control group. Then they were studied for over five years. (The study was done in China because the Chinese did not have screening mammography or physical exams to complicate things at that time, so the only way for a woman to be diagnosed with breast cancer to find it herself). The women in the instruction group were given intensive training in breast self-examination. The other women, the "controls," were not. All women were followed up for the development of breast diseases and for death from breast cancer. Approximately equal numbers of breast cancers were detected in the two groups (331 in the instruction group and 322 in the control group). The breast cancers detected in the instruction group were not diagnosed at a significantly earlier stage or smaller size than those in the control group. The death rates from breast cancer in the two groups were also virtually equal. What most people miss, however, is the fact that the women in the control group *found their own cancers* as well. They found them while showering or lovemaking or moving their arms or any of the other ways we tend to touch our bodies without even thinking about it. They just did not find the cancers doing a formal breast self-exam. Interestingly, there was even a downside to formal BSE. The women in the instruction group detected more benign lesions (1,457 versus 623) than did those in the control group. This means that formal BSE not only failed to benefit the women in the instruction group by finding cancers earlier, but led them to be subjected to more biopsies than were those in the control group.

When the 2009 U.S. Preventative Services Task Force (USP-STF) guidelines came out, they recommended that doctors stop teaching formal breast self-exam.[2] This was misconstrued to mean that women should not do it, or indeed should not even explore their breasts. What it really meant was that since formal breast self-exam was no better than women's normal acquaintance with their breasts, it was not worth having health care professionals spend their limited time teaching it.

BREAST PHYSICAL EXAM

What may make a difference, however, is that health care professionals routinely examine women's breasts during their yearly checkups. Yet this process (known as clinical breast exam) has never been studied in terms of its usefulness in detecting breast cancer. I've always wondered about that. You'd think it would be worth researching, since it's so ubiquitous. Or, if it didn't have any value, we could then save time and energy for busy medical professionals, as well as sparing patients the mild discomfort and embarrassment involved. And if it did have value, we could make certain every medical professional was trained in it. In any case, the result of this great oversight is that what we know comes from information in other studies.

A study done in Canada looked at whether, in older women, mammograms added anything to a well-performed medical physical exam.[3] After a seven-year follow-up they found that in women between 50 and 59 adding mammography didn't decrease mortality anymore than physical exam alone. This is good to know, but it doesn't really address medical examination in itself.

One problem is that most doctors haven't been trained to do clinical breast exams. The breast has always been considered the property of the general surgeon. So hardly any gynecologists and primary care doctors have formal training in the breast. Yet most women with breast problems go to their gynecologists or primary care doctors rather than surgeons. A colleague of mine, William Goodson, reported on an interesting study in 2009. Researchers developed a form for primary care doctors to document their findings on clinical breast exams.[4] Just adding this reminder not only increased the number of exams done but also increased the number of lumps found. There has been a tendency with all the available imaging to stop paying attention to physical examinations. Nonetheless, many cancers that are not detectable on imaging will be picked up this way. So we need primary care doctors to be well trained in breast examination. Then every woman will have access to a good clinical breast exam as part of her yearly checkup. It's a very helpful, low-tech tool.

MAMMOGRAPHY

There have been eight randomized controlled trials of mammography over the past 40 years, which is an impressive number. The findings are very striking. All eight studies consistently show a 20 percent reduction in death from breast cancer in women between 50 and 69. (This means that a fifth fewer breast cancer deaths occurred in women who were screened.) These benefits far outweigh the risks in having mammography (see below). However, mammography is not perfect, and a mammogram that shows nothing unusual is no guarantee that the woman doesn't have cancer.

What is so magical about age 50? Nothing, except that 50 is a surrogate for menopause. Before menopause, breast tissue tends to be denser because your breasts have to be ready to make milk. After menopause breasts go into retirement, and breast tissue is replaced by fat. Cancer shows up well against fat tissue but not against dense breast tissue. As mentioned in Chapter 8, it's like looking for a polar bear in the snow. Not surprisingly, mammographic sensitivity is directly related to the density of the breast tissue. That is, the ability of a mammogram to find a cancer is 48 percent in an extremely dense breast compared to 98 percent in a fatty breast. Further, breast cancer becomes more common with age and more likely to be slow growing—the kind that mammography is good at finding. These two factors combined make mammography more accurate in postmenopausal women.

Although in the United States we have leaned toward annual mammography in women over 50, many other countries support screening programs with mammography every two years.[5] Studies comparing the two screening schedules show no difference in the diagnosis and survival from breast cancer.[6] The 2009 U.S. Preventive Services Task Force reviewed all of the data and then used a variety of computerized models to see what the differences would be between the two schedules. They concluded that the most efficient screening strategies are those that have a two-year interval. In other words the breast cancer deaths prevented outweigh the harm from false positives, overdiagnosis, and treatment. The consequences of this overtreatment with surgery, radiation, and chemotherapy can be significant, from heart failure to second cancers caused by the therapy (see Part 5).

In a recent study looking at screening programs internationally, the authors were able to estimate that 30 percent of breast cancers found on mammography screening overtreated and would go away by themselves if left alone and therefore could be considered overtreated. While many women find this hard to believe, it makes some sense if we go back to our cells in the neighborhood metaphor. Possibly a change in the woman's lifestyle such as stopping HT or losing weight could cause a tumor to resolve or at least become dormant. It will be great when we figure out which ones will resolve and how, and consequently we can avoid harsh therapies. For that you may have to wait for the next edition.

The message that was lost in the media screening presentation and resulting firestorm was that the overall guidelines depend on the goal. If the goal of a national screening program is to reduce mortality in the most efficient manner, then programs that screen biennially from age 50 through 79 demonstrate the most benefits per screening examination.[7] The goal for an individual woman may be different and may depend on her risk of developing breast cancer. The decision is ultimately hers.

The second controversy involves women under 50. The USP-STF recommends against *routine* screening mammography in all women aged 40 to 49 years. It went on to say, however, that the decision to start regular screening mammography before the age of 50 years should be an individual one and take into account patient risk, including the patient's values regarding specific benefits and harms. The benefits seen with starting at age 40 are small and may take over 10 years to show up—in other words, when the woman is already in her fifties. In the most optimistic analysis of studies not designed to answer this question, there would be one less death from breast cancer per 1,904 women screened in their forties versus one less death per 1,339 women screened starting in their fifties.[8]

The risks, on the other hand, include false positive results, false negative results, unnecessary biopsies, and overtreatment. The study did not take into account the risk from having radiation every year from age 40, and this is unfortunate. Other studies have estimated that the risk is real, although low. One model estimated that a decade of annual two-view mammographic screenings before age 40 would result in a net increase in breast cancer deaths, and that starting at age 40 could end up with the risk equaling the benefit.[9] This risk is estimated to be lower with digital mammography, and so any young woman who has to undergo screening should make sure to have this type of exam.

Summary data from five of the eight trials show a trend toward reduced breast cancer mortality (about 16 percent) but as mentioned above, only after a follow-up period of 10 or more years. In these studies many of the women began mammography in their late forties and continued to have mammograms after age 50. Consequently, we can't be sure if the women who benefited from mammography in these studies would have had the same benefit if they had started having mammograms at 50. The one study designed to answer this question found no statistically significant improvement in survival after 10 years of follow-up.

The USPSTF 2009 report suggested that the number of additional deaths averted by screening women between 40 and 50 is small, while the potential harms could be significant. Thus the report did not recommend a public policy of mammography at this age. It did not say that women under 50 cannot get a mammogram or that there may not be reasons to do so (such as a family history). It just said it should not be public policy.[10] This matches the conclusions of a study done by Armstrong for the American College of Physicians.[11]

It is unfortunate that this discussion got caught up in the politics of health care reform at the end of the decade, since it is just the kind of discussion we should be having. Remember, the arguments regarding screening refer to the value of recommending frequent mammography *as a public policy*: the benefit to the individual woman may be different. In a Cochrane review, an international effort to review all the studies comparing mammography screening to no mammograms, the authors estimated that the absolute reduction in the risk of dying of breast cancer for an individual woman is 0.05 percent.[12] At the same time, screening mammography also leads to overdiagnosis and overtreatment, which creates an estimated 30 percent increase, or an absolute risk increase of 0.5 percent. This means that for every 2,000 women screened for 10 years, one will have her life prolonged. At the same time, 10 healthy women, who would have not have been diagnosed if there had not been screening, will be diagnosed as breast cancer patients and treated unnecessarily.[13] Further, more than 200 women will experience important psychological distress for many months because of false positive findings. The important message is that mammography screening is the best tool we currently have to decrease breast cancer mortality, but we should be putting more effort into preventing women from getting breast cancer in the first place.

OTHER SCREENING TECHNIQUES

Although mammography is the only imaging tool that has been approved for breast cancer screening by the USFDA, other modalities are under study. Some of them are approved for diagnostic purposes and include MRI, ultrasound, scintimammography, thermography, and electrical impedance imaging.

MRI

As noted in Chapter 8, MRI is significantly more complicated than mammography or ultrasound. You need to schedule it during the first half of the menstrual cycle. It takes about 45 minutes and requires you to have contrast dye injected intravenously. Some claustrophobic women require sedation, which may or may not be offered. And finally, it is important that you have a radiologist who is experienced in breast MRI.

Screening studies have been limited to high-risk women, and the impact on breast cancer mortality has not been determined. Nevertheless, every study demonstrated that MRI has a higher sensitivity to breast cancer than do mammography, ultrasound, or both. In other words it finds more cancers. The largest study (1,909 women) was done in the Netherlands. It compared three screening methods and found that the sensitivity (cancers found) of clinical breast exam was 17.9 percent, while mammography was 40 percent and MRI 71 percent. The specificity (how many abnormalities were really cancer) was 98 percent for clinical breast examination, 95 percent for mammography, and 89 percent for MRI. The authors noted that MRI screening led to twice as many unneeded additional examinations (420 versus 207) and three times as many unnceded biopsies (24 versus 7) as did mammographic screening.[14]

Furthermore, MRI is expensive and the injection of the contrast material is fairly invasive. This means it is not a good screening test for the majority of women. Currently it is recommended only for women with a very high risk of breast cancer, although the critical question has yet to be answered: Does it make a difference in survival?[15] It is not a good tool for most women with moderately increased risk, and it shouldn't be done at all in women with a risk less than 15 percent.

An interesting study in late 2009 showed that women are not as eager to have MRIs as was once thought. In a study of screening techniques for those at high risk, women were invited to participate in an MRI substudy. Of the 1,215 women eligible, 42.1 percent declined to participate. Reasons included claustrophobia (18.2 percent), time constraints (12.1 percent), financial concerns

(9.2 percent), a decision, made by themselves or their doctors, that it was unnecessary (7.8 percent), objection to an intravenous injection (5.3 percent), leeriness toward biopsies or extra procedures that might be needed afterward (4.1 percent), and a handful of other reasons.[16]

MRI will have to become less expensive, more accurate, more convenient, and more acceptable to women to ever become a universal screening test.

Whole Breast Ultrasound

Ultrasound is a very useful tool for investigating palpable lumps and abnormal mammograms, which suggests that it might be used for screening as well. A recent study looked at this in women with dense breasts. (They explored only the number of cancers found, not mortality rates, which is very important in terms of its value to patients.) They found that ultrasound uncovered an additional 4.2 cancers per 1,000 studies. Unfortunately there were also a lot of false alarms. Only 9 percent of the lesions recommended for biopsy turned out to be cancer, while 91 percent were benign. Given the added physical and mental disadvantages of biopsies, ultrasound, at least in its current state of development, is not a worthwhile approach for screening.[17]

Other Techniques

Breast scintigraphy,[18] PET scan,[19] electrical impedance,[20] and thermography[21] are still being developed for diagnosis and screening, and are generally not used outside of studies. They have been studied only in conjunction with mammography.

SCREENING RECOMMENDATIONS

Most countries have government-sponsored mammography screening programs that start when a woman turns 50. In the United States we do not have this, but our government does have guidelines suggesting that every woman over 40 be screened. I think this should be viewed with some skepticism: the truth is we have nothing better to offer and want to make younger women feel secure. If we had a screening technique that really worked well in younger women, we would not be recommending a limited tool such as mammography.

If you're very young you should begin getting acquainted with your breasts, not in a rigid breast examination but in comfortable awareness of how your breasts look and feel. Have your doctor examine your breasts during your regular checkups; after 40, make sure to have this done at least once a year. Consider getting a mammogram every couple of years between 40 and 50. After 50, make sure you have a mammogram every two years. (See Chapter 8 for a description of the procedure.)

Many doctors stress the importance of a baseline mammogram—in other words, your first mammogram. What's more important is that you have serial mammograms once you're in your fifties a year or two apart so that we can compare each mammogram against the previous one. Often that's how we catch a cancer: this year's mammogram has something that wasn't there last year and the year before. There are people who believe they can get one mammogram and that's it. Much as I oppose overdoing mammography, underdoing it is just as bad.

This discussion of mammograms has focused on screening for women who have no symptoms but want to get checked out. Before 50, get to know your breasts, have physical exams during your yearly checkups, and discuss with your doctor whether you need a mammogram every couple of years. Mammography, whatever its limitations, is still the best tool we have for detecting breast cancer or determining the nature of a lump in women without dense breast tissue. We need to make full use of it while we search for something better. And as noted in Chapter 8, it has specific uses as a diagnostic rather than a screening tool.

Part Four

DECISIONS

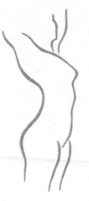

Chapter 10

Introduction to
Breast Cancer

THE FIRST THING MOST WOMEN THINK WHEN THEY'RE DIAGNOSED with breast cancer is, "Will I die?" This is quickly followed by, "Will I lose my breast?" Clearly breast cancer has a major psychological impact. Whenever you find a lump, get a mammogram, or have a biopsy, you rehearse the psychological work of having breast cancer. Although most women don't die of breast cancer and most do not lose their breasts, these fears remain.

How does a woman react to this terrifying diagnosis? In my experience, women go through several psychological steps in dealing with it.

First, there is shock. Particularly if you're relatively young and have never had a life-threatening illness, it's difficult to believe you have something as serious as cancer. It's doubly hard to believe because, in most cases, your body hasn't given you any warning. Unlike, say, appendicitis or a heart attack, there's no pain or fever or nausea—no symptom that tells you something's going wrong inside. You or your doctor have found a painless little lump, or your routine mammogram shows something peculiar—and the next thing you know you're being told you've got breast cancer.

Many women find this to be the worst part of their situation. The initial shock can leave you feeling confused and not sure how to proceed. Your mind is seesawing between numb denial and terrified comprehension. But once you get the medical information and need to make decisions, things get better. Once those decisions have been made, things get better still.

You also feel anger—even fury—at your body, which has betrayed you in such a deceitful fashion. The thought of losing a breast is almost unbearable, and at the same time your anger can incite you toward mastectomy. In spite of the horror you feel at the thought of losing your breast, often your first reaction is a desire to get rid of it. As one patient cried out to me, "Take the damn thing off and let me get on with my life!"

As an immediate emotional response, this makes perfect sense. As an active decision, it doesn't. Getting your breast cut off will not make things go back to normal; nothing can ever do that. Your life has been changed, and it will never be the same again. You need time to let this sink in, to face the implications cancer has for you, and to make a rational, informed decision about what treatment will be best for you both physically and emotionally.

Because patients are so vulnerable when they receive their diagnosis, in my surgical practice I didn't like to list their options at the same time I told them they had cancer. I preferred to tell a woman she had cancer and that there were a number of treatment options to discuss the next day at my office.

But ideally the process starts earlier than that.

When a patient came to me with what I thought might be a malignancy, I started talking with her right away about the possibilities, from the most hopeful to the most grim, and asked her to consider what it would be like for her in the worst possible scenario. We used the scary word: cancer. We discussed the general range of treatments available. Then we'd talk about going over the results of her biopsy, so she could decide where she would be and who would be with her. I was taught in medical school that you should never tell a patient anything over the phone, but I found that it often worked better if I did. If the patient didn't have cancer, why keep her in suspense? And if she did, I preferred that she find out in her own home or in whatever environment she'd chosen beforehand.

Then if it was bad news, she didn't have to worry about being polite because she was in my office and there were all these other people around. She could cry, scream, throw things, deal with the blow in whatever way she needed to. She wouldn't have to lie awake all night hoping I wouldn't tell her something awful the next day but knowing that I would. So I would tell her on the phone and then make an appointment to see her within 24 hours. By that time, the shock would have worn off a bit, and she could absorb information about her options a little better. Even when it's done this way, a patient can have a hard time taking it all in. For this reason I suggest that you bring someone with you when the doctor explains your options—a spouse, a parent, a close friend. Sometimes a friend is best: someone who cares a lot about you but isn't as devastated as you are by the news. The person is there partly to be a comfort and support, but also to be a reference later. So it's good if it's someone detached enough to remember everything that was said at the meeting, or even just someone to take notes and tape the conversation while you are busy trying to absorb as much as possible. Such a friend is also good for asking questions you may be afraid to ask.

These days, this approach isn't all that unusual. In the past, surgeons were very paternalistic: they told a woman she had cancer and she had to have a mastectomy and when it was over she'd be cured and everything would be fine from then on. It was a lie, of course, but the patient usually believed it because she wanted to—who wouldn't?—and for the time being at least, she was reassured.

At that time, they didn't have much else to offer. Progress has also occurred in the form of complex options, with results that are better—less mutilation, more aesthetic outcomes. These are the upside. The downside is that it takes time and patience to wade through the pros and cons of all the options. You have to take the time, and you have to have a doctor who will travel this road with you, along with your local reputable breast cancer support organization.

WEIGHING THE OPTIONS

Today there's much more emphasis on doctor and patient sharing the decision-making process, and there are more choices. There's also a lot more knowledge available—there are articles about breast cancer and survival rates in both the medical and the popular press and on the Internet; you know you have no guarantee that everything will be fine once "daddy doctor" makes you better. All this is good, but it's also very stressful. In the long run, I'm convinced you're better off when you consciously choose your treatment than when it's imposed on you as a matter of course. But in the short run, it's more difficult. The end result is more anxiety ahead of time while you are trying to make decisions about your treatment, but fewer regrets afterward.

Of course, different patients have different needs. Some women still want an "omniscient" doctor to tell them what to do. I was involved in a pilot study on how patients decide their treatments and what kinds of decision making had the best psychological results. I expected to find that women coped better when they got a lot of information from their doctors and learned all they could about their disease, its prognosis, and the range of available treatments. But we found this wasn't always the case. Far more important was whether the doctor's style matched the patient's. Some women preferred to deny their cancer as far as possible, and have their doctor take care of it for them. They did better with old-fashioned paternalistic surgeons who told the women what was best for them, giving them minimal information. Others liked to feel in control of their lives and wanted to know all they could about their illness and its ramifications. They did better with surgeons like me, who wanted to discuss everything with them. Still others wanted a great deal of information but deferred to the doctor for decision making. There is no right or wrong style, so don't feel guilty if your needs are not the same as those of your friend or neighbor. Remember, it's about what style works best for you.

I experienced this when I was in practice. I had a colleague who was a well-respected breast surgeon when I was at the Faulkner Breast Centre in Boston. He was much more in the taciturn, old-fashioned mode, and he and I would lose patients to each other all the time; sometimes we referred patients to each other. It worked out very well, and we were both happy about it, since we were both able to help people while remaining true to our own styles and philosophies.

Sometimes I would get a patient who clearly preferred not to know a lot, and over the years I learned to recognize the signs and respect them. I'd give such a patient enough information, but not in as much detail as I usually did, and then try to hear what she was choosing and say something like, "It seems to me that you're leaning toward mastectomy, and maybe that's the best decision for you." I still wouldn't tell her what to do, but I'd give a little more guidance than usual.

While the style matters, so does the knowledge and experience of the doctor. You may need to do some research to find the most knowledgeable doctor available. In many urban areas this will be a surgeon who specializes in breast cancer or even a multidisciplinary breast center. In more rural areas you need to find the general surgeon who does a lot of breast surgery. Sometimes asking a mammographer or oncologist or operating room nurse who is the most experienced can be a good idea. Or contact a breast cancer advocacy organization.

So if the first stage is shock, the second is investigating your options. (Sometimes, however, it works in reverse, and these stages can vary in order and intensity.) How extensive this investigation is varies enormously among women. Some of my patients simply went over what I told them, reviewed the tape they had made, and discussed it with a friend. Others did research in medical libraries and on the Internet, and then went for second and third and fourth opinions. You can't take forever, but you don't want to hurry yourself either. In my experience, most patients are able to assimilate the information and make their decisions in a month, including any second opinions they may need.

When you're exploring the options, you should reflect seriously on what losing a breast would mean to you. Its importance varies from woman to woman, but there is no woman for whom it doesn't have some significance. Although many women say, "I don't care about my breast," deep down this is probably not true for most of us. A mastectomy may be the best choice for you, but it will still have a powerful effect on how you feel about yourself. Often the loss of a breast creates feelings of inadequacy—the sense of no longer being "a real woman." In her book, *First, You Cry*, Betty Rollin talks about the first party she went to after her mastectomy.[1]

Although she knew she looked pretty with her clothes on, she felt like a "transvestite," only playing at being a woman.

The fear of feeling this way may start long before the mastectomy—indeed, it plays a part in how the woman copes with her breast cancer from the first. In the early 1980s, Rose Kushner surveyed 3,000 women with breast cancer and concluded that most women "think first of saving their breasts, as a rule, and their lives are but second thoughts."[2]

My experience was different. The first reaction of most of my patients was, "I don't care about my breast—just save my life." Later, when the first shock had worn off and they'd had time to think about it, their priorities remained the same, but they realized they did in fact care very much about their breast. Many women feel robbed of their sexuality when they lose a breast. Holly Peters-Golden points out the importance of distinguishing between the distress caused by mutilating surgery and the distress that comes from having a life-threatening disease.[3] Certainly in my experience with patients, the latter far outweighs the former. Still, the fear of losing a loved one can stress a relationship and affect one or both members sexually. It is also important to be clear what you want rather than try to please a spouse, partner, or adult child. As I used to say in the early days of breast conservation, "Husbands may come and go but you are stuck with your body forever."

Sociologist Ann Kaspar studied 29 women between the ages of 29 and 72, 20 of whom had mastectomies, and 9 of whom had lumpectomies.[4] While, as she hastens to explain, she had no illusions that 29 women constituted a definitive study, her findings are interesting. Most of the women with mastectomies had been deeply concerned before surgery that the mastectomy would "violate their femininity." Yet, with only one exception, they reported that after the surgery it was much less traumatic than they'd anticipated, and that they'd realized that being female didn't mean having two breasts. "They got in touch with their identity as women, separate from social demands. Even the ones most determined to get reconstruction didn't feel that the plastic surgery would make them real women—they knew they already were real women," Kaspar says. She did find that anxiety was higher among the single women in her study, especially the single heterosexual women, who worried that "no man will ever want me." Those already in relationships usually found their partners were still loving and sexual, and more concerned with the women's health than their appearance.

Although the experience of the young, single, heterosexual women in this study is consistent with my patients' experience, I've also had many other patients who had different reasons for wanting to keep their breasts. Middle-aged women approaching or just past menopause can have very strong feelings about their breasts. They've experienced the loss of their reproductive capacity with menopause; often their children are leaving home and they are rediscovering their relationship with their spouse. This is no time for a woman to experience yet another loss around her womanhood. Many elderly women too want breast conservation. They're already experiencing loss and may not want to add the loss of their breasts, which have been a part of them for such a long time. Nothing makes me angrier than hearing of an elderly woman who has been told by her surgeon, "You don't need your breasts anymore; you may as well have a mastectomy." Different choices may make sense at different stages in a woman's life. Your choice should be based not only on the best medical information you can gather but also on what feels right to you. Don't let generalizations about age, sexual orientation, or vanity get in your way.

Many studies have been done comparing conservative surgery and mastectomy with or without immediate reconstruction, looking for differences in psychological adjustment. Interestingly, the important factor often appears to be the match between the woman and her treatment.[5] That is, the way she feels about her body, about surgery, about radiation, about having a say in her treatment, and about a multitude of other factors affects how she reacts to this new and enormous stress.

Most importantly, a woman faced with these decisions cannot make a "wrong" choice. If you are given options it's because these are reasonable options in your situation. When a mastectomy is a better option, your surgeon will say that. In most cases both mastectomy and lumpectomy with radiation work equally well (see

Chapter 12). It is not as though if you choose wrong you'll die, and if you choose right you'll live.

Along with the fears and stages of recovery, there are also a number of related issues that come up for people with cancer. One of these is the tendency to feel guilty for having cancer—a sense that you've somehow done something wrong. People have a way of blaming themselves for being ill anyway, and, irrational though she knows it to be, a woman often feels she has betrayed her function as a caregiver by getting breast cancer.

In this connection, the holistic perspectives that I'll discuss in Chapter 18 can have their negative side. The mind-body connection is real, and its validation is important, but it's not the only force at work in any disease.

Most of the studies on the relation between stress and cancer have been done on rats and are equivocal at that—some studies show that stress is a factor in cancer, others that it's a factor in preventing cancer. In my opinion it probably has little effect in most women. I wish there were some simple, clear cause of cancer so I could say, "Don't do this and you won't get breast cancer." Unfortunately it doesn't work that way. We don't have total control over our own bodies; we don't always, to use the popular New Age phrase, "create our own reality." You didn't give yourself breast cancer, and you won't help your healing by feeling guilty.

FINDING SUPPORT

Having explored the options and their feelings, most women move into a "get on with it" stage. You know all you want to know, you've decided what you want to do, and now you're ready to do it. This is the time to make your decision—you understand that you have cancer; you know the pros and cons of the different treatments; you're not happy about it but you're not paralyzed with shock.

The duration of treatment depends on what the treatment is. If you're getting a mastectomy without immediate reconstruction, it may just be one or two days.

If you have reconstruction, it will be several days in the hospital and a few weeks recuperating at home. If you're having wide excision and radiation, it will go on daily for six weeks, and if you're having chemotherapy in addition to your other treatments it can go on for another four to eight months. However long the treatment process lasts, it's important to have a lot of support around you, and it's important to allow yourself to feel lousy. Cancer is a life-threatening illness, and the treatments are all emotionally and physically stressful; you need to accept that and pamper yourself a bit. You don't have to be Superwoman. Get help from your friends and family—throughout the treatment. Often, when you're having chemotherapy, the people who were supportive in the beginning start to drift off. At that point, you may want to get into a breast cancer support group, where there are women who are going through, or have been through, similar experiences. It can be of enormous help to you. (Check with the Social Services Department or cancer center at the nearest hospital or branch of the American Cancer Society.) In some parts of the country, away from big cities, it can be hard to find breast cancer groups per se, and you may not be certain about whether a mixed-gender, mixed-cancer group is appropriate for you. It's worth checking, though; sometimes such groups can work well, and often many of the members are women with breast cancer. You can check it out by calling the leader and getting the rundown on who is in the group, asking if your situation allows you to relate to the others in the group. This call would also be a good idea if you have found a breast cancer support group. In that case, you would want to ask the leader about the other women in the groups, specifically where they are in their breast cancer experience. Some women feel most supported and helped in a group where there are women with all stages of breast cancer; others are upset by the stories of women with metastatic disease and would not do well in a mixed-stage group. Also, you can join a support group on the Internet or a bulletin board community.

As stressful as the treatment period can be, it's an improvement over the earlier stages; you're actually doing something to combat your disease. (This feeling is often stronger when you're also doing meditation, visualization, diet changes, or one of the other techniques we'll talk about in Chapter 18.) But when the treatment period is done, you're likely to find yourself in a peculiar sort of funk. This is what I see as the fourth stage, what some call the "posttreatment blues." This stage lasts at least as long as the treatment itself. You're experiencing separation anxiety because the experience and preoccupation you've lived with so intensely is over, and where are you now? The routine established during your treatment has helped you feel supported, protected, and active against your cancer. Losing that feeling is hard. It's a little like leaving a job—even one you didn't like. Rationally you're glad it's over, but emotionally you feel lost. The caregivers (nurses, doctors, and technicians) you've come to depend on are no longer a daily part of your life.

The data that lifestyle changes, including low-fat diet, exercise, and weight loss, can affect recurrence (see Chapter 7) give women something they can do for themselves after the doctors are finished.

Compounding the situation is a reasonable fear. There's no more radiation going into your body, no more chemotherapy; without them, is the cancer starting up again? It's a scary time. This anxiety may well progress into depression, which is quite common and can sneak up on you when you're least expecting it. You find yourself feeling sad and anxious; you can't sleep or you want to sleep too much; you've lost interest and pleasure in people and activities that you used to enjoy. These symptoms are normal. Often they last only a few weeks or months; but if they seem to drag on, you may want to see a counselor or therapist to help you get unstuck and go on with your life. Barbara Kalinowski, a former colleague of mine who ran two support groups at the Faulkner Breast Centre in Boston, finds this one of the most helpful times for a woman to get involved with a support group. She says, "Sometimes it can be too much for a woman before this: she's working at her job, she's taking care of her kids, and she's going for treatment. Adding the extra time commitment of a support group can create even more stress. But when it's done and the depression sets in, you may really need the group."

Such groups can be especially helpful when, as often happens, you feel a little apart from the people you love. You're going through something they can't really understand—only somebody else who's been there can. You'll meet other women who are at various stages of the disease—including some who had it 10 or 15 years ago and are living happy, healthy lives. Often the only people you've known with breast cancer were in an advanced stage. The ones who get better seldom talk about their disease with anyone. Knowing long-term survivors can help you to realize that you're not necessarily doomed. And knowing other women who are at your stage can give you a sense of shared problems, of comradeship with people who understand what's happening to you because it's also happening to them. Indeed, you may want to look into a group before your treatment. Hester Hill Schnipper, an oncology social worker and breast cancer survivor (author of *After Breast Cancer: A Commonsense Guide to Life After Treatment*), has had women join her group before they have surgery, so they can learn about it from those who have already been through it.

Many women find that this period of intense feelings can be a time of emotional growth. They reevaluate their lives; they know their mortality in a new way. How are they living? Are they doing what they want to do for the rest of their lives? I've witnessed fascinating changes in my patients' lives during this period. One finally left a bad marriage she'd stuck with for years. Conversely, another decided it was time to make a commitment she'd avoided before—she married the man she'd been living with for a long time. A minister who lost her job because of her cancer left the ministry and got a job selling medical equipment. Another, a breast cancer nurse, left her job to work with a holistic health center. A patient whose husband once had Hodgkin's disease had her first child; faced with life-threatening illnesses, the couple wanted to confirm their faith in life and bring a new life into the world. Several of my patients began psychotherapy, not only to deal with their fears about cancer but to look into issues they'd been coasting along with for years. They wanted to make the best of the time they had left, whether it was 5 years or 50.

This period of preoccupation and inwardness can last a long time. It's not that you're always completely depressed; you're just tired, a bit listless. Your body and mind haven't fully healed yet.

For many women the cancer never returns, and they begin gradually to rebuild their lives. But sometimes cancer does return. Because the emotional issues of recurrence are so profound and complex, I devote a separate chapter to addressing them.

COPING: WHAT TO TELL YOUR CHILDREN

A particularly trying issue people face is the question of what to tell their children. Again, it's an individual decision, and there are no hard-and-fast rules. I do think, in general, it's wiser to be honest with your kids and use the scary word "cancer." If they don't hear it from you now, they're bound to find out some other way—they'll overhear a conversation when you assume they're out of the room, or a friend or neighbor inadvertently says something. And when they hear it that way, in the form of a terrible secret they were never supposed to know, it will be a lot more horrifying for them. By talking about it openly with them, you can demystify it. In addition, if all goes well your children learn about survival after cancer. Kids need to know they can trust you—you don't want to do anything to violate that trust. It's a two-way communication; remember to listen to their fears. If you find it difficult to bring up the subject, there are children's books that can help you begin.

How you tell them, of course, depends on the ages of the children and their emotional vulnerability. With a little child you can say, "I have cancer, but we were lucky and caught it early, and the doctors are going to help me get better soon." What younger kids need to know is that you're going to be there to take care of them, that you won't suddenly disappear. They also need to know that the changes in your life aren't their fault. All kids get angry at their mothers, and they often say or think things like, "I wish you were dead." When suddenly Mom has a serious illness, the child may well see it as a result of those hostile words or thoughts. They must be told very directly that they did not cause the cancer by any thoughts, words, anger, dreams, or wishes. There are other ways your children will also be affected. You may be gone for a few days in the hospital and will need to rest when you come home. You may be getting daily radiation treatments, which consume a lot of your time and leave you tired and lethargic. You may be having chemotherapy treatments that make you violently sick to your stomach. Your children need to know that the alteration in your behavior and your restricted accessibility to them aren't happening because you don't love them or because they've been bad and this is their punishment. The summary statement is that your children need honest, age-appropriate information and assurance that it is okay to talk—or not—about your breast cancer.

Some surgeons encourage their patients to bring young children to the examining room. I found that it could be very helpful for a daughter in particular to see me examining her mother. If you're being treated with radiation or chemotherapy in a center where your children are permitted to see the treatment areas, it's a good idea to bring them along once or twice. The environments aren't intimidating, and a child who doesn't know what's happening to you in the hospital can conjure up awful images of what "those people" are doing to Mommy.

It is also important to be careful about changes in your older children's roles at home. You don't want to lean too heavily on them to perform the tasks you are unable to do; instead, you want to give kids things they can do that make them feel useful while not overwhelming them. Wendy Schain, a psychologist and breast cancer survivor, and David Wellisch, a psychologist I worked with at UCLA, did a study on daughters of women who had had breast cancer. They found that the daughters who had the most psychological problems in later life were the ones who had been in puberty when their mothers were diagnosed. This was in part because their own breasts were developing at a time when their mothers' breasts were a source of problems. But interestingly enough, that wasn't the major reason for their distress. Far more damaging was the fact that they were expected to perform many of the mother's traditional household tasks. They were physically capable of this work, but they were not psychologically able to cope with the responsibility and they felt guilty about their resentment.[6]

Hester Hill Schnipper points out that it is important not to make promises that you may not be able to keep. It is a mistake to promise kids, for example, that the cancer won't kill their mother. Instead, if your child asks, "Will you die?" you can reply, "I expect to live for a very long time and die as an old lady. The doctors are taking good care of me, and I am taking good care of myself, and I hope to live for years and years."

Judi Hirshfield-Bartek, a clinical nurse specialist in Boston, usually recommends to couples that the partner take the kids out for some special time together. This gives them a chance to ask questions they may be afraid to ask their mother and know they'll get honest answers. A close relative or friend can also do this.

Frightening as it can be for kids to know their mother has a life-threatening illness, if you're honest and matter-of-fact with them, chances are it won't be too traumatizing. One of my patients decided when she learned about her breast cancer that she would demystify the process for her seven-and ten-year-old daughters by showing them a prosthesis (artificial breast) and explaining what it would be used for. The next day she came into my office for her appointment. When I asked her how her experiment worked, she started to giggle. "Well, they certainly weren't intimidated by it. They listened very carefully to my explanation—and then started playing Frisbee with it!"

Breast cancer has particularly complex ramifications for a mother and her daughter. Aside from the normal fears any child has to deal with, a daughter may worry about whether this will happen to her too. It's not a wholly unfounded fear. As I explained in Chapter 6, there is a genetic component to breast cancer. You need to reassure your daughter, explain to her that it isn't inevitable but as she gets older she should learn about her breasts and be very conscious of the need for surveillance.

Often teenage daughters of my patients came to talk with me about their mother's breast cancer and their fears for themselves. It can be very useful to a girl to have her mother's surgeon help her put the dangers she faces into perspective, and it may be worth asking your surgeon to meet with your daughter. This may also be useful years later, if your daughter does develop problems; she's already built a good relationship with a breast specialist, and she's more likely to seek treatment with confidence and a minimum of terror.

Often daughters find themselves feeling angry at their mothers, as though the mother created her own breast cancer and thus made her daughter vulnerable to it. Mothers often react the same way; their feeling that they caused their own cancer expands into guilt over their daughter's increased risk. Often a patient said to me, "What have I done to my daughter?" These feelings need to be faced and dealt with. Without openness, the cancer can become a scapegoat for all the other unresolved issues between the mother and daughter, putting the relationship at risk.[7]

It's a good idea to let the people at your child's school know about your illness. That way if the child begins acting out or showing other problems, the school knows what's going on.

Coping: Fears of Your Loved Ones

Husbands or lovers of women with breast cancer also have feelings that need to be acknowledged. They worry that she might die; they worry about how best to show their concern. Should they initiate sex, or would that be seen as callous and insensitive? Should they refrain, or would that be seen as a loss of sexual attraction to her?

The cancer is affecting your whole family, not just you. While you're in treatment, you focus chiefly on yourself. But as soon as possible you need to deal with how it's affecting those closest to you. They too are feeling frightened, angry, depressed, maybe even rejected, if all your attention is going to your illness, and they may not have as much support for their feelings as you do for yours. It's crucial to communicate with one another at this time, to work through the complex feelings you're all facing. Sometimes couples or family therapy can help.

Searching for Information

Since many women these days want to know as much as possible, I've set up a website, www.drsusanloveresearchfoundation.org, where I post new information as it emerges. The Internet in general is a wonderful source of information, but you need to be a savvy surfer. If you are searching the Internet, make sure you follow a few guidelines.

1. Know the site's sponsor and whether it has anything to gain from the information given. For example, a site sponsored by a pharmaceutical company may have good information but may be biased toward its own drugs. Some of the sites pushing alternative therapies are also selling them.

2. Know who is answering questions or giving medical advice. Is it someone you have heard of? What are her or his credentials? Is she or he an expert in breast care? You can get good advice from other women with breast cancer on the bulletin boards, but you don't know if their experience is standard or if they have an ax to grind.
3. Check who wrote the information on the site and when it was last updated.
4. Look to see if the information is backed up by references in scientific journals.
5. If information that you get on a site disagrees with what your doctor says, print out the page and bring it to your doctor for discussion.

The same provisos can be applied to books and articles.

WHAT TO LOOK FOR IN A DOCTOR AND MEDICAL TEAM

As women we are socialized not to question authority, especially when we're sick. A good place to begin is to put together a questionnaire that will help you assess your potential doctor or medical team. This doesn't have to be an actual document, but if it helps keep your thoughts, questions, and needs organized and concise, there's nothing wrong with putting pen to paper. What are some of the things you will want to include? The items may vary a bit from person to person, based on insurance coverage (or lack thereof), diagnosis, and so on. The following questions will give you a good start:

Do they listen? We all know doctors are busy, pulled in many directions, and pressed for time. When you are dealing with people you may otherwise find intimidating, you may be a bit reluctant to make demands. But remember, they are people just like you, and you can bet they'd want someone to pay close attention if they were in your shoes. Never lose sight of this fact—and don't choose a doctor who has.

Do they sit down, look you in the eye, and connect with you? You should expect your doctors to hear you. As a way of showing they are listening and caring, it is not unusual for doctors to pull up a chair and sit face-to-face while discussing your diagnosis and treatment options. You need to feel that your doctor sees you as a person.

Do they solicit and answer your questions? If only one of you is doing the talking, there's a problem. You will want to make certain that your doctor not only answers any questions you may have but also provides you with information that allows you to make decisions or shows you where to look for the answers.

Do they show you your X rays and test reports and explain them if you ask? Each of us has a comfort level when it comes to facing what lies ahead in terms of surgery, adjuvant therapies, prognosis, and possibilities. You may want to know every detail. If this is the case, you should expect the doctor you select to explain tests and procedures you will be undergoing. However, you should decide in advance how much you really want to know. Some of us need the hard, fast facts; others just want a broad overview; still others want only the information needed to take their first step. One size does not fit all, so feel free to ask about anything that comes to mind.

Do they allow you to tape the visit? Because you may be nervous or frightened—or simply because you may be asking questions that require lengthy or complicated answers—you may want to tape-record conversations with your doctor. Don't be afraid to ask. This is a great way to make sure you aren't missing anything important. It provides you with an opportunity to review what you discussed, and also allows you to absorb what was said at your own pace, in your own time. If you run into a doctor who doesn't want to be taped, you should seriously consider whether this is someone you feel safe and confident with, or if it's time to move on.

Do they ask you about your use of alternative and complementary therapies? In this day and age, it is not uncommon for women with breast cancer to seek out therapies that may be considered outside the realm of Western medicine. A growing number of patients feel they need to approach the cancer on more than one level. You may try acupuncture, massage, Chinese herbs, Reiki therapy, vitamins, or many other therapies currently labeled alternative or complementary. Your doctor should want to know about them and may have useful advice about things such as combinations of herbs or vitamins and mainstream drugs that may be helpful or should be avoided. You want to pay close attention to reactions when you discuss any therapies you may be trying or want to try. If your doctor dismisses these therapies without evidence that they are harmful or ineffective, you may want to leave that doctor and find one who acknowledges that alternative treatments can help your physical and emotional well-being. Many women feel that having the option of an alternative therapy provides them with a sense of control when everything else seems to be out of their hands. (However, always be skeptical of practitioners who promise a cure, ask for large amounts of money for treatment, or make statements that sound too good to be true. See Chapter 18.)

Do they suggest additional sources of education and support? Ideally, your doctor will present you with brochures, pamphlets, and the names of books and other resources designed not only to assist you in making decisions about your treatment options, but also to help you regain your equilibrium. You are going to need information that allows you to ask questions when you need to, talk to other women who have faced what you are going through, educate yourself about your specific type of breast cancer, and even have a shoulder to cry on once in a while. You should see a red flag if you are given a diagnosis, told you need surgery, and then sent home to prepare without any of the resources mentioned here.

Do they seem to feel threatened when you bring information from the media to discuss? While not every bit of information you retrieve from the Internet, magazines, newspapers, and so on, may be relevant, it's imperative that your doctor be willing to evaluate what you find, discuss it with you, and assist you in making decisions. Procedures, drugs, and information are changing so rapidly that you may stumble on an article, web page, or even information in a chat room that could have a profound effect on your treatment—and that your doctor may not have heard about. A good doctor won't be threatened by this sort of information but will want to help you interpret it.

Do you feel that they are partners in this process? Although no one else can travel the emotional, physical, or psychological path you will be following, it is important that your doctors convey a sincere aura of understanding, support, and partnering. You should feel that any decision you reach is one both of you can agree on, discuss honestly, and then act on in a spirit of hope and possibility.

Do they discuss clinical trials? A clinical trial (sometimes called a protocol or study) is designed to decide whether a new drug or procedure is an effective treatment for a disease, or has possible benefit to the patient. These trials give doctors and researchers an opportunity to gather information on the benefits, side effects, and potential applications for new drugs, as well as help them determine which doses and combinations of existing drugs are most effective (see later in this chapter).

Do they clearly explain how they, or someone covering for them, can be reached 24/7? Do they tell you whether they prefer phone calls or emails and approximately how long you may have to wait for a response? You need to know how to reach them or their associates and not have to worry whether you are annoying them. Clearly establishing the best means of communication is critical to your care.

You may also want to review the Wellness Community Physician/Patient Statement in Appendix C and discuss it with your doctor.

SECOND OPINIONS

Exploring the options often means getting a second opinion. Some women assume this is just a confirmation of the treatment plan chosen. Often patients came to see me with their surgery scheduled for the next day and became upset if I disagreed with their doctor's plan. But that is the risk you take. As anyone reading this book knows, the treatment of breast cancer is far from straightforward. If you go for another opinion, you may well get one. When the second opinion is different from the first, a patient often assumes that this new opinion must be the right one. Further, having to think about what both doctors have said and decide between them can be extremely stressful. You feel very insecure because your life is on the line and no one seems to know what to do. But the truth is that there are choices. There are different ways to approach the problem and there is no one right answer. It's really your decision: either the first or second opinion can be right. Even getting a third opinion may not prevent the uncertainty. You would like to believe that there is some objective truth: one right way to treat your disease. But this is often not the case. You have to explore all of the possibilities until you find the one you're comfortable with.

Sometimes patients are shy about seeking a second opinion— as though they're somehow insulting their doctor's professionalism. Never feel that way. You're not insulting us; you're simply seeking the most precise information possible in what may literally be a life-and-death situation. Most doctors won't be offended— and if you run into a doctor who does get miffed, don't be intimidated. Your life, and your peace of mind, are more important than your doctor's ego.

Treatment Studies:
Clinical Trials and Research Protocols

When you know what your general prognosis is, the next step is to figure out how to improve it. This is where the treatment studies come in. It is important to understand how studies are done and the terminology used in describing these results if you are going to make sense of the next chapters.

The most important studies in the treatment setting are clinical trials. These types of studies (also known as interventional studies or research protocols) are prospective trials that evaluate a new treatment by having one group of subjects get the treatment while another group, known as the control group, gets the standard treatment. This is where we actually test the hypothesis that a treatment has an effect. The people are followed closely for a given period of time, after which researchers compare the two groups. For example, let's say a new drug (or an older drug used for a new purpose, such as tamoxifen) was now being considered for prevention rather than just treatment. In the study the experimental group would be given the treatment and the control group would be given a placebo (an inert pill), and no one would know which group was which. If 20 percent of the women who received the drug developed breast cancer, and 40 percent of those who got the placebo did, we'd know that the treatment did some good. Not all clinical studies use placebos. If there is a standard therapy, the new treatment will be compared to it. In the studies of the new aromatase inhibitors, for example, the inhibitors were compared to tamoxifen, the standard therapy (see Chapter 17).

These studies are usually randomized. This means that each subject's treatment is picked at random, usually by a computer, so there is no possibility that subjects will be chosen based on situations they're already in. If, for example, all of the women with atypical hyperplasia are put on one treatment regimen to prevent breast cancer and all the women without it are put on another, the second treatment will end up looking an awful lot better than it really was.

It's important that neither the researchers nor the subjects know who's getting the new treatment and who's getting the placebo (or the standard treatment). That way the subjects won't be tempted to alter their behavior based on the treatment they're getting or unconsciously misreport symptoms, and the researchers won't be tempted to treat one group differently or interpret the results differently. Because neither researcher nor subject knows who's getting the treatment until after the study is completed, these studies are called double-blind.

The controlled study that is prospective, randomized, and double-blind has the fewest potential flaws, and so it's the most reliable. It's still not perfect because people who decide to participate in a study like that may not be like most of us—usually people prefer to know what treatment they're getting and don't want to risk being given a new drug that may not work as opposed to the tried-and-true treatment. But it's the closest we can get to good data.

An example is the Veronesi study, comparing radical mastectomy to quadrantectomy (see Chapter 12) for early breast cancer.[8] Surprisingly, this form of extensive lumpectomy had better medical results than mastectomy. (This study is also an example of an occasion when it isn't possible to include a double-blind approach.)

An example of the problems that can arise when a study is not randomized is the clinical acceptance of high-dose chemotherapy with stem cell rescue after initial studies in the early 1990s. These studies compared women who had undergone this very toxic therapy to what we call historical controls—women with similar cancers that had been treated in the past. The findings suggested that the high-dose chemotherapy was better and appeared to confirm the largely accepted hypothesis that more was better and that killing all the cancer cells was key.[9] When the randomized controlled studies comparing high-dose chemotherapy to standard chemotherapy were later completed, they showed no benefit from the high-dose regimen.[10] How could this happen? We don't know for certain, but probably the women in the original study were screened extremely well to make sure that they had no microscopic spread of their disease before they were enrolled, while the historical controls were not.[11] Also, treatments in general had improved over time; so the new therapy looked better than it actually was. It took the later, randomized study to bring out the truth. Thus the main job of randomized controlled trials is to correct or confirm the results of nonrandomized studies.

What, then, is the good of nonrandomized studies? They are a valuable first step for medical scientists. Randomized studies are difficult and expensive. So we do one only if we have good reason to believe it will contribute to our understanding of the disease. An early study might rule out the use of a randomized study. If, for example, those first studies on high-dose chemotherapy with stem cell rescue had shown no improvement, we could have ruled out the treatments without undertaking larger studies. We are lucky because approximately 200 randomized controlled studies have been done on breast cancer treatments, and our current approaches exist thanks to women who were willing to be randomized. This is a significant benefit to women who are diagnosed today. Ongoing and future studies will continue to improve treatment for women with breast cancer.

End Points of Clinical Trials

So that you can evaluate information from available studies and understand the figures your doctor may quote you, we need to spend a moment looking at what the numbers mean. Research studies about cancer therapy can be confusing. The first thing to look at is a given study's end point. End points represent the outcome that is being compared in the two treatments. For example, one study may be looking at whether a cancer came back in the breast, which is very important, but you yourself may be more concerned with whether it prevents the spread of cancer to the rest of the body.

The most important endpoint to most women is overall survival (OS). The time frame is the beginning of the subject's entry into the study to her death from any cause. This may seem odd—if someone who has had breast cancer dies of heart disease, why is that relevant to the study? It may not be—but it is possible that the treatment which cured her breast cancer caused the disease that eventually killed her. An example of this is the postmastectomy radiation therapy that was used in the 1970s. Although the women had fewer recurrences, those treated on the left had more heart disease twenty years later (see Chapter 16). This end point also takes into consideration the treatment for any recurrence. But the question then arises, how long do you follow a woman to measure overall survival? (This is where arbitrary numbers like five years come in.)

Since we want to evaluate the studies as soon as possible, we have other end points as well as OS. Disease-free survival (DFS) measures the time from randomization to the first evidence of recurrence or death. This figure reflects the number of women at a particular time who have no recurrence of breast cancer in the breast, chest wall (after mastectomy), or elsewhere in the body. It presumes that the more women who are disease free, the better. Local recurrences (see Chapter 20) aren't always as serious as disease that spreads to the rest of the body.

As a result, this is sometimes further modified in a third end point, distant disease–free survival (distant DFS), which indicates the time until the first recurrence outside of the breast. Here we are looking at how many women are alive without metastases at a particular point in time.

All of these end points have their limitations. DFS is a good measure of primary efficacy of the treatment, but it doesn't consider what happens to the woman after she has a recurrence. Although it usually translates into OS eventually, a treatment could put off recurrence but cause such serious side effects that the woman would die sooner than someone whose cancer recurred sooner and lived for a long time with her recurrence. Two treatments might not show a difference in overall survival, yet one might prolong the time the woman is symptom free—something valuable to the woman with cancer. Although lengthening the time to recurrence isn't a cure, it is important. For example, let's say you were diagnosed with a breast cancer that, with the old treatment, would have killed you in one year. A new treatment increases your time to recurrence, or disease-free survival time, by three years and so you die four years after your diagnosis. Your survival at five years would be zero either way, but you have had three extra years of quality time. Improving DFS or OS does not guarantee that the woman will not die of breast cancer eventually; it just makes it less likely to happen within the time frame of the study. Still, a longer life may be worth the side effects of the treatment, even if it is not ultimately lifesaving.

When studies are reported in the medical literature, they are often viewed as survival curves. This is the percentage of women alive in each arm (treatment) of the study at set time periods (see Figure 10.1). This graphically shows you the difference between the two curves in general and the absolute difference between them at any one point in time. The overall difference may be that in one arm of the study a large number of women die in the first few years but then anyone who gets past that has a good chance of survival, whereas on the other arm the benefits decrease much

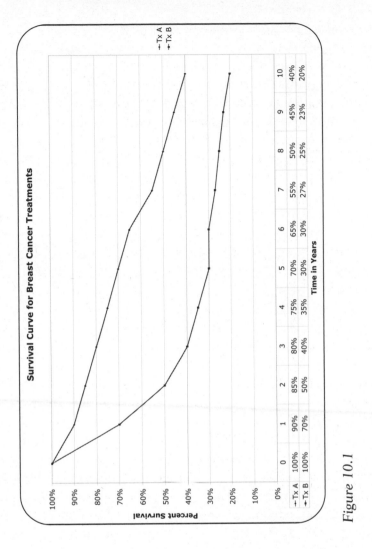

Figure 10.1

more gradually (see above). The absolute difference would be the difference in survival at any one point in time. In this figure, the absolute difference in survival at three years may be 40 percent, while at 10 years it may be 20 percent because the patterns of the curves are different.

Another way data are presented is in terms of a hazard ratio. You see the risk of a recurrence at a particular moment in time for a woman who is still surviving, depending on which of the two treatments she took. You then see the risk for a surviving woman taking the other treatment. These two are compared in the form of a ratio. Using our example above, the hazard ratio at three years would be 40/80 or .5; in other words, only 50 percent of women with treatment B are alive versus those with treatment A. At 10 years, this would also be 20/40, or .5, or 50 percent. Although this is useful for scientists (and drug marketers), it is less so for the woman with cancer. It tells you only that one treatment is relatively better than the other, not whether either is especially good. What is better for you is to look at the absolute difference in the treatments at a point in time. That time needs to be long enough for at least half of the women in the study to have reached it. On our survival curves, the absolute difference at 3 years is 40 women while at 10 years with the same hazard ratio, it is 20 women. All they say is that A is twice as good as B, but by 10 years neither one is that good.

Unfortunately not all studies are reported that way. Some studies refer to the "percentage reduction in mortality." This refers to the percentage of patients who died compared to the number of deaths that were expected. For example, if a study showed that eight patients died in the control group and only six in the study group, there were two fewer deaths than would normally be expected. This is then reported out as a 25 percent reduction in mortality, or two divided by eight. A similar study with more patients might show that 40 patients died in the control group compared to 30 in the study group. The reduction of 10 deaths over a possible 40 is still 25 percent. In the second study, 10 patients' lives were saved, while in the first it was only two. You should always try to get the absolute benefit rather than the relative one if you are comparing treatments. If your oncologist or surgeon does not know the absolute figures, he or she can get them on the Internet at (www.Adjuvantonline.com) and print them out for you.

Even here there are limitations. In the study we are analyzing, women who died of cancer within 10 years on treatment A still may have had their lives prolonged by the treatment. A way to get at this is to compare median DFS and OS. That is the time that half of the patients in the study had had recurrences or had died. In a study of one particular chemotherapy, the median time to recurrence was 3 years in the control group and 11 years in the chemotherapy group. The difference in median survival was 8 years and 15 years respectively. Clearly there were some women who benefited from a longer time before their cancer recurred who were not measured by looking at the data at 15 years.

Another important study tool is the meta-analysis. Sometimes a study is too small to show an effect. For example, let's say that 20 women are studied, 10 on the new treatment and 10 on the old. It appears that there is no difference. But if the study had included 100 in each category, 5 more women would have been seen to survive on the new treatment. By combining many studies looking at the same question, a meta-analysis can come up with more precise figures. The Early Breast Clinical Trialists' Collaborative Group combines studies looking at chemotherapy and hormone therapy for a large analysis about every five years and has come up with statistics that none of the small studies found individually. The data from the 2000 analysis reported in 2005 are included in Chapters 17–18.[12]

Understanding the value of various treatments will help you understand what your doctor is suggesting, and why. It will also help you decide the treatment you want—and they may or may not be the same thing. If, for example, the treatment has comparatively little chance of keeping you alive for a substantial length of time, you might decide that painful chemotherapy will ruin the time you have left to live and that you'd rather risk a shorter, more comfortable lifespan. The writer Audre Lorde, who died in 1992, explained her reasons for making this choice in her book *A Burst of Light*: "I want as much good time as possible, and their treatments aren't going to make a hell of a lot of difference in terms of extended time. But they'll make a hell of a lot of difference in terms of my general condition and how I live my life."[13]

On the other hand, a year or two may feel like "a hell of a lot of difference" to you. You may decide that the possibility of living a little longer is worth the limited suffering chemotherapy entails. There are no right or wrong decisions here; there is only your need, and your right, to have the most accurate information possible, and to decide based on who you are, what choices make the most sense for you.

Becoming Part of a Study

Learning what studies mean is vital for every woman who is considering using a study as part of any decision she makes. But you can also take a further step and become part of a study—helping others and very possibly helping yourself.

When you participate in a clinical study, you join a protocol—a program designed to answer specific questions about the effectiveness of a particular approach. The questions can be about methods of diagnosis, types of treatment, dosage of drugs, timing of administration of drugs, or type of drugs used. Let's say you're involved in a protocol for breast cancer treatment to compare two new hormone therapies. You'll be one of a large group of patients who fit the criteria, and randomized to take one drug or the other. Both groups will be followed just as rigorously. What makes it a protocol is the fact that it is asking a question, for example, will the women receiving drug A do better than the women on drug B? By participating in such studies you and the other subjects will get reasonable treatment and at the same time help us figure out the answer.

If you're considering taking part in a study, you have a right to know everything about it. Ask the researchers what exactly they're giving you; find out the possible side effects; find out what they know and don't know. You have to sign an informed consent form, which is often very long. (The form for the study of high-dosage chemotherapy was 27 pages.) Read it thoroughly; it's worth the effort. Write out your questions. Sit down with the doctor, go over questions about anything that's unclear. Also ask to speak to another woman with breast cancer who has gone through the same program ahead of you, if the study has been ongoing.

There are safeguards in most trials. In addition, there is a human subjects protection committee (often called institutional review board, or IRB) in every hospital that that does research. This committee reviews each protocol to make sure it is safe and well designed, that the informed consent is readable, and that the potential benefits of the study outweigh its risks for the subjects being studied. Of course, you'll always be given the choice. It's both unethical and illegal for a doctor to put you on a protocol treatment or clinical trial without your full and informed consent, and you have every right to refuse. If you're in a study and become convinced that it's harming you, you can leave it. You and your doctor both have the right to take you off the study at any time.

There are very good reasons for participating in a protocol. Aside from its usefulness to women in the future, studies assure the patient that she will get the most up-to-date care. For these reasons many women are eager to be part of studies.

One woman who was diagnosed in 1990 with a stage 3 cancer became involved in a phase II study using far higher doses of chemotherapy than the standard—the dose was adjusted upward as far as the patient's tolerance allowed. Along with the treatments in the hospital, which occurred every three weeks, she gave herself nightly injections of a material that stimulated the growth of bone marrow destroyed by the chemotherapy.

She had a difficult time with the treatment, throwing up so often that she slept on the bathroom floor for weeks. "They called me the nausea queen," she recalls ruefully. But her experiment paid off. Although in this study the patients went straight into chemotherapy without having surgery or radiation beforehand, they had been warned that they would probably require both when the chemotherapy course was over. But this woman's tumor shrank so dramatically that she did not need either. "I feel that the only reason I'm alive is because I did that trial," she says. One of the other women in the trial, who became a close friend of hers, survived in spite of the fact that she had aggressive inflammatory cancer.

Some studies are actually begun by patients themselves. You can get a group in the community together and initiate a study on your own terms. For example, if you want to research lesbians and breast cancer, you can go to the local medical school or a researcher and say, "This is a study we want to see done. We'll supply the participants—do you have anyone who can work with us?" A number of recent studies have begun that way. As you'll recall from Chapter 5, for example, a group of women in Long Island were disturbed at the high level of breast cancer in their community. They lobbied the National Cancer Institute and got a study that investigated a possible relationship between environmental pollutants in Long Island and breast cancer. Women on Cape Cod set up a similar study for Massachusetts.

So far, we haven't done enough to encourage women to participate in studies. Only about 3 percent of breast cancer patients in the United States participate in protocols, much lower than in Europe. But we can't wholly blame the patients for this. Many hospitals or doctors don't offer protocols. If you're being treated at a research hospital or major cancer center, you'll usually be offered protocols if you qualify, and large numbers of patients there do participate. Women who choose such hospitals for treatment tend to be those who seek out the most advanced, sophisticated treatments. They feel safer in an environment where the major purpose is to study and fight cancer. But the ability to offer protocols isn't limited to these hospitals. There is now a mechanism allowing community hospitals to offer participation in protocols through a program called CCOP (Cancer Center Outreach Program) that links community hospitals with large medical centers and allows you to participate in the same studies in your local area. Participation ensures that your doctor is keeping up-to-date and that you're getting the best medicine has to offer.

If you're a patient, please think seriously about joining a study. If you ask about trials and your doctor doesn't know of any and doesn't want to bother finding out, you can check out www.breastcancertrials.org or call 1 800 4 CANCER at the National Cancer Institute or check its website at www.cancer.gov. You can obtain a list of every clinical trial you're eligible for. You'll also find out the trial locations so you'll know whether or not a given study is being conducted near you. Then you can go with that information to your doctor and work with it from there.

The financial aspects of studies vary greatly depending on the nature of the study. For a study that offers no benefit and some inconvenience to the subject, payment may be offered as an incentive—those are the studies college kids often get into to earn a few hundred dollars. (I participated in a study of DES as a contraceptive to help pay my tuition when I was in medical school.) Studies that might benefit the subject or cause the subject no inconvenience involve no financial exchange at all. Occasionally a study of a treatment that can benefit the patient will offer a reduced fee for the treatment, like an asthma and visualization study my coauthor participated in. Finally, as is the case with the chemotherapy studies comparing drugs already approved by the FDA, the patient (or the insurance company) pays the full price for the procedure. When new drugs are being tested, the drug company generally pays for the treatment. Many hospitals will not allow studies involving an experimental drug or device in which the patient must pay. Political action has led some states to mandate insurance coverage and Medicare for standard cancer care as part of a clinical trial.

Unfortunately, even when they're offered protocols, only a small percentage of women accept the offer. Here too there are a number of reasons. Some women are afraid of being randomized. They want to get the best treatment and they find it hard to believe that the medical profession doesn't know what that is. Or they have strong feelings about getting a particular treatment and they don't want to experiment with anything else.

Often women don't want to be in studies because they will not be able to decide which group they'll be in. "I'll be in a study comparing chemotherapy and an aromatase inhibitor," a woman will tell me, "if I can choose which one I'll get." That can't be done in a study, since the treatments need to be chosen randomly for the study to be valid.

Some women don't participate in clinical trials because they think we already have the answers. For example, they assume that the standard treatments will save their lives, and they don't want to rock the boat with something new. But it's precisely because the standard treatments don't always work that we do experiments. The courageous women who participated in the phase 1 and phase 2 trials of Adriamycin and Taxol benefited not only themselves but the many women who followed them.

Some women fail to understand the whole idea of a study. They want to choose their own treatment rather than participate in a protocol. After the treatment is finished, they want that treatment and its effects on them to be studied. But of course, that isn't the way it works. For a study of a treatment to give us clear information, it must be done under controlled circumstances, defined by the researchers and strictly followed. For instance, if women whose overall health was best were most likely to choose the experimental drug, the results of the study would be skewed. After-the-fact statistics have their use, but we can never get the same level of information with this kind of observational study that we can with randomized control studies.

Ironically, some women swing to the other extreme. Once in a while a highly publicized experimental procedure comes along that people think is the miracle we've been searching for. Then the attitude toward being in a study turns around. Instead of fearing being part of an experiment, people demand what they think will be their share of the miracle.

After learning what protocols are available, you may decide that none of them offers the treatment you want. But you owe it to yourself and other women to find out what protocols you are eligible for and what they involve, before you decide. My patient who took part in the high-dose chemotherapy experiment says that if she had a friend newly diagnosed with breast cancer she would strongly urge her to look into protocols. "I'd tell her not to jump into anything," she says, "but to explore everything. Find out what's there; weigh it in your mind. 'Latest' isn't always best, and it may be that what you find isn't right for you. But there's a very good chance that you'll find that what's best for you is in a clinical trial."

Whether or not you decide to become part of a clinical trial in terms of your treatment, there's another way you can contribute to breast cancer research and do yourself a favor as well. If you have any surgical procedure—whether a biopsy, a wide excision, a mastectomy, or even breast reduction—make sure tissue removed from your breast is deposited in a tissue bank. This is becoming more and more possible because one of the things we're pushing for politically is regional and national tissue banks. You can also have this done through the Love-Avon Army of Women. Both benign and cancerous tissue are useful in medical studies.

We have no guaranteed cures—if we did there'd be no need for trials. But trials ensure that we are doing all we can to help women in the future. Already we see some of the trial results. Not too long ago a woman with breast cancer had no choice but to lose her breast. But a number of women participated in the first breast conservation studies and were randomized to get either mastectomy or lumpectomy and radiation. They were very courageous women, going against the standard thinking to see if there was an alternative. Thanks to them, thousands of women today have saved their breasts. As you make the complex, difficult decisions about your own treatment, keep those women in mind—the brave experimenters and all of us who have benefited from their courage.

Chapter 11

What Kind of Breast Cancer Do I Have?

MOST OF YOU ARE READING THIS BECAUSE YOU OR A LOVED one has been diagnosed with breast cancer. Face it, most people don't pick up this book out of idle curiosity or for a good beach read. You need to know what's going on with your cancer.

So the first thing you'll need to figure out is what kind of breast cancer you or your loved one has. This chapter will help you sort out your pathology report and will also discuss the key questions you'll want to ask your doctors, so you can sort out the decisions you will need to make. Then in Chapter 12 we'll expand on the ramifications of the possible decisions. A lot of new vocabulary will be coming at you. Don't let that intimidate you. You'll only have to read what is relevant to your situation. My plan is that after reading the next two chapters you will be able to understand the nature of your cancer and the options available to you.

What Kind of Breast Cancer Do I Have?

First, get the pathology report from your core biopsy and ask your doctor for a copy of it for your records (see Appendix D). If the doctor doesn't give it to you, call the pathology department in the hospital where you had the procedure and ask for a copy. Once you have it, sit down with the next section of this book: it will help you translate your report from "medicalese" into English. There will be a second pathology report after your surgery (lumpectomy or mastectomy and sentinel node or node dissection). It too will be worth obtaining and reading.

How to Interpret a Pathology Report

A pathologist is a doctor who specializes in looking at tissue under the microscope. Your surgeon should select a pathologist who has had a lot of experience in diagnosing breast cancer. The language of a pathologist's report can be puzzling and intimidating, and for this reason you should always discuss the report with your surgeon. The pathologist normally directs the report to the referring or treating physician and not the patient. But if you still have questions, you can ask the pathologist to answer them. Don't be shy about this: addressing patients' questions is part of any doctor's job.

Some reports, as noted in Chapter 8, start with a summary, but most begin by describing what the pathologist received from the surgeon. It includes measurements and comments on the appearance of the tissue. We call this a "gross description," not because the tissue is disgusting but in the sense of the word that means "obvious"—we need to see how the fresh tissue looks to the trained naked eye. The gross description is different from the microscopic description, which tells how the tissue looks magnified 40 to 400 times under the microscope after it has been chemically processed and placed on glass slides.

Examining the tissue that has been removed, the pathologist can usually tell whether or not breast cancer is present and, if it is, what kind of breast cancer you have. I say "usually" because sometimes the core gets only a small piece of the lesion. In this situation the pathologist can report only on what is there. It is important to remember this when reading a pathology report. The pathologist may say that the tumor is "widespread," creating an alarming image of a cancer throughout your breast. But in fact, it

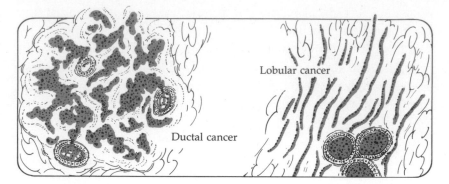

Figure 11.1

just means the tumor is widespread *in the small piece of tissue* that's under the microscope. On the other hand, the pathologist may say that the tumor is small or "focal"; this reflects only what is in the tissue piece removed, which is usually, but not always, representative of what is in the breast.

Further, there are limitations in terms of the kind of cancer the pathologist sees in that one piece of tissue. Most breast cancers are heterogeneous—several different types of breast cancer can coexist. The cells are not all alike. It is possible for the biopsy to look like one type of cancer and the lumpectomy or mastectomy to show that other types are also present in the same tumor. When you read your pathology report, remember that a report based on a biopsy may not tell the whole story. Still, it can usually tell if you have cancer—and that is where we will start.

All breast cancer begins in the lining of the milk ducts. Some cancers originate from the duct cells themselves and others from the lobules that populate the ends of the ducts like leaves at the ends of tree branches. Thus your cancer will probably be described as either ductal carcinoma or lobular carcinoma (Figure 11.1), indicating whether the cells look like they came from the duct or the lobule. Some cancers contain elements of both ducts and lobules and are considered mixed cancers. Next, the report will say whether or not the cancer is invasive. If it is not invasive, it is called *intraductal carcinoma* or *ductal carcinoma in situ* or *lobular carcinoma in situ* or even *noninvasive carcinoma* (Figure

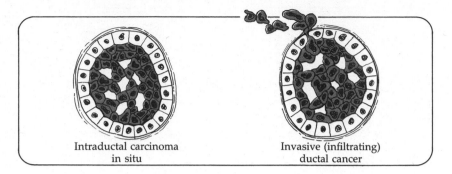

Intraductal carcinoma
in situ

Invasive (infiltrating)
ductal cancer

Figure 11.2

11.2). As mentioned earlier, noninvasive means the cells are contained and have not grown outside the duct or lobule where they started and into the surrounding tissue. Invasive, or infiltrating, means they have gotten out of the duct or lobule. In this case the report will read either "invasive ductal (or lobular) carcinoma" or "infiltrating ductal (lobular) carcinoma." This can sound scary— has your cancer spread to the rest of your body? But that isn't what it means. The pathologist has only a piece of breast to look at and is describing only that small piece. Sometimes both cancer and noninvasive material are present in one lump, and the report may read "infiltrating ductal carcinoma with an intraductal component." It is important to remember that the initial biopsy may only show part of the cancer—for example the in situ component—and it is not until the cancer is entirely removed that the pathologist can fully describe the whole tumor.

Since lobules and ducts are kinds of glands and the medical term meaning "related to a gland" is *adeno,* sometimes these cancers are called "adenocarcinomas." People can be confused by this term, thinking it's a different kind of cancer. In reality, it's just a broader category—like calling someone from Los Angeles a Californian.

An infiltrating ductal cancer forms a hard lump because scar tissue (fibrosis) around the cells causes a lot of reaction. This scar reaction is called *desmoplasia.* Infiltrating lobular cancer, on the other hand, is sneaky. It sends individual cells in little fingerlike

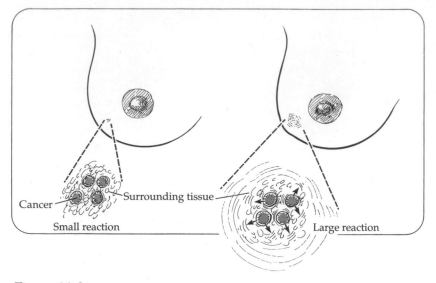

Figure 11.3

projections (cells extending in a line, single file) out into the tissues without inciting a lot of desmoplastic reaction around them, and so you may feel it as a little thickening rather than a hard lump or you may not feel it at all (Figure 11.3). For this reason it's harder for surgeons to tell if they've got all the lobular cancer out: the little projections can't be felt as easily as a hard lump. Because lobular cancers elicit less scarring, they tend to grow to larger sizes (average 5 cm) than ductal carcinoma (average 2 cm) before they are detected. The prognosis has been based on size, not type, of cancer, although this is changing. Aside from that, however, one form is no worse than the other; neither has an inherently better or worse prognosis. Infiltrating lobular cancers are almost always sensitive to hormones and seem to be more common in women who have taken hormone replacement therapy. In addition, there's a slightly higher tendency for lobular cancer to occur in the other breast at a later time. Although an infiltrating ductal cancer has about a 15 percent chance of occurring in the other breast over your lifetime, a lobular cancer has about a 20 percent chance—an increase in risk but not an overwhelming one.[1]

Other names for cancers may also appear on the pathologist's report. For the most part they're variations on invasive ductal can-

Table 11-1.   Types of Breast Cancer and Frequency

Infiltrating ductal	70.0%
Invasive lobular	10.0%
Medullary	6.0%
Mucinous or colloid	3.0%
Tubular	1.2%
Adenocystic	0.4%
Papillary	1.0%
Carcinosarcoma	0.1%
Paget's disease	3.0%
Inflammatory	1.0%
In situ breast cancer	5.0%
ductal	2.5%
lobular	2.5%

*There can be combinations of any of these types.

Source: Henderson C., Harris J.R., Kinne D.W., Helman S. Cancer of the breast. In DeVita V.T., Jr., Helman S., Rosenbert, S.A., eds., *Cancer: Principles and Practice of Oncology,* vol. 1, 3rd ed. Philadelphia: J. B. Lippincott, 1989; 1204–1206.

cer, named by the pathologist according to the visual appearance of the cells under the microscope. *Tubular* cancer, in which the cancer cells look like little tubes, is very unusual—1–2 percent of breast cancers—and generally less aggressive. *Medullary carcinoma* resembles the color of brain tissue (the medulla), though it has nothing to do with the brain. *Mucinous* (or *colloid*) *carcinoma* is a form of infiltrating ductal cancer that is gluey-looking ("colloid" is the Greek word for glue). *Papillary carcinoma* has cells that stick out in little fronds (fingerlike projections). (See Table 11.1) These special cancers tend to have a better prognosis than do typical invasive ductal or lobular cancers, but they are treated according to the same principles. Other types of cancer, such as inflammatory or cystosarcoma phylloides, are a different matter. They are examined in Chapter 13.

After deciding what kind of cancer you have, the pathologist studies the appearance of the cells further to predict how aggressively the particular type of cancer will behave. This isn't 100 percent accurate, however; it's like the old saying "You can't tell a book by its cover." Sometimes appearances can be deceiving even

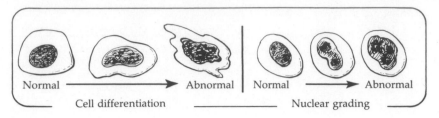

Figure 11.4

under the microscope. This is why it is combined with an analysis of the molecular biology of the tumor, as you will see in a bit.

Similarly, the pathologist who sees wild-looking (poorly differentiated) cells will know that such cells are usually more aggressive, while the cells that look more normal (well differentiated) are usually less aggressive (Figure 11.4). The cells in between are called "moderately differentiated." But poorly differentiated cells aren't a sign of doom—the fact that they look wild doesn't guarantee they'll act that way or can't be treated. Most breast cancers are either moderately or poorly differentiated, but many women who have these cells do fine.

Another thing the pathologist looks for is how many cells are dividing and how actively they're doing it: this is known as *mitotic rate* or activity. The most aggressive cancers tend to have a lot of cells dividing at the same time because they're growing rapidly. Less aggressive cancers tend to have fewer dividing cells. Another feature indirectly related to tumor growth and differentiation is the *nuclear grade*. The nucleus of the cell is the part that contains the DNA, so the grade gives you an idea of how abnormal the DNA is. Pathologists usually grade on a scale of 1 to 3 or 1 to 4, with the higher number being the worst.

The pathologist will also look for cancer cells inside a blood vessel or lymphatic vessel. If there are any, it's called vascular invasion, lymphatic invasion, or lymphovascular invasion, and suggests that the cancer is potentially more dangerous. In addition, the pathologist sometimes counts the number of blood or lymph vessels associated with the tumor. This is because tumors secrete substances that cause blood vessels to grow, a process called *angiogenesis or lymphangeogenesis* (growth of new lymphatics). A lot

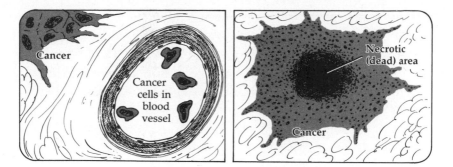

Figure 11.5

of blood vessels may indicate that the tumor is growing rapidly and thus is especially aggressive. I noticed that if I was operating on a lump I thought was benign and there was significantly more bleeding than I would have expected, it was often the tip-off that the lump was cancerous. Another ominous sign can be "necrosis," or dead cells. This usually means the cancer is growing so rapidly that it has outgrown its blood supply (Figure 11.5).

Checking all of these factors gives the pathologist as much information as possible about the cancer. All help determine the nature of the cancer cells, but none are 100 percent perfect at predicting behavior. Usually all of these observations are combined as a score. One commonly used scoring system is the Nottingham histologic score, otherwise known as the modified Bloom Richardson score. (I know, it's hard enough to take in even one name, and then they have to go around and invent a second one. It reminds me of one of those medieval novels where there's a guy named Edgar, duke of Buckingham, and you're never sure who he is because one moment they're talking about Edgar and on the next page they're talking about Buckingham and you have to stop and figure out who Buckingham is.) The score is based on three features: degree of tubule formation (well-formed tubules are better than poorly formed ones, as you might expect), nuclear grade (regularity in the size, shape, and staining character of the nuclei, with small being better than large), and mitotic activity (no or few mitoses are good and many mitoses not as good). Each of these gets a score of 1, 2, or 3, with the higher number reflecting poor tubules, large nuclei, and high mitotic rate. The scores are then added up: 3–5 is grade 1, 6–7 is grade 2, 8–9 is grade 3. Grade 3 is the highest and supposedly the most aggressive. Unfortunately all of these features are very subjective. A comparison of different pathologists' Nottingham or Bloom Richardson scores on the same cancer showed they agreed only 75 percent of the time. If you see a Nottingham or Bloom Richardson score on your report, you will know what it is and you will also know that it is just a way to quantify how the tumor looked.

The pathologist should indicate if there's cancer at the margins of the tissue that was removed. This is less relevant if you have had a core biopsy since, by definition, it is sampling the lesion and not trying to remove the whole thing. On the other hand if you are reading the pathology report from your lumpectomy or mastectomy this will be a key point. Margins are evaluated by a fairly imprecise technique. Ink is put all around the outside of the sample before it is cut up and fixed, and slides are made. If the slides show cancer cells next to the ink, this means there's cancer on the outer border and presumably some left in the patient. If there are cancer cells only in the middle, away from the ink, there is a "clean margin" (Figure 11.6). So the report might say, "The margins are uninvolved with tumor," or "The margins are involved with tumor," or "The margins are indeterminate." If the lump has been taken out in more than one piece, we usually can't tell if the margins are clean or not. Some surgeons will remove the lump or area in question and then remove an extra rim of tissue at each

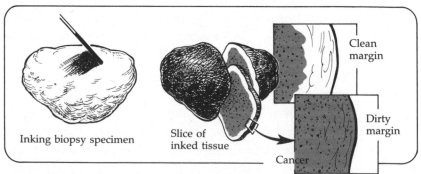

Figure 11.6

edge as if the tumor were a cube. They will send these additional pieces to the pathologist labeled as superior (toward the head), inferior (toward the feet), medial (toward the middle), lateral (toward the side), anterior (toward the skin), and posterior or deep (toward the chest wall). The pathologist will comment on these sections separately in the report. The idea is that if a margin is involved, the surgeon will know where to go back and take more tissue. It is important to realize that there are enormous sampling problems with this approach. We can do only representative sections of the margin; to get them all, we'd have to make thousands of slides. So when we say the margins are clean, we're only making an educated guess—we can't be 100 percent sure. (See Chapter 13 for a discussion of margins and DCIS.) Margins are often misunderstood as a black-and-white type of test rather than simply a predictor of the amount of cancer that may remain in the patient's breast. Thus a lumpectomy that shows just one spot of cancer at a margin suggests that not a lot of disease is left behind, while one with a lot of cancer throughout it and one dirty margin probably indicates that there is more disease left in the patient. The importance of positive margins has different significance in the setting of DCIS than it does with invasive cancer.

If the pathology report includes the sentinel node biopsy or axillary dissection (see Chapter 12), then it will describe how many nodes were received as well as their size and shape. If there are cancer cells seen in the node they will be described by size. If the pathologists are not sure whether the cells they are seeing are cancer, they may do special stains to see if they can confirm it. This too will be described. Sometimes pathologists will use the words "metastatic focus" or "metastatic disease" in describing a lymph node. Don't panic if you see this. Strictly speaking, the word metastatic means that there are breast cancer cells outside their organ of origin. Clinicians, however, are more likely to use the term when the disease has spread outside its region: not in the adjacent lymph nodes or chest wall but in the liver, lungs, or bones. But the pathologist sees only the biopsied tissue, none of the other parts of the body. Also the mere presence of cancer cells in a lymph node is no cause for alarm. Lymph nodes that contain single isolated tumor cells or small clumps of tumors cells, so called micrometastases, may not signify any worse behavior than if they are completely negative.[2] The summary will also say how many nodes were positive for cancer and how many altogether were removed.

Some of the things I've described aren't easy to see on the slides. Identification can be somewhat subjective: are these cells bizarre looking enough? Are they invading other structures? It's worth getting a second opinion. Often the pathologist will ask other pathologists on the staff to look at the slides and give their opinions. If you live in a small town with a small hospital, you may want your slides sent to a big university center, where someone sees a lot of breast pathology. You can call the university hospital's pathology department and arrange to have them look at your slides, then call your hospital and have the slides sent. Make sure it is the slides themselves they send, since that's what the second pathologist needs to see—not just the first pathologist's written interpretation. You need to get the best information possible to decide what course of treatment to embark on.

In the digital age, getting a second opinion can be facilitated by having your original slides scanned into virtual slides and sent anywhere in the world through the Internet. Centers are emerging with this capability.

BIOMARKERS

The pathologist's work doesn't end with these slides. The next step is studying and reporting on the *molecular markers*. These tests often take longer to do than looking at the slides, and so they may come back later than the original report informing you that you have cancer. Although most of these markers are done only on invasive tumors, we are increasingly using them in the treatment of noninvasive tumors as well. The markers are classified into three categories: (1) ones that are used to help determine the prognosis of a particular cancer (how life-threatening it is), (2) ones that are used to predict that a cancer will respond to a certain treatment, and (3) ones that do both. I'll discuss the biomarkers that are most frequently reported and used in all three categories.

The most common analysis is one that explores the estrogen and progesterone receptors, to find out whether the tumor is sensitive to these hormones. The report will tell you that the tumor is estrogen receptor positive or negative and progesterone receptor positive or negative. More often than not, the report will include the percentage of positive cells. Tumors lacking both estrogen and progesterone receptors are not sensitive to those hormones.

The implications of the hormone receptor tests are both prognostic and predictive. In general, tumors that are sensitive to hormones—that have receptors—are slightly slower growing and have a slightly better prognosis than tumors that aren't.[3] Generally, postmenopausal women are more likely to be estrogen receptor positive and premenopausal women are more likely to be estrogen receptor negative. Why premenopausal women who have a lot of estrogen get estrogen receptor negative tumors and why postmenopausal women who have reduced estrogen get estrogen receptor positive tumors is one of the great mysteries that remain unanswered. Further, the test tells whether the tumor can be treated with some kind of hormone blocking therapy. As long as there are some positive cells, such therapy will have some response. If it's not sensitive to hormones, it rarely responds to hormone-blocking treatments (see Chapter 12).

Another biomarker is overexpression (too many copies) of the Her-2/neu (also known as erb-B2) oncogene (see Chapter 4). Her2/neu is one of the dominant oncogenes that contribute to cancer by telling cells to grow. Instead of being mutated, however, Her-2/neu is frequently overexpressed and amplified: in other words, there are too many copies of the oncogene so the intensity of the message telling the cells to grow is increased.[4] This occurs in about a fifth of invasive cancers. Having your tumor tested for the Her-2/neu receptor is important because the test can function not only as a prognostic indicator (Her-2/neu positive tumors tend to be more aggressive) but also as an indicator of the best treatment. There are several tests that can be used for Her-2/neu overexpression. One, *immunohistochemistry* (IHC), assesses the overexpression of the Her-2 protein while the other, *fluorescence in situ hybridization* (FISH), assesses whether there are too many copies of the actual gene. It is the difference between measuring the effect or the cause. Initially IHC was used, but later work indicated that FISH may be more precise in certain categories (2+ on IHC).[5]

Generally tumors will first be tested by IHC as it is less expensive. If it is positive (3+), then the woman knows that her tumor is Her-2/neu positive. If the IHC test is negative or 1 or 2 plus out of a possible three it will usually be sent for FISH, which is more precise, to confirm that it is positive. If the FISH is negative (not amplified), then the cancer is considered negative for Her-2, regardless of the IHC score. Many medical centers do both tests, IHC and FISH, in all breast cancers because one test can serve as a check on the other.

Trastuzumab (Herceptin) is currently used in women with (Her-2 positive) metastasis, and it is also useful for women as an adjuvant therapy for Her-2 positive cancers (see Chapter 12). Almost all DCIS is Her-2/neu positive, but this does not mean it should be treated with chemotherapy or Herceptin.[6] It is still precancer, growing only within the duct and not worth the risks of the drug.

Next, we try to figure out how rapidly the breast cancer cells are dividing (we call rapid division *proliferative*), based on the idea that the more they divide the more aggressive they must be. We measure these features by *flow cytometry,* measuring the amount and type of DNA.[7] If the tumor cells have the normal amount of DNA, they're called *diploid;* if the amount of DNA is abnormal, they're called *aneuploid.* Aneuploid tumors account for about 70 percent of all breast cancer tumors. Diploid tumors behave much less aggressively because they are less abnormal. In addition, we can measure the percentage of cells that are in the process of dividing at any one time. This is called the S *phase fraction.* If there are a lot of cells dividing (high S phase fraction), the tumor may behave more aggressively than if there are only a few cells dividing (low S phase fraction).[8] The problem is that S phase fraction is usually measured on fresh or frozen tissue, although it can be measured on fixed tissue, and so is logistically more difficult. As a result, Ki-67 is being used more recently for this purpose. Ki-67 is an antibody for a protein found in the nucleus of proliferating cells. While no one is sure of what the protein does, it is a reliable marker that can be measured in fixed tissue. The higher the Ki-67, the more proliferative the cancer. These measures are a way of quantifying the number of dividing cells, which the pathologist can also see under the microscope. More biomarkers are being discovered but none is yet ready for prime time.

When all these tests have been done, your tumor will be characterized in a description something like the following: This is a stage 2: T2 centimeter, node negative, estrogen receptor positive, Her-2/neu amplified tumor.

STAGING

The microscopic aspects of the tumor that the pathology report addresses are combined with clinical features of the tumor in a staging system. This classification system, known as TNM (tumor, nodes, and metastasis), categorizes cases so that we can keep statistics and determine likely long-term survival rates that various treatments can create. The system is still used, but it is actually a holdover from the past. It doesn't fit very well with our current knowledge of biology because it is based only on the size of the tumor in the breast, the number of lymph nodes involved, and clinically detected spread to other organs. It is a static system based on a snapshot in time; yet we know that cancers are a dynamic disease in evolution. It is like looking at the students who cut classes in high school and predicting that they will grow up to be irresponsible in the workforce. Obviously other determinants of behavior (e.g., parenting, peer pressure, and health) also influence future performance. Similarly, other determinants of tumor behavior, such as the molecular biology of the tumor or its rate of growth (did it spread to the lymph nodes while small or after it had been around awhile?) are not reflected in the TNM classification system but are important in predicting prognosis and response to therapy. However, since the TNM system is still being used and you will probably be exposed to it, I'm including a summary of it here. Just keep its limitations in mind.

The system has been changed various times over the years. In an attempt to make it more relevant, a seventh version was introduced in 2010.[9] The major changes have to do with sentinel nodes and smaller tumors. I will provide a general overview of how it works and take a look at the large classifications. In the appendix you'll find a check sheet to help you classify your own tumor.

In this new system (Figure 11.7), the tumor size is first judged clinically, based on the surgeon's exam or an imaging modality such as mammography, ultrasound, CT scan, or MRI scan. If it's between 0 and 2 centimeters, it's T1; between 2 and 5 centimeters, T2; above 5 centimeters, T3 (one centimeter is .39 inch). Each of the T classifications can be further subdivided. If it's ulcerating through the skin or stuck to the chest wall, it's T4. Although the original tumor staging is based on the clinical estimate, it is further refined once it has been removed surgically and examined pathologically so that the full extent of the cancer can be determined. This is called the pathological T stage and is based on the size of the invasive tumor only, without regard to its possible in situ component. If there is more than one tumor in the same breast, the largest is used for determining the T size. As we are diagnosing smaller and smaller tumors, subclassifications have been developed. T refers to the in situ or noninvasive tumors as well as Paget's disease (see Chapter 13), while T1mic refers to microinvasion 0.1 centimeter or smaller in the tumor's greatest dimension; T1a tumor between 0.1 centimeter and 0.5 centimeter; T1b tumor between 0.5 centimeter and 1 centimeter; T1c tumor between 1 centimeter and 2 centimeters.

Then the lymph nodes are examined by the surgeon or by an imaging test such as CT scan or ultrasound. If there are no palpable nodes, it's N0; if the surgeon feels nodes but thinks they're negative, it's N1a; if they're positive it's N1b. If they're large and matted together, it's N2; if they're near the collarbone, it's N3. Nodes that cannot be accurately accessed are termed N_x. Nodes too are reclassified once they are removed. With the increasing use of sentinel node biopsy, this has been incorporated into the new staging system. For example, if only one or several clumps of cells of breast cancer are found in a lymph node based on IHC staining only (see Chapter 12) or RT-PCR only, and they measure less than 0.2 mm they are considered isolated tumor cells and the nodes are still considered negative (pN(i+). This is because we think a few cells may be dislodged during the procedure but have

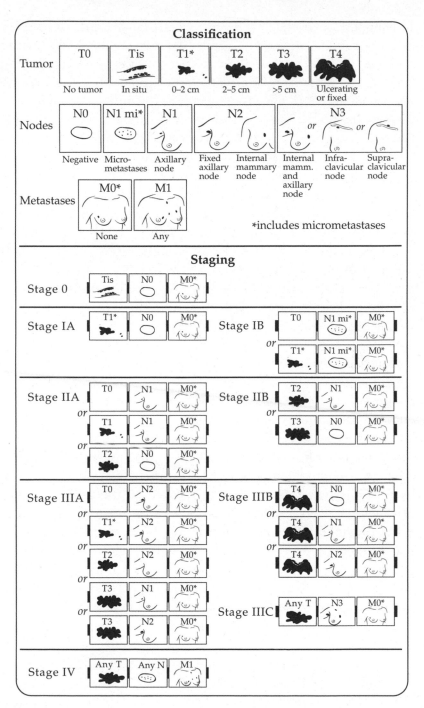

Figure 11.7

no long-term consequence. Only cells that make it to the nodes on their own seem to count. Cancer deposits greater than 0.2 millimeters but less than 2 millimeters are considered micrometastasis and are termed pN1mi, while any bigger than 2 millimeters are considered pN1. The other change in the newer system is subdividing the nodes based on the number that are positive: pN1a 1 to 3 positive nodes; pN1b 4 to 9 positive nodes; and pN1c more than 10. These breakdowns are as much to help researchers collect data as they are to improve survival prognostications.

Finally, if an obvious metastasis has been discovered by any of the tests I'll describe shortly, it's M1: otherwise it's M0; if we can't tell whether there is metastasis, we designate it M_x.

Then this information is combined into stage numbers. Stage 1 is a T1 tumor with no lymph nodes. Stage 2 is either a small tumor with positive lymph nodes or a tumor between 2 and 5 centimeters with negative lymph nodes. (Sometimes this is designated as stage 2A.) Tumors between 2 and 5 centimeters with positive lymph nodes or tumors larger than 5 centimeters with negative lymph nodes are also stage 2, but these latter types are designated stage 2B. Stage 3 is a large tumor with positive lymph nodes or a tumor with "grave signs" (see below). Stage 4 is a tumor that has obvious metastasis.

The complexity of this system suggests that we still don't completely understand breast cancer. As you will see later in this chapter, the new techniques of DNA analysis are beginning to help us differentiate breast cancers based on the specific mutations in each cancer and on which genes are either over- or underexpressed, and thus to determine more accurately both prognosis and treatment. We are now in a transition between molecular biological and the traditional TNM classification. But in spite of its limitations, the TNM system gives us a conceptual framework for categorizing each case of breast cancer so that different treatments can be compared in the same types of patients.

Has It Spread?

One obvious way to predict a poor prognosis is to find cancer cells in other organs. When the first edition of this book was written, all newly diagnosed women would undergo tests to look for cancer cells in their liver, lungs, or bones. The problem with that approach, however, was that the imaging tests we had, and indeed still have, are useful only for finding chunks of cancer (1–2 cm), not isolated cancer cells, and they often show other things that are probably not cancer but need to be checked out to be certain. So we don't do those tests now unless we have reason to think the cancer is likely to have spread because it is large or aggressive.

By the way, a cancer that starts out as a breast cancer remains a breast cancer, wherever it travels, and treatments used for the cancer are breast cancer treatments, not liver cancer or lung cancer treatments (very few cancers travel *to* the breast, by the way). Often you'll hear someone say, "she had breast cancer, but now it's metastasized and it's liver cancer." But it isn't; it's breast cancer within the liver. It's a bit like what happens when a Californian moves to Paris. She's living in a new environment, but her language, her personality, her basic approach to life are still those of a Californian. She hasn't become a Parisienne.

Based on our current knowledge of breast cancer biology, a great percentage of breast cancer patients are thought to have micrometastases either in terms of circulating tumor cells (CTCs) or disseminated tumor cells (DTCs). But we don't understand the significance of these cells, and certainly their mere presence does not mean that breast cancer cannot be cured. Most patients with breast cancer are successfully treated initially. Some will get recurrences later on and some will never get them. The cells can remain dormant for the rest of your life, even if you live for a very long time.

To screen for metastatic disease, we can do a chest X ray or a CT scan to find cancer in the lungs. We can do a blood test and/or an ultrasound to see if the cancer has spread to the liver. To learn if the cancer has spread to the bones, we do a more complicated test called a bone scan, one of a group of tests we call *nuclear medicine tests*. A technician injects a low level of radioactive particles into your vein, where they are selectively picked up by the bones. After the injection, you wait a few hours while the particles travel through the bloodstream; then you go back to the examining room where you are put under a large machine that takes a picture of

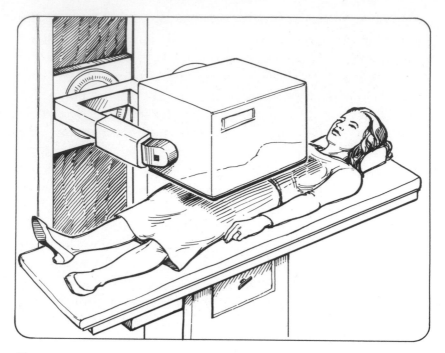

Figure 11.8

your skeleton (Figure 11.8). The machine whirs above you, reading the number of radioactive particles in your body. (The husband
of one of my patients used to wear a Geiger counter, and right after
her bone scan it started clicking whenever she came near it.)
In the areas where the bone is actively metabolizing—doing
something—the radioactive particles will show up much more
strongly than in the more inert areas.

This doesn't necessarily mean that what the bone is doing has
anything to do with cancer, however. It can mean there's arthritis
(which most of us have in small amounts anyway), a healing fracture, or some kind of infection. All the scan tells us is that something's going on. If the scan is positive, the next step is to x-ray the
bone. This will help tell us what it is. We could just x-ray the bone
to begin with, but we don't want to expose you to any more radiation than we have to. Another experimental test looks in the blood
or bone marrow for evidence of circulating cancer cells. Although
this sounds like the perfect test to predict the spread of breast

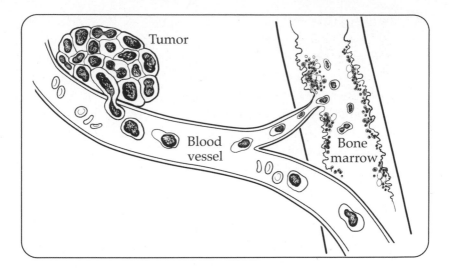

Tumor

Blood
vessel

Bone
marrow

Figure 11.9

cancer, it has a lot of limitations, not the least of which is the fact that we don't have a specific marker on breast cancer cells that we can focus on. This means we are looking for cells that *could* be cancer cells. It's like knowing that the criminal is blond and looking for all the blonds in town.

There are some blood tests for women with breast cancer—CEA, CA 15-3, CA 27.29. All of these are nonspecific markers found in the blood. They can be followed over time and will often go up if metastases develop. It was initially hoped that these tests would detect the presence of a few cancer cells that had spread before they were visible on a scan. Unfortunately, we've found that they're neither specific nor sensitive enough for that. But since they tend to go up in people with extensive metastases, they're useful in following women with metastatic disease because they help us adjust treatment.

Some researchers have done aspirates of the bone marrow to see if cancer cells are found there.[10] In addition many studies have looked at the blood for circulating tumor cells (Figure 11.9). While one might think this would be the most accurate at finding cells that have "gotten out," the question is whether it has significance. For a cancer to spread it needs not only to get out of the breast and into the bloodstream but to find a neighborhood in another organ that will take it in and support it. Packing up and getting into the car does not mean you will find a place to live at the other end. Many of the CTCs spontaneously undergo cell death. Neither test is recommended outside of a research setting.

The significance of breast cancer cells in the bone marrow, so-called disseminated tumor cells (DTCs), is hotly debated. In a recent study, 30.6 percent breast cancers had DTCs.[11] Other recent studies have suggested that it is not the presence of DTCs that is significant but their nature and composition—if they are stem cells or not.[12] Remember that all tests have limits. A negative finding doesn't give you a clean bill of health; it simply tells you that there are no large chunks of cancer in those organs. Most people who are newly diagnosed don't have a spread of this magnitude. So we no longer do these tests in the usual stage 1 or stage 2 breast cancers. If you have stage 3 or locally advanced breast cancer, or if you have symptoms in any of the organs breast cancer typically spreads to—like low back pain that started right after you found your lump and hasn't gone away—we may do these tests. But we no longer do them routinely.

Most doctors currently recommend that all women who are diagnosed with breast cancer undergo a history and physical exam, tests of liver function and bilateral mammography.

In most women without advanced disease (palpable matted lymph nodes in the armpit or above the collar bone, tumor in breast growing into the chest wall or skin, inflammatory breast cancer) there is no reason to do any additional staging until after surgery, if at all. Women with tumors larger than 5 centimeters and positive nodes as well as women with tumors 2–5 centimeters and positive nodes or those with high-risk tumors as indicated by biomarkers may undergo bone scan, liver ultrasound or CT, and chest X ray or CT.

PUTTING IT TOGETHER

The reason you want to know what kind of breast cancer you have is to figure out how best to treat it. Since there's no foolproof method for determining early (microscopic) stages of a cancer's spread, we have to approach the question differently than we do

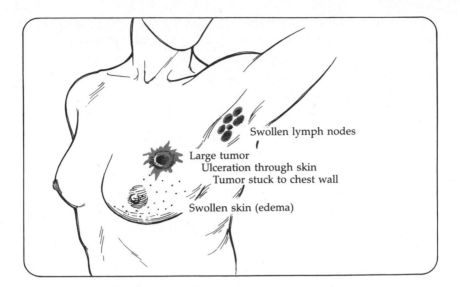

Swollen lymph nodes

Large tumor
Ulceration through skin
Tumor stuck to chest wall

Swollen skin (edema)

Figure 11.10

looking for later stages. We do have a number of methods of esti-mating the likelihood of early spread—sort of like trying a case on circumstantial evidence. We do this by looking for other condi-tions that are often associated with cancer spread. If these condi-tions exist, we can guess that the cancer has spread; if they don't, we can guess that it hasn't. We go through a series of tests in dif-ferent sequences to try to determine what the chances are.

The first level is based on how the cancer appears at diagnosis. Certain signs and symptoms statistically indicate a higher chance of microscopic cells being elsewhere. These have been incorpo-rated into stage 3 (T4 lesions) of the TNM system. Cushman Haagensen first described what he called the "grave signs"—findings on physical exam that indicated the likelihood that mi-croscopic cells had spread to other areas of the body (Figure 11.10).[13] His work was done in the 1940s before chemotherapy was used to treat early-diagnosis cancer. Haagensen's plan was to determine which women would really benefit from a radical mas-tectomy. If there was no hope of saving a patient's life, he didn't want to cause needless suffering and destroy the quality of what-ever life she had left. His system is still useful in a general way.

The question is no longer whether a cancer has spread but rather the likelihood of what has spread growing as a metastasis. Evidence is emerging that large primary tumors have more of a stem cell component, suggesting that they have more potential to recur and metastasize.

Another danger sign is swelling of the skin (edema) in the tumor area. As the skin swells, ligaments that hold the breast tissue to the skin get pulled in, and it looks like you've got little dimples on the area. Because this can look like an orange peel, it's known as *peau d'orange* (Figure 11.11). If the tumor is ulcerating through the skin, it's ominous. If it's stuck to the muscles underneath so it doesn't move at all, that's also a bad sign. If there are lymph nodes you can feel above your collarbone (superclavicular nodes) or walnut-size lymph nodes in your armpit, that's also dangerous. And if the skin around the lump appears red and infected, it can indicate inflammatory breast cancer (see Chapter 13), which is also likely to spread.

Any one of these signs suggests a high probability that microscopic cancer cells elsewhere in the body can grow and develop into a metastasis. In that setting, we plan a systemic treatment (see Chapter 12) as well as a local treatment for the cancer. These tumors are called "locally advanced" and are often treated with chemotherapy rather than surgery as a first step (see Chapter 13).

Most people don't have any of these grave signs, but we still need to figure out the likelihood of microscopic cancer cells exist-

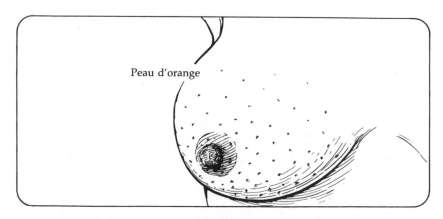

Peau d'orange

Figure 11.11

ing and growing in other organs. The way we do this is to remove some axillary (armpit) lymph nodes. There are between 30 and 60 lymph nodes under the arm. We try to sample the ones most likely to show cancer cells under the microscope and then examine them. (See Chapter 14 for this surgery.) We look at these lymph nodes because they are a good window into what is going on in the rest of the body. If they reveal cancer cells, we assume there's a high probability that there are microscopic cancer cells in other parts of the body. If they don't show cancer, it means there is a lower probability. We do this by a procedure called a *sentinel node biopsy*, which involves finding if the few nodes that are most likely to have cancer cells present do in fact have them, and if they do, examining them very thoroughly. (Sentinel node biopsy is discussed in detail in Chapters 12 and 14.)

The lymph node evaluation, however, doesn't give us a perfect answer either. Positive lymph nodes don't necessarily mean that there are microscopic cells elsewhere with the ability to grow. In fact, they don't in about 30 percent of cases. Conversely, even if the lymph nodes are negative, it does not mean that the cancer has not spread—20–30 percent of breast cancers with negative lymph nodes have spread elsewhere.

To a certain degree, though, the number of positive lymph nodes gives us a sense of the probability of having microscopic breast cancer cells elsewhere in the body. With one or two positive nodes, you're less likely to have metastatic potential than with 10 or 15, and this is reflected in the new TNM system, which separates N_1 into a, b, and c categories based on the number of positive nodes. However, because with any positive lymph nodes there's a pretty high chance that there are cancer cells elsewhere capable of growing, we almost always treat women with positive nodes with either hormones or chemotherapy or both (see Chapter 17).

In women with negative nodes, it's trickier. What we want is a way to identify the 20–30 percent who have microscopic cells elsewhere and not overtreat the other 70 percent. At present we don't have a direct way to do this. However, we do it indirectly by examining the primary tumor for the features described earlier in this chapter. We look at the biomarkers. More recently we have begun to analyze the tumors for molecular changes that can predict the risk of recurrence as well as the best therapy.

Molecular Classifications

As I noted in Chapter 4, it is becoming clear that not all breast cancer is the same. While we had suspected this for a long time, we had assumed that it all started with the same mutations and that the difference occurred over time when some tumors became more aggressive. We now know that there are at least four kinds of breast cancer that are different from the start, based on their molecular biology. There are probably more or subgroups that await our discovery—and we're searching for them. Identifying these different kinds of cancer has allowed us to better determine the prognosis of each tumor, and even more importantly to match the treatment to the type of tumor. This growing ability to personalize treatment means that it will both work better and limit the potential side effects.

The most important tool in this regard has been the cDNA microarray analysis. This is done with a wonderful tool that new technology has enabled us to create. The *microarray* is a cDNA chip that gives researchers the astounding ability to look at the expression of hundreds of genes in hundreds of tumors at the same time. What we are actually looking at is the levels of messenger RNA, the signal from the DNA to the protein that determines the expression levels of genes (see Chapter 4). When this tool is applied to the tumors of patients who participated in previous research, the patterns of gene expression can be associated with what we know has happened within the participant's body in the years since her study. The four main kinds of breast cancer identified by cDNA analysis correlate pretty well with the combinations of biomarkers noted earlier in the chapter. It is important to keep in mind that these analyses are looking at *all* the cells in the tumor, which include both the cancer cells and the cells around it. Together they give us a picture of the conditions in which cancer has occurred.[14]

The most common types of breast cancer in Western countries are the luminal subtypes, so called because their genetic pattern is close to that of cells lining the lumen, the hollow center of the duct. The group is subdivided into luminal A and luminal B and all are sensitive to estrogen. The rare occurrence of breast cancer in men (see Chapter 13) includes almost exclusively luminal A and B.

Luminal A tumors generally have high levels of estrogen receptors, are Her-2/neu negative, and have little cell division. They comprise about 30–40 percent of breast tumors, and they generally have a good prognosis. Although we have not yet figured out the risk factors for the specific subtypes of breast cancer, it seems that most of the traditional hormonal risk factors (see Chapter 5) are predictors for the luminal A kind.[15] Luminal A cancers generally have a well differentiated pathology. Many are the tubular cancers described earlier in this chapter.

The luminal B tumors are less common, about 20 percent of breast cancers, and are still estrogen positive, although less so than the luminal A's. They also have more cell division and tend to be moderately or poorly differentiated.[16] Some classifications have designated a luminal C classification. These tumors correspond to infiltrating lobular carcinomas.

Her-2/neu overexpressing tumors can be estrogen receptor positive or estrogen receptor negative, and they have their own group. The Her-2/neu overexpressing estrogen receptor negative tumors have high rates of cell division and are more aggressive looking. In the pre-Herceptin era these tumors had a poor prognosis. Fortunately, targeted therapy using Herceptin has changed all that (see Chapter 12).

Another molecular subtype is the triple negative breast cancer. These estrogen negative breast cancers include, but are not limited to, the basal carcinomas. Just to demonstrate how complicated this really is, in the mRNA analysis of the basal subtype of tumor we find low levels of the hormone receptor positive luminal genes and low levels of Her-2/neu but high levels of the proliferation genes that drive cell division. Moreover, they have their own unique additional cluster of genes, which gives it its name, the basal cluster. Eighty percent of women who carry the mutation in BRCA 1 and develop breast cancer have the basal type of cancer. However, most basal breast cancers are *not* in women with BRCA

1, which suggests that the BRCA pathway may be disrupted by acquired mutation rather than inherited. Interestingly, these tumors are more common among African American women of all ages and premenopausal women of all races. Though very aggressive, these tumors are also very sensitive to chemotherapy.[17] Generally the basal type of tumor is characterized by being triple negative (estrogen receptor negative, progesterone receptor negative, and Her-2/neu negative), but not all basal tumors are triple negative.[18] Their defining characteristic is that extra unique basal cluster. I should also point out that this key cluster is a research finding and is not routinely looked for in clinical practice because we don't have an easy way to do it. So don't expect to see it mentioned on your pathology report. Finally there is the overlapping triple negative group, 70 percent of which will not have the basal cluster. Both of these groups at represent a therapeutic challenge because they do not offer specific molecular targets. Luckily they respond very well to chemotherapy.

Obviously this is not only complicated stuff but still a work in progress. I would not be surprised if there were several more groups or subgroups that are uncovered over the next five years. I spent some time delineating them because you will start to hear these terms and need to recognize where they come from. They are helpful not only in estimating your prognosis, but, as you will see in the next chapter, they play a key role in predicting which treatment will be best for you. Once you have reviewed the three main markers (ER, PR, and Her-2/neu) in your pathology report, you will have a pretty good idea of whether you have a Her-2/neu overexpressing tumor, a triple negative tumor or a luminal one. While this may sound hopelessly arcane to you now, it will help you sort out the decisions ahead of you.

Commercial Tests

Another approach to identifying different types of tumors and matching the therapies has come from commercial tests of patterns of gene expression based on a limited sampling of genes, whereas the molecular classification discussed previously are based on an analysis of 10,000 genes. While there are overlaps with the types of tumors, these tests have actually been validated and in some situations actually can predict the best therapy.

The first such test to be clinically available, Oncotype DX, is from Genomic Health.[19] Scientists selected 21 genetic markers that held promise for both prognosis and prediction. They then developed a method to analyze these genes in fixed tissue (leftover tissue from a removed tumor that had already been used to make diagnostic slides). They first tested the genes on the tissue from a completed NSABP (National Surgical Adjuvant Breast and Bowel Project) study on women with estrogen positive, node negative tumors who were randomized between tamoxifen and placebo.[20] Since this study had been completed, they knew which women had cancer that recurred within the 10-year follow-up. Their test was able to distinguish high-risk, low-risk, and intermediate-risk groups from supposedly good prognostic tumors. The high-risk group had a 30 percent chance of recurrence, while the low-risk group had a 6 percent chance. This recurrence score was more predictive of outcome than age or tumor size. In fact they found some very small tumors that had a high chance of recurrence and some larger ones that did not. Interestingly when an independent researcher applied the cDNA microarray and the Oncotype DX to the same group of tumors, they found that 50 percent of the luminal A tumors had low recurrence scores while only 2 percent of the luminal B tumors did.[21] The value of the test was increased with their second report at the San Antonio Breast Cancer Symposium in December 2004. By applying their test to women who had received chemotherapy in addition to tamoxifen, they showed that the high-risk group benefited significantly from chemotherapy while the low-risk group did not. The benefit from tamoxifen was examined using this test in another retrospective study and showed that women with a low recurrence score and high estrogen receptor score got the biggest benefit from tamoxifen, while the women with a high recurrence score got none.

Oncotype DX is currently clinically available through Genomic Health. If you are interested, ask your doctor to order it or your pathologist to send the fixed tissue or slides. Check in advance to see if your insurance will cover it.

More recently, and to my mind more exciting, are the data from node positive, estrogen receptor positive women. The old "the worse the disease the stronger the treatment needs to be" theory would suggest that these women all needed chemotherapy. However, when the Oncotype DX test was applied to these women their prognosis looked just like the node-negative women's.[22] The ones with a lower recurrence score did better and responded very well to tamoxifen, while the ones with a high recurrence score had both a higher rate of recurrence and a better response to chemotherapy—suggesting that the biology of the tumor is more important at predicting prognosis and the best treatment than the stage of the cancer. It reminds me of infections and antibiotics. Before we knew about bacteria, we would talk about tuberculosis and streptococcal pneumonia as if they were the same disease because they were both lung infections. In fact they are very different requiring different treatments and having different outcomes. We would not treat a really bad streptococcal pneumonia with a higher dose of a tuberculosis drug and expect it to work. Similarly, if a breast cancer is one that has a low recurrence score that indicates that it's very sensitive to hormones, it makes no sense to give the woman chemotherapy which it is not sensitive to.

Some of you might wonder about the women with an intermediate recurrence score. To date we don't know the right approach for these patients, but a large clinical trial, Tailor RX, is being conducted to answer that question. Furthermore, the current test does not address risk of recurrence in estrogen receptor negative cancers. An additional combination test from Europe (Mammaprint), based on the cDNA microarray discussed earlier, combined 70 genes to predict which women with stage 1 or 2 breast cancer who had not received chemotherapy developed metastases 14 years later. It has been validated in a randomized controlled trial in Europe called Microarray in Node Negative Disease May Avoid Chemotherapy (MINDACT) study.[23] The advantage of this test is that there is no intermediate group, allowing the results to be more clear-cut. Although it has been approved by the FDA, it has to be done on fresh or frozen tissue and so is less convenient for the logistics of pathology in the United States than the Oncotype DX test.

Both of these tests are available today, although you may have to ask your surgeon or oncologist to have the tissue sent for analysis. They can be very helpful in decision making. An older friend of mine called me to say that she had been diagnosed with estrogen positive, node positive breast cancer and was worried about getting chemotherapy since she had a history of heart disease. I was able to tell her to have her tumor tested for Oncotype DX. Her oncologist balked, saying that the test was valid only on women with negative nodes. My friend was able to direct this oncologist to the latest study on node positive women and the test was done. It came back with a low recurrence score, indicating not only that she had a relatively low chance of recurrence but that chemotherapy would not help and hormone therapy was just fine. She was delighted. I think most women with hormone positive cancers should consider this test although at the time of this writing there is still some controversy in the oncology community. Several randomized studies are under way that should sort this out. Meanwhile, if the test comes out with a high recurrence score, then you can feel some reassurance that chemotherapy is worth it.

Statistics

Even considering the different types of breast cancer, it is impossible to tell what is going to happen with any one woman. Two women may have the same genetic mutations, but the factors affecting the microenvironment (neighborhood) in which those cells live will vary. This explains why a doctor can say that someone with advanced metastatic disease can still "beat the odds." All our prognostications are of necessity based on large statistical groups of patients. Table 11.2 shows five-year survival rates with only a mastectomy as treatment. This does not mean everyone died at year six or, as some wishfully think, that all who make it to five years are cured. It just means that the researchers checked to see who was alive at year five. These prognostications have some use—as long as you realize they don't absolutely predict the course of your particular disease.

A five-year survival without recurrence, for example, is significant but not definitive. In the earliest editions of this book I

Table 11-2.   Five-Year Breast Cancer Survival Rates According to the
Size of the Tumor and Axillary Node Involvement

Tumor Size (cm)	Patients Surviving 5 Years		
	Negative Nodes (%)	1–3 Positive Nodes (%)	4 or More Positive Nodes (%)
< 0.5	269 (99.2)	53 (95.3)	17 (59.0)
0.5–0.9	791 (99.3)	140 (94.0)	65 (54.2)
1.0–1.9	4,668 (95.8)	1,574 (86.6)	742 (67.2)
2.0–2.9	4,010 (92.3)	1,897 (83.4)	1,375 (63.4)
3.0–3.9	2,072 (86.2)	1,185 (79.0)	1,072 (56.9)
4.0–4.9	845 (84.6)	540 (69.8)	727 (52.6)
> 5.0	809 (82.2)	630 (73.0)	1,259 (45.4)

Source: Carter C., Allen C., Henson D. Relation of tumor size, lymph node status, and survival in 24,740 breast cancer cases. Cancer 63 (1989): 181. With permission.

downplayed its importance. However, a recent analysis of several studies has shown that I was probably missing an important point of biology. According to Don Berry, Ph.D., a statistician from Texas, the factors we use to determine prognosis (nodes, tumor size, etc.) have an effect only initially.[24] This suggests that if you have positive nodes and larger tumors and your cancer hasn't recurred within five years, your risk of recurrence is probably the same as everyone else's with breast cancer: you are no longer considered high risk for recurrence. Although this doesn't assure you of long-term survival, it does give you reason for cautious optimism.

There are several software programs that add more factors to the survival data shown above. You can go to my webpage (www.drsusanloveresearchfoundation.org) and look under Decision Tools to see what factors each one addresses. Or you can ask your physician to go to Adjuvantonline.com and print out a chart for you. This kind of evaluation of the cancer is what we're currently using to decide what seems to be the most medically sound course of treatment because it encompasses as much as we know to date about the natural history of the disease and the biology of the tumor. Keep in mind that these statistical tools apply only to populations and so can only give you an overall picture of what is likely. What happens to you may not fit the norm.

So, none of this gives us absolute knowledge. All we do is look at large groups of patients and say, "The majority of women with these signs have this prognosis, and are likely to have this response to this treatment." But you, the individual patient, may or may not fall into the majority category. This has several implications. If 80 percent of patients in your cancer category survive, that's very hopeful. You'll probably be in the 80 percent. But it's not certain. You may be in the 20 percent who don't survive. You need to be optimistic but cautious. Do everything possible to keep your advantage—careful follow-up and perhaps some of the adjunct, nonmedical techniques discussed in Chapter 18 to complement your treatment.

By the same token, if 80 percent of women in your category die, that doesn't mean you will. While it would make sense for you to think seriously about the possibility of your upcoming death and how you'd want to prepare for it, it also makes sense to think in terms of being part of the 20 percent who survive. Again, you may find it worthwhile to look into nonmedical attitudinal and nutritional therapies to complement your treatment and improve your odds as much as possible.

Chapter 12

DECISIONS REGARDING TREATMENT

FOR MANY WOMEN THE THOUGHT OF HAVING BREAST CANCER IS so appalling that their first thought is, "I don't want to deal with this—just remove the breast, get the cancer out of me, and let me go on with my life." It's not unreasonable to feel that way; a cancer diagnosis can turn your world upside down.

But if this is your reaction, don't follow through on it right away. Spend a day or two reflecting on the new reality you're facing. When your panic subsides, you may decide on a less drastic treatment than your original horror dictated. Whatever you choose, you'll have to live with your decision for the rest of your life—and that life won't be shortened by giving yourself a little time to think it over. Obviously, if you've got cancer you want it taken care of as soon as possible. But the week or so you give yourself won't kill you, and it will help you make the clearest decision possible.

In the past, it was common to make the decision—or rather, allow the doctor to make it for you—before the cancer was even diagnosed. You'd sign a consent form before your biopsy, agreeing to an immediate mastectomy if cancer was found. Fortunately that's much less common now, though it still sometimes happens. It's a terrible idea. No woman should be put to sleep without knowing whether she'll still have her breast when she wakes up. If your doctor wants you to sign such a form, don't do it. What you think you'll want when you're not sure if you have cancer may or may not mirror what you really want when you have a definite diagnosis.

Part of the sense of urgency comes from the way we used to think about the disease before we had the numerous options we have today. Now, you have choices. Any given procedure or combination of procedures may or may not be right for you, depending on the kind of cancer you have, the location of the cancer in your breast, its size, and, very importantly, your own thoughts and feelings. This chapter contains an overview of how different types of breast cancer relate to the different available treatments, and in subsequent chapters I'll explain how particular cancers are treated in particular situations. Finally, in Part 5 we'll consider each different treatment and what it entails.

GOALS AND DECISIONS

Treatment for breast cancer involves both killing cells and changing their neighborhood or environment. Surgery kills cells indiscriminately. Radiation therapy kills both healthy and malignant cells. Some cancer cells seem to be resistant to radiation therapy, and research suggests that these cells may have their own pattern of mutations that gives them immunity from radiation attacks.[1] Chemotherapy kills cancer cells in many different ways, among them by causing fatal mutations in the cell's DNA. In general, the effects of chemotherapy are quite similar to those of radiation therapy; both interfere with the cancer cells' growth. But here too, the process harms healthy cells, changing the environment along the way.

Hormone therapy, whether it is tamoxifen, an aromatase inhibitor, or even ovarian ablation (removing or blocking the ovaries), targets specific cancer cells, altering cell functions needed for survival and/or cell growth. At the same time it also changes the environment. Thus it causes a different hormonal

milieu in the whole body, including the breast and the neighborhood directly around the tumor.

Tamoxifen is a great example of how changing the neighborhood can have a lasting effect. It blocks the estrogen receptor in
the cells and the neighborhood, preventing estrogen from getting
to them. You would think that stopping it would stop its effects.
But the effect persists long after a woman stops taking it. One
study showed that taking tamoxifen for only a year provided benefits that lasted for at least 15 years.[2] The longer a woman takes it,
for a period of up to five years, the greater the benefit. Undoubtedly it kills some cancer cells, and also affects the stromal environment they live in. It may even put some of the cancer cells to
sleep. The idea of living with cancer cells remaining in your body
may seem alarming, but it shouldn't be. If you are feeling fine and
ultimately die of a stroke at 95, will you care that there were
sleeping cancer cells in your body? Probably not.

The newer, targeted therapies probably have mixed effects.
Herceptin is an antibody that blocks Her-2/neu, the growth factor
receptor that spurs cancer cells on (see Chapter 4). Does it kill
cells or change the environment? Probably both. It alters one of
several key processes that are necessary for the cancer cell's survival and/or growth. These processes exist in normal cells, too,
but are much less prominent. Herceptin kills and may block
growth factors that signal to the cancer cell, and that signal
causes the cancer cell's neighbors to respond differently. It's as if
the nasty grocer in the neighborhood has a nonfatal heart attack
and changes his ways, encouraging the entire neighborhood to become more friendly. Avastin, which blocks the growth of new
blood vessels into a tumor, changes the environment by preventing the cancer from getting nutrients and thus starving it to death.

Finally there are all the complementary and lifestyle approaches. How do stress reduction, weight loss, or increased
physical activity prevent recurrence? My bet is that they change
the environment of the body and thus maintain the cancer cells in
a more dormant state.

So, we can take advantage of all the approaches to help you
achieve a long life. Most initial treatment plans, as we will see, reduce the amount of cancer through surgery and radiation (local

therapy) and then add one or more systemic therapies (chemotherapy, hormone therapy, and/or targeted therapy) to kill or control any remaining cells. This is what the doctors do. You can add the lifestyle changes that will support this approach (see Chapter 18).

When you are newly diagnosed with breast cancer, you'll have to make two sets of decisions based on the kind of cancer you have (see Chapters 11 and 13) and your personal situation. The first is what will be done to treat what we call the *local* area—the breast and lymph nodes under your arm. This is usually a combination of local therapies, including surgery and radiation. The second is what will be done to treat the rest of the body. And these won't be simple, cut-and-dried decisions. More than one factor must be considered. For example, we know now that a recurrence in the breast or lymph nodes increases the chance of dying of cancer. In addition, we know that tamoxifen and chemotherapy not only treat microscopic cells elsewhere in the body but also reduce local recurrences. This can be overlooked because the local decisions are determined with the help of a surgeon and radiation therapist while the systemic ones are the province of the medical oncologist. Still there can be some coordination if you see the doctors your surgeon usually works with or go to a breast center with a multidisciplinary team. As a surgical colleague, Lisa Bailey, reminded me, "It is often the surgeon who determines the referral to the medical oncologist and radiation oncologist. This can affect the potential for neoadjuvant therapy, as well as adjuvant therapy. For example, I know that some medical oncologists almost always recommend chemotherapy while others are more thoughtful, or that some radiation oncologists offer partial breast radiation while others only recommend whole breast radiation therapy. So, I can influence what treatment a patient gets by who I refer them to." This is a good thing if you trust your surgeon, but may not be if you are uneasy with the surgeon's manner or approach. Always remember, you are the patient and have to make the decision that works for you. If you feel uncomfortable or uneasy with your doctor or team, get a second opinion.

And remember that while this chapter focuses on the benefits of various treatments, there are side effects from every approach.

I encourage you to read through the entire treatment section to be sure you understand ahead of time what you are getting into.

SURGERY AND RADIATION

For years, most surgeons began any treatment course with mastectomy, assuming that this drastic procedure was the most effective way to save lives. But studies have proven them wrong. As we have seen again and again in breast cancer treatment, more is not necessarily better. The main goal of surgery to the breast is to prevent breast cancer from coming back in the specific area in which the cancer appears. This can be done by taking out just the cancer and necessary lymph nodes and letting radiation destroy any remaining cells: we call this breast-conserving therapy, as it does not remove the breast itself. (Less formally, it's called lumpectomy, wide excision, or even partial mastectomy—they all mean the same thing.) The cancer can also be removed by a mastectomy, which in small tumors usually takes out enough tissue to prevent recurrence, eliminating the need for radiation. Finally, with very large tumors we use both mastectomy, to remove as much of the tumor as possible, and radiation therapy, to take care of leftover cells. The best choice is generally dictated not only by the biology of the tumor but also by the choice of the patient.

Most women naturally conclude that the more drastic treatment will be better and that having a mastectomy will remove not only the breast but any possibility that cancer will return. But that isn't always the case. Breast cancer can come back in the scar, chest wall, or axilla (armpits) after a mastectomy, just as it can after a lumpectomy. In fact, all things being equal the local recurrence rates are the same for mastectomy alone (6 percent) and lumpectomy followed by radiation (6 percent).[3] The first women treated with breast conservation compared to extended radical mastectomy showed no difference between the two treatments in terms of cancer in the other breast, distant metastases, or new cancers in the area of the same breast after 20 years.[4]

In June 1990 the National Cancer Institute Consensus Conference concluded: "Breast conservation treatment is an appropriate method of primary therapy for the *majority* of women with

Stage I and II breast cancer and is *preferable* because it provides survival equivalent to total mastectomy while preserving the breast" (emphasis mine). What amazes me is that 20 years later we are still doing so many mastectomies rather than breast conservation. Recent studies have shown that only 57.8 percent of women are receiving breast conservation.[5] And even this number varies geographically. The overuse of mastectomy holds true especially when the tumor appears more aggressive, suggesting that even after 20 years of data to the contrary many people still think of breast conservation as less aggressive therapy—though, as I'll explain later, it isn't. This may be due in part to the American tendency to think that more is always better in virtually any situation. If it hurts more or it's a bigger operation, it must be the best. Many of the women I counsel in regard to this decision have that attitude. And too often their surgeons don't try to dissuade them. In Los Angeles and nationwide, growing numbers of women are having bilateral mastectomies for cancers that could be treated as well with breast conservation. The surgeons say it is the patient's choice, but I wonder how often the surgeon just agrees with woman's initial preference rather than take the time to explain that it does not necessarily guarantee a better chance of survival. When you are considering your options, be aware that more is *not* necessarily better. Your doctor has an obligation to discuss all the options with you, not to just agree with your first choice. If your doctor does not explain all the options, then it is wise to get a second opinion. Scary as it may be, you need to take the time to become educated in the options, risks, and complications before you decide which path will work better for you.

In some cases, lumpectomy plus radiation is as important medically as it is cosmetically. If your cancer is right near the breastbone, the best mastectomy won't allow the surgeon to get a normal rim of tissue around the lump. But radiation will treat the surrounding tissue.

On the other hand, mastectomy is sometimes the best medical choice—for instance, if you have a large cancer in a small breast or extensive ductal carcinoma in situ (a form of noninvasive cancer). Even then it may not be the best option; sometimes a woman with a large cancer in a small breast can have chemotherapy or hormone therapy before surgery to shrink the tumor and thus allow breast conservation (see Chapter 17). In short, there are both medical and cosmetic implications to whatever course you choose, and you should be fully informed about both.

PREOPERATIVE MRI

Studies suggest that the most important factor to achieving local control is getting most of the tumor out with surgery. "Most of the tumor" does not mean every speck of cancer. When we started doing breast conservation, many studies were done extensively examining breasts that had been removed, looking for small cancers that might have been missed if the woman had had lumpectomy. One study showed 40 percent of breasts had other spots of cancer more than 2 centimeters from the original tumor.[6] This number corresponds closely to the recurrence rate in women who are treated with lumpectomy *without* radiation therapy,[7] and to the identification of unsuspected cancer in women who undergo MRI before their surgery.[8] Radiation has been proven very good at treating these secondary lesions, since the local recurrence rate when radiation is added to lumpectomy is significantly lower than 40 percent. These recurrences are usually at the site of the original lesion, not elsewhere in the breast. Despite what you might think, these tiny spots of cancer elsewhere in the breast do not have to be removed because they can be treated with radiation therapy. Systemic therapies will affect them either by killing them off or changing their environment.

The other argument for preoperative MRI is that it will benefit surgery planning and reduce the chance that a surgeon would have to do a second operation to ensure the tumor is removed. While this sounds reasonable, studies have not supported the premise. One report by Hayes and his group in Michigan reviewed more than two dozen recent studies and found that there is little evidence to support the routine use of MRI in newly diagnosed patients.[9] They found that 11.3 percent of patients have more extensive surgery than initially planned, and 8.1 percent of women who had been planning breast conservation had mastectomies. And yet a randomized controlled study in the United

Kingdom demonstrated that the reexcision rates (number of times the surgeon had to reoperate to get clean margins) were the same whether women had a preoperative MRI or not.[10] The assumption is that preoperative MRI will lead to lower recurrence rates, but no data support it. Dr. L.J. Solin from Pennsylvania showed essentially identical outcomes after eight years in women who had breast conserving surgery without a preoperative MRI and in those with it (96 percent versus 97 percent).[11] A study from Fox Chase Cancer Center showed that women who had a preoperative MRI were almost twice (1.8) as likely to opt for a mastectomy whether something was found or not, just because they did not want to have to go through another MRI, and/or potential additional biopsy.[12] I tend to recommend that women avoid having routine preoperative MRIs. This sensitive test will only show up other spots and lead you on a wild goose chase. Unfortunately, it is being widely done. Once a hospital or breast center has purchased a machine, doctors want to use it. And everyone can think of one case where it was useful. Yet you are allowed to say no.

Different opinions regarding preoperative MRI remain. Lisa Bailey from Oakland told me she orders MRIs on many patients, and has found that sometimes there is a delay to getting to surgery because of false positive results. But occasionally the surgery has been significantly changed based on the MRI results. Ben Anderson from Seattle says his group agreed that it was reasonable to perform MRIs on all newly diagnosed patients for study purposes. He points out that 3 percent of women with one breast cancer will have another on the other side. However, he admits that having no MRI is better than having a bad MRI. The big problem is that the technique has not been standardized, so if a patient has a positive MRI at one institution and then decides to go to another, the MRI must be repeated because of varying injection and imaging protocols.

Luckily a large study has been funded to look at this issue in the community setting and settle it once and for all. What should you do in the meantime? You need to realize that you will have to make a decision based on inadequate information, as is often the case in this disease. You can follow the advice of your medical team combined with your own feelings about the issue. Just remember that

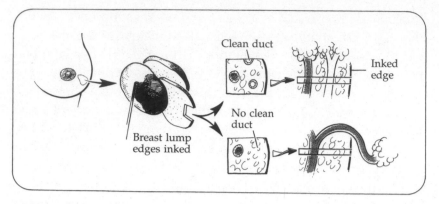

Figure 12.1

the key to curing breast cancer is not just finding spots in the breast but also treating the body as a whole.

Local Control

We determine whether we've removed the majority of the tumor by evaluating the margins of the tissue (see Chapter 11). If they're free of tumor, breast conservation is fine. This can be affected by the tumor's pathology. Breast cancers have tentacle-like protrusions stretching out into the breast tissue from the original lump. Ductal carcinomas with lots of DCIS (also called *extensive intraductal component,* or EIC) associated with them can reach much farther out. When this occurs, the margins may not be clean on the first try (the surgeon can't see or feel the "tentacles") (see Figure 12.1). A reexcision, which removes additional breast tissue, sometimes takes care of it. But in some cases even a reexcision won't get clean margins, and a mastectomy, the ultimate wide excision, is necessary to get it all out. Infiltrating lobular carcinomas also have a tendency to be sneaky and difficult for the surgeon to find and get around (see Chapter 13). These too need a wider excision and clean margins if they are to be treated with breast conservation, and may still end up requiring a mastectomy. New surgical approaches, termed oncoplastic surgery, apply plastic surgery techniques to cancer surgery (see Chapter 15). This allows larger areas to be removed while maintaining a reasonable-appearing breast and then reducing the other breast to match. If you prefer breast conservation you should ask your surgeon if she or he is skilled in oncoplastic techniques, and if not, find someone who is.

If the cancer is a distinct lump with short "tentacles," then just removing it with lumpectomy is fine. Sometimes the margin is just barely involved in one spot and is otherwise clear. This may still be acceptable for radiation therapy.[13] The key is determining the likelihood of cancer being left behind. In the usual type of cancer, the chance is very low, and radiation therapy can get rid of whatever cells may remain. When we first employed lumpectomy with radiation in Boston, we it didn't know that margins were important and we just took the tumor out. Reviewing this data in retrospect, we found that in tumors without EIC or lobular carcinoma our recurrence rate was only 4–6 percent over more than 10 years, even though we did not have perfectly clean margins.

Overall there are five situations that exclude a patient from being a good candidate for breast conservation with radiation therapy.[14]

1. The woman has two or more primary tumors that cannot be removed in a lumpectomy (although a recent small study questioned this proscription[15]) or diffuse microcalcifications throughout the breast.
2. She has a history of previous therapeutic radiation to the breast region (i.e., Hodgkin's disease) that combined with the proposed treatment would result in an excessively high total radiation dosage.
3. She is pregnant. However, in many cases it may be possible to perform breast conserving surgery in the second and third trimester and treat the patient with radiation after delivery, or give chemotherapy to shrink the tumor and perform the surgery and radiation after delivery (see Chapter 13).
4. There are persistent positive margins after reasonable surgical attempts. A very small sign of cancer in one place on a margin (focally involved margin) may not rule out breast conservation, however.

5. The presence of specific active autoimmune diseases, particularly scleroderma or lupus, which can result in severe short-term and long-term complications in the presence of radiation.

In addition, there may be other reasons for not having breast conservation therapy. For example, if the area that needs to be removed is very large compared to the breast itself there will not be enough breast tissue left after a lumpectomy to make it cosmetically worthwhile. If the woman is a carrier of the BRCA 1 and/or 2 gene (see Chapter 6) and has a high risk of other cancers developing in the remaining breast tissue, she may want to consider bilateral mastectomy. However, lobular carcinoma in situ (LCIS; see Chapter 13), once considered a contraindication for breast conservation, is no longer believed to be one.

If the patient has a mastectomy, breast reconstruction (see Chapter 15) can be done immediately after mastectomy or later, when and if she wants it. Commonly a surgeon will leave a large envelope of skin (skin sparing) when reconstruction is planned for the plastic surgery to fill. Nipple sparing is also being tried more recently, although the spared nipple is usually numb. Even with these possibilities, however, it makes no sense to me to remove a breast and try to reconstruct it when it can be preserved in a cosmetically acceptable way with the same risk of recurrence and same chance of cure and still have fairly normal sensation.

Sometimes a woman will choose mastectomy over breast conservation because she has been told that if she had breast conservation and the cancer recurred later, she would be unable to have reconstruction at that time. This is silly for several reasons. To begin with, only about 6 percent of women will develop a local recurrence (cancer coming back in the breast or lymph nodes) in the breast and require a mastectomy. Further, although it is harder to do reconstruction with an implant (see Chapter 15) in this situation, studies have shown that patients who undergo reconstruction with a pure myocutaneous flap (skin and muscle taken from another part of the body) following postmastectomy radiation have the same outcome as women who have not had radiation therapy.[16]

With mastectomy, we usually don't do radiation because the tumor has been removed. But studies have shown that in certain situations even after mastectomy there is a higher risk of recurrence in the skin or lymph nodes. Women with four or more positive axillary lymph nodes, a tumor over 5 centimeters, close margins (cancer cells at the edge of the mastectomy), and significant invasion of the lymphatic or blood vessels in the breast tissue (called lymphovascular invasion) may well benefit from postmastectomy radiation therapy. A patient who does not quite fit these criteria, but because of young age or aggressive tumor type, may still be advised to consider radiation after mastectomy.

Postmastectomy radiation reduces the chance of local recurrence from 5–10 percent to 3–5 percent. If the chance of recurrence is higher, as in the situations mentioned above, the benefit is also higher. If a woman has negative nodes, the five-year local recurrence rate after mastectomy is 6 percent and goes to 2 percent with radiation. If she has four or more positive lymph nodes, the five-year local recurrence rate is 23 percent without radiation therapy and 6 percent with it. Although there is no difference in survival in node negative women, women with positive nodes will improve their survival rates by 5 percent when they add radiation therapy.[17]

Why, then, shouldn't everyone who has a mastectomy also have radiation? Because radiation has its own risks. Studies show that people who had cancer on the left side and got radiation had an increase in heart disease, although this risk has decreased substantially as radiation techniques have improved[18] (see Chapter 16). In addition, recent studies have shown a doubling of the risk of lung cancer 10 years after postmastectomy radiation therapy.[19,20] (This risk is related to smoking history as well as the amount of lung that has been treated and, interestingly, does not apply to radiation therapy after breast conservation.) As with all the decisions related to breast cancer treatment, it ends up being a balance of risk versus benefit. When the risk of local recurrence is high enough after a mastectomy, radiation is worthwhile. Most specialists now agree with the idea presented above—that patients with four or more positive nodes or tumors that are larger than 5 centimeters should be treated with radiation.[21,22,23] More

controversial is the question of the patient with up to three positive nodes.[24] Until we have good data to support treating women
with fewer positive nodes, it is probably better to forgo it. Talk to
your doctors and consider your own feelings; then make the decision that feels best for you.

Integrating postmastectomy radiation therapy with potential
reconstruction can be complicated. Postmastectomy radiation,
whether given before or after reconstructive plastic surgery, substantially increases the risk of capsular fibrosis (scarring around
the implant) as well as other complications following reconstruction with a silicone prosthesis in most studies (see Chapter 15).
Implants are easier to do than the tissue flap procedures and
therefore are more widely available. And not all women will have
problems. One approach is to treat patients with radiation either
before or after implant reconstruction, recognizing that some
women will need a flap reconstruction if there are problems later.
Another common path is to do expander reconstruction immediately (if the patient wants reconstruction), and overexpand during
radiation therapy. That seems to reduce capsular contracture. The
patient can then have a permanent implant or a free flap at a later
time. The second problem arises when a woman who may be a
candidate for postmastectomy radiation therapy wants reconstruction with a microvascular flap. In this case having the radiation after the reconstruction results in a substantial increase in
complications. One way to solve this has been termed the delayed
immediate approach. The mastectomy is done and a skin expander is placed to maintain the skin envelope. As soon as the
pathology is available, the decision regarding postmastectomy radiation is made. If she does not need it, she can go on to have her
flap done in the same hospitalization and if she does, she can
have the radiation therapy first with the skin expander in place.
Tissue flap reconstruction can be done four to six months later.

Partial Breast Radiation

Partial radiation is an area of recent study. If local recurrences arise
after lumpectomy alone, they almost always arise near the primary

tumor. So perhaps we can just irradiate the bed of the tumor, sparing the rest of the breast. Further support for this idea comes from the observation that 10 years or so after lumpectomy with radiation therapy, the risk of a new cancer elsewhere in the breast is about the same as the risk in the other breast. So irradiating the whole breast does not seem to decrease the risk of a new cancer developing elsewhere in that breast. Limiting radiation to the tumor bed allows the treatment to be shorter and should limit side effects.

Based on this line of thinking, several techniques have been developed to deliver radiation locally: interstitial brachytherapy, limited external beam irradiation, intracavitary brachytherapy (balloon catheter), and intraoperative limited radiation therapy. The most commonly used, the balloon catheter, delivers radiation to the site of the lumpectomy twice a day for about five days. This approach uses a balloon to fill the biopsy cavity (see Figure 12.2). As we will see in Chapter 16, women who undergo oncoplastic surgery are not candidates for this type of partial radiation. Because the balloon and brachytherapy techniques require additional breast procedures and equipment that is not universally available, efforts have been made to figure out how to use the standard linear accelerator to deliver localized radiation using a technique called 3D conformational radiation therapy or limited external beam irradiation. Computerized planning and multiple beams can allow the same area to be treated that the balloons do, in about 4 to 10 days. These will be described in Chapter 16. Limited but encouraging reports of these techniques have shown local recurrence rates similar to those with standard six-week treatment, and also fewer side effects. The American Society of Therapeutic and Radiation Oncology (ASTRO) recommends this approach for women over 60 with tumors less than or equal to 2 centimeters, positive estrogen receptors, and no lympho-vascular invasion.[25] The American Association of Breast Surgeons has more liberal guidelines. It is important to recognize that guidelines like these (from both organizations) are the consensus of the group, since there are as yet no data. This means the radiation therapists might be more conservative about changing the way they have always done things while the surgeons might be eager

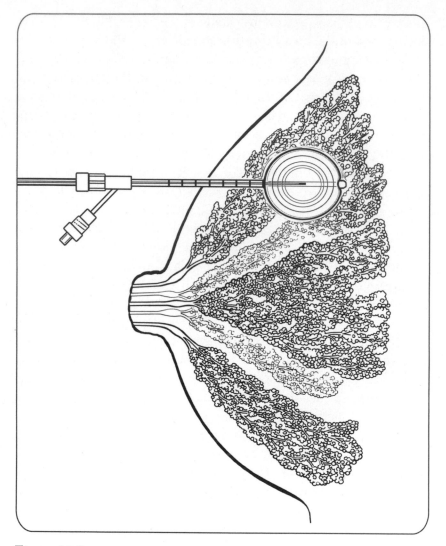

Figure 12.2

to get more involved in this aspect of care, which can be lucrative, and thus have more liberal recommendations. Over the next five years, we can expect data to be reported and the path to become clearer. This is another area where you are stuck making a decision based on inadequate information. Review your own feelings: are you a risk taker who loves the newest thing or a conservative who doesn't believe it is worth changing an approach with a long track record of what works? Then talk to your doctors and think about getting a second opinion.

Intraoperative radiation therapy is the most convenient method of receiving radiation, as it is given in a single dose at the time of surgery. As we went to press a large, randomized study showed that in selected patients it is as good as six weeks of radiation in preventing local recurrences.[26] However, it requires specialized equipment and is therefore offered only at a few centers as part of a clinical trial. Several randomized clinical trials comparing standard radiation therapy to newer techniques are under way. These studies will give us the safety data we need before such approaches become more widely adopted. If you think you are a candidate, ask your surgeon for a referral.

Ongoing Research

With the success of figuring out different kinds of breast cancers using DNA analysis discussed in Chapter 11, some researchers have asked whether this same approach can be used to figure out which women's cancers are more likely to recur even with radiation therapy. A preliminary study suggests that it can. Granted it was a small study of only 80 women, but researchers were able to distinguish between the women who had a local recurrence despite radiation therapy and those who didn't, at least in the estrogen receptor positive cancers and less so but still potentially in the estrogen negative ones.[27] It is highly likely that by the time of the next edition we will be able to tell who needs what in terms of local therapy, just as we are beginning to be able to do for systemic therapy.

AXILLARY SURGERY: CHECKING THE LYMPH NODES

Along with getting rid of the cancer, we usually try to discover if there are affected lymph nodes in the armpit area (axilla). Women do better when these lymph nodes are treated. The improvement in survival has been calculated to be about 5 percent in women whose axilla are routinely treated than in women whose axilla are just observed and left alone unless a lymph node appears cancerous to the touch.[28,29]

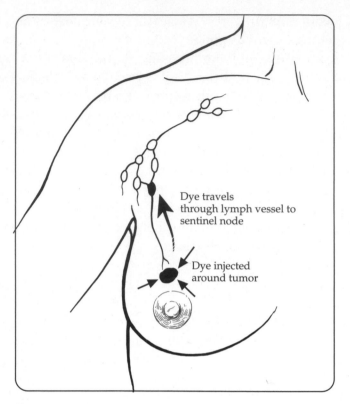

Dye travels
through lymph vessel to
sentinel node

Dye injected
around tumor

Figure 12.3

Aside from preventing recurrence in the armpit, the other purpose for doing axillary surgery is to help decide the stage of the
breast cancer. If a woman has palpable (feelable) lymph nodes in
her axilla, an ultrasound directed fine needle aspirate or core
biopsy should be done to determine whether those nodes represent cancer. If they do, a full axillary dissection is done. If not, or
if there are no palpable nodes, a *sentinel node biopsy* is the preferred choice (see Figure 12.3).

The concept of sentinel node biopsy is pretty straightforward. It
is based on the theory that there are one or more nodes to which a
breast cancer is most likely to spread.[30] During or just before surgery the surgeon injects a small amount of blue dye and radioactive
tracer into the breast and follows it as it travels up to the lowest
draining lymph node or nodes. These nodes are then removed for

examination with the thought that they would be the first stop on the cancer's way out of the breast and into the body (see Chapter 14). If these nodes are found not to have any cancer, the rest of the axilla is left alone. This is another example where more is not better. We find the one or two nodes that are most likely to have cancer, so we don't worry that we may miss a node that's hiding in a corner somewhere. And since the pathologist knows that this is the node to check, it will be checked more thoroughly than the many nodes in a regular node dissection (see Chapter 14). Thus there's less room for error. About 50 percent of women found to have a positive sentinel node will have other positive nodes in the axilla. As this book was in production, results from a randomized study were announced demonstrating that even women with positive sentinel nodes may not need full dissection with all the consequences thereof. The Memorial Sloan Kettering Cancer Center (MSKCC) has developed a nomogram that helps a surgeon and patient determine which women with positive sentinel nodes will need a full axillary dissection.[31] The exception is when there are just a couple of isolated cancerous cells or the cells are identified only with special staining or there is only a very small area of the lymph node with cancer (less than 0.2 mm) that is considered node negative. In this situation many surgeons will not do a full dissection. In women found to have micrometastases of 0.2–2.0 millimeters there is an advantage to undergoing a full axillary dissection and receiving adjuvant therapy (see Chapter 17).[32,33] Because the surgery is less extensive, sentinel node biopsy is also associated with fewer complications. No axillary drain is inserted, and there is less patient discomfort, decreased incidence of lymphedema (a swelling of the arm that can follow surgery), and less chance of inadvertent damage to nerves and blood vessels (see Chapter 14).

Sentinel node biopsy can be used effectively in all age-groups with breast conservation surgery or mastectomy at the time of primary excision or reexcision in bilateral breast cancer, after long-interval reduction mammoplasty (see Chapter 2), and with breast implants. Its safety is not clear in women who are pregnant or lactating because a little radioactive tracer is used, although one small study has shown no radioactivity in the pelvis with the dose of tracer used to find the sentinel node.[34] The technique is also effective with most types of tumors, including those treated with chemotherapy to shrink them before surgery (examined later in this chapter). An interesting new approach that is being explored is mapping the lymphatics in the arm to help prevent the surgeon from inadvertently injuring the arm and causing lymphedema (see Chapter 14).[34]

Infrequently the sentinel node is not in the patient's armpit but in her chest, beneath the breastbone (sternum), and here the radioactive tracer has a definite advantage. The absence of radioactivity in the armpit leads the doctor to check for it elsewhere. The usefulness of removing lymph nodes from under the breast bone is controversial, and surgeons need to weigh the pros and cons. It is not clear that it will change a woman's survival rate, but if it shows positive nodes it may affect her decision about whether or not to have chemotherapy or perhaps radiotherapy to the internal mammary nodes. In general, at this stage it should be done only as part of a study.

Guidelines for Local Control

In 1996 we published the first practice guidelines for breast cancer treatment.[36] Since then more have been developed. The most all-inclusive are those of the National Comprehensive Cancer Network (NCCN), which can be found free in a patient-friendly version in English and Spanish at www.nccn.org. In general, every woman should be considered a candidate for breast conservation unless she strongly prefers mastectomy or has a clear medical reason for it. As I mentioned earlier, I do not think the science thus far warrants preoperative MRIs. Many of my colleagues in practice disagree with me, however.

The first step for local control is definitive surgery. This means either wide excision or mastectomy, using sentinel node biopsy to determine if axillary dissection is called for. If the margins are clean after surgery, the patient is a candidate for radiation therapy without further breast surgery, although she may still need an axillary dissection if her sentinel node was positive. Any woman whose cancer was picked up with microcalcifications on a mammogram should have a careful study, preferably including a postbiopsy mammogram to make sure that all of them have been removed. If she has a lumpectomy and the margins are involved in more than one spot or the postbiopsy mammogram shows residual disease, or if she has EIC or infiltrating lobular carcinoma, the surgeon usually suggests a reexcision. This step gathers further information on the cancer. If the new margins are clean, she is a candidate for radiation therapy; if not, she may need a mastectomy. If the tumor is too large compared to the size of the breast for lumpectomy, she may be a candidate for neoadjuvant therapy or chemotherapy before surgery, to shrink the tumor before the operation. All women who choose mastectomy should be offered the option of reconstruction, either immediately or, if they prefer, at a later time.

Choices About Mastectomy

What are some of the factors that may influence your choice? There's a tendency to think that mastectomy is more aggressive because it's more mutilating. Actually, the combination of lumpectomy and radiation is more aggressive. Lumpectomy and radiation treat all the breast tissue. The field of radiation may encompass all the tissue that even extensive surgery misses. Some women choose mastectomy because they do not want to make daily trips for radiation therapy; others may want to get it all over with as soon as possible and get back to their lives as though it never happened. That is always a very individual decision; but you need to remember that, as I said earlier, it *has* happened, and you can never go back to your life exactly the way it was.

There are important drawbacks to mastectomy. It's less cosmetically appealing except with the very best reconstruction. And even with reconstruction (see Chapter 15), you are left with no sensation in the breast or breast area. Lumpectomy and radiation leave you with a real breast that retains its physical sensation.

Some women choose mastectomy because they don't want to take more time off from a demanding profession than is necessary. This makes sense, but now they can also consider one of the partial breast irradiation (PBI) studies, which will allow them to be treated in one or more days.

The availability of one kind of treatment or another is also a factor. In some areas radiation is not offered. In others, it is available but is not especially good. A radiation oncologist has to know the technique to get good results. For some women, however, their breasts are an integral part of their sexuality and identity and they are willing (and able) to go to great inconvenience to save them. One of my patients lived in a small town in the Central Valley of California, too far to commute to my breast center in Los Angeles. So she and her husband drove down in their van and lived in the hospital parking lot for six weeks until her treatment was completed. I've had patients whose cancer recurred after lumpectomy and radiation, and even though they finally had a mastectomy, they were grateful for an extra few years with both breasts.

Regardless of the medical facts, however, you need to feel safe with your choice. Some of my patients who had lumpectomy and radiation would wake up every morning sure that the cancer had come back. Even though this is unlikely, they may have been better off with mastectomies in the first place.

Remember above all that it's your body and no one else's. Don't decide on the basis of what anyone else thinks is best. By all means talk to your friends and your family and your husband or lover, and think about what they say. But make your own decision. As I said earlier, husbands and lovers come and go, but your body is with you all your life. A truly caring mate will support whatever course you think is best for you.

The next issue that may come up in the decision-making time is whether to have a *prophylactic mastectomy* on the other breast at the same time. This is not usually necessary or even contemplated unless the woman is a carrier of a BRCA 1 or BRCA 2 mutation, and even then it's certainly not mandatory (see Chapter 6). Women with a new diagnosis of breast cancer and a family history suggestive of a BRCA 1 or 2 mutation could choose to have a lumpectomy and lymph node surgery, then undergo testing and have chemotherapy while waiting for the genetic test result (it can take 3–8 weeks). If the test is positive they can, if they wish, undergo bilateral mastectomy with or without reconstruction following the completion of chemotherapy. If the test is negative they can go on to radiation following chemotherapy. Remember, there is no urgency over prophylactic mastectomy and you may want to get the cancer therapy taken care of first; then, when the timing is convenient, if you still want it, you can have your breasts removed. It is important to remember that BRCA mutation carriers are also at increased risk of ovarian cancer. In these women, prophylactic removal of the ovaries can reduce the risk of breast cancer as well as ovarian cancer.

The risk to the other breast in nonmutation carriers averages about 0.8 percent per year and an estimated 2–11 percent over a woman's lifetime,[37,38] A recent nonrandomized study compared 1,072 women who had undergone prophylactic mastectomy to 317 who had not. After 5.7 years of follow-up, 2.7 percent of women who had not had the preventative surgery developed a second cancer, compared to 0.5 percent of the women who had it.[39] This suggests a benefit from the surgery; however, prophylactic contralateral (on both sides) mastectomies did not affect the 10.5 percent of women who developed metastatic disease or the 8.1 percent who died. And the current use of hormone therapy in most women with hormone sensitive tumors has the added benefit of reducing the risk of cancer in both breasts by at least 50 percent. It is important to be realistic about the risks and benefits in your own case before jumping to extra surgery in an effort to do "everything possible."

Some plastic surgeons encourage removing both breasts at once because breast reconstruction surgery is easier when they don't have to match an existing breast. While this is worth considering, I don't think it should be the main factor in making the decision, unless you're a Playboy model.

Finally, neither reconstruction nor prophylactic mastectomy has to be done immediately. Sometimes all the decisions you have to make are overwhelming and it helps to leave a few for later. A woman I was counseling recently had dirty margins and a positive sentinel node. She needed a mastectomy and axillary dissection on her right breast and was agonizing on whether she should have a prophylactic mastectomy and immediate reconstruction at the same time. Once she realized that she did not have to make that decision right away, she was quite relieved. She decided to go ahead with the mastectomy and axillary dissection and then chemotherapy, while getting genetic testing (she had a family history of breast cancer) to find out what the risk really was to the second breast. After her systemic therapy was over, she went on

to consider prophylactic mastectomy on the other side and research the best type of reconstruction for her.

SYSTEMIC THERAPY

After you decide about local treatment, and usually once you have
all the pathological information that the nodes and breast tissue
can give you, there will be a discussion regarding systemic therapy. Systemic means something that creates its effect by circulating throughout your body; local treatments are applied only to the
area in question. Systemic treatments include chemotherapy
(drugs that selectively kill cancer cells and are known as cytotoxic
drugs) and targeted therapies such as hormone therapies (treatments that are hormones or affect your body's hormones) and
newer drugs. These latter include both antibodies administered to
the patient and small molecules that interfere with one or several
key processes that are vital to the survival and/or growth of the
cancer cell. They can also include alternative and complementary
therapies (see Chapter 18).

Adjuvant Chemotherapy

Drugs given at the time of diagnosis when there is no known
metastatic disease are called adjuvant treatment. If they are given
before surgery, they are called neoadjuvant. The same drugs are
just called "treatment" when metastatic disease is clearly present.
The reason for adjuvant therapy is the fact that breast cancer
deaths do not occur because of what is in the breast. You could
have a lump as big as a basketball and it would not kill you. What
kills people with breast cancer are the breast cancer cells that
spread into other, more important parts of the body such as the
lungs, liver, bone, or brain. This became all too clear in the 1930s,
when the 10-year results from a radical mastectomy study revealed a 12 percent survival. Needless to say, this was well before
the days of mammography and most tumors were larger than
those we deal with today. However even in modern times 20–30
percent of women with negative lymph nodes at the time of diagnosis and 75 percent of women with positive ones will die of their

disease within 10 years if they are treated *only* with surgery or surgery and radiation alone. Obviously many women have undetectable microscopic cells in other parts of their bodies at the time of diagnosis. Adjuvant therapy is an attempt to treat these cells either by killing them or changing the environment in which they exist or both. The success of this approach is the fact that we currently can cure over 80 percent of breast cancers.

Although the first randomized trial of adjuvant therapy was in 1948, when ovaries were removed to change the hormonal environment, only recently has it become a mainstay of treatment. Initially adjuvant therapies were given to all women with positive nodes. As newer drugs have been developed they have been added to the mix, and often given to women with negative nodes as well. As we have figured out the different types of breast cancer we have become better able to match the treatments to the patients both in terms of their risk of recurrence and the potential benefit of the therapy. This is important because none of the systemic therapies are without side effects, some of which can be quite significant. If a drug has prolonged your life you may well put up with secondary heart problems or surgery for uterine cancer. If, on the other hand, you really did not need or benefit from chemotherapy, then developing leukemia as a result would be tragic. Although we are better nowadays at matching treatment with patient, there still is a gray zone. How much risk of recurrence is enough to justify a treatment? Physicians frequently use the threshold of greater than 90 percent disease-free survival at 10 years with local therapy alone to define the women whose prognosis is too good to justify systemic therapy. Depending on your age, general health, and outlook on life, this might be what you would choose as well. However, it is worth taking the time to think about what you are willing to undergo for a statistical improvement in your odds. It is after all a bit of a gamble. For example, if we consider that chemotherapy reduces the risk of recurrence by about a third, that means that the higher the chance of recurrence, the more beneficial the chemotherapy is likely to be for you.[40] If you have a 60 percent chance of recurrence, a one-third risk reduction means chemo will reduce that chance by 20 percent, but if you have a 9 percent chance of recurrence the one-third reduction is only 3 percent, although these effects are not perfectly linear.

This concept is important to understand when you are weighing risks and benefits. In Chapter 11, I noted that it is always better to look at the absolute benefit of chemotherapy. This can be estimated in Table 12.1.[41] In other words, if your chance of dying in 10 years were 50 percent and you had a treatment that reduced the risk of mortality by 40 percent, your absolute benefit at 10 years would be 16 percent. And of course you also need to take your age into consideration (see Table 12.2).(Remember that chance of recurrence is not the same as absolute reduction.) Another way to further break down the benefits to women with negative nodes is to look at whether you are at low, medium, or high risk of recurrence. This is determined by all of the biomarkers discussed in Chapter 11. (See Table 12.2.)

The table shows hypothetical breast cancer risks of death for pre- and postmenopausal women. Taking into consideration the other causes of death, we see the 10-year benefit on mortality for adjuvant chemotherapy in the premenopausal women and tamoxifen in the estrogen receptor positive postmenopausal women. The table is dated, having been created before we had the current data on the aromatase inhibitors discussed later in this chapter, but it is still not far off.

Not all oncologists agree with this way of looking at the figures, and there is a bit of wishful thinking in their approach to chemotherapy. They want it to work and so they start believing it works better than it does or they just don't understand statistics. And they make their income by giving chemotherapy. In a 1994 study by S. Rajagopal, oncologists were presented with certain scenarios and for each one were asked whether or not they'd give chemotherapy.[42] Then they were asked what percentage of improvement in survival they thought the patient would have. Overall, they estimated a three times greater improvement than was justified by the available evidence. Thus you need to pin your oncologist down so that you are realistic about the benefits of chemotherapy in your case. If your oncologist is not sure of the absolute benefits, you can suggest she or he go to www.adjuvant online.com. This program allows your physician to put in your

Table 12-1.   Absolute Reduction in Mortality at 10 Years per 100
Women Treated

	Hypothetical Proportional Reduction in Mortality Due to Treatment				
Estimated 10-yr Death Rate with No Therapy	50%	40%	30%	20%	10%
70% (several positive nodes)	25	19	13	8	4
50% (5 cm tumor, neg nodes)	21	16	12	7	4
30% (avg tumor diameter, neg nodes)	14	11	8	5	3
10% (< 1 cm tumor, neg nodes)	5	4	3	2	1

Source: Osborne C.K., "Adjuvant endocrine therapy," Chapter 53 in Harris J.R., Lippman M.E., Morrow M., Osborne C.K., eds. *Diseases of the Breast*, 3rd ed. Philadelphia: J.B. Lippincott, Williams & Wilkins, 2004, p.868.

Table 12-2.   Survival Estimates at 10 Years by Age and Risk of Breast
Cancer Death, With and Without Adjuvant Therapy

Hypothetical risk* of breast cancer	*Natural mortality without breast cancer, next 10 yr (%)*	*No adjuvant therapy*	*Adjuvant therapy[†]*	*Absolute benefit*
40 year old				
10% (low risk)	2	88	90	2
28% (intermediate risk)	2	71	77	6
57% (high risk)	2	41	51	10
65 year old				
9% (low risk)	19	73	75	2
26% (intermediate risk)	19	58	63	5
54% (high risk)	19	34	43	9

*Values shown are derived from three different risk estimates and assume exponential death with a constant hazard ratio. The differences between 40 and 65 years of age reflect deaths from other causes.

[†]Based on a 25% annual reduction in the odds of death, a reasonable estimate of the benefits of chemotherapy in premenopausal patients and tamoxifen in an estrogen receptor-positive postmenopausal patient.

Source : Osborne C.K., Ravdin P.M. Adjuvant systemic therapy of primary breast cancer. In Harris J.R., Lippman M.E., Morrow M., Osborne C.K., eds. *Diseases of the Breast*, 2nd ed. Philadelphia: J. B. Lippincott, Williams & Wilkins, 2000, p. 625.

information regarding the stage and type of cancer and your age and health. Then it generates statistics about how many women like you will die of breast cancer within 10 years with no systemic treatment. It also tells you your chance of dying from a condition other than breast cancer, something we all seem to forget about. Finally, it estimates the benefits you would receive from chemotherapy, hormone therapy, or both. I have found that this helps many women gain perspective on their odds and the benefits they can expect. It does not, however, include the potential side effects of the therapy, a point too often glossed over. I will examine this at length in Chapters 17 and 19.

Systemic therapy does not guarantee that your cancer will be cured. It may simply prolong the time to recurrence. But that in itself is a worthwhile goal. A few years ago a sixty-eight-year-old woman with an estrogen receptor negative tumor called me for advice. Her oncologist thought she should be on chemotherapy because her chance of dying in the next five years was 15 percent without it. So she thought she might try it. I asked if the doctor had told her what her chance of dying in the next five years was even if she did take chemo. He hadn't. "I assume it means I have a 100 percent chance of surviving the next five years," she said. I told her that wasn't accurate: her chance of dying from breast cancer, with chemo, was 13 percent. She paused. "Then forget that!" she said finally. "I don't want to go through that for a 2 percent better chance!" However, studies have shown that some women will choose chemotherapy even for a 1 percent improvement in survival. What matters is that each woman has accurate knowledge to work with.

Types of Chemotherapy

The effectiveness of chemotherapy depends on which drug or drug combination you use. Chemotherapy treatment generally includes more than one drug and is given over a period of 3 to 6 months (see Chapter 17 and Appendix A). Although anthracycline regimens appear to be better than CMF-type therapies, they also have more toxicity, and that has to be taken into account. The anthracycline doxorubicin (Adriamycin) is commonly used in the United States, while epirubicin (E) is used more in Europe. These drugs are often given in combination as FAC or FEC or AC. More recently studies have suggested that adding a taxane (T) (paclitaxel or doxcetaxel) either before or after the anthracycline regimen provides additional benefit. Currently there is discussion about whether or not some of these drugs work better with specific types of breast cancer. For example, some early data suggest that using a non-anthracycline regimen may be possible in some circumstances. Women who will be receiving Herceptin for a Her-2 positive cancer may do as well with a non-anthracycline regimen (Taxotere/Carboplatin/Herceptin) as with a more "typical" Adriamycin regimen. It is worth asking about, since what we know in this field changes quickly. There may be other reasons that you would want one drug rather than another. Cyclophosphomide is more likely to cause premature menopause in young women who may still want to have biological children. Anthracyclines are more likely to cause heart problems and may not be a good choice for women with, or at risk for, heart disease. Women who receive taxane chemotherapy followed by an aromatase inhibitor have four times more problems with their joints.[43] As we become more successful in treating breast cancer, the side effects of the various therapies become more important and need to be weighed in your risk versus benefit equation. Make sure your oncologist discusses with you the short- and long-term side effects of the therapy being proposed so that you will not be surprised later.

Drug intensity and drug dosage are also issues. Dose intensity refers to how high the total dose can be over a set period of time, while dose density refers to how short the time in which the same dose can be given. Investigators have studied the dose of given drugs being received over a period of time. While studies have shown that dose intensity is important, they have indicated that individual agents have a threshold dose that must be achieved. Dose reduction below that threshold appears to be associated with poorer outcomes, but dose escalation beyond the threshold increases side effects to the patient while contributing no added cancer benefit. High-dose chemotherapy with stem cell rescue is a good example of this. So-called bone marrow transplant was an attempt to improve the benefit to women at high risk of recurrence. Patients were given such high doses of chemotherapy that their bone marrow was wiped out and they needed stem cells to reconstitute it. Multiple randomized studies showed it to be more toxic but no more effective than standard regimens.[44,45]

Because high dose was not better, researchers started to look at the schedule the drugs were given on. The standard program has been to give three different drugs with three different mechanisms of action simultaneously. This works but is limited somewhat by the combined toxicities of the drugs, restricting the maximum doses that can be given of any one drug. In the dose dense model, the interval between two courses is shortened, while the dose of each course may be increased, decreased, or made equivalent to a standard dose so that the dose per unit of time is higher. In one study, the drugs were given every two weeks instead of every three. Preliminary results showed that after three years there was a 4 percent improvement in disease-free survival and a 2 percent improvement in overall survival compared to the three-week version.[46] This schedule of chemotherapy, however, required that women receive GCSF (granulocyte-stimulating factor), a drug that stimulates the bone marrow to recover faster from the chemotherapy. Further, the treatments were more difficult for some women to take because there was little down time. The fact that they ended sooner made up for that among some patients.

Since there are choices to be made among different chemotherapy drugs, it's especially important for the patient to enter into the decision-making process. Ask why your doctor has chosen a particular treatment regimen and ask to see studies that back it up. Find out exactly what the differences are in efficacy and side effects. For example, as I explained earlier, some drugs are more likely to put you into menopause and thus render you infertile than others (see Chapter 17). Some, like doxorubicin (Adriamycin), can be more toxic to the heart. So you may prefer to stick with the CMF or you may be willing to take a slightly higher risk, hoping that the stronger drug will be better. If you don't feel you are getting straight answers from your oncologist, get a second opinion. If a clinical trial is available, consider participating in it so that we will get some answers (see Chapter 10). You can get accurate numbers for your own case in a several ways. There are two programs available to oncologists (Adjuvant! at www.adjuvantonline.com or Numeracy at www.mayoclinic .com/calcs from the Mayo Clinic) and one for patients from Nexcura (this can be found on the homepage of my website www.dr-susanloveresearchfoundation.org under Decision Tools) that can calculate more precise numbers for you. Ask your oncologist to provide you with the data from the Adjuvant! and Mayo Clinic sites. You are smart enough to take control of this decision.

Timing of Chemotherapy

Classically, chemotherapy treatment follows local treatment. But another course is *neoadjuvant* (or *preoperative*) chemotherapy. This means that chemotherapy is given before surgery, after a diagnosis is made with a core or needle biopsy. Because chemotherapy is the most important treatment, dealing with the life-threatening element of the cancer, some of us thought that giving it first might make a difference in survival. Unfortunately none of the studies have shown this to be true. However, we have found two advantages. First, we can see whether or not the chemo works. If the tumor starts melting away, we know the chemotherapy is working. If it's not working, we can turn to a different one. The National Surgical Adjuvant Breast and Bowel Project (NSABP) study of neoadjuvant chemotherapy found an 80 percent reduction in the tumor size, and in 36 percent of women the tumor completely disappeared.[47] This allowed doctors to do lumpectomies in 8 percent of women who would otherwise have needed mastectomies (67.8 percent versus 59.8 percent). The issue is that if chemotherapy is going to be needed at some point in the treatment process (high-risk cancer, Her-2 positive, ER negative, palpable nodes), then perhaps giving the chemotherapy first can offer improvement in the surgical management and the information we get about the tumor biology. Today, most surgeons will consider preoperative chemotherapy for tumors over 3 centimeters in women who wish to have lumpectomy. If the tumor is smaller, which would allow a lumpectomy anyway, and if the doctors are not certain before surgery whether chemotherapy will be required, it is better to wait until after the surgery.

The caveat to this recommendation is that preoperative chemotherapy may not shrink the tumor enough to prevent mastectomy, particularly those tumors like lobular cancers that are estrogen sensitive. On the other hand, estrogen receptor positive cancers in postmenopausal women have been effectively treated with neoadjuvant hormonal therapy, particularly aromatase inhibitors. The American College of Surgical Oncology group is doing a trial of neoadjuvant hormone therapy with aromatase inhibitors. It is great to have a drug clinical trial sponsored by surgeons.

Combinations of Systemic Therapy

We can classify most cancers into one of the four categories discussed previously and from there come up with the likely combination of drugs. Women with estrogen receptor negative tumors will be offered chemotherapy with the addition of trastuzumab (Herceptin) if their tumor shows high levels of Her-2/neu. Women with an estrogen receptor positive tumor that is over a centimeter will be offered hormone therapy and possibly chemotherapy, depending on their risk (see Chapter 11 for a discussion of Oncotype DX and Mammaprint). If the tumor is also Her-2/neu positive, then chemotherapy and trastuzumab will be added. Although early studies suggested that chemotherapy worked better in premenopausal women, it now looks like the hormone receptor status of the tumor is also important, and these combinations are recommended across all ages. There is a caveat, however, for women over 70. Generally they have not been included in the studies and therefore we do not have good data for them. If you are over 70 and in good health, it is probably reasonable for you to undergo the same regimen as a younger woman. It is not your numerical age but any other conditions and life expectancy that should affect your decision to undergo toxic therapy for small improvements in survival.

TARGETED THERAPIES

Hormone Therapy

Since 1890, doctors have been interested in the hormonal manipulation of breast cancers. In fact, the first adjuvant therapies were based on changing the body's hormonal milieu. If a premenopausal woman had a "bad" cancer, her ovaries were removed in an attempt to decrease the total amount of estrogen in her system. The idea was good, and recent studies show a survival difference between women who had ovarian ablation and those who did not. This difference is as great as or greater than that with chemotherapy.[48]

Now we can actually predict who is likely to benefit from adjuvant hormone therapy by using the estrogen and progesterone receptor test described in Chapter 11. In women with hormone-sensitive tumors, we can use a hormone treatment as adjuvant therapy—though it is useless and even potentially harmful in women whose tumors are not sensitive to either estrogen or progesterone.

We are also are starting to understand how these hormone therapies work. What they probably do, at least in part, is change the environment around the cell, resulting in control or even death of the cancer cell (see Chapter 4). This can happen in a number of different ways. Currently we have two different adjuvant hormone approaches: reducing the production of estrogen or blocking the estrogen receptor on the cell.

Tamoxifen

You sometimes hear that tamoxifen throws premenopausal women into menopause. Actually, it's more complicated than that. Tamoxifen stimulates the ovaries to make more estrogen. While blocking estrogen receptors in the breast, it is acting *like* estrogen in other organs, such as the bone and uterus. (See SERMs, Chapter 7.) This trait is responsible for both its negative side effects, such as uterine cancer and blood clots, and its benefits, such as increased bone density and lower cholesterol. Tamoxifen is still the hormone treatment of choice for premenopausal women, with or without ovarian ablation (see below). Sometimes women and doctors act as if it is not as good as some of the newer drugs because it is old and has been around a long time. This is certainly not true. In fact because it is an old drug, we know a lot more about it. We know all about its side effects as well as its benefits. We have a lot less experience with some of the newer aromatase inhibitors. (An added benefit with tamoxifen is financial: because it's been around so long it has become a generic drug.)

The 2004 overview of treatment for early breast cancer found that tamoxifen doesn't help with estrogen receptor negative tumors.[49] But with estrogen receptor positive tumors, it has a benefit across the board. The reduction in the odds of recurrence is 29 percent, and the reduction in the chance of death is 24 percent in women between 40 and 49. This means that while women are on tamoxifen, one of every three recurrences and approximately one of every four deaths are prevented. Looking at absolute reductions, we find an 11 percent decrease in recurrence and a 6.8 percent reduction in death at 10 years for premenopausal women who have taken tamoxifen (with or without chemotherapy as well) for 5 years. For postmenopausal women it is 15 percent decrease in recurrence and 8.2 percent reduction in death at 10 years. As I pointed out earlier in the chapter, the absolute benefit depends in part on the risk and may not be proportional. By that I mean that the benefits may not be as good for the high-risk woman as for the low-risk one. The aromatase inhibitors are a fairly recent addition for postmenopausal women and will be discussed below.

When I lecture, women often come to me and say they're taking tamoxifen but having side effects, and they want to know if they need to continue on it. I suggest they check with their oncologist about why they're taking it. The tendency now is for oncologists to put every estrogen receptor positive premenopausal woman on it because it benefits everyone. But it benefits by different amounts, and if you're in a category in which the benefit is only 1–2 percent and it's making your life miserable, you may not want to stay with it. On the other hand, if you're in the 11 percent category, the suffering may be worth that chance. So it's important to ask your oncologist what benefit tamoxifen offers you, given your specific breast cancer scenario.

Though tamoxifen is the best studied drug for women whose tumors are sensitive to hormones, we don't know yet whether it is the best *working* drug. One area of active study is whether all women metabolize tamoxifen the same way. Endoxifen, the active metabolite of tamoxifen, is lower in women who carry a specific variant of a gene known as the CYP2D6 gene. This genetic variant is present in 7 percent of white women and even more in women of Asian descent. Other women (5 percent of whites) have multiple copies of the gene, which can lead them to ultra high metabolism of the drug and higher levels of the active ingredient. These variations in metabolism may be responsible for the range of tamoxifen's side effects. As of this writing, the data are not clear enough to make recommendations—but stay tuned for more information on this front.

Ovarian Ablation

Blocking the estrogen receptor is one way to deprive the breast cancer cell of estrogen; another is to remove the source of the hormones. In premenopausal women this is the ovary. There are three ways to do this: surgery, radiation, or hormonal manipulation—all of these are known as *ablating* the ovaries. Unless you are a carrier of the BRCA 1 or 2 gene and therefore at higher risk of subsequent ovarian cancer, surgery probably is not the best way of doing this. The surgery is irreversible: if it doesn't help with the cancer, we can't return your ovaries to you. So you're stuck with all the consequences of having no ovaries—a condition that recent studies have shown increases overall mortality.[50]

Sometimes doctors can irradiate ovaries instead of removing them, saving the patient the pain of surgery. The problem here is that it's hard to aim precisely at these small organs, and intestines in the area can also get radiated, causing possible problems. Further, like surgery, it's permanent.

Today we can use gonadotropin-releasing hormone agonists (GnRH), originally developed for endometriosis, that block the ovaries and essentially put you into a temporary menopause. This approach seems to work as well as surgery or radiation and has the advantage of being reversible.

The most thoroughly tested drug for doing this in breast cancer is goserelin (also known as Zoladex). In a 1998 study, women were put on goserelin for three to five years to see if it had the same effect as oophorectomy, and it did.[51] In the study, premenopausal node-positive and estrogen receptive positive women were randomized to take CMF chemotherapy or goserelin for two years. With 7.3 years of follow-up there has been no difference between the two groups. Most interesting to me was the fact that most of the women on goserelin got their periods back after the therapy was completed and yet did just as well as the women on CMF, who stopped menstruating permanently. In other words, just as with tamoxifen, a short time (2–3 years) of decreased estrogen production was enough to change these women's prognosis. On the other hand, the estrogen positive women who did not become menopausal on CMF did significantly worse than those who stopped menstruating.[52] Obviously part of the benefit of the chemotherapy was that it put these women into menopause. Further studies have shown that adding tamoxifen to the goserelin is even more effective.[53]

This leads me to believe that ovarian suppression may help women who are still menstruating after completing chemotherapy and are estrogen receptor positive. Tamoxifen is a good alternative in these women as well. Women who stop their periods can consider the aromatase inhibitors if hormone therapy is indicated—so we'll talk about them next.

Aromatase Inhibitors

Removing the ovaries or blocking them with drugs has much less effect on women who are already postmenopausal: their main source of estrogen is no longer their ovaries. Instead, the precursors of estrogen, such as testosterone and androstenedione, are produced in the ovaries and the adrenal glands and then secreted into the blood stream, where specific organs pick them up and convert them into estrogen through an enzyme called aromatase. This enzyme has been found in the adrenal glands, fat, breast, brain, and muscles, and is responsible for much of the local estrogen in postmenopausal women. (Other enzymes such as sulfatase may also be important in this regard.) In addition, fairly recent studies show that postmenopausal women with breast cancer have aromatase in their breast tissue, giving the breast its own supply of estrogen.[54] So to reduce estrogen levels in the tissues of postmenopausal women we need to block aromatase. A class of drugs called aromatase inhibitors (AIs) can do this with minimal side effects.

Three drugs that block aromatase are available clinically. Anastrozole (Arimidex) and letrozole (Femara) work by reversibly blocking this enzyme, while exemestane (Aromasin) binds to the enzyme and inactivates it permanently. These drugs were first tested in women with estrogen positive metastatic disease. All of them had favorable effects (see Chapter 19). Anastrozole was then studied head to head against tamoxifen and showed a small advantage. Randomized trials have shown that initial treatment with an aromatase inhibitor and the sequence of tamoxifen followed by an aromatase inhibitor are acceptable strategies. Unlike tamoxifen, aromatase inhibitors have no estrogenic effects. This gives them a whole different set of side effects, including bone and joint pain, and, more significantly, increases in fractures. Interestingly, the women who took both tamoxifen and anastrozole at the same time did no better than the women who took only tamoxifen. One theory is that tamoxifen acts more like estrogen when total body levels of estrogen are low.

Because of the way they work, aromatase inhibitors have no current role in the treatment of premenopausal women with estrogen positive tumors. Although some doctors have suggested using goserelin to temporarily induce menopause in premenopausal women so that they can take an AI, this has not been demonstrated to be better than goserelin plus tamoxifen.[55] As yet we have no data on the safety of aromatase inhibitors in women rendered postmenopausal with chemotherapy, so we probably should not use them without further ovarian suppression, since many of these women still have significant estrogen levels. It is also not clear that the results would be the same in women with menopause induced by GnRH agonists like goserelin, although this is actively being studied.

Nonhormonal Targeted Therapy

Trastuzumab (Herceptin). In addition to the efforts to destroy cancer cells or change their hormonal milieu, there is a new form of drug designed to attack a target on the cancer cell in hopes of reducing its malignant potential. Trastuzumab is the first drug of this category in clinical use. It is the antibody to the Her-2/neu oncogene, which is overexpressed in 20 percent of women with breast cancer. It was first tested in women with metastatic disease and shown to have a beneficial effect, both alone and with chemotherapy.[56,57] Subsequent studies have shown its benefits as an adjuvant therapy, and it also can reduce recurrence by one-half at three years after administration. All women with tumors over 1 centimeter or positive nodes whose tumors overexpress Her-2/neu are now given one year of trastuzumab, unless there is a contraindication, such as cardiac disease.[58] Some doctors may recommend trastuzumab for even smaller tumors, based on new data that indicate Her-2 positive tumors pose a significant risk for spreading, even when caught early.[59] Ongoing studies are evaluating shorter and longer durations of therapy. Trastuzumab can be given at the same time as some drugs but not others, depending on the specific drug and possible interactions (see Chapter 17).

Bisphosphonates. Another way to change the environment to make it less supportive of cancer is the use of bisphosphonates. Bisphosphonates are drugs like alendronate or Fosamax, commonly used to treat osteoporosis and prevent bone loss. Since they function well in conditions where bone is being absorbed, they were first used to treat bone metastases and had some success. Studies were then launched to see if they could prevent bone metastases as well. This goal was combined with the consideration of preventing bone loss in women on aromatase inhibitors in the studies known as Z fast and ZO fast, in which post-menopausal hormone positive women took up-front zoledronic acid, a bisphosphonate, to prevent them from losing bone right away, or only if needed. Data showed a lower recurrence rate in the women who received the zoledronic acid (also known as Zometa) up front (1.1 percent versus 2.3 percent).[60,61] Two more large studies that are awaiting completion will indicate whether they will have the same effect in postmenopausal women who have estrogen receptor negative tumors and who are receiving chemotherapy. And of course there are side effects. The more serious are kidney failure and areas of exposed and necrotic (dead) bone in the jaw. Both of these are uncommon, but women should be tested for kidney function and have all needed dental work prior to starting this regimen. Bisphosphonates are not yet standard in care for all patients (and are not covered by many insurance programs) but may be worth pursuing for the highest-risk patents, until definitive data emerge.

LIFESTYLE CHANGES

Accumulating data suggest that lifestyle changes can also have an adjuvant effect. The ones that have been studied the most are weight loss, diet, and physical activity. The influence of excess weight on breast cancer outcomes was recently examined in a group of 14,709 women with localized disease. Being overweight increased the chances of metastases, second cancers in the other breast, and decreased overall survival. In the Nurses' Health Study higher weight at diagnosis was associated with decreased survival, and another study of 3,924 women with localized breast cancer showed that women with a body mass index over 30 were more likely than lean women to die of their breast cancer.[62] Several other studies have confirmed this effect, but to date there have been no prospective randomized studies. The LISA study being conducted out of Canada will help determine whether weight loss decreases the risk of cancer recurrence in breast cancer survivors, but until then it is probably prudent for women who are newly diagnosed and overweight to try to lose that weight. In this case the side effects are minimal and the improvement in overall health significant. The exact diet appears to be less important than we would like to think, although randomized studies have not been done. The other recommendation is for physical activity. Here the data are similar. Several studies show that women who participate in physical activity for at least 30 minutes a day have a lower likelihood of recurrence than couch potatoes. The more activity, the better the outcome. While randomized studies have not been done yet, the risk is low, and it's something virtually everyone can do.

SYSTEMIC TREATMENT: SUMMARY

This chapter has described the menu of adjuvant treatments. At this point you and your doctor need to consider it in relation to your situation and particular kind of breast cancer (see Chapters 11 and 13). We are moving into the era of personalized medicine, rather than one size fits all. So the global recommendations that you may have found in previous editions of this book have given way to descriptions of particular scenarios. That being said, I will try to summarize where we are in general, so that you have a place to start.

Women with positive lymph nodes are generally given chemotherapy regardless of their hormone status. However, the Oncotype DX test can be used in postmenopausal women to forgo chemotherapy if the recurrence score is low (see Chapter 11). If the tumor overexpresses Her-2/neu, you will be given Herceptin for one year. If you are estrogen receptor positive, you will also probably receive a hormone regimen such as tamoxifen, ovarian ablation, and/or an aromatase inhibitor.

A 2008 analysis of all the studies of estrogen negative women who received chemotherapy versus those who did not demonstrated a decrease in recurrence as well as a decrease in mortality at 10 years. The decrease is higher in the woman under 50, with a decrease of recurrence of 12 percent and death 8 percent. In women between 50 and 69 the decrease is 10 percent for recurrence and 6.0 percent for mortality.[63] Of course, these numbers are based on older chemotherapy treatments that were less targeted. Now we can better categorize your tumor and target the therapy, which should result in better outcomes.

All this means that deciding whether or not to have systemic treatment, and if so which one, is complicated. You may want to look at the practice guidelines from the NCCN online at www.nccn.org to give you a guideline. And you certainly will want to discuss with your doctor all the prognostic information you can (Oncotype DX testing if done, Her-2 status, grade of tumor, etc). This can all be helpful in understanding your individual risks and benefits.

Finally, lifestyle changes and complementary treatments (the subject of Chapter 18) are actually a form of systemic treatment and should be considered by everyone.

SECOND OPINIONS

It's always wise to consider getting a second opinion, no matter how much you trust your surgeon or oncologist's advice. The preference for a treatment is always somewhat subjective, and you're entitled to consult with more than one expert. Furthermore, special kinds of cancer may require a different approach than your doctor's, and different institutions may be involved in different research with new treatments you may be interested in.

Several breast centers in the country have multidisciplinary programs, in which you can meet with all the specialists involved in your care at the same place. And there is currently a National Approval Program for Breast Centers (NAPBC), which will be able to assure you of a certain level of quality. In most of them you can be self-referred—you don't have to be referred by a doctor. I would recommend that any woman with breast cancer research the possibilities of hooking up with one of these centers.

If looking to a multidisciplinary program for a second opinion doesn't sound optimal for you, try a single expert who knows the field and specializes in breast cancer. Either a breast surgeon or medical oncologist specializing in breast cancer is more likely to be able to talk to you about chemotherapy and radiation therapy than a general surgeon.

And don't be afraid of hurting your original doctor's feelings. Most doctors welcome another point of view—and if yours doesn't, you should probably be looking for another doctor anyway.

This field is changing constantly. Yesterday's answer may be passé today. I suggest you supplement the information in this book with other sources and especially the Internet. On my website, www.drsusanloveresearchfoundation.org, or on the NIH website, www.cancer.gov, you can find the latest studies and up-to-date information to add to the overview given here.

Chapter 13

SPECIAL SITUATIONS AND POPULATIONS

So far, I've been discussing breast cancer in general, the overall benefit of various treatments, and the overall risk of getting the disease. But as I have been repeating throughout this edition, all breast cancers are not the same. There are different types based on molecular biology, on the way they are diagnosed, or even on the people who get them. In this chapter I am going to become bit more specific. I wish we could tell you exactly how we'd treat your ER positive Her-2/neu positive cancer when you're a forty-year-old vegetarian who has had her ovaries removed and had her first child at 20. In other words, I'd like to be able to give each one of you a prescription for the best treatment for you. But since that's not possible, I'll do the next best thing and at least hone in on some aspects of various specific forms of breast cancer.

NONINVASIVE CANCER: DCIS AND LCIS

In ductal cancer in situ (DCIS) and lobular cancer in situ (LCIS), you have cells that look like cancer cells and even have the molecular changes of cancer cells but are completely

363

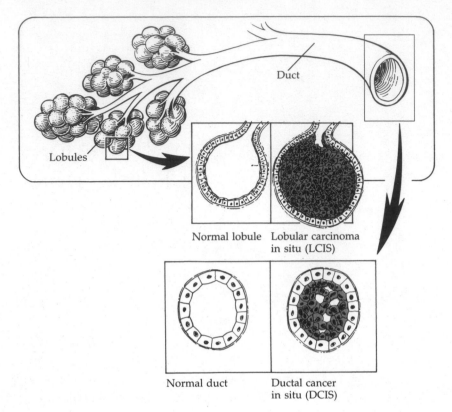

Figure 13.1

contained within the lobule or duct (Figure 13.1). These tumors are called noninvasive breast cancer because they have not spread outside of their normal territory into the stroma. And until they do that, they cannot enter a blood vessel and spread to the rest of the body. Current thinking is that it is not the cells that develop the ability to break out of the duct but rather the neighborhood that allows or even invites them out (Figure 13.2). Think of a prison surrounded by ferocious guards keeping the inmates inside the walls. Then someone comes around with a jug of whiskey and gets the guards drunk, and before you know it they are inviting the prisoners out. How this happens is not totally clear, but what *is* clear is that not everyone who has DCIS or LCIS will go on to develop invasive cancer. The treatments, as I will explain at length later, include either strengthening the

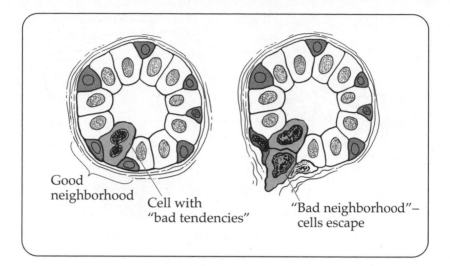

Figure 13.2

neighborhood cells with tamoxifen and/or removing the mutated cells so that they can't cause trouble.

While we have worked out the differences in breast cancers in respect to the invasive tumors, we are only just beginning to apply this understanding to the noninvasive lesions. Are they, like invasive cancers, different from each other? Should they be dealt with differently? Maybe. This is a particularly active area of research these days. Studies of DCIS have found many of the types of cancer that are seen in invasive disease, although not in the same distribution. For example, DCIS shows a higher percentage of luminal B and Her-2/neu positive tumors and somewhat less luminal A and basal than invasive ductal cancer (see Chapter 11). Consequently there may not be a direct route from one to the other, as if, for example, all luminal A DCIS that grew into cancer became luminal A invasive ductal cancer.[1] An intriguing study by Craig Allred from Washington University in St. Louis suggests that at least a third of DCIS showed a combination of types.[2] He proposes that only the most aggressive or "fittest" cells or types go on to become invasive. What makes these types is so interesting is that that they may direct therapy in the future for these lesions, just as they do for invasive cancer.

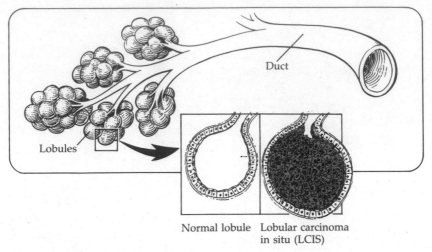

Normal lobule   Lobular carcinoma
                in situ (LCIS)

Figure 13.3

And they also may give us some clues about the causes of the disease.

I have debated whether to discuss these "noninvasive cancers" in the section about prevention or in the section about cancer. Since most women who are diagnosed with LCIS or DCIS consider themselves as having cancer, and indeed in medicine we've tended to move from the language of "precancer" to "noninvasive cancer," I have settled on discussing them as a special type here. Still I like the word "precancer," which is much less formal sounding than noninvasive cancer, so I will use both terms.

Lobular Cancer in Situ

Under the microscope, LCIS appears as a bunch of small, round cells stuffing the lobules, which normally don't contain any cells (Figure 13.3). Such clusters of cells have been termed "multicentric" because they can be scattered throughout both breasts. However, no one has tied them to one ductal system, as we have with DCIS. We may not always be accurate in this: since the lobules are at the periphery of each ductal branch, the LCIS could appear scattered while actually being part of the same branch of ducts.

We thought we knew the natural history of LCIS based on studies by Cushman Haagensen in 1978, but recent work has challenged our previous ideas. The old theory was that LCIS doesn't grow into cancer but signals a possible danger—the way, for example, an overcast day warns you it may rain. Because of this, many experts believed that lobular carcinoma in situ wasn't a true precancer but more of a risk factor. Recent data, however, suggests that this may not be the case. The first piece of evidence that LCIS can actually progress to invasive lobular cancer came from a 2004 analysis of 180 women who had participated in a study of the National Surgical Adjuvant Breast and Bowel Project (NSABP).[3] Overall they found after 12 years of follow-up that nine (5 percent) invasive breast cancers developed in the same breast as the original lesions, and eight of these (89 percent) were invasive lobular cancers—in the same area as the original LCIS. A second piece of evidence was a study of women who had both LCIS and invasive lobular cancer in the same breast. The pattern of mutations in the involved cells was very similar, suggesting that one had indeed evolved from the other.[4] More recently molecular studies have shown that both LCIS and infiltrating lobular cancers are estrogen positive and Her-2/neu negative, and they lack expression of the protein E-cadherin,[5] which helps cells stick together. Its absence may help explain why lobular cancers don't cling together in a nice lump but march cell by cell through the stroma in single file lines forming a diffuse pattern that is often difficult to detect.

Three other studies have been published since 1996, including one of 214 women with LCIS, which suggest a continuous 1 percent per year risk of developing invasive breast cancer.[6,7,8] This risk can be compounded by other risk factors for breast cancer (see Table 12.1).

What can you do if you have lobular carcinoma in situ? Basically you want to prevent yourself from getting invasive breast cancer. There are a number of options; the most drastic is bilateral prophylactic mastectomy. Why bilateral (both breasts)? Because the risk occurs in both breasts. In the NSABP study mentioned above, there was a 5 percent chance of getting an invasive cancer in the same breast and a similar 5 percent chance of getting an invasive cancer in the opposite one.

Some women choose bilateral mastectomies because they want to know they've done everything possible. That way if they do get breast cancer, they feel that at least it isn't their fault. If they hadn't had this surgery and then developed the disease, they'd always wonder if they could have prevented it. In the mid-1980s a patient told me, "I knew instantly what my decision should be. I was astounded to see how greedy for life I was." This woman was in a high-risk group because of her family history; she had relatives with breast cancer and was determined to do all she could to avoid suffering with it herself. She was uncomfortable with the studies about monitoring, which she thought were too recent, while mastectomy had been around a long time. She was helped by the knowledge that she could then have breast reconstruction, which we'll look at in Chapter 15.

The alternative to surgery is close monitoring—follow-up exams every six months, with a yearly mammogram or MRI for the very high-risk woman. That way if a cancer does develop you're likely to catch it and can decide then if you want to have a mastectomy or a lumpectomy and radiation (see Chapter 14). If a cancer doesn't develop, you've been spared the ordeal of major and disfiguring surgery. This approach is what most surgeons, including myself, recommend and is supported by the NSABP group. Most of my patients have opted for this course.

Another alternative to mastectomy is the practice of taking tamoxifen or raloxifene (in postmenopausal women) for five years to prevent the future development of breast cancer. These estrogen-blocking drugs have been shown to decrease the chance of getting breast cancer by 56 percent in women with LCIS. Remember this means that the risk becomes half of the original risk—about 0.5 percent a year as opposed to 1 percent per year. All of the drugs have side effects that must be taken into consideration (see Chapter 17). In addition, they are not safe to take if you are trying to get pregnant; tamoxifen taken during pregnancy can cause birth defects. However, not all the side effects are bad. In postmenopausal women, both tamoxifen and raloxifene can help prevent fractures. This is a decision that, like so many, depends a lot on how you personally weigh the pros and cons.

If you're diagnosed with LCIS, give yourself time to think about what you want to do. LCIS doesn't call for an immediate decision. A woman called me once in a panic because she had been diagnosed with LCIS and was told by her oncologist that she should start on tamoxifen immediately. She was appropriately uncomfortable with this. He was treating it as if it were cancer and not a precancerous or noninvasive lesion. The risk of developing invasive cancer is 1 percent per year, so there is no rush to begin a treatment. I suggested to this woman that she take the follow-up route initially, and see how she felt about it in six months or a year. If she was comfortable living with it, then she could continue this course for the rest of her life, or until a cancer occurred. You can always decide on tamoxifen or mastectomy later, but you can't undo a mastectomy, and you may not be able to undo some of tamoxifen's side effects. However, if a woman finds herself living in a constant state of anxiety, waking up every morning thinking, "This is it—this is the day I'll find the lump," then maybe a bilateral mastectomy is best for her. Invasive lobular cancers are much more common in women who take hormone therapy, so HT is not a good idea for women with LCIS.

Radiation and chemotherapy are not necessary treatments for LCIS because it's not really cancer. As we reconsider the data on its ability to progress to cancer, we are also rethinking our treatment. Should we, or even could we, remove it all? Usually LCIS is scattered throughout an area of the breast. (Remember that the lobules are like the leaves on a tree.) Wide excision is probably not realistic and therefore not worth attempting.

Sometimes when a patient has a lump that turns out to be cancer, the pathologist will find LCIS in the adjacent tissue. What does this mean? In essence it suggests that the patient was at a higher risk of getting breast cancer and, sure enough, she got it. A number of studies show that women with LCIS associated with their invasive cancer who get a lumpectomy have the same risk of local recurrence and contralateral breast cancer as those without LCIS.[9,10,11,12]

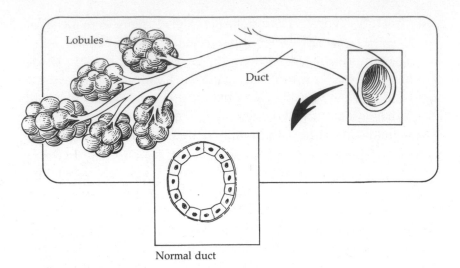

Figure 13.4

Ductal Carcinoma (DCIS) in Situ

DCIS is more common than LCIS, and it is more likely to grow into an invasive cancer. DCIS rarely forms lumps, but it does sometimes form a soft thickening (caused by the pliable ducts becoming less pliable because they're filled with cells; see Figure 13.4). DCIS is now found far more frequently because of mammograms, where it appears as little specks of calcium or microcalcifications. A full 20 percent of malignancies detected by screening mammography are DCIS. In fact, it's probably very common. Autopsies done on women who died from all kinds of other causes show that between 6 and 16 percent had DCIS.[13,14] This suggests that many of us have it unknowingly; it is probably not, as we used to believe, a rare condition.

In the past, standard treatment was a mastectomy of the breast with the lesion. That worked most of the time, but it might not have been necessary. Since the breasts had been removed, we had no way of studying what happened when a breast that had DCIS *wasn't* removed.

A few small studies, however, have given us a clue. Two studies followed women who were biopsied and thought to have something benign. These studies, in which the biopsied tissue was examined years later, have led us to believe that about 20–25 percent of women with untreated low-grade DCIS will go on to get invasive cancer up to 25 years after the initial biopsy, and in the same area of the breast in which that biopsy was done.[15,16] Since the studies together add up to only 78 patients, they may not be representative. Furthermore, the lesions were on the border between atypical hyperplasia (see Chapter 6) and DCIS or they would have been diagnosed initially; the studies don't address the situation of women with obvious DCIS. What is clear from these studies, however, is that untreated DCIS can go on to invasive breast cancer but in the majority of women apparently doesn't.

Unfortunately, we don't know how to tell which cases will become invasive and which won't. There's a lot of research going on in molecular biology seeking a marker that clearly shows which lesions are on their way to becoming invasive and which will never do so. The other critical question is whether DCIS is confined to one "sick duct"[17] or represents changes that are going on throughout the whole breast (multicentric). This is important not only in terms of our scientific understanding of DCIS but in an immediate way for patients diagnosed with the disease. If it were multicentric, it would lend itself to the argument that you may as well have mastectomies in both breasts because it is only a matter of time until the second breast gets cancer. But if DCIS is actually unicentric, the wiser treatment would be to remove the one affected section of the affected breast.

Most high-grade lesions tend to be continuous and well marked by calcifications that are visible on a mammogram. Low- to intermediate-grade lesions, however, can be more sneaky, with discontinuous intraductal spread, often having gaps of up to 1 centimeter between areas of involvement.

What we currently do is a wide excision based on our best guess of the extent of disease. We arrive at this guess by looking at the preoperative mammogram and magnification views, and then studying the tissue we remove from the breast. Although over 80 percent of DCIS is diagnosed by the presence of microcalcifications on a mammogram, some parts of the DCIS may not have

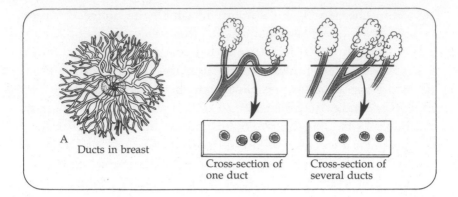

A
Ducts in breast

Cross-section of
one duct

Cross-section of
several ducts

Figure 13.5

microcalcifications and so are essentially invisible to the surgeon. That can make it tricky to know exactly how much breast tissue to remove (Fig 13.5).

In deciding what to remove, we look at the margins (see Chapter 11) and look for a normal rim of tissue (1 mm) around the diseased area. This is not perfect, however, so when there's a "recurrence" of DCIS, it's often not a recurrence at all; it's DCIS that we left behind in the first place, in spite of what we thought were clean margins. This doesn't happen frequently, but often enough (about 10–20 percent of the time) to make it significant. That's why surgery is often followed with radiation therapy. And also why mastectomy, though imperfect, tends to give a lower recurrence rate—it's the widest excision possible.

It is also important to look at a postbiopsy mammogram. This is usually done about a month or so after surgery. Since DCIS usually shows up on the mammogram as calcifications, it is important to make sure that all suspicious calcifications have been removed with the surgery. As already noted, however, DCIS can be present without calcifications.

The goal of treating DCIS is prevention. When the lesion is completely removed, it can neither come back nor become invasive. The question is how much surgery is necessary. Reasons for mastectomy are the same for DCIS as they are for invasive cancer: if the extent of the lesion is too large to allow a cosmetic excision then a mastectomy (with or without immediate reconstruction—see Chapter 14) is indicated. This can sometimes be predicted before the operation when there are extensive malignant-appearing calcifications throughout the breast. In other cases, several attempts are made to excise all the disease but the margins remain positive.

Since DCIS can fill a whole ductal system, some of which take up a third of the breast, these lesions can be fairly extensive in their reach. Monica Morrow from Memorial Sloan Kettering found that about 33 percent of women with DCIS ended up needing mastectomies, while women with stage 1 invasive cancers forming very discrete lumps required mastectomy only 10 percent of the time.[18] While you might think that MRI would be as good as or better than mammogram at predicting the extent of disease, this has not proven to be the case for DCIS.[19,20]

Although mastectomy is sometimes required, lumpectomy is a reasonable choice to treat DCIS, when the margins of resection are clear (see Chapter 11). Lumpectomy is usually followed with radiation therapy. Four randomized controlled studies have compared wide excision alone to wide excision and radiation for DCIS.[21,22,23,24] All of these studies found that the addition of radiation therapy reduced the risk of recurrence by 50–60 percent. In the NSABP B 24 trial, the twelve-year rate of an invasive recurrence was 18 percent, which was reduced to 8–9 percent with radiation therapy.

The second question is the use of tamoxifen. In the same study tamoxifen was shown to be beneficial for women with estrogen receptor positive DCIS, further reducing the risk of recurrence when combined with radiation by 2–3 percent. As with all other treatments, the higher your risk, the more you stand to gain.

Can we predict which women with DCIS can do without radiation? After all, 75 percent of the DCIS never recurred in those biopsy-alone studies mentioned earlier. The predictors of recurrence after breast-conserving surgery have been extensively studied. One attempt to make this distinction is to look at the architecture of the DCIS. Researchers have discovered three general patterns (Figure 13.6). One is called *micropapillary*: the cells fill the duct with a finger-like mass sticking out into the

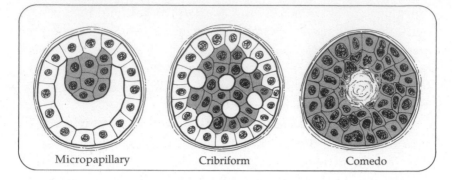

Figure 13.6

duct's center. A second is called *cribriform*: it also fills in the duct but there are punched-out holes like Swiss cheese. These are low-grade patterns sometimes referred to avs *noncomedo*. The third is called *comedo* for its resemblance to a closed comedo, which is a whitehead pimple. This is the high-grade pattern. The cells are stuffing the duct, and some of them are necrotic (dead). There is also a lot of apoptosis (cell death), and there are very aberrant cells. If the tissue around the duct is squeezed, white, cheesy material comes out, exactly as if you were squeezing a pimple. And of course these patterns do not exclude each other, so there can be combinations of the above.

The two key features that appear to be predictive of recurrence are whether the cells are high-grade and necrotic. In addition, younger women have a greater rate of local recurrence than older ones. There is no reason to remove lymph nodes for small areas of DCIS because noninvasive cancer can't spread at this stage. But if the lesions are big (greater than 5 centimeters), some experts think they may hide microinvasion and recommend removing the lymph nodes as well. (Sentinel node biopsy, discussed in Chapter 12, is a good option here; most experts agree that removing all the lymph nodes is not necessary, unless the sentinel node contains cancer.) On the other hand, many surgeons will forgo lymph node surgery in this group as well, since even with microinvasion the chance of having positive nodes is very low.[25] The new NCCN guidelines recommend not doing a sentinel node biopsy with breast conservation for DCIS. If the wide excision demonstrates invasive carcinoma, the surgeon can go back to the few patients with invasion, rather than create a risk of lymphedema (see Chapter 19) if there is no invasion.

Treatment Options for DCIS

What does all this mean for you? How should you proceed? First, if your routine mammogram has shown a cluster of microcalcifications, you'll need to have a core biopsy. This will determine whether you have DCIS. If the core biopsy does show DCIS, make sure your pathology report includes information regarding the grade, presence of necrosis, and estrogen receptor status. Then you've got the four choices described above: wide excision alone, wide excision and radiation, a combination of those with tamoxifen, or mastectomy.

Most surgeons will recommend a wide excision. This means taking out the area with a centimeter-wide rim of normal tissue around it. Sometimes this has been done on the first operation and other times it is necessary to go back and remove more tissue (a reexcision). This will usually be followed by radiation therapy. You can add five years of tamoxifen to any of the choices above if the DCIS is estrogen receptor positive (a bonus of doing this may be not in treating the DCIS but in preventing an invasive cancer or one in the other breast).

Mastectomy, as noted earlier, is the ultimate wide excision. Most of the time this will be more than adequate, but there have been reports of DCIS recurring in the remaining breast tissue.[26,27] It happens in about 2 percent of cases. Generally we do a mastectomy only if the DCIS is so extensive that it's the only choice or if the patient strongly wants it.[28]

One final alternative to the above standard treatment options for DCIS includes a plan of "watchful waiting" for low-risk DCIS. Shelly Hwang at UCSF is evaluating women with DCIS who have chosen to decline surgery and instead choose to take either tamoxifen or an aromatase inhibitor. We will wait to see whether this approach can safely prevent the need for mastectomy or even surgery altogether in some women with DCIS.

As we were putting the final touches on this chapter, an important study came out suggesting that there are molecular markers that can predict which DCIS will recur locally and which are most likely to go on to invasion. These markers will be studied on the original biopsy specimen much the way the Oncotype DX markers are. The DCIS that was detected as a lump rather than only on mammogram or is triple positive (p16, COX-2, and Ki-67) had a 19 percent risk of invasive disease over eight years, compared to 4 percent for those who were triple negative and found on mammogram. On the other hand about 5 percent of DCIS cases have characteristics that predict a local recurrence, including being estrogen negative, Her-2/neu positive, and Ki-67 positive or p16 positive, COX-2 negative, and Ki-67 positive. This work by Thea Tlsty and Karla Kerlokowske promises to be a major advance in the clinical options for women with DCIS by predicting who truly is at risk for local recurrence and therefore needs a mastectomy and who on the other hand is at risk of developing invasive disease and needs tamoxifen. If you have just been diagnosed with DCIS, it may be worth asking to have your sample tested for estrogen receptor, Her-2/neu, as well as COX-2, Ki-67, and p16.

LOCALLY ADVANCED BREAST CANCER

Once in a while, a breast cancer isn't discovered until it's fairly big—a stage 3 cancer. It is larger than 5 centimeters (2 inches), with positive lymph nodes. Or it has one of the other features that we think give it a bad prognosis, like swelling (edema) of the skin or a big, matted cluster of lymph nodes. It may be stuck to the chest muscle or ulcerating through the skin. In this situation the diagnosis of cancer is made with one or more core biopsies. These can be used to determine the type of cancer as well with such biomarkers as hormone receptors, Her-2/neu, and nuclear grade (see Chapter 11). Tests such as mammogram, ultrasound, and often an MRI are done to rule out obvious spread and determine the size of the tumor as a baseline. Sometimes even moderate-size tumors (3–5 cm in a small breast) may behave like locally advanced tumors and respond best to a combined approach.

The clinical indications, however, suggest that the cancer is likely to have spread elsewhere in your body, at least microscopically. When we find locally advanced breast cancer, we often go straight to neoadjuvant systemic therapy to destroy those cells and try to shrink the tumor. Surgery and radiation therapy then follow chemotherapy or hormone therapy, though this is done more often in Europe than the United States. Some women are nervous about leaving the tumor in the breast and want a mastectomy right away. This is a bad idea for two reasons. First, the tumor often shrinks with the chemotherapy or hormone therapy, making it more possible for doctors to do breast conservation surgery rather than a mastectomy. Even if lumpectomy is not possible after chemotherapy, it is more likely that all the cancer will be removed with negative margins. Second, the tumor's response to the chemotherapy can be a test of whether this tumor responds to a particular combination of drugs and allows them to be changed if it does not (see Chapter 17). This approach results in major shrinkage of the tumor for 75–95 percent of patients.

The group at MD Anderson Hospital has the most experience with this approach and has found that giving two different regimens of chemotherapy before surgery maximizes the response.[29] They usually start with four cycles of FAC (5-fluorouracil, Adriamycin, and cyclophosphamide) and follow with four cycles of a second taxane-containing regimen. If the tumor does not seem to be responding to the FAC after a cycle or two, an alternate chemotherapy such as Taxol can be tried sooner. Whether all the chemotherapy is given at once or one regimen before and another after does not seem to alter the outcome. If the tumor overexpresses Her-2/neu, Herceptin is added preoperatively.[30] The potential problem with surgery can be finding the tumor. In 30 percent of women treated with chemotherapy and up to 60 percent who receive Herceptin, the tumor can't be seen on exam and imaging. For this reason a clip often needs to be placed in the tumor under imaging prior to starting the systemic therapy.

Although chemotherapy is most often used for neoadjuvant therapy, occasionally hormone therapy (tamoxifen or an aromatase inhibitor) may be used, especially in older women with hormone receptor positive tumors who may not tolerate the chemotherapy well. It is also capable of shrinking the tumor and allowing less surgery. Recent data suggest that women with tumors over 3 centimeters who have a low recurrence score on Oncotype DX or Mammaprint (see Chapter 11) and/or are estrogen receptor positive with low-grade, low-proliferative tumors have a low chance of responding with neoadjuvant chemotherapy (7 percent) but do well with hormones. On the other hand, tumors that were estrogen receptor negative, high grade with high proliferative markers did well with chemotherapy given up front, with 45 percent having no apparent tumor when the area that had been involved was removed. So yet again it is important to know the biology of the tumor rather than just the size.[31]

After neoadjuvant therapy, surgery alone, radiotherapy alone, or a combination of both are currently recommended. Surgical therapy may be a total mastectomy or only a wide excision for the breast, and sentinel node biopsy or axillary dissection for the lymph nodes. The criteria for breast conservation therapy include complete resolution of skin changes, decrease in tumor size, absence of extensive lymphatic vascular invasion, and absence of extensive microcalcifications or multicentricity. In this setting the local recurrence rate and 10-year overall survival rate after breast conserving therapy are equivalent to those of early-stage disease.[32]

If the tumor has shrunk, we do a lumpectomy; if there is no change, we do a mastectomy. Even when the tumor seems to have disappeared—we can't feel it or see it on a mammogram—there may still be some cancer cells present. So we always want to do a lumpectomy at least on the spot where the tumor had been to see what's actually left. (This procedure is rather imaginatively called a ghostectomy.) If the ghostectomy is clear or shows clean margins, the patient is a candidate for radiation. Similarly, if we can do a lumpectomy and get clean margins because the lump is small, following that with radiation is sensible. If there is still a large lump or a lot of cancer at the margins, it may be best to do a mastectomy with or without immediate reconstruction. In the case of an ulceration that doesn't leave enough skin to sew together, breast reconstruction provides medical as well as cosmetic benefit, since reconstruction usually takes skin from another part of the body (see Chapter 15). At this time the lymph nodes are also checked. Although the significance of negative nodes is not the same after someone has received chemotherapy, it is still a prognostic marker of the likelihood of recurrence. Finally, after either form of surgery, the woman will have radiation therapy to reduce the chances of cancer coming back in the breast or chest wall. And if the tumor tested sensitive to hormones, either tamoxifen or an aromatase inhibitor will be given for five years.

Locally advanced cancers usually fall into one of two categories, though both are generally treated the same way. Sometimes a very aggressive cancer seems to come up overnight as a large and evidently fast-growing tumor (although it's been there undetectable for a while). At other times, the tumor has been present for several years and the woman has tried to pretend it wasn't there, until it's gotten huge or begun ulcerating through the skin, and she finally gets to a doctor. This latter case we call a neglected primary—it's not an especially aggressive cancer, just an especially frightened woman. Patients with a neglected primary cancer often do better than you may expect. If you've had an untreated cancer for five years and it hasn't killed you or obviously spread anywhere, it's clearly a slow-growing cancer.

If you've been putting off seeing your doctor about a lump that's been growing, or if you're suddenly faced with a new large or ulcerating tumor, don't ignore it and assume you're dying—get it diagnosed and start your treatment right away. Your prognosis may not be as good as it would be with a smaller tumor, but the cancer may very well be curable, and the sooner you begin to take care of it, the better your chances are.

INFLAMMATORY BREAST CANCER

One kind of locally advanced breast cancer is termed inflammatory, as the first symptoms are usually the rapid development (within 6 months) of redness and warmth in the skin of the breast, often without a distinct lump. Frequently the patient and even the doctor mistake it for a simple infection, and the woman is put on antibiotics. But it doesn't get better. It also doesn't get worse, and that's the tip-off: an infection always gets better or worse within a week or two—it rarely stays the same. If there's no change, the doctor should biopsy the underlying tissue to see if it's cancer. Two of my patients who have had this cancer had similar stories. One had been breast-feeding and developed what her doctor thought was lactational mastitis (see Chapter 3). It never cleared up and didn't hurt much; there was no fever or other sign of infection. In six months it hadn't gone away or gotten worse. The other patient, not breast-feeding, noticed that one breast had suddenly become larger than the other, and there was redness and swelling. Here too, the doctors at first thought it was an infection. So if you have such symptoms and they continue after antibiotic treatment, you should ask for a biopsy of the breast tissue and the skin. With inflammatory breast cancer, you have cancer cells in the lymph vessels of your skin. The skin is red because the cancer is blocking the drainage of fluid.

Although inflammatory breast cancer accounts for only 1–5 percent of all breast cancer cases in the United States, it constitutes as much as 24–40 percent of locally advanced disease.[33] Women with inflammatory breast cancer tend to be significantly younger than those with other breast cancers, and African Americans with this cancer tend to be younger than whites. Most of the tumors are estrogen and progesterone negative, but many overexpress Her-2/neu. Currently inflammatory breast cancers are treated with a neoadjuvant therapy protocol: three or four cycles of AC followed by paclitaxel or docetaxel. Then we'll do local treatment—usually mastectomy followed by radiation. Tumors that overexpress Her-2/neu can also be treated with Herceptin. If the tumor is sensitive to hormones, then either tamoxifen or an aromatase inhibitor will be added to the mix. Serious though it can be, inflammatory breast cancer is an extremely variable disease. It can be especially scary to have inflammatory breast cancer because it is so rare. I would strongly suggest that any woman with this diagnosis check out the two websites dedicated to the disease: www.ibcsupport.org and www.ibc research.org for up-to-date information and support. This disease is serious, but great progress is being made and the prognosis is much more positive than it was when I wrote the first edition of this book.

This type of cancer has seen a remarkable improvement in overall survival since the use of combination therapy. A study published in 1998 shows an increase in survival of 10 percent (42 percent survival versus 32 percent earlier), while other forms of breast cancer survival increased only 5 percent (from 80 to 85 percent). A recent report followed 61 women with inflammatory breast cancer who had received multimodality (several types of treatment) and found that the five-year survival rate was 47 percent with over 50 percent of the women who received trimodality (chemotherapy, radiation, and surgery) free of disease at five years.[34] This is doubly encouraging, since if this type of aggressive cancer does not recur in five years, the woman generally has a good chance of being cured.

Since inflammatory breast cancer is less common than most others, you should be treated at a cancer center, preferably one that conducts research on this disease, such as MD Anderson. This way you not only have the best chance of survival, but you help us make progress in treating and curing this aggressive type of breast cancer.

THE UNKNOWN PRIMARY

"The unknown primary" may sound like the title of a murder mystery, but it's the name we give another kind of mystery—a cancer that has spread to a lymph node in the armpit without an obvious primary tumor. In women this type of tumor (also called occult primary) almost always originates in the breast.

This is a rare form of breast cancer, accounting for less than 1 percent of cases. Someone shows up with an enlarged lymph node, usually in the armpit. A biopsy finds breast cancer cells, but there are no breast lumps. Sometimes we call this "axillary presentation of breast cancer," and it is staged as T0 and either N1 or N2 (see Chapter 11). Modern imaging techniques have helped in finding the original tumor. A woman in this situation is first sent for a mammogram and ultrasound. Looking for a cancer that we suspect is there is different from screening, and many tumors are found on repeat study. If that doesn't show a tumor, then an MRI is done.

As you remember from Chapter 8, MRI is very sensitive but not that accurate. Although this does not make it a good general screening test, it does help in this situation. Recent studies have shown that MRI can detect the missing tumor in the breast in 70–95 percent of women.[35] If the doctors can find the primary cancer, then the patient has the option of getting a lumpectomy and radiation rather than a mastectomy. Several years ago, a woman called me to ask for advice. She was 68 and had been diagnosed with an unknown primary. Her surgeon was insisting that she have a mastectomy, but she really didn't want it. I suggested an MRI and spoke to her surgeon about it. He was reluctant because she had implants and he felt that imaging techniques wouldn't work. I told him that MRI actually worked very well with implants. This was a fairly recent discovery, and he was glad to hear it. She had an MRI and it revealed the cancer—a 4 centimeter tumor that had draped itself around the implant. This position necessitated the mastectomy after all. But at least the woman knew that the operation was indeed necessary, and not a possibly fruitless hunting expedition.

When no breast lesion can be found, the treatment is more controversial. There's no doubt that a mastectomy would get rid of a cancer if it's there, but we have to ask if it's necessary, given that the primary cancer is so tiny we can't even detect it. It can be devastating to a woman to have a mastectomy and then learn that the primary cancer didn't show up in the tissue after all, and she had her breast removed for nothing. Three studies have now reported on using radiation for occult primary (T0N1) breast cancers. All showed a decreased local recurrence rate (18 percent in the irradiated group versus 54 percent in the breasts that did not undergo irradiation in the MD Anderson group).[36] In all of the studies, however, survival was the same whether the woman got radiation or not. Obviously it is not the local options that are the most important here but the systemic, and doing nothing to the breast is also an option. The local options when the primary can't be found, therefore, are radiation alone or mastectomy, coupled with axillary dissection and chemotherapy.

Systemic therapy is given according to the type of tumor. Contrary to what you may expect, the survival rate in cancers that show up in the nodes but not in the breast is actually a bit better than it is for cancers that show up as both a breast lump and an enlarged node.[37]

If you have this kind of cancer, you should think about what treatment you'll be most comfortable with. If your surgeon comes down with a hard line and tells you there's one sure way to deal with it, be suspicious and insist on a second opinion.

PAGET'S DISEASE OF THE BREAST

Dr. James Paget (1814–1889) has gotten his name on any number of diseases: there's a Paget's disease of the bone and a Paget's disease of the eyelids, as well as a Paget's disease of the breast. The diseases have no relation to one another, except for their discoverer. In the breast, Paget's disease refers to a form of breast cancer that shows up in the nipple as an itchiness and scaling that doesn't get better.

As I was researching this section, I was amazed to find that the first description of this rare type of breast cancer was by John of Arderne in 1307. John described a nipple ulceration in a male priest, which over several years without treatment (there weren't many treatments available in 1307) went on to become full-fledged breast cancer.[38] Luckily we can now do more than just observe someone with Paget's.

There are two theories about this type of breast cancer. One is that the cancer cells start in the lactiferous sinus (see Chapter 1) and travel up to the nipple openings. This explains why the nipple itself rather than the areola is the first spot of irritation noted in Paget's, as well as the fact that people with Paget's disease often harbor cancers with similar cell types elsewhere in the breast.[39] The other theory is that the cancer cells actually originate in the nipple openings. This correlates with the fact that some women with Paget's disease have no sign of cancer elsewhere.[40] Further study will tell us whether either or both theories are correct.

Usually Paget's disease presents as redness, mild scaliness, and flaking of the nipple skin and gradually goes on to crusting, ulceration, and weeping. It can be itchy, hypersensitive, and painful. It's often mistaken for eczema of the nipple—a far more common occurrence. Paget's disease is almost never found in both breasts, so if you have itching and scaling on both nipples, you probably have a harmless skin condition. In addition, the fact that Paget's usually starts in the nipple and not the areola can be a telling sign. However, if it doesn't get better, you should get it checked out, whether it's on one or both nipples, or even on the areola.

First, the skin on the nipple will be biopsied. This can be done in the doctor's office with local anesthetic; either a nipple scrape or a "punch biopsy" can make the diagnosis. If it's Paget's, the pathologist sees little cancer cells growing up into the skin of the nipple—that's what makes the skin flake and get itchy. Then you will need a mammogram to look for cancer in the breast itself. As with the unknown primary tumors described above, you may want to have an MRI if the mammogram is negative. MRI can be especially useful in making sure that there is no other area of disease besides the nipple. If these imaging tests detect something, then a biopsy of that lesion is necessary. Paget's can indicate the possibility of a further breast cancer. Carolyn Kaelin, a Boston breast surgeon, combined several studies of Paget's disease and found that out of 965 cases, 47 percent had a breast mass as well as the nipple symptoms and 53 percent had no mass. Of the women with a mass, 93 percent had invasive carcinoma of the breast and 7 percent had noninvasive cancer. Among those with no mass, 34 percent had invasive cancer, 65 percent of the women had DCIS, and 1 percent had only Paget's disease with no cancer in the breast.[41]

The treatment of Paget's disease depends on whether it is associated with DCIS, invasive cancer, or neither. In and of itself Paget's disease is low grade and not aggressive. If there is an invasive or a noninvasive cancer near the nipple, a lumpectomy that includes the nipple and areola can be performed, followed by radiation. Sentinel node biopsy can be added if it is invasive. If the invasive cancer lump is far from the nipple, a mastectomy may be necessary to get both areas out; otherwise wide excision and radiation make up a reasonable alternative. If just the nipple is involved, then removing the nipple-areolar complex and adding radiation has an excellent result.[42]

As you might guess, Paget's disease that involves only the nipple has a better prognosis than other types of breast cancer.[43] Usually the lymph nodes turn out to be negative. Because of its rarity, most doctors do not see many cases of it, and many assume that it requires a mastectomy. They seem to think that if you can't keep your nipple, your breast doesn't matter. Most women, of course, know better.

This has been a campaign of mine, and a few years ago some of us managed to convince the rest of the medical establishment that removing the nipple and areola is sufficient treatment, and that many women prefer to keep the rest of the breast.[44,45] True, your breast looks a bit funny after the nipple has been removed, but it is still there. A plastic surgeon can make an artificial nipple (see Chapter 2), though many women don't mind the breast's appearance, as long as they look natural in a bra. Some of my patients with this kind of Paget's disease chose plastic surgery and some didn't bother with it.

CYSTOSARCOMA PHYLLOIDES

This is another rare type of breast tumor, occurring less than 1 percent of the time. The most dramatic thing about this cancer is its name. It's usually fairly mild and takes the form of a malignant fibroadenoma (see Chapter 3). It shows up as a large lump in the breast—it's usually lemon-size by the time it's detected. It feels like a regular fibroadenoma—smooth and round—but under the microscope some of the fibrous cells that make up the fibroadenoma are bizarre-looking and cancerous. It's not very aggressive and rarely metastasizes; if it recurs at all, it tends to do so only in the breast. In the past it was usually treated with wide excision, removing the lump and a rim of normal tissue around it.[46] Today it is simply scooped out. It doesn't require radiation, and we usually don't check the lymph nodes, since when it does metastasize it is usually to the lungs and not the nodes.[47] A patient once came to see me because her cystosarcoma phylloides had recurred three times, and her surgeon told her she'd have to have a mastectomy because it kept coming back. I told her I thought we should wait and see if it did come back, and in the six years I followed her, it didn't recur. Chemotherapy is almost never recommended for these tumors. In the extremely rare case of metastatic cystosarcoma phylloides the type of chemotherapy used for sarcomas (a cancer of the connective tissues) rather than breast cancer is used.

The medical literature sometimes talks about a "benign" versus "malignant" versus intermediate cystosarcoma phylloides, based on a subjective interpretation of how cancerous the cells appear. The implication is that malignant cystosarcomas behave more aggressively. About 95 percent are benign, and the 5 percent that metastasize and ultimately kill the patient are hard to predict accurately in advance. Most surgeons suggest a more aggressive approach (mastectomy) if the pathologist feels that it's malignant. These cancers are sufficiently rare that you should definitely get a second opinion on the pathology from a specialist at a major medical center before embarking on a more aggressive therapeutic approach. Recent research has focused on finding a biomarker that will predict this better.

CANCER OF BOTH BREASTS

Once in a while a woman is diagnosed as having cancer in both breasts at the same time. Typically she finds a lump in one breast, gets a mammogram, and learns there's also a lump in the other breast. Biopsy shows both to be cancer. Although the woman can despair, thinking her situation is twice as bad, that actually isn't the case. The prognosis is based on the stage of the more aggressive of the two tumors. And the "more aggressive" isn't always very aggressive. A recent review from Milan reported that these tumors are more likely to be small, invasive lobular, low grade, and sensitive to estrogen.[48] Such tumors are thought to reflect a situation in which a woman's particular hormonal environment is conducive to developing cancers. Or maybe there is some external environmental risk/cause.

Does one cancer spread from the other? Most studies have found noninvasive cancer associated with each of the two tumors, suggesting that it is not. They're both treated the same way: a lumpectomy or mastectomy and lymph node dissection on one and then the other side. Usually the surgeon first looks at the lymph nodes on the side that appears worse. If the nodes are positive and require chemotherapy, the other nodes won't necessarily have to be dissected if the second cancer has a low likelihood of spreading to the nodes. Unfortunately the surgeon's guess isn't always right. Many years ago I had a patient with three cancers: she had a lump in the top of her right breast, and the mammogram showed two densities in the bottom of the left breast. They'd all been biopsied with needles. Since she wanted to keep her breasts, I did a wide excision of the right breast and sampled the lymph nodes, which were fine. Then I did a wide excision of the two cancers in the left breast, and on the left side she had positive lymph nodes and went on to receive chemotherapy. For this reason many surgeons will do bilateral sentinel nodes.

You can have radiation treatment on both breasts at the same time, but the radiation therapist has to be very careful that the treatment doesn't overlap and cause a burn in the middle area. It isn't necessary to do the same treatment on both breasts. You may decide on a mastectomy on one side and wide excision plus radiation on the other, for example.

Cancer in the Other Breast

Sometimes a woman who has cancer in one breast turns up later with cancer in her other breast. Usually this isn't a recurrence or a metastasis; it's a brand-new cancer and the likelihood of finding yourself in this situation is estimated to be about 0.5 percent per year. It's possible for breast cancer to metastasize from one breast to the other, but it's rare. A new primary cancer has a different significance than a metastasis. It suggests that your breast tissue, for whatever reason, is prone to develop cancer, so you developed one on one side and then several years later the other side followed along. As with any new cancer, it's biopsied and removed, your lymph nodes are checked, and you're treated. Your prognosis isn't any worse because you developed the second breast cancer; rather, as with cancer of both breasts, it's only as bad as the worse of the two. You can still have breast conservation; you don't have to have a mastectomy if you don't want it. People who have second cancers are more likely to have a hereditary predisposition to breast cancer, so women in this situation should ask their doctor about whether they should go to a genetic counselor (see Chapter 6). Some women with cancer in one breast are so scared of getting cancer in the other one that they consider having a prophylactic mastectomy to prevent it, and more and more women are choosing this option (see Chapter 12). However, in women without a genetic mutation that causes breast cancer, prophylactic mastectomy has been shown to improve the chance of not dying from breast cancer only in young women with very early disease (see Chapter 12).

BREAST CANCER IN VERY YOUNG WOMEN

As noted earlier, breast cancer is most common in women over 50, and there are many cases in women in their forties. It's rare in women under 40, but it does occur. We tend to be particularly shocked when it occurs in a young woman. Usually in this situation it's detected as a lump, since we generally don't do screening mammography in young women for the reasons discussed in Chapter 9.

Often a young woman gets misdiagnosed. She detects a lump or a thickening, and she's told it's just lumpy breasts, or "fibrocystic disease," and it's followed for a while until doctors realize it's serious. The vast majority of lumps in women under 35 are benign, and the risk of cancer is very low. Still, it's important for doctors to be vigilant and bear in mind that young women can develop breast cancer.

The youngest patient I ever diagnosed was 23. She was on her honeymoon when she discovered a lump. We diagnosed the cancer; she had a positive node, and she underwent lumpectomy, radiation, and chemotherapy. Ten years later she developed a local recurrence that required a mastectomy.

Breast cancer in younger women is more likely to be hereditary.[49] If you've inherited a mutation (and you need only one or two more mutations to get cancer), you're one step closer and likely to get there sooner, whereas if you haven't inherited any mutations, you still need to get all of the mutations for cancer to develop. That doesn't work all the time. Like older women, the majority of younger women with breast cancer have no family history of it. But if you have a BRCA mutation in your family, you're more likely to get breast cancer at a younger age than if you don't. It is advisable for very young women with breast cancer to have genetic counseling and consider being tested for the BRCA mutations, particularly if they feel that the result would affect their treatment decisions.

Overall, there is no evidence that breast cancer in a woman under 35 matched for prognostic features (see Chapter 11) is any more aggressive than a cancer in an older woman.[50] Cancers in younger women do, however, have a higher incidence of poor prognostic features such as negative estrogen receptors, poor differentiation, and high proliferative (growth) rates. And they are more likely to be triple negative.

Both lumpectomy with radiation and mastectomy have special implications for younger women. There has been some reluctance to do breast conservation in younger women. The concern is twofold. One is that we don't know what the long-term (40–60 year) risks of radiation are. The other is that there appears to be a higher local recurrence rate reported in young women who get lumpectomy and radiation than in women in their forties and fifties.[51] Recent data have suggested that younger women benefit significantly from a radiation boost (see Chapter 16), which reduces this risk considerably.[52] No evidence exists to suggest that mastectomy in young women is better for survival than breast conservation, probably because the risk of metastatic disease is higher than the risk of local recurrence. Nor are double mastectomies necessarily indicated in nonmutation carriers. Yet many young women have been choosing this. The incidence of breast cancer in the other breast is about 0.8 percent per year, which usually maximizes out to about 10–15 percent. However, women with BRCA 1 or BRCA 2 mutations (about 6 percent of women under 36) can have a much higher chance of developing a second breast cancer in the same or other breast. Since younger women have many more years to get cancer in the opposite breast, their risk is slightly higher than that of older women. Both chemotherapy and hormone therapy reduce this risk.

Generally, the systemic therapies for younger women are the same as for older women, depending on the type of breast cancer. Women with tumors that are not sensitive to hormones do well with chemotherapy and Herceptin when indicated. Controversies arise with the hormone-positive tumors. An interesting study done by the International Breast Cancer Study group evaluated the treatment outcome for very young women compared with that for older but still premenopausal women who received chemotherapy but no hormone treatment.[53] The women under 35 who had estrogen positive tumors did worse than older premenopausal women with ER positive tumors and older and younger women with ER negative tumors. This surprising finding led to three reviews, all of which found the same result.[54,55,56] In recent years it has become clear that in patients with ER positive disease the beneficial effects of chemotherapy are the result of a complex mixture of cell killing and hormonal changes. An interesting study done in Europe compared chemo alone to chemo plus 24 months of goserelin (which puts you into temporary menopause) or goserelin alone. Women with estrogen negative disease did better with the chemotherapy alone, while those with estrogen positive disease who had either chemo or goserelin alone did about the same, and the combination was much better in the very young women.[57]

For some very young women endocrine therapy alone may be enough. Studies looking at tamoxifen suggest that it is not as effective in younger women, possibly because it stimulates the ovaries. In young women with metastatic disease and hormone sensitive tumors, however, combining tamoxifen and ovarian suppression seems superior to either treatment alone. Despite this data the tendency is still to offer younger women chemotherapy for six months with the mistaken belief that the side effects will be fewer. Also, the ovarian suppression lasted for two years, not for life. In the goserelin study the women under 40 returned to their premenopausal status at six months after finishing treatment while the ones given chemotherapy were still having hot flashes. There is an ongoing study of different approaches to endocrine therapy comparing tamoxifen, tamoxifen plus ovarian suppression, and an aromatase inhibitor plus ovarian suppression that should help us sort out the best approach. Meanwhile my colleague Craig Henderson from UCSF says that ovarian ablation is probably the best form of hormone treatment for premenopausal estrogen positive women. He gives all his premenopausal women who do not get chemotherapy or do not go into menopause with chemotherapy, ovarian ablation, usually with goserelin and tamoxifen, especially if they are under 40.

Fertility is a problem with both chemotherapy that can put you into menopause and/or ovarian suppression. This plays out in two ways. First, breast cancer treatment with all the components can take several years. Herceptin is usually given for a year following the six months of chemotherapy, and tamoxifen can be given for five years. During this time when pregnancy is dangerous because of the drugs, a woman's fertility will already be declining because of age. Often chemotherapy will prompt premature menopause even when it does not bring it on directly. The risks of menopause range from 10 to 90 percent depending on the drugs, the age of the woman, and the definition used for menopause. Although this sounds odd, some studies say that you are in menopause if you do not have a period for six months to a year. But many women get their period more than a year later. Even blood tests like FSH are not that accurate at predicting whether your menopause is temporary or permanent (see Chapter 11).

If you desire to have a biological child in the future, advise your doctor of this very early in your consultations. Especially ask about the statistics for the treatments being recommended so that you have a realistic assessment of the risk. In the end you will decide what matters most to you, and you may want to try a regimen that is more likely to preserve your fertility. Go back to the discussions in Chapter 12 regarding the absolute benefit you will receive from adjuvant therapy so that you have a realistic idea of the risks versus benefits.

The likelihood of chemotherapy-induced menopause has led some women to consider freezing eggs or ovarian tissue before the treatment so they can have children later. Both of these strategies have had only limited success to date and their safety is not known. So far the success of egg preservation has been three or four times lower than that of embryo preservation.[58]

Another problem is that a lot of hormones must be administered to make the eggs grow for harvesting. Doctors are often reluctant to give those high doses of hormones to women who have cancer, especially those with hormone receptor positive tumors. Attempts have been made to retrieve eggs without hormone stimulation, and recently tamoxifen has been used to help harvest eggs from 12 women prior to chemotherapy. Two of the seven women in the tamoxifen group and two of five women in the no-stimulation group conceived.[59] Femara is used to stimulate the ovaries. Ovarian tissue cryopreservation (freezing) would theoretically solve this problem, since there would be high numbers of eggs available. At this time, however, only two live births have been achieved with this approach, which also has many technical difficulties. Cryopreservation of embryos is a more standard path but requires a male partner or sperm donor and hormones for egg stimulation.

This is obviously a moving target. Again, if this is an issue for you, make sure you check out your options *before* undergoing chemotherapy. The website www.youngsurvival.org or www.fertile hope.org are a good sources for up-to-date information on this topic. And remember there are other ways to parent. Losing your fertility does not mean losing all chances to be a parent.

CANCER DURING PREGNANCY

Once in a very great while a patient develops breast cancer while she's pregnant or breast-feeding. The studies are contradictory. Most show that, stage by stage, it's no worse than any other breast cancer. The problem is that when you're pregnant, your breasts are going through a lot of normal changes that can mask a more dangerous change. For one thing, breasts are much lumpier and thicker than usual. Similarly, when you're breast-feeding, as I explained at length in Chapter 1, you tend to have all kinds of benign lumps and blocked ducts, and you may not notice a change that otherwise would alarm you. Infections are common when you're breast-feeding and can mask inflammatory breast cancer, so the physician may also find diagnosis of inflammatory breast cancer difficult.

Studies have found that women who were diagnosed with breast cancer while pregnant or within the four following years did indeed have a higher mortality rate.[60] As more women are having later pregnancies at the age when breast cancer becomes more common, this may become a bigger issue.

Treatment is also a problem. What we can do about your cancer depends on what stage of pregnancy you're in. If you're in the first trimester, you may want to consider terminating the pregnancy, depending on your beliefs about abortion and how much this particular pregnancy means to you. Aborting the fetus does not in itself cause a better prognosis, but treatment becomes easier. If you continue with the pregnancy, treatment options can be planned around the pregnancy and there is no evidence that the prognosis will be different. Radiation in the first trimester can injure the fetus. The fetus's organs are being formed at this time, and the data from other cancers suggest a high rate of fetal malformation with chemotherapy in the first trimester. Although less of a concern, general anesthesia is usually avoided during the first trimester if possible. We can do a biopsy or a wide excision under local anesthetic. But if further treatment is called for, we usually try to wait until the second trimester.

In the second trimester, since the fetus's organs are already formed and it's safer to use general anesthetic, we can still do operations that require general anesthesia. We would rather not risk radiation. In recent years, studies have shown that chemotherapy can be used safely in the second and third trimesters. So far, in these studies the babies have appeared healthy, but we won't know if complications will appear later in the child's life. If you're in your third trimester, we can do a lumpectomy, or, if need be, a mastectomy, then wait for further treatment like radiation and/or tamoxifen until after the child is born. We can begin chemotherapy if it's important to get going right away. If you are close to your due date, your obstetrician can induce labor as soon as the baby can be expected to survive well outside the womb (as early as 33–34 weeks if needed), or do a cesarean section, and then start you on chemotherapy and radiation after delivery. Sometimes the due date can be moved up with medication to increase the lung maturity and allow earlier delivery.

A neighbor of mine in Los Angeles was diagnosed with breast cancer when she was pregnant with her seventh child. Her physicians told her to abort and she had trouble convincing them that she wanted her seventh child just as much as the first. She underwent a mastectomy in the second trimester and did well. Because she had many positive nodes, she received chemotherapy during her third trimester. Her delivery went well, and she said for years afterward that this seventh child was the smartest of all, which she attributed to chemotherapy. Unfortunately she developed metastases several years later and died of breast cancer.

In the mid-1990s I saw a woman who had been diagnosed 20 years earlier, when she was seven months pregnant. She had undergone a radical mastectomy and then had radiation with cobalt (a chemical used in the mid-twentieth century) while she was pregnant. She said she had to have a dose monitor in her vagina to keep track of the amount of radiation her fetus was receiving. Nonetheless she carried the baby to term and both were fine 20 years later.

BREAST CANCER DURING LACTATION

Breast cancer during lactation isn't quite as complicated, since you can always stop breast-feeding and start your child on formula. Radiation will probably make breast-feeding impossible, and you won't want to breast-feed if you're on chemotherapy, since the baby will swallow the chemicals.

There are some misconceptions about cancer and breast-feeding that need to be addressed. The first is that a child who suckles from a cancerous breast will get the cancer. This theory is based on a study of one species of mouse, which does transmit a cancerous virus to its female offspring through breast-feeding. At this time, it hasn't been found in any other species of mouse or in any other animal.

Another notion is that a baby won't accept milk from a cancerous breast. Normally this isn't so. If a breast has a lot of cancer, it probably won't produce as much milk, so the baby will, quite sensibly, favor the milkier breast. There's nothing wrong with this. Many babies simply prefer one breast to another, even with a healthy mother.

We're not sure yet if lactation affects the cancer. I've had two patients whose breast cancer showed up while they were lactating. Both were treated, both stopped breast-feeding, and both did well without a recurrence for several years. After much debate both women decided to get pregnant again. One had a recurrence during the second pregnancy; the other had a second primary develop in the other breast while she was lactating. This leads me to wonder whether, if a cancer shows up while a woman is pregnant or lactating, there is a higher risk of a recurrence in another pregnancy. However, I have no data for this. Obviously we can't do a randomized study, and it's too unusual an occurrence to draw any conclusions. Our evidence is purely anecdotal. For now, all I can suggest to someone who has developed breast cancer while pregnant or lactating is to consider seriously not having another pregnancy, in case it affects the chance of a recurrence. An article by the late breast surgeon Jeanne Petrek in 1997 discussed pregnancy after breast cancer.[61] She looked into a number of published series (articles by doctors reviewing their own cases over a period of time) and found that breast cancer survival didn't change with a subsequent pregnancy. But because there were a number of possible biases (see Chapter 15), the results are inconclusive. It's possible that the doctors selected their patients by telling only the women who were likely to be cured that pregnancy would be safe, and discouraging the others. Or it may be that getting cancer while you're pregnant has a different effect on your body than getting it afterward.[62,63,64] Petrek's point, wisely, is that we don't really know the answer yet.

BREAST CANCER IN ELDERLY WOMEN

Just as very young women can get breast cancer, so can women over 70, and they share some issues. Neither end of the extreme always fits our general models. There are studies showing that older women aren't treated as aggressively. There's a tendency to restrict the options for treatment: "Well, they're old; they don't really want chemotherapy."[65] I think a special effort has to be made to ascertain what the patient wants and what is appropriate for her cancer, and not permit physicians to act on their own assumptions alone.

In addition, there's a tendency to do mastectomies on older women without offering them breast conservation treatments, assuming that elderly women don't care as much about their looks. Some doctors tell an older woman that six weeks of radiation therapy will be too much for her, making mastectomy sound less arduous than lumpectomy plus radiation. But radiation isn't really all that hard to go through. As I noted in Chapter 12, for some older women, just as for their younger friends, it's preferable to the emotional trauma of mastectomy.

Not only do many doctors neglect to mention lumpectomy and radiation, they also neglect to offer reconstruction to the older woman on whom they've urged mastectomy, again assuming that she won't care enough about her looks to want it. And again, that assumption is totally off base. I remember one patient in her mid-eighties with large, droopy breasts, who had always wanted to have a reduction but thought it was too dangerous. She got a cancer at the upper end of one of her breasts. She wanted breast conservation; she didn't want a mastectomy. But it seemed foolhardy to us to radiate this entire breast when most of it showed no cancer. So after discussing it with her, we did a lumpectomy and bilateral reductions, and then did radiation. She was delighted; when the radiation was done she went off on a cruise and found a new boyfriend.

So you can't make any assumptions.

The recommendations for older women, of course, have to consider their overall health. As with younger women, larger tumors can be treated with systemic therapy in an attempt to shrink them enough to allow breast conservation. This can be done with an aromatase inhibitor or, if the woman is fit enough and the tumor is not sensitive to estrogen, with chemotherapy. If the tumor is small, then breast conservation with sentinel node biopsy and mastectomy are both options. The use of systemic therapies after local treatment again depends on the woman's health. If she has a hormone negative tumor and can tolerate chemotherapy, it certainly should be an option. But if she has other serious health problems, it may not be wise. Hormone therapy is easier to take and should probably be used in most women with hormone positive tumors.

In one of the few studies directed specifically to women over 70, patients who had undergone lumpectomy were randomized to have either tamoxifen alone or tamoxifen plus radiation therapy. There were no differences between the two groups, suggesting that radiation therapy may not be necessary in this situation.[66] One would suspect that similar results would be obtained with an aromatase inhibitor.

Part of the problem in studying women over 70 is that we really can't evaluate long-term survival, since elderly people die from many illnesses. But not all elderly women are frail. I had a ninety-five-year-old breast cancer patient in Boston who was very active. I did a lumpectomy and put her on tamoxifen. Unfortunately she couldn't tolerate the tamoxifen and dropped it. She was fine for about a year and a half; then her cancer recurred locally. I did another lumpectomy, and this time I really tried to get her to stick with the tamoxifen, and she did for a while. The last I heard she was still going strong. So when we look at how to treat elderly women, we need to look at how frail they really are: people vary greatly. Those who live into their nineties tend to be healthy, or they wouldn't live to that age. We can't just assume, as many doctors do, they'll be dead in a year or so and forget it—sometimes they live to over 100. Some ninety-year-olds are healthier than some women at 60.

WOMEN WITH IMPLANTS

There's no evidence that women with implants have a higher vulnerability to breast cancer than other women, and some evidence that it may actually be lower.[67] Sometimes cancer is detected on a mammogram, and sometimes the lump is palpable. It's diagnosed in the same way as any breast cancer—with a biopsy. We may be able to do a needle biopsy, depending on where the lump is. We don't want to stick a needle into the sac and release the silicone or saline into the breast.

The treatment options are the same. You can have lumpectomy and radiation.[68] You can radiate with the implant in place.

There is a higher incidence of encapsulation (see Chapter 2), but other than that there's no problem. You may think that cutting into the breast would break the silicone cover, but there are a couple of ways around that. For example, we can use the electrocautery instead of the scalpel, and that can't cut into the implant.

If you had silicone injections back in the 1960s when they were legal, the same applies. They make detecting cancer on mammogram more difficult, since it's hard to tell what's silicone and what's something else. So you need to go to a high-quality center where you can be carefully monitored. It's very important to have the mammograms serially, comparing one year's to the next, because that's what can tip you off: one of these lumps that you were calling silicone is growing. You can have lumpectomy and radiation.

BREAST CANCER IN MEN

This book addresses breast cancer in women because it is the most common malignancy in women. Among men it accounts for less than 1 percent of all cancers. Overall there are 1,500 cases a year in men and over 200,000 in women. Many of the men who get it seem to have a family history on their father's or their mother's side.[69] Not surprisingly many men who develop breast cancer are also carriers of mutations in the BRCA genes, most commonly BRCA 2. It is therefore a good idea to be tested for yourself and even more so for your female siblings and offspring. There's also a theory that it's connected to gynecomastia— female-like breasts (see Chapter 1), either now or during puberty, but so far we have no proof of this. We do have proof that men with Klinefelter's syndrome, a chromosomal problem in which not enough testosterone is produced, are susceptible to breast cancer.[70] Interestingly, risk factors for women such as early exposure to radiation[71] and higher estrogen exposure in utero also seem to be relevant to men.[72]

For a time there was concern that men who got estrogen treatments for prostate cancer were more vulnerable to breast cancer, but this doesn't seem to be the case. Rather, prostate cancer can metastasize to the breast.[73] (Remember that it remains prostate cancer, not breast cancer.)

Breast cancer in men shows itself in all the ways it does in women—usually as a lump—but it tends to be discovered later because men aren't usually very conscious of their breasts. The treatments are the same as well. Men can undergo sentinel node biopsy[74] (see Chapter 14), and either lumpectomy and radiation or mastectomy. There is a tendency to overtreat men with post-mastectomy radiation because surgeons see these cancers so rarely. Breast cancers in men more frequently involve the skin or chest wall, probably because of the relatively small amount of breast tissue, and this can be an indication for radiation. Recent data demonstrate that local recurrences in men are rare even in stage 3 disease and that the same indications should be used that are employed in women (see Chapter 16).[75]

One issue that is often not addressed, however, is the fact that the cosmetic implications are somewhat different for men. On the one hand, they don't tend to regard breasts as crucial to their sexuality the way women do. On the other hand, their naked chests are more likely to be visible. It can be more awkward for a man to have a scar, to lack a nipple, or to have a deformed chest, than it is for a woman. So, like a woman, a man might prefer lumpectomy and radiation to mastectomy. The one extra consideration is hair. After radiation therapy a man loses most of his chest hair on that side. If he is very hairy, a mastectomy with the scar hidden in hair may prove more cosmetic. Depending on where the tumor is, the nipple can often be conserved. If he loses the nipple, a plastic surgeon can give him an artificial one. When I worked at UCLA, a golfer with a small breast cancer came to me. He was distressed that the only option he had been given was a mastectomy. After a lumpectomy and radiation, he was very happy and felt normal on the course.

Treatment in terms of chemotherapy and axillary nodes is exactly the same as for women. As mentioned earlier, most breast cancers in men are estrogen receptor positive, either of the luminal A or B type. Interestingly, tamoxifen works in men with estrogen receptor positive tumors. Recent reports suggest that the aromatase inhibitors work as well.[76,77]

DCIS (ductal carcinoma in situ) is even rarer in men than is breast cancer. In 1999 the Armed Forces Institute of Pathology did a study on male DCIS. Researchers found 280 cases of pure DCIS and 759 of invasive.[78] They studied the pure DCIS cases and found older rather than younger men. It was different from DCIS in women (see Chapter 12) in that it was more frequently the low-grade papillary version than either cribriform or the high-grade comedo kind. High-grade DCIS was especially rare. Occasional cases showed necrosis. The men were treated with wide excision alone without radiation for this low-grade DCIS.

Several years ago I received email from a man who had DCIS. He had a mastectomy and then radiation. Then he was told he had to go on tamoxifen. He wanted to know if tamoxifen could harm him. It's unlikely that it would. There are lots of data on men taking tamoxifen, and it doesn't harm them. They can get hot flashes or increased blood clotting, but they can't get vaginal dryness or endometrial cancer, or any male version of those. But this man didn't need it. He probably needed a mastectomy without radiation. The only data for tamoxifen with DCIS show a very small benefit, and that occurs only with women who had lumpectomy and radiation, not mastectomy. The doctors were probably inexperienced in male breast cancer and thought it wisest to use every treatment possible.

Usually, however, when a man has a breast lump, it isn't cancer but unilateral gynecomastia, which can happen anytime in a man's life, especially if he's been on some of the drugs used to treat heart conditions or hypertension or smokes marijuana. It's never a cyst or fibroadenoma—men don't get those.

OTHER CANCERS

When I arrived at UCLA in 1992, within the first week or two I got a call to see a patient who had a breast lump. It was soft and smooth, and on the side of her breast. It felt like a cyst, but I was unable to aspirate it. Then she had a mammogram and an ultrasound, which confirmed that the lump was solid. We took the lump out under local anesthesia, and indeed it was malignant. When I talked to her afterward, I broke one of my cardinal rules—never make absolute promises. I told her that although her tumor was malignant, it was small, and I could guarantee that she wouldn't have to get chemotherapy. Since she was elderly, the most she'd need would be tamoxifen.

Then we looked at it more closely under the microscope, and found that it wasn't a breast cancer at all but lymphoma, a lymph node cancer, showing up in the breast. Lymphoma is treated with chemotherapy. The tale has two morals. One, never break your own wise rules. And two, things aren't always what they seem. It's ironic that my first breast cancer patient at UCLA didn't have breast cancer. (I'm glad to report that she responded well to the treatment and when last I saw her she was in her nineties and doing fine.)

Occasionally other kinds of cancer occur in the breast. Since the breast contains several kinds of tissue besides breast tissue, any of the cancers associated with those kinds of tissue can appear in the breast. In addition to lymphoma (since there are lymph nodes), these include a cancerous fat tumor (liposarcoma) and a blood vessel tumor (angiosarcoma—occasionally found in patients who have had radiation). You can also have a melanoma—a skin cancer. Connective tissue in the breast, as elsewhere, can become cancerous. Usually these cancers are treated the same way they'd be treated in any other part of the body—the tissue is excised, followed by radiation and chemotherapy (the chemicals are different from those used to treat breast cancer).

When another form of cancer shows up in the breast, we know it isn't breast cancer from the pathologist's report. As I noted earlier, each kind of cancer has its own distinct characteristics, and we rarely mistake one kind for another. We choose treatment for the particular cancer rather than breast cancer treatment. We didn't, for example, do an axillary section on my lymphoma patient.

Having breast cancer doesn't immunize you from other forms of cancer. You have the same chances as anyone else of getting other cancers, though perhaps a bit higher if you have a BRCA mutation. I've had a couple of patients with breast cancer who were also heavy smokers. They were treated for their breast cancer, continued smoking, and ended up with lung cancer. A bout with any kind of cancer can provide a useful time to consider altering your lifestyle in ways that promote overall health.

Part Five

TREATMENT IN THE AGE OF PERSONALIZED MEDICINE

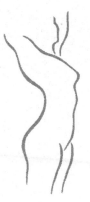

Chapter 14

SURGERY

ALMOST EVERY FORM OF BREAST CANCER INVOLVES SURGERY AS part of treatment—occasionally for the initial biopsy (when a core is not feasible) and usually a lumpectomy or mastectomy as well as surgery on the lymph nodes. It's always a frightening prospect, but demystifying the process can be helpful. I've already discussed some general aspects of surgery in Chapter 12. In this chapter we will go over what you can expect from your surgeon and your operation for breast cancer. I'll also go into the likely side effects and the recovery process. Be warned: I will be fairly explicit because I think the more information you have, the less scared you will be. If you find surgical details unpleasant, just skip those parts.

When I was in practice, I would talk with the patient a few days ahead of time and explain exactly what I'd do in the operation, and what risks and possible complications were involved. I'd draw her pictures and show her photographs, so she'd know what to expect. (If your doctor doesn't do that, you can check my website and others for photos and descriptions.) At Boston's Beth Israel Deaconness Medical Center, my former colleague Susan Troyan, MD, and Judi Hirschfield Bartek, RN, often encourage women to read Peggy Huddleston's book *Prepare for Surgery, Heal Faster*, which helps women learn techniques to feel in control.

As with any operation, patients are asked before the surgery to sign a consent form. This can be a little scary, especially if you read all the fine print, because it asks you to state that you know you can die from the surgery or suffer permanent brain damage from the anesthetic. This doesn't mean that either is likely to happen, or that by signing the form you're letting the doctors off the hook if something *does* happen. Rather, it's an acknowledgment that you've been told about the procedure and its risks and that you still want to have the operation. (Obviously you have to balance for yourself the risks involved in the operation against the risks of not having it.) You've probably seen many similar forms, since virtually any medical procedure—including flu shots—uses them.

It's very important to know the risks. Never permit yourself to be rushed through signing the consent form. You should be given the form well before you go in for surgery; it's hard to read small print when you're about to be wheeled into the operating room. You need to have plenty of time to ask the surgeon questions about risks and complications. If anything confuses you, be sure to ask for clarification.

For the bigger operations involving long or extensive procedures such as mastectomies with flap reconstruction (see Chapter 15), some surgeons may recommend that the patient donate a couple of pints of her own blood a week or two prior to the procedure. Transfusions are rarely necessary in breast surgery, but it's a nice, secure feeling to know that if you do need blood you can get the safest possible—your own. The Red Cross is more than happy to assist in this procedure. Blood donation is not recommended if you have anemia or have recently completed chemotherapy, as it can suppress the body's ability to form new blood cells. Keep in mind that directed donor blood has not been shown to be safer than blood bank blood, so if you or your family don't give your own, trust the blood bank. You should discuss this with your plastic-reconstructive team to determine if they think blood transfusion may be needed.

Your surgeon will tell you to stop taking aspirin, aspirin-containing products, and vitamin E and some herbs/supplements at least 7–10 days before surgery. All of these interfere with clotting and cause more bleeding in surgery. If someone has taken a drug of this type we do a "bleeding time" (a test that tells how fast your blood clots) prior to surgery to make sure it's safe to proceed. If not, we postpone the surgery for a week or two until the clotting returns to normal. It is important to tell both your surgeon and anesthesiologist about all drugs, vitamins, and herbs you are taking so they can check for interactions or consult with your primary doctor if you are taking blood thinners.

ANESTHESIA

There are several anesthetics we can use in various procedures: local anesthesia, general anesthesia (described below), and a kind that falls between, called conscious sedation. It puts you into a sort of limbo in which you're somewhat aware of what's happening but you don't much care.

Other anesthetics that are midway between local and general—nerve blocks, epidurals, and spinals—don't work well for major breast surgery, although some surgeons use a thoracic epidural (like the block used in childbirth but higher up on your body) to decrease the amount of general anesthesia needed. This is particularly helpful for tissue flap reconstruction procedures. Local anesthesia doesn't work for extensive breast surgery, since the amount of local anesthesia you'd need to block out the pain can be toxic.

In recent years, general anesthetic has become a complex, sophisticated combination of drugs. The first element in any general anesthetic combination is something to induce sleep quickly—usually propofol. This drug is given intravenously and puts you out immediately. Its effects last about 15 minutes, and it's followed with a combination of other drugs. Sometimes the anesthesiologist uses a mixture of narcotics to prevent pain, gas to keep you unconscious, and a muscle paralyzer to keep you from coughing or otherwise moving during the operation. Since the muscle paralyzer prevents breathing, it's necessary to put a tube down your throat and into your windpipe to keep your airway open and hook you up to a breathing machine to ensure that you get enough oxygen into your body during the operation. Sometimes doctors skip the paralysis and run a tube called an LMA into your throat. (LMA stands for a laryngeal mask airway, although I must admit that until I looked it up for this book, I thought it was "Ella May"; my coauthor thought it was "Louisa May Alcott." Both interpretations are prettier, but, alas, inaccurate.) This tube makes sure your airway stays open so that you continue to breathe on your own. Instead of narcotics, sometimes they use inhalational anesthesia, or gas that can keep you asleep and get rid of pain. Finally there is a wonderful drug called Versed that makes many patients feel amnesic on awakening; this state is sometimes called "twilight sleep." Also, antinausea drugs can be given, and propofol reduces nausea in addition to being a really good drug for general anesthesia or sedation.

Doctors decide which of these various agents to use, and in what combination, only after consultation with the individual patient. Your medical history will make a big difference here. If you have asthma, for example, a drug that opens up the airways is more suitable so that you don't have an attack under anesthesia. If you have a heart condition, a drug that has a calming effect on the heart will be chosen.

Since anesthesia and its administration are so complicated, most hospitals will have you talk with an anesthesiologist before the operation. This is usually done during a preoperative screening appointment. For some less complicated operations you will see the anesthesiologist the morning of surgery rather than earlier. Anesthesiologists are highly trained doctors who have gone through at least three years of specialized training after internship. They often work with nurse anesthetists who are equally experienced. The anesthesiologist will take your medical history, looking for information that may suggest using, or not using, various anesthetic agents—for example, chronic diseases you may have, past experiences with anesthetic, and so on. After thoroughly exploring all this with you, the anesthesiologist will decide what to use in your operation. If you have previously undergone surgery and had trouble with the anesthesia, try to bring a copy of your anesthesia record from the hospital where the surgery was performed. But remember drugs and procedures may have changed a lot since then. Your interview with the anesthesiologist is very important, since the risk of an operation lies as much in the anesthesia and its administration as in the surgery. When you talk to the anesthesiologist, ask questions and give any information you think may be important. While you may have a different anesthesiologist for your operation, you can be assured that all the pertinent information will be available.

PROCEDURE

On the day of surgery you will be checked in and asked to change into a gown and taken to the holding area. Here your doctor or an assistant will ask you which side is being operated on and mark it with an X. This is not because they have forgotten but to confirm that the record is correct and ensure no errors are made. The nurses in the holding area will again ask you your name and what operation you're having, just to make sure that you are the patient they think you are. An IV will be put into a vein in your arm. If you are having lymph node surgery, the IV will be placed in the side opposite the lymph node operation; patients with lymph node surgery on both sides will usually have the IV placed in the foot or neck to avoid risk of lymphedema.

If you receive a sedative in the holding area, you may be asleep before you get into the surgery suite, or if you're awake you may not remember all the preliminaries. Once in the surgery suite, you will be hooked up to a variety of monitoring devices. There's an automatic blood pressure cuff that feels very tight when it's first inflated, but don't worry. As soon as it registers how big your arm is, the amount of pressure used on subsequent inflations is less. There's an EKG monitoring your heart rate. And a little clip or piece of tape is put on your finger, toe, or earlobe to measure the amount of oxygen in your blood. If the operation is a lengthy one, as when it includes reconstruction, a catheter is put in your bladder to measure the amount of urine output and make sure you're not dehydrated. Thus your bodily functions are all carefully monitored. Large pads are placed over your lower body to maintain your body temperature during the process. You'll probably wear pneumatic boots—plastic boots that pump up and down

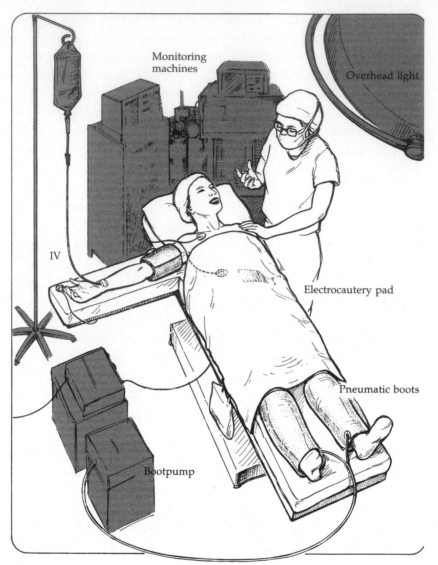

Figure 14.1

massaging your calves during the operation to prevent clots from
forming during long operations (Figure 14.1). A grounding plate is
put on your skin to ground the electrocautery and protect you
from shock. During this time, your surgeon may or may not be
with you. Some surgeons prefer making personal contact before
surgery; others maintain a professional distance. Then the surgeon goes out to scrub (wash hands).

Then you're given propofol and go right to sleep. Many people who haven't had surgery for 30 or 40 years remember the old days of ether and are nervous about the unpleasant sensations they recall while going under. But sodium pentathol (which is almost never used anymore) and propofol work differently, and most patients report it as a very pleasant experience. You may experience a garlic taste at the back of your mouth just before you go under, and you may yawn. Propofol may burn as it goes into your arm. Pretreatment of the vein with local anesthetics before the propofol is injected helps this considerably, but if you feel it, it is only for a second or two before you go to sleep, and you probably won't remember it. Then you're asleep. People are often reassured to know that they don't talk under anesthesia, even sedation: your deep dark secrets remain safe. With MAC (monitored anesthesia), you may tersely answer a direct question, but you won't chat, and the questions won't be any more personal than "Do you feel this?"

After scrubbing, the surgeon returns to the operating room. The area of your body that's going to be worked on is painted with a disinfectant, and drapes are put around you to prevent infection. A fairly new addition to the procedure has been borrowed from the checklist approach for airplanes, where everything is reviewed before take-off. It is called a time-out. Once the patient is asleep and prepped but before the first incision is made, everyone stops—surgical team, anesthesia team, and nursing team. They turn off the music, the anesthesiologist reads the name of the patient and identifies the surgical issues, reporting that the antibiotic has been given and reminding the surgeon about any drug allergies and also whether the patient is on a particular medication such as a beta blocker. (This is significant, because if you forget to put a patient back on her beta blocker postop, she can have cardiac complications.) Then the surgeon announces what operation is going to be performed, which side, estimated operating time, and estimated blood loss. The circulating nurse is meanwhile reading directly from the consent form to verify that everything is correct.

After this thorough review the operation is under way. Most surgical operations have traditionally been done with a scalpel or scissors. More recently, electrocautery (a type of electric knife) has been used with less blood loss. Once the surgery is over and your wounds have been dressed, you are allowed to wake up.

How you wake up from the operation will depend, again, on the drugs that were used. For some drugs an antidote can be given to end the effects. For example, if you've been given a muscle paralyzer, a drug can restore your muscle mobility. But if you've been given gas to put you to sleep, you have to wait slightly longer till it wears off. As soon as they think you're awake enough to breathe on your own, the tube is removed. Occasionally you'll be vaguely aware that this is happening, but usually you're still too out of it to notice. You stay a little fuzzy for a while. When the surgery is over, you're taken to the recovery room, where a nurse remains with you, monitoring your blood pressure and pulse every 10 or 15 minutes until you're fully awake and stable.

Patients used to feel cold when they first woke up, but now every patient is covered with a heating blanket, and temperature is monitored. Although some of the drugs can create nausea, patients for whom anesthesia tends to create nausea can be given antinausea drugs, including propofol.

You may wake up crying or shivering, but only rarely do patients wake up in great pain. You'll probably fade in and out for a while, and then you'll be fully awake. But expect to be groggy and out of it for a while. Most of the drugs take several hours to exit your system, and it's a day or more till they're all gone. If it's day surgery, you'll probably want to go home and go to bed; if you're still in the hospital, you'll sleep it off there.

Even apart from the surgery, anesthesia is a great strain on your body, and it will cause some degree of exhaustion for at least four or five days and sometimes up to a month. People often don't realize this, especially if the surgery is very painful; they attribute their exhaustion to the pain of the operation. But anything that puts great stress on your body—surgery, a heart attack, an acute asthma attack, or anesthetics that interfere with your body's functions—has a lingering effect. Your body seems to need all its energy to mobilize for the big stress and doesn't have any left over for everyday life for a while. You need to respect that and give yourself time to recuperate from the stress of both the surgery and the anesthetic. I also think it has some effect on brain chemistry that we don't yet understand. Previous experience is not a good guide to how it will affect you the next time, even if the same drugs are used. So don't assume that because you felt fine after your last surgery, you'll feel fine after this one. You may or may not.

There are, of course, risks involved with general anesthetic, but it's important to keep them in perspective. With the refinements in anesthesia in recent years, the risks are extremely low.

Depending on how complicated the operation is, you will usually have surgery the same day you're admitted to the hospital, and you may have day surgery or 23–24 hour stay surgery. Hospitals often have special wings with nurses trained in postop care to serve these patients. Many surgeons tend to do lumpectomy with axillary dissection on an outpatient basis, so the patient has two hours of surgery, spends another few hours in the recovery room, and then goes home. Since the rate of infection is twice as high among women who stay in the hospital, I think leaving as soon as possible is a good idea. (I understand the concerns of many patients that managed care companies try to save money by sending people home too soon, but in some cases, leaving the hospital as soon as possible really can be best for the patient.) Remember you will need to have someone drive you to the hospital and home since you will not be allowed to drive yourself home even if you feel fine.

Although many women prefer going home right away, others feel more comfortable staying in the hospital for a couple of days. A patient who has a mastectomy and immediate reconstruction will be in the hospital for two to five days. If your surgeon wants to send you home earlier than you feel comfortable with, discuss your problems with him or her and see if you can arrange a longer stay.

One thing that keeps people in the hospital after mastectomy is learning how to manage a drain. If possible, ask your doctor to show you and your family the drain and how to empty it at the preop visit. The other reason to stay in the hospital is advanced age or pain control if you remain in a high degree of pain. As soon as you can take oral pain pills, you can go home and not be awakened at 2:00 A.M. for your blood pressure check! When the surgery is being done under general anesthesia, all the preop procedures are the same, however long your hospital stay.

All of the procedures I've just described are done regardless of what kind of operation you're having. Now I'll describe what happens in each different breast cancer operation, starting with the simplest and moving on to the more complex. (Biopsies are described in Chapter 8 and breast reconstruction in Chapter 15.)

SENTINEL NODE BIOPSY AND AXILLARY DISSECTION

Sentinel Node Biopsy

As explained in Chapter 12, sentinel node biopsy has become the standard of care since the last edition of this book for women who have no abnormally palpable lymph nodes or whose lymph nodes are not otherwise found to be positive. When worrisome lymph nodes are noted on an examination, a woman can undergo an ultrasound. If an abnormality is observed, then it will be sampled by either fine needle aspiration or core biopsy. If the node is positive, then she will have an axillary lymph node dissection and if not, a sentinel node biopsy.

The usual practice is to do the sentinel node biopsy before attending to the breast. That way the dye and/or radioactive protein is injected into an intact breast. This also allows the pathologist to examine the sentinel nodes removed and see whether they harbor cancer cells while the lumpectomy or mastectomy is taking place. If the sentinel lymph nodes are shown to be positive during the surgical procedure, then a full axillary dissection can be done at the end of the surgery. Unfortunately the techniques that are used for this type of immediate diagnosis are not perfect and occasionally when the final pathology is completed and all of the nodal tissues are examined, a patient is found to be node positive, and she will likely need to go back for a second procedure to have a completion node dissection.

In order to identify the nodes most likely to be involved, two different types of tracers are usually injected. Most commonly these include a radioactive protein and blue dye. The radioactive protein is usually injected two hours before surgery or up to the afternoon before for early morning surgery. The injection of the radioactive tracer can be done by a surgeon or a radiologist or a trainee. Make sure you ask for EMLA (an anesthetic cream) to apply to your breast an hour before the injection to reduce the pain. In addition you can request Ativan (a drug used for anxiety) ahead of time if you think you will be queasy or are very sensitive to pain. The radiation is very low dose so you don't have to worry about becoming radioactive or exposing others to harmful effects from your injection.

The blue dye is usually injected in the operating room once you are asleep followed by a five-minute breast massage prior to operating. There are several different blue dyes that are commonly used. Isosulfan blue has a very low but real risk of allergic reactions, but your surgical team will be right there and looking out for it. A colleague of mine routinely pretreats all women with a combination of diphenhydramine (Benadryl), famotidine (Pepcid), and hydrocortisone intravenously prior to anesthesia. One study[1] showed fewer allergic reactions with this cocktail, while another showed the same number of reactions but less severity. Although anaphylactic reactions are uncommon, she feels they are better avoided altogether. The other dye, methylene blue, does not cause allergies but has been noted to occasionally cause a superficial ulceration around the injection site. There is less reaction if you dilute the methylene blue, but then it's harder to see the dye in the node. More minor but potentially alarming is the fact that both dyes can turn your breast blue, which can take several weeks to months to fade completely. There is also a transient change in the color of your urine (blue) and stool (greenish). (See Barbara's story below.)

As mentioned in Chapter 12, some surgeons are investigating an approach that they hope will reduce lymphedema. Called reverse axillary mapping, it involves injecting 2 cubic centimeters of lymphazurin under the skin of the upper inner arm and massaging it a little. A large bright blue splotch appears on the arm, but it is gone in a day or two, unlike the residual often seen when injected into the breast. This may allow the surgeon to differentiate the lymphatics related to the breast from those of the arm, which can then be protected.[2] Hypothetically, this should reduce subsequent lymphedema, although it is still under investigation.

The low-level radioactive materials can be injected in the tissue around the tumor, in the skin overlying the tumor, or the peri-areolar area. The radioactive protein is detected by waving a handheld gamma detection probe in concentric circles over the breast. It identifies where the sentinel nodes are most likely to be and can also indicate when the drainage is in an unusual and un-expected direction, such as under the middle of the rib cage, sug-gesting a different approach. Usually, however, the drainage is to the armpit and a short incision is made (just below the hairline) over the area with the strongest signal. The tissue is carefully dis-sected looking for the blue dye in the lymphatic vessel, which will lead to the blue sentinel node or nodes (see Figure 14.3). Al-though we call this a sentinel node biopsy, it is really more than a biopsy and often involves more than one node, since all the nodes that are radioactive and/or blue (usually two to four) are then re-moved and sent to pathology for examination. The nodes can be evaluated during surgery with either a "frozen section" or a molec-ular study. These tests generally take about 30 minutes to per-form, and they are about 90 percent accurate. If the nodes are negative, the incision is sewn closed without a drain. In some centers, the nodes are not evaluated at the time of surgery. If this is the case and a positive sentinel node is found, you may be ad-vised to have additional nodes removed in a separate operation (see "Full Axillary Lymph Node Dissection," below). Very rarely, even if the frozen section shows a negative node, the final pathol-ogy report may show some cancer cells. Often this situation will require a discussion with your surgeon or oncologist to determine whether additional lymph nodes need to be removed.

Barbara, a flight attendant I met when she volunteered for my nipple fluid studies, was happy to have the sentinel node biopsy first, even though she later needed a full axillary dissection. She knew that with sentinel node biopsy as part of the process, doc-tors would remove fewer lymph nodes. Barbara was particularly concerned, since she was afraid that with many nodes removed, she was likely to have lymphedema, which would probably be ex-acerbated by the constant changes of air pressure involved in her job. So far she has had no swelling since the procedure. Her doc-tor injected the radioactive dye before the surgery. "I lay on the table, and the camera doing a lymphoscintigraphy scan came down at me. It looked like a huge diving bell," she said. "When the nuclear medicine was shot in, it was painful." The doctor waited five minutes after the anesthetic and then put the dye into one breast. Because both breasts were affected, the procedure took about an hour. She was lying on a gurney, and every 10 minutes the camera took another picture to see if the tracer had moved to a lymph node yet. "This diving bell camera was practically in my face, and I couldn't move at all," she said. "But at least it wasn't as bad as the MRI, where I *really* couldn't move. Here at least I could scratch my nose if I had to in between pictures!"

The surgery lasted several hours, and she stayed overnight in the hospital. "At 9:00 P.M., I had to go to the john, and the nurse helped me. My pee was a bright cobalt blue. I had known about it, but the poor nurse hadn't and she was really shocked." There was also some blue in her breasts, which took about a month to clear out. Rarely the dye can tattoo the breast for a year; this is still normal and happens when the dye is taken up by the lymphatics in the skin.

The operation on her nodes left her with several weeks of discomfort. "I felt like I had a wad of scotch tape under each armpit," she recalls. "For about two weeks, I couldn't stand my arm and chest skin meeting." By the end of a month the discomfort left, and it was never bad enough to make her take the painkillers the doctors had given her.

Full Axillary Lymph Node Dissection

A full axillary dissection is done because either there are palpable nodes that have been shown to contain cancer or a positive node was found on sentinel node biopsy.

If a sentinel node has already been done, the surgeon can go through the fresh incision and extend the dissection. If the procedure is a mastectomy, then the axilla is approached through the mastectomy incision.

If the report comes back later that a node is positive and the procedure is done separately, the surgeon makes an incision about two inches across the armpit and removes the wad of fat in the hollow of the armpit, which should contain most of the lymph nodes. The lymph nodes, as I said earlier, are glands. Sometimes they're swollen and big, but usually they're small and embedded in fat. This lump of fat is defined by certain anatomical boundaries and usually contains at least 10–15 lymph nodes. We hope, but can't be sure, that we've included in this fat all the significant lymph nodes. The tissue is sent to the pathologist, who examines the fat and tries to find as many of the lymph nodes as possible. The pathologist then cuts each node in half, makes slides, and examines each of them for cancer.

Some women have more nodes than others. Occasionally a patient asks me, "How come you got 17 lymph nodes in me and only 7 in my friend?" We are all built differently. This difference was brought to my attention once after I did a routine axillary dissection. A new pathologist was dissecting out the nodes and amazed me by finding 40 in a specimen that usually would contain 15. She just looked harder than usual.

However, the total number of nodes is less important than the number positive. It is important for the surgeon to remove the tissue that probably contains the nodes. Studies have shown that the chance of missing a positive lymph node if we remove the tissue in the lower two levels of the armpit is less than 2 percent.

Some surgeons put a drain in the axillary incision afterward, and some do not. The operation takes from one to three hours. You'll go home with a small dressing on your incision. Depending on the surgeon, there may or may not be sutures to be removed, but in any case, most surgeons like to see their patients ten days to two weeks after the surgery to monitor their progress. An earlier visit can be scheduled to discuss pathology results.

Side Effects

The good news is that most studies have shown that the sentinel node biopsy has significantly fewer immediate and delayed complications than a full axillary dissection.[3] Nonetheless, since the surgery is in the same area of the body, the potential complications are the same: axillary pain, numbness, paresthesias (abnormal sensations), and arm swelling (lymphedema).

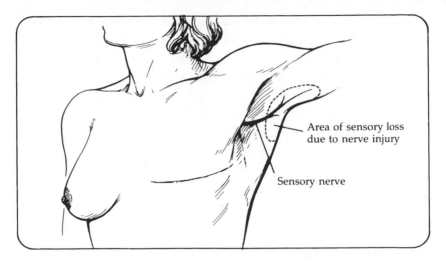

Figure 14.2

One problem is fluid under the armpit (seroma). Most women have some swelling, but sometimes a woman will get so much that it looks like she has an orange in her armpit. Usually the fluid is aspirated by the doctor in the office.

Very rarely a patient gets a hematoma (collection of blood) from surgery. If a hematoma is recognized soon after surgery, the surgeon may decide to return to the operating room to find the source of bleeding. A hematoma that develops days after surgery will generally improve on its own, without the need for additional surgery. You may, however, be black and blue for a few weeks. The surgical dressing tape may cause a rash known as tape burn.

Damage to a sensory nerve or nerves that pass through the middle of the fat that is removed may be longer lasting. This nerve gives you sensation in the back part of your armpit, though it doesn't affect the way your arm works. If that nerve is cut, you'll have a patch of numbness in the back part of your arm (Figure 14.2). Most breast surgeons and many general surgeons try to save the nerve. Even so, it may get stretched and cause decreased sensation either temporarily or permanently. If the sensation is gone for more than a few months, the loss is probably permanent. This problem is less common after sentinel node biopsy but is certainly not eliminated. (If this happens to you, you may want to give up shaving your armpits, or use an electric shaver rather than a razor, which is more likely to cut the skin and cause bleeding.)

Another early problem can be phlebitis in an arm vein. This usually shows up three or four days after surgery. The woman says, "I felt wonderful after the operation and now I have this tight feeling under my arm that goes down to the elbow and sometimes even to the wrist. And I can see a cord. The pain is worse and I can't move my arm nearly as well as I could before." This has more recently been called axillary web syndrome and is very common, but is also temporary, typically resolving within six to eight weeks.[4] I have always felt that it is an inflammation of the basilic vein, but others think it is just a general inflammation from the dissection or even a clogged lymphatic. It's not serious but it's bothersome. The best treatment is ice and aspirin or an NSAID (nonsteroidal anti-inflammatory drug) such as ibuprofen. It will go away within several days to a week. It's important to move your arm and keep it from stiffening. Ellen Mahoney, a breast surgeon I admire in northern California, tells her patients to keep their hand behind their head while reading or watching TV postoperatively to stretch the scar. If the symptoms don't improve, physical therapy will usually help the problem.

Both lymph node operations result in a variety of new and often unpleasant sensations in the area of the surgery. These have been recently reported in an article entitled appropriately "Eighteen Sensations After Breast Cancer Surgery: A 5-Year Comparison of Sentinel Lymph Node Biopsy and Axillary Lymph Node Dissection." The eighteen sensations include tender, sore, pull, ache, painful, twinge, tight, stiff, prick, throb, shoot, tingle, numb, burn, hard, sharp, nag, and penetrate.[5] Although certain sensations are far more prevalent in full dissection than sentinel node biopsy in the initial period after surgery and five years later, some sensations are still present five years after sentinel node. Tenderness remained in 33 percent of women after five years with sentinel node and 40 percent after full dissection.

The major complication, but fortunately an uncommon one, is swelling of the arm, a condition called *lymphedema,* which we'll consider in Chapter 19. Suffice it to say, the risk of lymphedema ranges from 3 to 5 percent after sentinel node biopsy compared to 15 to 20 percent after full axillary dissection.[6]

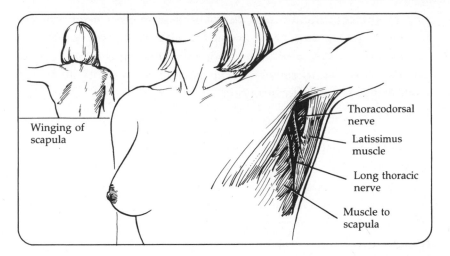

Figure 14.3

A rare complication of full axillary dissection involves the motor nerves (nerves that go to muscles and control movement). Two motor nerves can be injured by lymph node surgery, as can the nerve to the pectoralis. When injured, the pectoralis atrophies over time. One of them—the long thoracic nerve—goes to the muscle that holds your shoulder blade against your back when you hold your arm straight out. If the other two nerves are injured, your shoulder blade, instead of remaining flat, will stick out like a wing when you hold your arm out. Hence the deformity is called a winged scapula (Figure 14.3). (There are other causes of winged scapula as well; sometimes it's a congenital condition.) If you're not athletic, it probably won't affect your daily activities, but it affects things like serving in tennis or pitching a baseball.

Permanent winged scapula cases are extremely rare; if the condition is temporary, it should go away in a few weeks or months. Physical therapy can help, especially if an athlete—even a golfer—is affected.

The other nerve is called the *thoracodorsal nerve*, and it goes to the latissimus muscle. Damage to this nerve is rare and less noticeable than the winged scapula. It is likely to produce a sensation of tiredness in the arm, which won't work quite as well as it did before. Sometimes pushing a door open away from you may become more difficult. This could be a problem for an athlete, since the latissimus dorsi is involved in chin-ups, overhead tennis serves, golf drives, and swimming. Also, damage to the thoracodorsal can lead to atrophy of the muscle, limiting its utility for some types of flap reconstruction.

PARTIAL MASTECTOMY

Partial mastectomy, lumpectomy, wide excision, segmental mastectomy, and quadrantectomy are all names for procedures short of mastectomy and are used virtually synonymously (Figure14.4). What each term means precisely depends on the surgeon who's using it. Except for quadrantectomy, none of the terms suggests how much tissue will be removed, and often surgeons use quadrantectomy when they don't necessarily mean they'll remove a fourth of the breast. With a partial mastectomy, the part removed can be 1 percent or 50 percent of the breast tissue. Lumpectomy depends on the size of the lump. Wide excision just says that tissue will be cut away around the lump—not how much will be cut. "Segmental" sounds like the breast comes in little segments, like an orange. But it doesn't, and the segment removed can be any size. Your surgeon will use whatever term appeals most to her or him. The goal of breast conservation is to excise the primary tumor with negative margins while maintaining a cosmetically acceptable breast.

Wire Localization

If your lesion cannot be felt, it must be localized preoperatively. Most of these lesions have been diagnosed by a stereotactic core biopsy (see Chapter 8) and a titanium clip has been left at the biopsy site. Although this can sound scary the clips are incredibly tiny, reaction to titanium is extremely rare, and failure to leave a clip can make correct localization in the breast quite difficult, or may be the reason that the wire localization misses.

If a wide excision needs to be performed, the clip will be localized for the surgeon with a guide wire (needle localization) in the mammography suite immediately before surgery. The radiologist

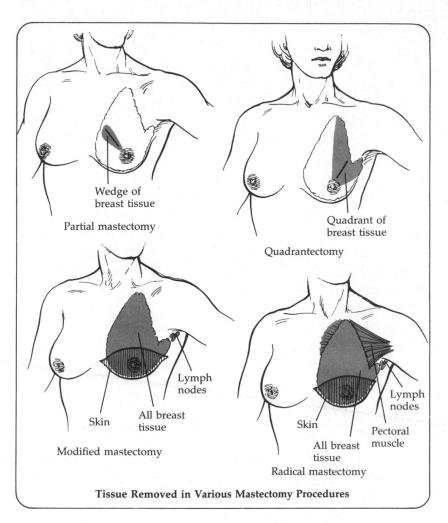

Wedge of
breast tissue

Partial mastectomy

Quadrant of
breast tissue

Quadrantectomy

Lymph
nodes

Skin   All breast
tissue

Modified mastectomy

Lymph
nodes

Skin

Pectoral
muscle

All breast
tissue

Radical mastectomy

Tissue Removed in Various Mastectomy Procedures

Figure 14.4

will give you a local anesthetic and put a small needle into your breast under X ray guidance, pointing toward the lesion (Figure 14.5). She will then pass a wire with a hook on the end through the needle, and then position the hook so the end of the wire is on the site of the calcifications or density. If the lesion encompasses an area of more than a centimeter or if it follows a linear pattern, more than one wire may be placed to outline the area that needs to be excised for the surgeon. Shelly Hwang, a surgical colleague at UCSF, likes to think of the wires as "brackets" or "parentheses" around the area to be removed. The wire or wires are left in the breast and you're taken to the operating room. After the tissue and wire(s) are removed, the specimen is sent to the radiology department. There they x-ray it to make sure it includes the calcifications or lesion and then send it to the pathology department where they make slides and look at it under the microscope. The X ray of the specimen will tell you if the surgeon got the calcifications or area that was seen on the mammogram. Since the surgeon can't see or feel calcifications, the surgery may miss them. In this case the X ray of the specimen will not show calcifications and you may need to get another biopsy.

Another technique that is sometimes used takes advantage of a side effect of the diagnostic core biopsy used for diagnosis. After any core there will be a small hematoma (collection of blood) in the breast where the tissue was removed. This can often be located with ultrasound, allowing a surgeon to identify the tissue he or she needs to remove without the insertion of a wire.[7]

A new method of localizing the breast tissue has been described by surgeons at the Mayo Clinic and involves placement of a small radioactive seed in the breast. The seed is removed at the time of surgery. In the future, this approach may allow surgeons to better localize the area to be removed, thus improving the likelihood that the right area is removed.[8]

The operation itself is pretty standard. If a sentinel node biopsy is going to be done, the radioactive tracer is injected before

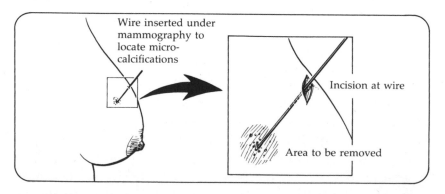

Figure 14.5

the patient arrives in the operating room, as previously described. In the operating room you will undergo carefully monitored anesthesia, either local with sedation or general anesthetic. If a sentinel node biopsy is going to be done, the surgeon will also inject blue dye prior to starting. The lumpectomy will be done after the nodes, while the surgeon waits for the result of the sentinel node biopsy. If a full axillary dissection is being done, then the lumpectomy usually comes first. If you're opting for such surgery, you need to make sure your surgeon explains precisely how much tissue will be removed, and what you're going to look like afterward.

As we gain more experience with breast conservation, improved surgical techniques are leading to better cosmetic results. The placement of the incision will take into consideration the cosmetic result as well as the area that needs to be removed. Once the surgeon makes the incision, going through skin, fat, and tissue to get to the lump isn't actually cutting; it's just spreading tissue apart until the lump is reached. The lump is cut away from the surrounding tissue and removed. Every effort is made to take the lump out in one piece so that the pathologist can determine whether there is tumor at the edges or margins (see Chapter 11). There's little bleeding from this excision because there aren't many blood vessels here, and the cautery takes care of the few there are. Prior to closing the incision four metal clips (like large staples) are often put in the four corners of the biopsy cavity to help the radiation therapist in directing the radiation postoperatively. The incision is then sewn up, usually in layers—tissue, then skin. The spot where the tissue was removed will fill with some fluid in the process of healing. The goal is to prevent a dent from forming in the breast when it heals (Figure 14.6). Most surgeons use dissolvable stitches that tend to leave less scarring.

The current trend is to do oncoplastic surgery, a combination of cancer surgery and plastic surgery. This involves using some of the techniques originally developed for reduction mammoplasties (see Chapter 2) to remove the tumor in such a way as to allow the breast to be reconstructed in a cosmetically pleasing manner.[9] This approach is most important when a large area is removed. If your surgeon says it's impossible to remove your tumor cosmetically, you may want to get a second opinion from someone who is

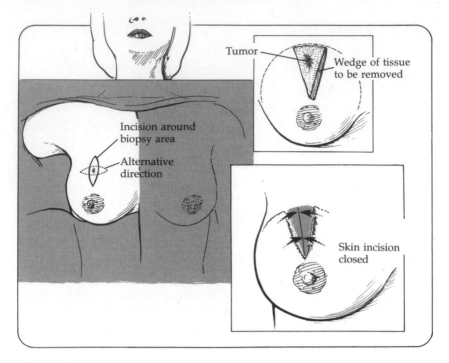

Figure 14.6

trained in oncoplastic surgery. Sometimes this approach looks great but the breasts won't be the same size. In that situation it is possible to reduce or lift the uninvolved breast to match.

After the operation the surgeon bandages the incision and will probably tell you when you can take the bandage off and when you can shower.

Once the tissue is removed, it is oriented for the pathologist and marked to indicate which side is toward the head and which is toward the middle of the body. This way the surgeon knows not only if there is tumor at a margin but also which margin. As explained in Chapter 8, the surgeon or pathologist paints the tissue with different color ink and then it is cut into small pieces (Figure 14.7). It goes through several stages. First it's dehydrated in different strengths of alcohol, then embedded in a block of paraffin wax. This is put on a microtome, a knife that cuts it into very thin slices. Each slice is then put on a slide, the wax melted away, and the tissue stained with different colors. This whole process takes between 24 and 36 hours.

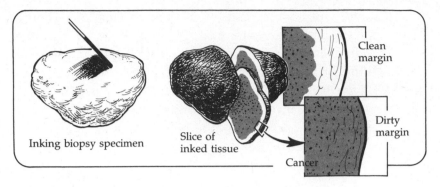

Figure 14.7

When the slides are ready, the pathologist looks at them and makes a diagnosis; this takes a few hours. The pathologist then dictates a report that is sent to the doctor, who will probably have it in a week. Some doctors wait till the report comes in, but others prefer to call the pathologist the day after the operation. This is what I used to do because I liked to let my patients know what was happening as soon as possible, and because for all patients the waiting and uncertainty can be terrifying. Whatever your doctor's practice, you'll know in a week or so what the biopsy has shown.

At Home After Partial Mastectomy and Lymph Node Surgery

Once you're home, you'll feel exhausted for a while. Respect that tiredness: you've just been through major surgery, anesthesia, and an emotionally difficult experience. The exhaustion often comes and goes suddenly: you'll feel fine and go do an errand; when you get home you'll suddenly feel completely wiped out and need to sleep. It may take a couple of weeks for you to feel fully recovered.

You'll have some pain but probably not a lot. Most doctors give their patients pain medication—usually Vicodin or codeine—when they go home, but the majority of women don't finish the prescription. Occasionally people have a lot of pain, and if that's the case it's a good idea to let the doctor know. It's often a sign of something wrong, like postoperative bleeding or a hematoma. Also be aware that if you were already taking pain medication before surgery for another condition, then you may need more medication than most patients.

After a lumpectomy, you should wear a strong support bra day and night for about a week—it hurts when your breast jiggles. Another trick my patients taught me, particularly my patients with larger breasts, is that if you want to lie on your side, you can lie on the side that wasn't operated on and hold a pillow between your breasts: the pillow cushions the breast that's been operated on (Figure 14.8).

Side Effects of Partial Mastectomy

As with any surgical procedure, there are sometimes complications in a partial mastectomy. The two most common are hematoma and infection. If a hematoma occurs it will usually be within a day or two of the procedure. Bleeding inside the area where the surgery was done causes a blood blister to form (Figure 14.9). It turns blue and forms a lump right under the skin. The body usually simply absorbs and recycles it, as it does with any bruise. But sometimes, before the body can do that, you'll bump into something or someone will bump into you, and it will burst

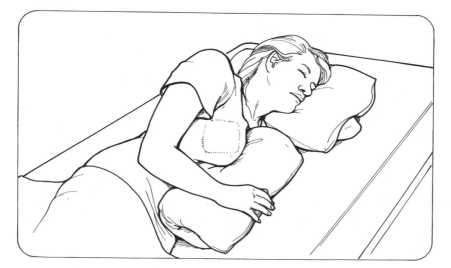

Figure 14.8

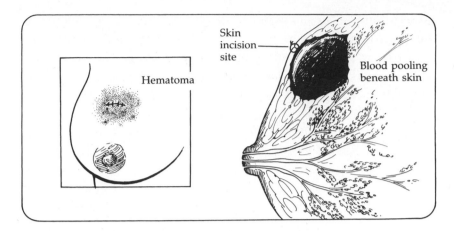

Figure 14.9

open, causing dark blood to come out. It looks gross and disgusting and you'll think you're dying, but don't worry—you're not. It's old blood; you're not bleeding now. What you need to do is go home, clean up the mess, and take a shower. You should also call your doctor and let her know what is going on; she will probably want to see you in the office to get it checked out. Unless there is ongoing, bright red bleeding, this is not an emergency and it will eventually get better on its own.

If an infection occurs, it will show up a week or two after surgery—there'll be redness and swelling and fever, and the doctor will treat it with antibiotics. Again, it's more of a nuisance than anything else. If the infection is slow to improve, you may need to be rehospitalized for a few days of IV antibiotics.

Sometimes you'll get a combination of infection and hematoma—the blood mixes with pus, like an abscess or a boil, and needs to be drained by the doctor. Sometimes when stitches are removed after breast surgery—either biopsies or cosmetic procedures—a small, nondissolvable stitch is overlooked and remains in the breast, which will then get infected, as was the case with one of my patients (no, I wasn't the surgeon who removed the stitches). It's easy to treat by prescribing antibiotics and removing the stitch.

There may be some loss of sensation in your breast after a partial mastectomy, depending on the size of the lump removed. If it's a large lump, there may be a permanent numb spot, but there won't be the total loss of sensation that results from a mastectomy.

Your breast may be different in size and shape than it was before and will probably differ from your other breast. How great the difference depends on how much tissue was removed and how skillfully the surgery was done. If your breasts have become asymmetrical to an extent that disturbs you, you can get partial mastectomy breast pads called shells to wear in your bra. Or you can have reconstructive surgery: a small flap of your own tissue is put in to fill things out (see Chapter 15). Or, depending on how large your breasts were to begin with, you can get the other breast reduced to create a more symmetrical appearance. Usually, however, that isn't necessary. If you have a small lump and medium or large breasts, it's often hard to tell which breast was operated on, except for the scar.

The pathology results are usually available within a week. The surgeon can then tell the patient what the margins were like and what was actually in her breast tissue and, most important, whether there was any cancer in the lymph nodes. On the basis of the pathology report, you'll discuss the next steps, and whether there is a need for adjuvant therapy.

TOTAL MASTECTOMY

In spite of the availability of partial mastectomy and radiation, which conserve the breast, most women in this country have total mastectomy as their initial therapy for breast cancer.

Total mastectomy should not be confused with radical mastectomy. The latter, once the norm, is now of interest for historical reasons only. The surgical procedure was basically the same as that for the modified radical (described below), but more extensive. In addition to trying to remove all the breast tissue, the surgeon removed the pectoralis major and pectoralis minor muscles (see Figure 14.10). All of the lymph nodes in the axillary area (up to the collarbone) were removed as well. It was far more deforming than the mastectomy we do now. Today we almost always use neoadjuvant chemotherapy to shrink very large tumors before surgery (see Chapter 12). If the tumor is stuck to the muscle, the

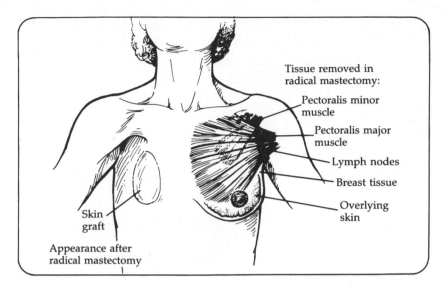

Figure 14.10

surgeon must remove the muscle in order to get to the tumor. (In very rare cases the cancer spreads into the muscle.) We used to do radical mastectomies in all of these cases, but now we just take a wedge of muscle under the tumor and leave the rest.

"Total mastectomy," the name usually given to the form of mastectomy used today, is a bit of a misnomer, since we can never be certain the operation is total. Our goal is to remove all the breast tissue, but we can't ever be sure we've achieved that. We remove as much of the breast tissue as we can and some of the lymph nodes. It usually takes between two and five hours.

The breast tissue extends from the collarbone to just below the inframammary fold and from the breastbone to the muscle in the back of the armpit. The surgeon wants to remove as much of it as possible and starts with an elliptical incision that includes the nipple and biopsy scar; exactly where it is depends on where your biopsy scar is (Figure 14.11).

With the increasing popularity of immediate reconstruction, surgeons have taken to removing as little skin as possible. We used to take out a large amount of skin when we did mastectomies in part because we liked the fact that this helped the scar

close neatly. If the surgeon leaves a lot of skin and scoops out all
the breast tissue, the skin looks wrinkled and baggy. Trimming the
skin creates a nice neat line across the chest. But now, as immediate reconstructions are being done, removing so much skin is being reconsidered. We've moved into the era of skin-sparing
mastectomy. Instead of removing a lot of skin around the breast,
surgeons remove only the amount that's needed to take the breast
off, unless the patient is absolutely sure she never wants reconstruction in which case it is still nice to be tidy. We've begun to

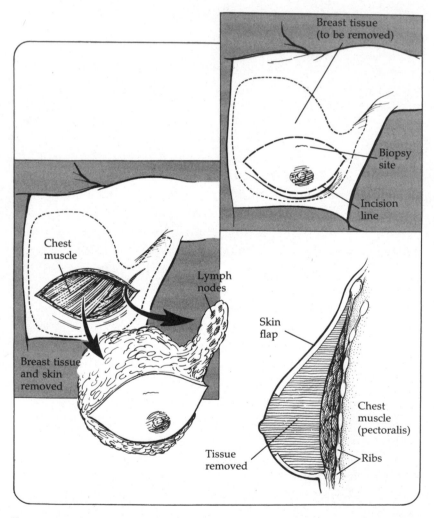

Figure 14.11

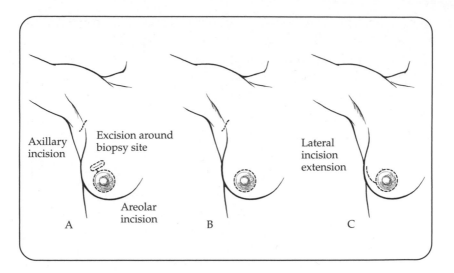

Figure 14.12

view mastectomy as a very wide excision. Removing every bit of breast tissue isn't possible or necessary: it's getting the tumor out that really matters (Figure 14.12). In some cases where the tumor is not near the nipple, the nipple may be spared as well. While there is some controversy over whether this gives as low a chance for recurrence as removing all the nipple tissue, several centers in the country are using it routinely for women who have breast reconstruction in order to preserve as much of the natural appearance of the breast as possible. Long-term results are not yet available, but so far, the results look very promising.[10]

Next we tunnel underneath the remaining skin all the way up to the collarbone, then down to just below the inframammary fold (see Chapter 2) from the middle of the sternum, and out to the muscle behind your armpit. Once the dissection is done, we peel the breast off, leaving the muscle and skin flap behind.

When the breast is fully removed, we reach up under the skin to the armpit and do an axillary dissection or sentinel node biopsy as described earlier. Most surgeons do the sentinel node biopsy first so that they will have the results of the pathological evaluation available when they finish the mastectomy. That way if the woman needs a full dissection they can go right ahead. If the mastectomy incision was very small, a separate incision is made in the armpit for the lymph node surgery.

We send the breast tissue and the attached fat with nodes to the pathologist, who examines it and begins the process of fixing it to make slides. Meanwhile we sew together the flaps of skin around the incision. You end up completely flat (or, if you're very thin, slightly concave), with a scar going across the middle of that side of your chest. The skin doesn't completely stick down right away; the body doesn't like empty spaces, so the area fills up with fluid. To prevent this, we insert some drains in soft plastic tubes with little holes in them, coming out of the skin below the scar (Figure 14.13). They help create suction that holds the skin down against the muscle till it heals. Fluid will come out of these drains—it's just tissue fluid, the kind you get in a blister. Initially there'll be a little blood in the fluid, but over time it will become clearer.

If you've decided to have immediate breast reconstruction (see Chapter 15), the plastic surgeon comes in after the mastectomy is finished but before the skin is sewn up and does the reconstruction. Alternatively, the plastic surgeon may be part of the team from the beginning, raising the tissue flap from the abdomen while the breast surgeon is doing the mastectomy. As with partial mastectomy, the pathology results will be available in four to five days.

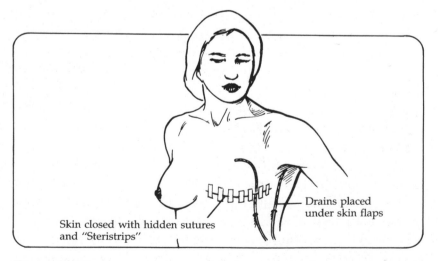

Skin closed with hidden sutures and "Steristrips"

Drains placed under skin flaps

Figure 14.13

Different surgeons have different styles in postoperative treatment. I usually put a big, bulky wraparound dressing on my patients because it helped them feel protected from the world for a while. My colleague Susan Troyan has switched to a light gauze dressing with a plastic covering so that the woman can shower and move more freely. You'll probably stay in the hospital at least overnight. When there's no longer much fluid coming out of the drains—in about 7 to 10 days—we remove them and change the dressing. We used to keep people in the hospital till all the drains came out, but nowadays patients usually go home and come back later to get the drains removed in the office.

One of my colleagues, Lisa Bailey, explained that she deals with the postoperative pain with a pump that delivers continuous local anesthesia into the space between skin and muscle. This has made a big difference, as patients have little or no pain, and therefore can get out of bed and walk faster, don't need narcotics and so have less nausea.

Some women want to see the wound right away; some prefer to put off looking at it for a week or two. Either way is fine; you need to decide what makes you feel best. But it's important that you look at it at some point. It's amazing how, if you're determined to avoid looking at your body, you can do so when you shower, get dressed, even when you make love. That's okay for a while, but this is the body you're going to be living with, and you need to see it and accept it.

Many of my patients liked me to be with them the first time they saw their scar so that I could offer emotional support and answer any questions they had. If you would like your surgeon with you when you first look at your chest, ask.

Others want to see it alone before showing it to their husband or lover. Again, there's no right or wrong way to face it, as long as you do. In my experience, most women are relieved when it doesn't look as bad as they feared it would.

Permanent numbness in the area around the mastectomy scar is an unfortunate result of the operation, since the breast's nerve supply has been cut. Some sensitivity remains around the outer borders of the area where your breast was located. Sometimes the breast area is not entirely numb; you can tell if someone is touching you. Unfortunately this usually isn't a pleasant sensation. It can be very uncomfortable, like the sensation you feel when your foot is asleep and starts coming back again, with a tingly feeling. This is known as dysesthesia, and it will lessen but will remain with you. Often people who have had mastectomies don't like their scars being touched because it brings about this sensation. Some women will recover sensation over a long period of time.

Some women also experience phantom breast symptoms—like the amputee who feels itchiness in toes that are no longer there. The mastectomy patient may feel her missing nipple itch or her missing breast ache. This means that the brain hasn't yet realized what's happened to the body. The nerve supply from the breast grows along a certain path in the spinal cord and goes to a certain area of the brain. The brain has been trained over the years that a signal from this path means, for example, that the nipple is itching. When the nipple has been removed, the signal may get generated in a different place farther along the path, but the brain cells think it should be coming from the nipple, and that's the information they give you. This will gradually improve as your brain becomes reprogrammed.

Audre Lorde described these feelings wonderfully in her book *The Cancer Journal*: "fixed pains and moveable pains, deep pains and surface pains, strong pains and weak pains. There were stabs and throbs and burns, gripes and tickles and itches."[11] In addition, some women feel tightness around the chest as the healing starts. This will ease up over time, and all the weird sensations will start to settle down.

Side Effects of Total Mastectomy

Like any operation, mastectomy has risks. In the process of removing the breast tissue, we sever a number of blood vessels. The only ones left are those that go the whole length of the flap of skin remaining when the tissue underneath is removed. These vessels can barely get to the ends of the flap. Sometimes this doesn't supply enough blood, and the wound doesn't heal right; a little area of skin dies and forms a scab (Figure 14.14). Once healing is complete, the scab falls off. It's usually not a serious complication. If a big enough area of skin is involved or an infection develops, the

Two possible complications . . .

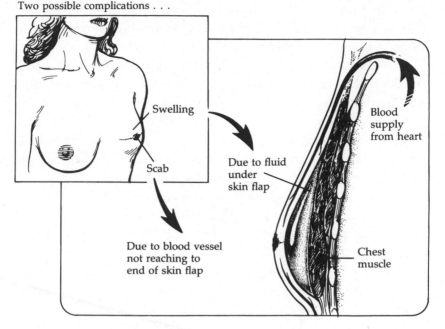

Swelling

Scab

Due to fluid
under
skin flap

Due to blood vessel
not reaching to
end of skin flap

Blood
supply
from heart

Chest
muscle

Figure 14.14

surgeon may have to trim the dead tissue so the body can heal the wound. Sometimes a skin graft to cover this area can speed up the healing process.

A second possible complication occurs when fluid continues to collect under the scar after the drains are removed. You'll know this is happening because there's a swelling under the skin below the incision; sometimes you'll hear a slosh when you're walking or you'll feel the fluid in your chest. If it's a small amount of fluid, it will eventually go away by itself. If there's a lot of fluid, it can be aspirated with a needle; it won't hurt because the area is numb, and it usually doesn't require local anesthesia. (We try to avoid too many aspirations, since there's always the slight risk of transmitting infection through the needle.) Again, this isn't a serious complication, but it can be annoying.

Exercise After Mastectomy

Exercise is important after your treatment, and not only in terms of lymphedema. After you've had a mastectomy or a lymph node sampling, your surgeon may tell you not to move your arm at all. There's a lot of controversy about how protective of the area you should be, and some doctors can be overrestrictive.

If you keep your arm very still at first, you'll probably have a stiff shoulder when you start moving around. Ben Anderson in Seattle tells me that all mastectomy and axillary lymph node dissection patients get an automatic referral to physical therapy where, at a minimum, they are taught basic exercises and also receive additional lymphedema education. As he rightly points out, physical therapy works better preventing than curing a frozen shoulder.

Certain exercises actually help your shoulder (Figure 14.15). Immediately after surgery, shoulder rolls are a good way to prevent your shoulder from getting stiff. Another exercise is called "climbing the walls." It involves walking your fingers up the wall, stretching a little bit farther each time. You can do it while you're watching TV or talking on the phone. Another good exercise starting a couple of weeks after surgery involves leaning over and making bigger and bigger circles with your arm. Swimming is also excellent exercise and will help maintain strength and range of motion.

If your arm remains very stiff after two or three weeks, ask your doctor to refer you to a physical therapist. It's very important to get your shoulder flexible again, and soon; otherwise you can end up with frozen shoulder, a condition that is difficult to treat successfully. If you already have shoulder problems, see a physical therapist preoperatively for advice.

Any sport or exercise you did before your cancer, you can do now—and you should, if you want to.

Long-Term Side Effects of Surgery and Radiation

Unfortunately your body doesn't always feel the way it did before your cancer began. Radiation can cause delayed problems. A certain side effect can occur between three and six months after you've finished your treatment. The muscle that goes above and behind your breast, the pectoralis major muscle (Figure 14.16), will get extremely sore, and it's worse if you grab it between your fingers. That's because the radiation caused inflammation of the

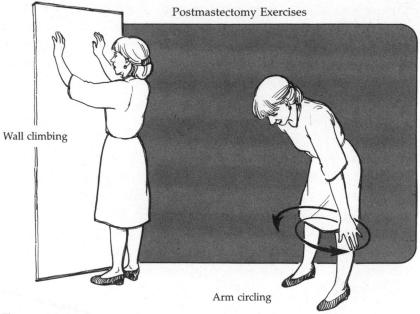

Figure 14.15

muscle, and as it begins to regenerate, it can get sore and stiff, just as it would if you threw it out during strenuous exercise. Most women think it's the cancer spreading—especially since the radiation has been over for months and they're not expecting new side effects from it.

Many women have a stiff or frozen shoulder a month after breast surgery. These arm and shoulder problems result from the lymph node dissection, not the breast surgery. When your armpit hurts, it's natural to try to protect it by keeping your arm immobilized. But when you don't use your arm, your shoulder muscles grow weak and the tendons and ligaments tighten. You may have difficulty reaching and feel pain when you raise your hand above your head. Not using your arm for a long time may lead to frozen shoulder—the joint becomes locked. Frozen shoulder can be more difficult to treat than a stiff shoulder, and it sometimes requires surgery. Bear in mind, however, that arm and shoulder problems are not an inescapable consequence of the procedure. They can be prevented or reversed by doing the exercises described above. The

YWCA has a wonderful exercise program, Encore, that focuses on helping women recover. Swimming is also good because it doesn't put weight on the arm. You can contact your local Y to see if they offer the Encore program. Over time, you can resume any exercise routine you enjoyed in the past.

If exercising on your own isn't successful, a physical therapist can assess what you are capable of doing and where you need help and then devise a program to increase your strength and flexibility. The therapist will train you to do exercises properly so that you don't get hurt when you do them. Insurance plans often cover physical therapy after breast surgery, so be sure to ask.

Massage has effects similar to those of exercise. It can help relax tight tendons to get your shoulder back in commission. Acupuncture is another possibility (see Chapter 18). Although it has been tested for only a few applications in Western medicine, acupuncture hasn't been demonstrated to cause harm or cause lymphedema. There is some evidence it can help relieve lower back pain, so it may also help shoulder stiffness. However, there are no scientific data about this.

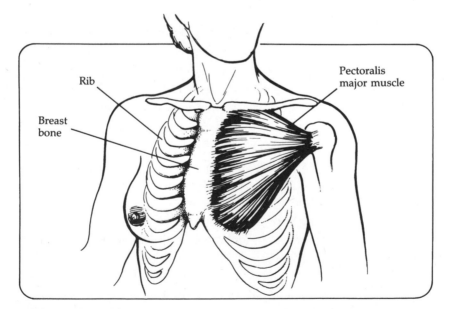

Figure 14.16

Scarring is an inevitable consequence of breast surgery, as it is for any type of surgery. Initially, many women are so intent on saving their lives that they don't think about how their body will look after therapy. Of course, the appearance of the scar depends not only on the extent of surgery but on your skin, your body type, the size of your breast, and the type of surgery you had. To avoid being surprised by your body's appearance after surgery, ask your doctor to show you pictures of women who have had a similar operation; you may also go to my website and look at the "show me" collection or read books on the subject. There are several things you can do to make the scar more acceptable to you, from working with the surgeon to prevent surprises to having plastic surgery.

After mastectomy, the incision can take more than a year to heal completely. It may be difficult to know whether a problem that arises is temporary or will be with you long-term. Either way, you should discuss problems that seem significant or unusual with your surgeon. Remember that you don't need to wait a year to have additional surgery or procedures to correct the problems. There is nothing wrong with being concerned about how you look.

The scar may be raised, seemingly filled with extra skin. This is a keloid scar and results from an overly aggressive effort by the body's immune system to heal the wound. The body keeps filling the scar with collagen long after the wound has closed. The tendency to form keloid scars is probably inherited and can't be prevented. A plastic surgeon may be able to improve the scar's appearance.

A mastectomy leaves a fairly large wound. When the surgeon pulls the skin and underlying tissue together to close it, the surface of the chest is drawn taut. In contrast, the surrounding tissue under the arm may seem baggy and excessive and hang over your bra. If fat is a major component of the extra tissue under the arm, it can be removed through liposuction. Excess skin can also be eliminated without increasing scarring.

Even a lumpectomy can change the appearance of the breast you've saved. It may look foreign and disturbing to you; it may have a dent, look shrunken, or appear to be pulled to one side.

If you are still troubled by the appearance of your breast months or years after surgery, you can always have a reconstructive procedure. A plastic surgeon can discuss various techniques to re-align nipples, reshape breasts, and make the breasts more symmetrical (see Chapter 15).

Other long-term problems may also result from the surgery. While most women experience some pain in the weeks after surgery, especially after mastectomy, many will have pain for years. It can even begin years after the operation. Forty-nine percent of patients who have operations for breast cancer say they have some sort of ongoing pain or change in sensation, and 10 percent say it interferes with their daily lives.[12] The biggest complaint is "aching," experienced by 44–47 percent of the women who say they have pain. Many others describe it as a "stabbing" pain. "Shooting," "sharp," "tiring," and "throbbing" are other descriptions. They feel the pain in the mastectomy scar, the arm, even the muscle under the breast. I've known a number of women with this problem and it affects their lives.

C. B. Wallace studied pain experienced a year after different kinds of breast surgery.[13] Lumpectomy alone resulted in pain among 31 percent of subjects. Mastectomy plus reconstruction caused pain in 49 percent of the women. Women who had breast reconstruction varied. Those who had implants under the muscle had pain in 15 percent of cases, whereas those who had them above the muscle had pain 21 percent of the time. Mastectomy alone caused pain through the armpit and arm; 82 percent of women had pain under their arms three months after a mastectomy, and in 16 percent, it lasted at least six months. Sometimes the pain was so bad the woman couldn't move her arm and developed frozen shoulder (described above). Women who had breast reduction suffered later pain in 22 percent of cases, and 40 percent of women who had breast augmentation had pain. One study shows that careful surgical techniques reduce the amount of chronic pain.[14] Researchers found fewer pain problems associated with operations performed in centers that do lots of surgery than in those that don't. It makes sense: an inexperienced surgeon is more likely to injure nerves.

Fortunately this kind of pain is not common and has been treated with *myofascial release,* a form of massage.[15] Among my patients acupuncture has helped a great deal. Another pain study suggests that antidepressants can relieve pain caused by damaged nerves. This has no relation to the patient's frame of mind but to the way such drugs work on nerves.[16] Most large hospitals have pain specialists on staff to consult with patients who experience long-term problems with treatment-related pain.

Cellulitis

Cellulitis is a skin infection occurring in places that have diminished access to the immune system, such as areas of swelling or areas that have been radiated. It can start from any small infection and spread rapidly, often with a red streak up the arm or redness of the arm and/or breast. Sometimes it can be accompanied by lymphedema. There is usually a fever as well. Although this type of infection can sometimes be treated with oral antibiotics, usually it requires hospitalization for intravenous drugs. Some women who are prone to recurrent attacks of cellulitis ask the doctor for a standing antibiotic prescription so they can start taking it at the least sign of impending infection. In a series of studies from Memphis, Tennessee, 1 percent of the lumpectomy and radiation patients had cellulitis of the breast.

Whatever your choice of surgery, it can be an emotional and difficult experience now. Fortunately, there are more options for women with breast cancer, and the options are more effective than ever before at maximizing cancer cure and reducing the side effects of cancer treatment. Use all the resources available to you to make a decision you will be able to live with comfortably. Your surgeon is a great resource, but it is important to try to connect with other women who have been through the experience as well. And make sure that you free up enough time and energy so that you can focus on making good decisions for yourself and your family.

Chapter 15

ONCOPLASTIC SURGERY, RECONSTRUCTION, AND PROSTHESES

FOR MOST WOMEN WITH BREAST CANCER THE FIRST CONCERN is maximizing their chances to live; a second important concern is how they will look after breast cancer surgery. As noted in Chapter 1, our breasts carry a lot of meaning and feelings and their appearance is important to many of us. The options for creating a cosmetically appealing breast or breast equivalent have increased significantly over the years. Your lumpectomy can be done with oncoplastic surgery. You can have postmastectomy reconstruction immediately or later. Or you can use a prosthesis in your bra after mastectomy or lumpectomy (Figure 15.1). Finally, there is always the option of simply not appearing to have two symmetrical breasts. In this chapter we will review all of the options, their pros and cons, and include some women's stories about what they have chosen to do.

PARTIAL RECONSTRUCTION AFTER LUMPECTOMY: IMMEDIATE AND DELAYED

Although we have better and better ways to apply the techniques of plastic surgery to lumpectomies, more women than ever are

444

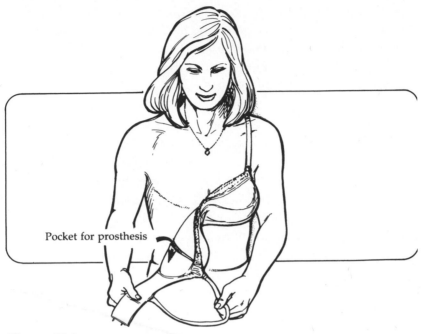

Pocket for prosthesis

Figure 15.1

choosing mastectomies as noted in Chapter 14. This has always seemed odd to me, especially since, the medical results of lumpectomy plus radiation are the same as those of mastectomy. Part of this may be the realization that, as breast conservation surgery became more common, surgeons started removing larger pieces of tissue to achieve clean margins, often at the expense of cosmetic results. I wonder if these women are fully aware that the reconstruction techniques associated with mastectomy are also available for lumpectomy. We can achieve an excellent aesthetic result while conserving most of the feeling in your breast. It has been reported that 20–30 percent of women who have lumpectomies have a poor cosmetic result.[1] Yet it needn't be that way. If the potential cosmetic effect plays a large part in your choice of cancer surgery, you should be reassured by the increased availability of reconstruction for either path. If your surgeon doesn't mention this, you should ask about it and then do some research yourself. Some breast centers have multidisciplinary teams that include a plastic surgeon in the planning and during the surgery. Other centers include surgeons who have taken special courses in oncoplastic surgery (a combination of cancer surgery and plastic surgery). If you are concerned about the cosmetic results of your operation, you should definitely get a second opinion from a surgeon or team that has a special interest in this approach.

Oncoplastic surgery can be done at the time of the original operation, in a week or so after the pathology has been reviewed, or at a later time to improve the appearance of your treated breast; however, doing it around the time of surgery is usually best. If a woman has medium or large breasts (C cup or larger), the defect from removing the tumor can be repaired by rearranging the breast tissue or applying techniques that were developed for reduction mammoplasty (see Chapter 2). Removing the tissue without repairing the defect until after radiation therapy often leaves a large deformity that requires the transfer of a flap similar to those used for total reconstruction (see below).

A team at MD Anderson Cancer Center in Houston, Texas, has looked at different applications of this oncoplastic approach.[2] Ideally, the patient comes in before the lumpectomy (also known as partial mastectomy) and radiation, enabling doctors to plan the approach. The critical factor is the likelihood of being able to remove the tumor with clean margins (see Chapter 14). Many women have distinct tumors without a lot of associated DCIS and therefore are likely to get clean margins in the first attempt to remove the tumor. These women can undergo immediate reconstruction before radiation therapy. On the other hand, women with extensive DCIS or lobular tumors may not achieve clean margins as easily and may need to have the tissue removed and then return for reconstruction once the status of the margins has been confirmed. Other issues include the size of the tumor, the size of the breast, and the amount of available skin.

Sometimes mastectomy and reconstruction may be a better choice; for example, if you have had a partial mastectomy with a negative margin but poor cosmetic results and have not yet had radiation therapy. In this setting the choices are dictated by the location, extent of tumor resection, and breast size. And once tissue has been radiated, it is harder to rearrange to fill in a defect. If the radiation was partial or localized, there are more options. A woman with a C or D cup can probably use her own breast tissue, while one with smaller breasts may need a tissue flap from the back to fill in the defect. Similarly, a woman who has already undergone surgery and whole breast radiation therapy may not be satisfied with her result. Although tissue rearrangement can be attempted it has a much higher complication rate because of the radiation therapy. The alternative is to use a tissue flap bringing unirradiated tissue into the area. While this can work, the flap is rarely the same color as the remaining breast tissue. Many women in this setting elect to do nothing or to have a completion mastectomy (have the rest of the breast removed) and reconstruction.

The size of the breast is important. The local procedures work for women with size C or D cup breasts but not for smaller women. The location of the tumor also plays a role. Fixing the involved breast often means surgery to the other breast to make it match. This is usually not done at the same time if there is still radiation to come, since the radiated breast may shrink a bit. After the radiation is done, the other breast may be reduced so that it matches. If the plastic surgery is done after radiation, then the reduction on the other side can be performed at the same time.

If all of this sounds like a lot of surgery, it is. But as you will see, mastectomy with reconstruction is also often a multioperation procedure. As you contemplate these approaches, make sure you find out how many operations will be involved and what you can expect at each stage. Talk to women who have been through this surgery and get their description of what is involved. I don't want to discourage you, but I do want you to have a realistic picture of what is involved so you can make an informed decision. Only you can decide what is most important to you.

RECONSTRUCTION AFTER MASTECTOMY

Reconstruction after mastectomy is the creation of a new and natural-appearing breast by a plastic surgeon. Breast reconstruction has made a big difference, both physically and emotionally, for many women who have had mastectomies. But it's important to understand the limits of reconstructive surgery before you decide to have it done.

What's constructed is not a real breast. It may look real, but it will never have full sensation, as a breast does. Any surgeon who says, "We're going to take off your breast and give you a new one, and it'll be as good as ever" is either naive or dishonest. The surgeon may tell you that the new breast "feels normal": at best, a half truth. It will feel normal to the hand that's touching it, but it will have little sensation itself. However, feeling is part skin sensation and part mental experience. You may have some slight "feeling" return, but it will never feel the same to you. As a patient told me, you need time to bond with your new breast.

Reconstruction can make your life a little easier—you can wear a T-shirt or a housedress and not worry about putting on a bra. If the doorbell rings while you're still in your bathrobe, you don't have to deal with whether or not you want the mail carrier to see your asymmetry. Wearing bathing suits and other revealing clothes is easier. In *Why Me?* Rose Kushner explains her decision to have reconstruction. She was alone in a hotel room one night, when she was awakened by a fire alarm and the smell of smoke. She jumped out of bed, threw on her clothing, grabbed her glasses, and ran. Downstairs in the lobby with the other guests, she realized that only she had gotten dressed; the others were in their robes. Then she realized why: "This 'well-adjusted' mastectomee wasn't going anywhere publicly with one breast."[3]

A reconstruction can help some women put their cancer experiences behind them. As one of my patients said, "When I was wearing my prosthesis every day, when I looked at my body and it was concave where there had been a breast, I felt that I was a cancer patient, that I was living with that every single day. With the reconstruction I feel that I'm healthy again, that I can go on with my life." Another patient says that after her mastectomy, "I always felt the hollows under my arm. After my reconstruction, I put my arms down, and something was there. That's when the tears came; it was splendid to have that back."

On the other hand, reconstruction isn't right for everybody. One of my patients regretted having it. Displeased with the appearance of her reconstructed breast, she also felt that the plastic surgery functioned as a form of denial. "It caused me to postpone the mourning I had to do over losing a breast," she says. "Instead of mourning the loss of a breast, I was thinking in terms of getting a breast. So it wasn't until the process was over, and I saw my new breast, which wasn't like my other breast, that it hit me that I'd lost a breast. If I had the decision to make now, I don't think I'd have reconstruction."

Another woman felt she had not really been given a choice. "I appreciated the option to reconstruct; however, it almost didn't feel like an option. There was definitely an assumption that I would reconstruct because of my age. I was 40. 'Here are the names of two great plastic surgeons.' I was coping with the shock and aftermath of a devastating breast cancer diagnosis. I was on autopilot." She followed the suggestion and felt all right about it in the beginning. "After I completed chemo and radiation, the reconstruction (with a flap from her stomach) didn't match the remaining breast but I really could not have cared less." In spite of her plastic surgeon urging her to "do some fine-tuning," she decided she had been through enough surgery. It really bothered the plastic surgeon. The patient had problems with discomfort from the surgery for years after. "I was an active woman who mountain climbed and kayaked. If I knew then what I know now, I would not have reconstructed. To quote Popeye . . . 'I yam what I yam.' I would have skipped the rest entirely."

Some dissatisfaction may result from the limits of the procedure. The best reconstructions look like real breasts, but others look real only through bras or clothing. It is important to be realistic about your expectations. What do you hope to get from having a reconstructed breast? Some women are very concerned about symmetry; many others aren't. Do you want to look good in your clothes, or is it important that a new lover won't even know you've had surgery? Do you want to have your remaining breast altered to achieve a closer match? These concerns are not foolish, and you should never hesitate to look for what you want out of guilt over "vanity." You've been through an unpleasant and life-changing experience; you're entitled to do what you can to make its aftermath as comfortable as possible. Talk with your plastic surgeon about all the possibilities and decide what's best for you.

Although most plastic surgeons strive to create symmetry in the nude, the most realistic goal and expectation is to obtain symmetry in a bra or clothing. Dr. William Shaw, a former colleague of mine, warned against looking for one universal operation that's best for every patient. "One of the mistakes surgeons and patients both make is to act as if breast reconstruction is some kind of product you can compare objectively—what's the best airplane? One thing I've learned over the years is that there's no one operation that's best for everyone."

When Should You Have Reconstruction?

You may not be sure at first whether you want reconstruction. Some premastectomy patients are too upset by the cancer and the prospect of a mastectomy to make yet another major decision at the time. When I come across this kind of ambivalence, I suggest the patient have her mastectomy, take whatever time she needs to deal with it, and then, when she feels ready, come back if she still wants reconstruction. (This, by the way, is equally true of surgery for lumpectomy.) You may also consider a consultation with a plastic surgeon just to obtain information, not to make any decisions.

Although plastic surgeons once were reluctant to do immediate reconstruction, it is becoming much more popular. I find some surgeons will actually recommend bilateral mastectomies with immediate reconstruction as the easiest way to achieve symmetry. It probably *is* the easiest for the surgeon, who doesn't have to worry about the cosmetic results of breast conservation. It is also easier for the plastic surgeon, who doesn't have to worry about matching the uninvolved breast. But it may not be easiest for *you*.

Make sure you think it through. Planning a mastectomy with immediate reconstruction will have to allow for any needed chemotherapy and radiation. This can mean using whatever team is available when you need it. The local plastic surgeon, however, may not be the one you want to do your reconstruction, especially if you want a free flap or a muscle-sparing approach (described below). If you delay reconstruction, you may have a greater choice of surgeons. If you are going to need postmastectomy radiation therapy, it also may be better to delay reconstruction because the acute effects of radiation lead to an increased incidence of local compli-cations regardless of the method of reconstruction.[4] However, if you are interested in implant reconstruction and will need radia-tion, delaying the reconstruction may prevent the possibility of an implant-only reconstruction. The breast skin can be expanded quickly prior to radiation, leaving you with an acceptable result (al-though the radiation usually tightens the tissues around the im-plant somewhat). After radiation, however, the skin is usually not amenable to expansion and a tissue flap is typically required.

There is a pervasive bias that immediate breast reconstruction improves patient quality of life, but the few studies available do not demonstrate such a benefit and instead suggest that breast re-construction, whether immediate or not, may actually impair quality of life.[5] It is well documented that surgical complications have a big effect on quality of life. A study that looked back on women who had undergone mastectomy and reconstruction found that dissatisfaction with the operation was associated with dissatisfaction with appearance, complications with reconstruc-tion, having prophylactic surgery, and increased level of stress.[6] Data from the Mayo Clinic demonstrate substantial postoperative complications after mastectomy with immediate reconstruction. This is in contrast to the much less common and less severe com-plications after breast conservation alone or mastectomy alone, which rarely require further surgery.[7] Delayed breast reconstruc-tion in general is associated with fewer postoperative complica-tions as well.

There is no time limit for reconstruction. In fact, current tech-niques have made it a better option than it used to be. If you had a mastectomy in the past and are now thinking about reconstruc-tion, you should feel encouraged. Even with a radical mastec-tomy, reconstruction is still possible. Or if you originally decided against reconstruction and now want to reconsider, that's also fine. (Some of my patients had their mastectomies in the winter and didn't want reconstruction but changed their minds in the summer, when they wanted to wear bathing suits and sun-dresses.) Women with bilateral mastectomies can have both sides reconstructed into any reasonable size they like. If you were an A cup and always wanted to be a C, now you can probably do it! Of course, you are limited somewhat by the amount of tissue and skin you have.

Types of Postmastectomy Reconstruction

Reconstructive surgery is done in a number of ways. It has at least two components: reconstruction of the breast mound and reconstruction of the nipple areolar complex. The reconstruction of the breast mound can be done with artificial substances, your own body tissues, or both.

Implants and Expanders

Of the 60,000 reconstructions done a year, 85 percent are done with either saline or silicone implants. Current options for implant-based reconstruction include immediate or delayed reconstruction with a standard or adjustable implant, two-stage reconstruction with a tissue expander followed by an implant, or reconstruction with the combination of an implant and your own tissue. One-stage implant reconstruction is gaining popularity, although the results are best in highly selected patients: typically a C/D cup patient with minimal droop who wants to be a cup size smaller and higher. In the right situation the results can be excellent.

More commonly, a tissue expander is placed under the muscle at the time of the mastectomy. After initial healing the expander is inflated over time with saline during weekly office visits. This process can be quite uncomfortable, as the tissues are stretched out over six to eight weeks. The expander can be used while you are receiving chemotherapy. Once the expansion is complete, the tissues are allowed to relax and adjust to the new position for another one to two months or until chemotherapy is finished. At that point the tissue expander is exchanged for the final implant in an outpatient surgical operation (Figure 15.2).

Recently a piece of acellular matrix (tissue without cells) termed Alloderm has come into use to cover the bottom of the implant like an internal bra. Alloderm is an option when placing the expander in the first operation. Some surgeons use it routinely, feeling that it reduces pain and capsular contracture rate. Other

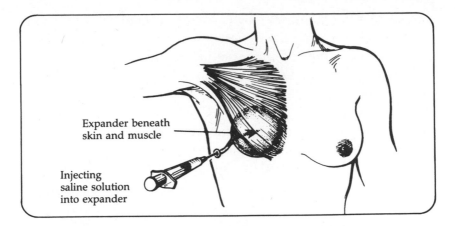

Expander beneath
skin and muscle

Injecting
saline solution
into expander

Figure 15.2

surgeons never use it because they do not want to add more foreign material and it is expensive. Still others use it selectively
when the muscles have been damaged in mastectomy. A surgeon
who knows that a woman has poor-quality tissues from radiation
or previous surgery may use a flap of back muscle to cover the expander with healthy tissue. In this case the flap is performed at
the same time as expander placement. It is always a good backup
option if an implant reconstruction fails.

This two-stage technique of expander-implant reconstruction
has become the most common approach to implant-based reconstruction. The final implant is either saline or silicone and is
placed behind the pectoralis muscle (Figure 15.3). The outer
shell is always silicone and can be either textured or smooth.
Most plastic surgeons think that silicone implants provide a
softer, more natural feel and maintain their shape better than
saline implants. Saline implants tend to be firmer and provide less
natural fullness in the upper portion of the breast, and they are
much more likely to produce visible rippling. Nevertheless, silicone implants are not without some drawbacks. If a saline implant ruptures, the fluid leaks out, your body absorbs it, and it is
immediately obvious. If a silicone implant ruptures, you may or
may not detect it, and the silicone can spread into the tissues
around the implant. Although this is not necessarily harmful,

surgery to remove a ruptured and leaking silicone implant is certainly more traumatic than surgery to remove a saline implant. Most silicone implant manufacturers recommend screening MRIs every few years to monitor for silicone implant rupture. Your plastic surgeon may or may not agree with this, and will likely recommend a different protocol. Make sure you are comfortable with this issue before deciding on silicone implants.

Generally the expander/implant reconstruction will take four steps (depending on whether you count a tattoo as one of the steps) to complete. Stage 1 is the immediate reconstruction with an expander, stage 2 is converting it to the final implant, stage 3 is nipple reconstruction, and stage 4 is the areola tattoo. In terms of advantages, this approach is simple and most plastic surgeons are comfortable with it, so they can do it without a special team. There are no scars elsewhere on your body as there would be if your own tissue were used. The disadvantages include the long time it takes to get a breast mound and the multiple visits to the

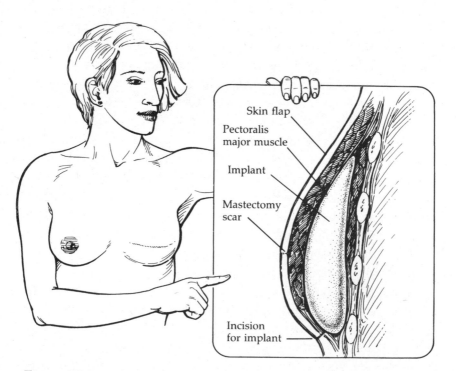

Skin flap

Pectoralis
major muscle

Implant

Mastectomy
scar

Incision
for implant

Figure 15.3

plastic surgeon for inflation. Early complications include bleeding (hematoma) and infection, the latter sometimes requiring implant removal. Although many patients mistakenly think that they are "rejecting" the implant, in most cases the problem is an infection around the implant or a capsular contracture. Surgery always carries the danger of postoperative infection. An expander or implant can make infection more difficult to treat. Since they are foreign to your body, an infection will not heal by itself. One of my patients developed a very bad infection and had to have the expander removed.

As many as 50 percent of women who undergo implants will need further surgery within seven years for leaks, deflation, pain, or capsule contracture (a firm scar that forms around the implant). Moreover, implants or expanders are more likely than other procedures to necessitate a procedure that makes the other breast match. They're going to give you a nice, perfect seventeen-year-old's breast, but you're probably not a nice, perfect seventeen-year-old woman. Since the reconstructed breast doesn't sag much, it may be higher than you want it to be. One of my patients found this particularly displeasing. "The reconstructed breast didn't look like my real breast, and it was much higher," she says. "I had to start wearing a bra, which I don't like at all." Thus you may need to have your other breast operated on for symmetry (augmentation mammaplasty, mastopexy, or reduction mammoplasty as discussed in Chapter 2).

So when a plastic surgeon tells you implants are the easiest form of reconstruction, requiring the least amount of surgery, it's true as far as it goes. But you need to consider that it may end up also involving surgery on the other breast.

It's important to let the plastic surgeon know what size you want to be. I had a relatively flat-chested patient who wanted an implant. She wanted to stay flat-chested; that was what she was used to. But the plastic surgeon, conditioned to think that all women want large breasts, kept trying to persuade her to let him give her a bigger implant and then enlarge her other breast to match it. Another patient had had cosmetic silicone implants, and the implant on one side encapsulated. But she liked the rock-like texture of that breast, and when she had a mastectomy on the other breast, she wanted the reconstructed breast to match the encapsulated one. The plastic surgeon had a hard time with that—it wasn't what women are supposed to want. If you know what you want and your plastic surgeon argues with you, argue back or change plastic surgeons. It's your body, not the surgeon's, and it's you who will live with that body.

Sometimes an implant can even have a bonus. One of my Facebook friends wrote that she had been "a large C," and she'd always wanted a reduction. "When I was diagnosed I decided to get what I wanted out of it. I had a reduction on the 'good' side, and expanders put in for my reconstruction during my mastectomy to make me a full B. The expander was removed, and a saline implant was put in after chemo through a small incision under the reconstructed breast before I started radiation. I haven't had any trouble, and the reconstruction looks great."

When the operation works well and the patient's expectations are realistic, implants can make a wonderful difference. As one of my patients says, "I forget it's there—it's a part of me now. It's a little harder than my other breast, but otherwise great. I don't have to worry about what I wear."

One caution: implants don't last forever. Even for the woman who has implants to enlarge her breasts, replacing them can be upsetting enough. For the mastectomy patient, it can be devastating— like losing the breast all over again. Such patients may require the flap reconstruction described below. Having problems with the implant suggests the likelihood of having more problems later on. Patients need to weigh the comparative ease of the implant surgery against the inconvenience and emotional consequences of possible later surgeries.

Flap Procedures

The breast mound can be reconstructed using your own tissue. In the *myocutaneous flap*, a flap of skin, muscle, and fat is taken from another part of your body and moved. It's your own tissue, and because you've got extra skin, it can make a bigger breast and a more natural droop. You may feel more normal since it's real tissue, skin, and fat, though it has little sensation. These flaps can come from the abdomen (transverse rectus abdominis muscle, or TRAM flap), back (latissimus dorsi flap), or buttock (gluteus maximus flap).

There are two different techniques for the myocutaneous flap. One is the pedicle, or attached flap (Figure 15.4). Here the tissue is removed except for its feeding artery and vein, which remain attached, almost like a leash. The site from which the tissue was removed is sewn closed. The new little island of skin and muscle is then tunneled under the skin into the mastectomy wound. Since the blood vessels aren't cut, the blood supply remains.

The more recent operation is the "free flap." In this procedure, the tissue is removed and the feeding artery and vein are cut. Then the tissue is moved to a new location and the artery and vein are sewn to an artery or vein in the chest or armpit; the surgeons use a microscope to help them reconnect the tiny blood vessels.

The pedicle flap can be done only from tissue close enough to reach to the breast and so is limited to the abdomen (TRAM) or back (Latissimus). The free flap is less limited.

The most common free flaps are from the abdomen, based on the lower blood vessels that feed the skin (inferior epigastric). Other free flaps include those from the infraumbilical area (SIEA, or superficial inferior epigastric artery flap) and the buttocks (SGAP or IGAP, depending on whether it's based on the superior gluteal artery perforator or the inferior one). Another procedure gaining some popularity is the TUG flap, or transverse upper gracilis flap. This flap takes one of the muscles in the medial thigh (gracilis) with tissue from the upper inner thigh. Sacrificing this muscle usually has no effect on leg function, and the flap can usually supply enough tissue for an A or B cup reconstruction. This means you can have a flap reconstruction even if your abdomen has been scarred and take advantage of whatever abundance nature granted you (Figure 15.5).

Another popular variation of the free flap, the so-called perforator flap, or DIEP, was introduced by Dr. Robert Allen of New Orleans. Instead of taking some muscle with the free flap, the surgeon dissects out the arteries that perforate the muscle to the skin, keeping them attached to the skin and thus sparing the muscle completely. If the surgeon can identify a sufficient number of

458

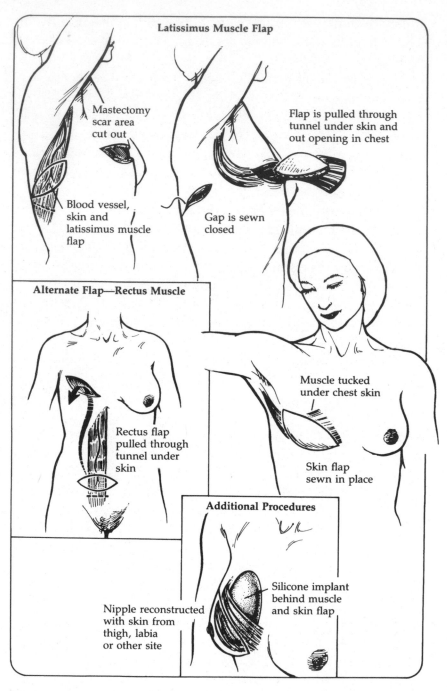

Figure 15.4

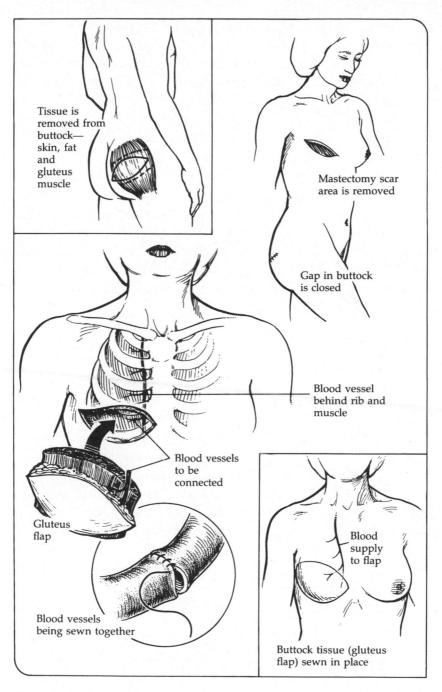

Tissue is removed from buttock—skin, fat and gluteus muscle

Mastectomy scar area is removed

Gap in buttock is closed

Blood vessel behind rib and muscle

Blood vessels to be connected

Gluteus flap

Blood vessels being sewn together

Blood supply to flap

Buttock tissue (gluteus flap) sewn in place

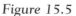

Figure 15.5

perforating arteries to support the skin and fat, there is no need to
take any muscle at all. While there may be obvious theoretical advantages in not taking any muscle, it does add additional tedious
dissection through the muscle and possibly a small risk of complications related to this portion of the dissection. Also, because the
surgeon still has to dissect through the muscle, which can damage
it, the benefit of trying to save a small amount of muscle is uncertain. Thus in the end, it becomes a practical decision. The concept
of the perforator flap has been very helpful in focusing our attention on the perforating arteries rather than the amount of muscle.
As a result, there's a tendency to take less and less muscle and do
a "muscle-sparing" free flap. When there are large perforators that
make dissection fairly easy, it is worthwhile to do a perforator flap.
This approach usually requires four procedures—the mastectomy
with immediate free flap followed by a nipple-sparing operation
and then a tattoo of the areola. Finally, you may need to have
something done to the other breast so that it matches.

The advantage of the pedicle flap over these free flaps is that
it's easier, so more plastic surgeons can do it. It still involves at
least three procedures (reconstruction, nipple, and tattoo) and
four if you need to modify the second breast to match. A disad-
vantage is that we can use tissue only from locations that can
stretch to the breast—the abdomen or the back. Another disad-
vantage is that in making the "tunnel" to the breast, we have to
disturb all the tissue en route, so we're disturbing a lot of your
body surface. This means that you'll have a lot of long-term complications that aren't serious but can be uncomfortable. If we take
it from the abdomen, your abdominal muscle will no longer be as
strong and you won't be able to do things like sit-ups as well as
you used to. One of my patients now has to wear a panty girdle all
the time to help support her weakened abdominal muscle. Another has found that since the operation the area around her upper abdomen is so sensitive that she can't wear anything with a
waistband. There is a 25 percent chance of getting a lifetime
bulging of the abdomen as well. I should add, however, that these
problems are relatively unusual, and most patients have had few
problems but much satisfaction from the procedure. If the tissue
is taken from your back, there will be fewer problems, although

the muscles may weaken somewhat. This may interfere with shoulder strength for special sports like mountain climbing or competitive swimming. You also may need more physical therapy. Some women have a lot of stiffness and pain after this flap because it throws their whole shoulder girdle off. In either case, you'll have a scar on the area from which the flap has been taken.

With the free flap, the surgeon has to be skilled at sewing blood vessels together under the microscope (Figure 15.6) or using the new coupler (a stapler-like apparatus to connect small blood vessels), and most plastic surgeons aren't. In expert hands, there are fewer complications than with the pedicled flaps because free flaps have a better blood supply. It's about five to eight hours of surgery, and you'll probably be in the hospital for four to seven days. If the blood supply is disturbed, part or all of the flap can die and further surgery will be necessary. The patient I mentioned earlier, who developed an infection from her silicone expanders, was unable to have either the latissimus (back) or rectus (abdominal) procedure because of medical problems in her back and abdomen. The free gluteus flap was the only alternative she had left. Though it was difficult surgery that involved a long healing period, she feels it was well worth the pain and inconvenience.

As I noted earlier, both versions of the flap procedure require not only highly trained plastic surgeons but specialized teams. You want a center where they do this a lot and the whole staff is comfortable with the procedure and with its potential risks and complications. Researching and talking to people is important to find the right place. It may be necessary to travel to find the surgeon and team that can best fit your needs.

The advantage of reconstruction with your own tissue includes a softer, more natural appearing breast mound, which will gain weight when you gain and lose weight. The disadvantages include the longer duration of anesthesia, greater blood loss, a longer recovery period, risk of losing part of the flap due to inadequate blood supply, and problems at the donor site. The risk of complications tends to be higher in older and more obese women as well as those with compromised vascular microcirculation, such as smokers or women with diabetes.

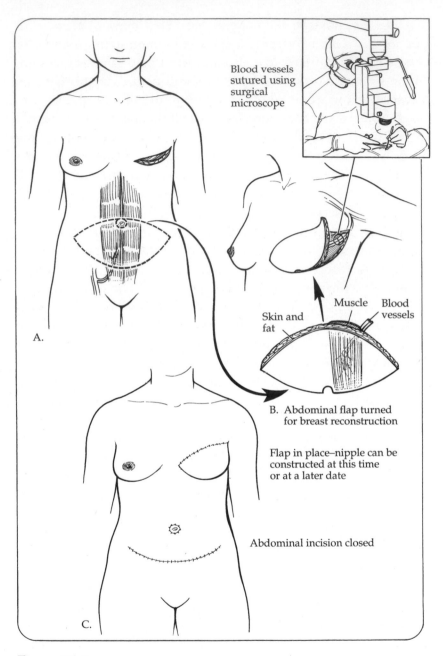

Blood vessels
sutured using
surgical
microscope

A.

Skin and
fat

Muscle   Blood
vessels

B. Abdominal flap turned
   for breast reconstruction

Flap in place–nipple can be
constructed at this time
or at a later date

Abdominal incision closed

C.

Figure 15.6

Free flap procedures have the advantage that less if any muscle is taken and so there are fewer problems at the donor site. They have better blood supply, although there is a small risk of the small blood vessel connections clotting, resulting in partial or complete flap loss.

In some cases the surgeon can do the mastectomy while the plastic surgeon raises the flap, an approach we used when I was still operating at UCLA. While I was doing a mastectomy, the plastic surgery team was working on the flap in the abdomen. (If the tissue was taken from the buttocks or back, I operated with the patient lying on her side.) By the time I finished the mastectomy, they were ready to start moving the flap up. This teamwork approach cut operating time to four or five hours.

When we were done, the patient was taken to the "flap room," a three-bed intensive care unit for the flap—not for the patient, for the flap. The concern was that the blood supply could get blocked, which would cause the flap to die. So they carefully studied the flap with various monitors. If the flap showed any signs of change, surgeons were alerted that the blood supply could be compromised.

After mastectomy and immediate reconstruction you come out of anesthesia feeling like a Mack truck just hit you. You've had hours of surgery on your breast and your abdomen, back, or buttocks. You have continuous pain medication through an IV with a button you can press to control the timing. You're kept in bed for one to two days, and you have a catheter so you don't have to go to the bathroom. By about the third or fourth day you can get out of bed and walk around a bit. You're usually in the hospital about four to six days. There are drains placed in the abdominal incisions as well as in the chest. You may have pain deep in your chest, which can also feel numb, as well as in your abdomen or other area the tissue has been taken from. So the double operation is certainly an ordeal. In addition, you'll need further operations for the nipple and other breast. Sometimes after the operation there is a little too much tissue in one place or another, so the surgeon does some fine-tuning. It won't hurt because the area is now numb.

But it's usually worth it and you do eventually recuperate. We've even done this surgery on elderly women with other medical problems, and it's worked for them.

If the free flap is the operation you want, you should take the time to research and find out who in your area can do it. If there's no one in your area and you still want a particular form of reconstruction, you can always wait, have the mastectomy first, and then go find the right plastic surgeon when your treatment is done.

Eric Halvorson is a plastic surgeon from Chapel Hill, North Carolina, who helped with this chapter. He says, "What I tell my patients is that implant reconstruction spreads the risk you take over your lifetime—there is less risk with the initial operation, but living with implants carries the risks of capsular contracture, rupture, infection, malposition, exposure. Tissue flap reconstruction puts all the risk up front—the surgery and recovery are longer, with risks of flap failure, wound healing complications, donor site complications, and so on—but once everything is healed they will rarely have other problems. Also, implant reconstructions tend to look worse with time, whereas tissue flap reconstructions tend to look better with time."

MAKING A DECISION

To decide what's best for you, you should discuss matters with your surgeon and, separately, with a plastic surgeon. Make sure you have thought about your goals for reconstruction and share them with both. Do you want to be higher, lower, larger, smaller? Some people assume that their only option is to look the same, but modern techniques have given women the option to change the appearance of their breasts. Some women are even happier with their breasts after mastectomy. Your surgeon will look at you, note how your body hangs together, and how your breasts look before your surgery, and tell you what kind of procedure she thinks would be best for you. Make sure you ask which procedures she is familiar with and perform regularly. Women have come to me after being told they're not a candidate for a flap, when in reality the plastic surgeon they saw just doesn't know how to do the operation. Get a second or even third opinion. Look at websites that discuss reconstruction.

The discussion of breast augmentation in Chapter 2 applies here as well. My former colleague Robert Goldwyn, who has done many reconstructions, points out something crucial: you should always be shown pictures of the best and the worst results your plastic surgeon has had. Some doctors will show only the best results—an act comparable to false advertising. It's important for you to know the limits of what the procedure can do for you and the risks you run of having far from ideal results.

Any of these procedures can be done immediately or at a later time. One advantage of doing it immediately is that you don't have another operation later. Your regular surgeon performs your mastectomy and then, while you're still under anesthesia, the plastic surgeon comes in and does the reconstruction. Also, when reconstruction is done immediately, the surgeon often performs a skin-sparing mastectomy (see Chapter 14), making it easier for the plastic surgeon to close the incision over the implant or flap. In my experience, though, many women don't have immediate reconstruction because they don't want to go through more surgery. The disadvantages are that it's a longer time in the operating room (usually about six to eight hours), and it's harder to schedule. Wound healing complications also tend to be higher with immediate reconstruction, although the cosmetic result can be better.

Once you have the new breast, you may want a nipple and an areola. We don't do it right away because the surgeon needs to be sure it's in the right place. There's a lot of swelling after reconstructive surgery, so we need to wait till that goes down and the reconstructed breast has had time to "settle down" due to gravity. The nipple can be created using skin from the breast or flap, but it won't be the same color as your original nipple. It can be tattooed. The areola can be reconstructed with a skin graft or a tattoo. Sometimes the skin from your inner thigh is used, since it's darker than breast skin. If the skin graft is not dark enough, it can be tattooed. Skin grafts tend to have more texture and thus are more realistic, but taking the skin graft will put one more scar on your body unless you take it from someplace where there is already a scar. Whether or not you want to bother with the nipple depends on why you want the reconstruction. If it's just for convenience to look symmetrical under clothes without having to bother with a prosthesis, you may decide against it. If you want the new breast to look as real as possible, you'll probably want the nipple. Again, it's your decision—you're the one who'll go through the surgery, and you're the one who'll live with the results. I've had a couple of patients who, before they had the nipple put on, showed their reconstruction to anyone who was curious. But once the nipple was on, they didn't want to show it. Somehow it felt more like a real breast, and displaying it seemed immodest.

THE UNACCEPTABLE RECONSTRUCTION

Sometimes reconstruction isn't entirely successful. It may not give you the look you want or it may be a source of pain or medical problems. It can cause unpleasant sensations ranging from pins and needles, to burning, to sharp pain. You may find it hard to adapt to the feel of an implant. An implant may seem solid, even rock-like to the touch. The breast's hardness isn't due to the implant but to the scar tissue that has formed around it, encasing it in a tough capsule.

Sometimes plastic surgeons may focus on crafting the "perfect breast," not on replicating the patient's natural breast. The result is often a breast that is, or feels, too big. Even when an implant matches the breast, the new breast is often heavier because the implant and scar tissue weigh more than breast tissue. Also, the new nipple may be higher or lower than the nipple on the other breast.

Because surgeons see women lying on an operating table, they see breasts from a different perspective than do the women, who usually see themselves standing before a mirror or looking down at their breasts. As a result a surgeon may misjudge the way a breast will fall when the woman is on her feet (see Chapter 3). If it is a good match for her other breast, which appears flatter when she is lying on her back, it will probably look smaller when she stands up. Most plastic surgeons are aware of this and will sit you up in the operating room to make sure things look symmetrical.

You don't have to simply resign yourself to such problems. A plastic surgeon can cut away hard scar tissue and replace implants, exchange an implant for a flap, reduce or enlarge a breast, or lift and reorient nipples. Technology is improving, and so are surgical techniques, as experience with the procedure—and the demand for it—grow. Get a referral to a plastic surgeon from a friend or your breast surgeon, explain your problem, and have the plastic surgeon outline a plan for correcting it. If possible, get a second opinion. Again, ask for pictures of the plastic surgeon's best and worst outcomes.

Occasionally, if the skin has been altered by radiation or is not elastic enough to make additional reconstructive surgery advisable, the best course may be to remove the implant and use a prosthesis instead.

Sometimes you can feel ambivalent. One woman on Facebook found the first reconstruction okay and not the second. "In 1996, I had a tram transplant. I was very happy with the end result as it was my own body being used rather than a silicone implant. The second was in 2004. This time we used the latissimus flap. Different result. As it turned out, by the time they wrapped the muscle around my torso there was little left for the breast pocket. The solution was to add an implant. I came within two days of getting on the table when I realized that I had put myself through all of this to avoid a external object in my body and canceled the procedure. So now I look odd to a first time viewer but I'm comfortable in my own skin." Some don't stop getting things fixed until they have it right. "I had both breasts reconstructed after BC . . . last change I made was to change implants & wanted silicone & try to get my real size back. Before OR asked doc to have 4 size options. Prior to anesthesia I sat up in OR & announced to all present that I wanted all 4 sizes tried out w the Doc sitting me up for all to see which suited me best. Had great ones put in & no bruising. "

Today, a reasonably good breast reconstruction can be achieved after mastectomy by any of these techniques, using expanders and implants or your own tissue from the abdomen, buttocks, back, or thighs. Achieving symmetry between the nonmastectomy breast and the reconstructed breast, however, sometimes requires reshaping, reducing, or enlarging the normal breast. A large, droopy breast on the normal side can be reduced to match the reconstructed breast. If the breast volume is satisfactory, then the breast can be reshaped by "mastopexy" techniques to lift the nipple and reshape the breast. A normal breast that is too small in relation to the reconstructed one may be augmented with an implant behind the muscle. This should be done cautiously because the implant-augmented breast tends to be firmer without the natural droop, thus presenting a potential problem for achieving symmetry if the opposite one is done with one's own tissue. Also, you should be careful about the potential problems in follow-up of this breast in terms of palpation or mammography. In high-risk patients, this would not be a good idea.

PROSTHESES

Many women don't get reconstruction because they are very comfortable with a prosthesis. It isn't invasive and can be removed at will. As I was writing this, a former patient of mine told me of her experience with a Beverly Hills surgeon "who tried to sell me a breast as if he was selling a car." When she explained that all she was looking for information and didn't know if she wanted reconstruction, he was appalled and demanded, "Why not?" She explained her reservations about getting additional surgery and said that she had come to learn more and discuss the pros and cons of reconstruction. Then he sent her to an office where she was shown the before and after photo album.

"It felt like it was a showroom and they were selling. I didn't buy any of it and have been quite satisfied with my prostheses for the past 16 years. Please remind women that they have choices and some (many?) of us are doing just fine 'au naturel' with prosthetics."

The option of wearing a prosthesis will probably be offered to you in the hospital after your surgery (unless you've had immediate reconstruction and obviously won't need one). In most areas of the country the hospital arranges for someone to visit you to talk about prostheses while you're still there. Your visitor will be from Reach for Recovery or a firm that sells prostheses. You can get a temporary prosthesis first and then shop around for a permanent one. The prosthesis fits into a pocket in a postmastectomy bra. You can shop for one in person or online, from catalogs, in medical supply houses, or in fancy lingerie stores. Each supplier has its advantages and disadvantages. You may be put off by the implications of mutilation or the wheelchairs and artificial limbs in medical supply outlets. In a lingerie store you may feel painfully reminded of the breast you no longer have. Your doctor or the American Cancer Society can help you find the stores, catalogs, or websites to buy your prosthesis, or you can ask friends who've had mastectomies. For a nominal fee, Y-ME, a volunteer organization of breast cancer survivors, will send you a prosthesis if it has your size in stock.

There are suppliers that will make a custom prosthesis for you; it's expensive and your insurance company may not pay for it, but you will have a precise match. (It's a good idea to check with your insurance company before buying your prosthesis anyway; different companies have different quirks, and you may want to be sure of what your out-of-pocket expenses will be.) Medicare pays for a prosthesis every year or two years—with a prescription. (Why you need a prescription for a prosthesis, I don't know—I've never met a woman who bought one for the fun of it. But the ways of bureaucracies are mysterious.) There are also specific forms for swimming, though most of the better prostheses are made of silicone and are waterproof.

Prostheses come in a range of prices and quality. If you don't have insurance to pay for one, or if you haven't decided between prosthesis or reconstruction, you'll probably want the least expensive form available, at least temporarily. Catalogs and many stores offer forms for as low as $20 and mastectomy bras for around $15.

Prostheses are made in different sizes and for different operations. If you have a radical mastectomy, you can get a fuller prosthesis. If you had a wide excision that's left you noticeably asymmetrical, you can get a small "filler," or shell that fits comfortably inside your bra. In the past, prostheses didn't have nipples, which caused problems for women whose remaining breast had a prominent nipple, (Betty Rollin in her book *First, You Cry* has a very funny description of her efforts to make her own "nipple" out of cloth buttons.) Fortunately any prosthesis you buy now has a nipple, and you can get a separate nipple to attach to it if your own nipple is more prominent than the one on the prosthesis.

Some situations may affect what makes a prosthesis right for you. Certain kinds of disabilities, for example, can make a particular form uncomfortable. Judith Rogers, an activist with Breast Health Access for Disabilities, has mild cerebral palsy, and she found that her first prosthesis caused problems. "It was good in terms of matching the size of my remaining breast," she says. "But it was bad for my shoulder: it was too heavy for me. It pulled down, harming my muscles and increasing the effects of lymphedema." When she got a lighter one, she had less pain. You need to take time to consider all the factors involving your body and mind when you choose a prosthesis.

Doing Nothing

Finally, there is a third option that a few women have embraced——not disguising the operation at all. If your lumpectomy doesn't create a dramatic lopsided look, you may decide just to ignore it. Even with the more noticeable change that comes with a larger lumpectomy or a mastectomy, some prefer doing nothing cosmetically. One of my patients early in my career thought about her options, then concluded that "a prosthesis sounded too uncomfortable, and reconstruction hasn't been around long enough to see what long-term effects it can have. And then I decided I was comfortable with the way I looked." She went to work dressed normally, jogged in a loose T-shirt, and felt that it was other people's problem if they were uncomfortable with it. Once in a while, she felt a need to look more "normal"—especially when she had important meetings with new business associates. Her solution was to stuff shoulder pads from her dresses into her bra.

For other women, refusing to create the illusion of a breast is part of their feminist beliefs. Artist Matuschka has created photographs of herself in a cutaway gown, showing not her remaining breast but her mastectomy scar. One photograph was on the cover of the August 15, 1993, *New York Times Magazine*. The effect is of harshness and defiance, showing the world what breast cancer does to a woman's body. Writer Deena Metzger, whose book *Tree* addresses her cancer, includes a photograph with a different approach: she softens the effect of the amputation by covering her scar with a beautiful, evocative tattoo of a tree, creating a new beauty where the beauty of her breast once was.[8]

Some people feel too conspicuous in public without a prosthesis, but they still don't like how the form feels. In that case there is another possible alternative: you can have both breasts removed. While this destroys a healthy breast, it does make it possible to wear loose shirts without self-consciousness. I had only one patient take this route, and she had to fight with her insurance company to get them to pay for the removal of the healthy breast. She told them that since they paid for reconstruction for symmetry they should pay for a contralateral mastectomy for symmetry.

Having the self-confidence to feel comfortable without the appearance of a breast shows wonderful courage, but most of us are products of our culture and still need to feel cosmetically acceptable to the outside world. In some cases there are actual penalties for failing to appear "normal." If nonconformity will cost you your job, for example, you're likely to want to have reconstruction or wear a prosthesis at least part of the time.

Recently a fashion designer, Hilary Boyajian, came up with an interesting line of tunic-style garments she calls "Chikara" for women with one breast or no breasts. The garment drapes loosely across the chest, so that unusual shapes aren't visible. "I get so many emails from breast cancer survivors thanking me for doing this," she told the reporter who interviewed her.[9]

As more women live and even thrive after a breast cancer diagnosis, more attention has been paid to the results of surgery. As with everything, it's your choice as to what road you want to take. The good news is that there are now lots of options and you can make a choice at the time of your diagnosis or years later. In a disease where you often feel out of control, this is one area where you can make the choice that works for you.

Chapter 16

Radiation Therapy

The idea of radiation therapy may make you nervous. After all, radiation can cause cancer, and the last thing you want is to find yourself in danger of even more cancer. But as you saw in Chapter 5, the doses given in radiation therapy rarely cause cancer and often cure it.

As a form of local control (treatment of an original cancer), radiation is more effective in some forms of cancer than others. Luckily it's been very effective with breast cancer.

Radiation in this case is ordinarily used in conjunction with surgery, so you may have had a lumpectomy (or even a mastectomy) before your radiation. It works best when it has comparatively few cells to attack; it's least effective on large chunks of cancer. So we try, if possible, to do the surgery first, getting rid of most of the tumor before cleaning up what's left with radiation.

In the old days, we used cobalt as a source of radiation. Now we use radiation generated by electricity in machines called linear accelerators. The edges of the beam from this type of machine are "sharper," sparing most of the adjacent tissue. Also, the treatment is planned more precisely, with newer planning machines called simulators. Further, it is aimed in tangents (at an angle) to the breast, so that it goes through the breast tissue of one breast and

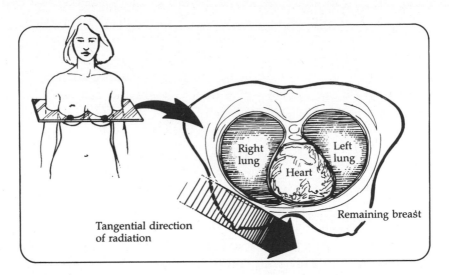

Figure 16.1

out into the air, with much less getting into the heart or lung (Figure 16.1). Even so, the radiation beam can be scattered once it enters the body and can affect other spots. Some women who were treated for Hodgkin's disease 10 or 15 years ago now have breast cancer (see Chapter 5). Unfortunate as that may be, radiation therapy is important. If the Hodgkin's had gone untreated, those women probably would have died long ago.

Like surgery, radiation is a localized treatment. (Chemotherapy, given by injection or in a pill, goes through your bloodstream and affects your entire body.) The radiation is aimed at a specific area and affects only that area. The linear accelerator, as you might guess from its name, accelerates charged particles and shoots them at a target that generates photons (forms of electromagnetic radiation). These photons are aimed directly at the body part they're intended for, as a beam. The beam is sharpened in the head of the machine to minimize scatter.

As I explained in Chapter 12, radiation complements lumpectomy as an alternative to mastectomy and may also be used with mastectomy. In the past 20 or 25 years, as adjuvant chemotherapy has improved survival, we're seeing more local recurrences. Chemotherapy, which is so good at stopping cancer that has spread outside the immediate area, doesn't help the immediate area itself. This has fueled the current trend to do more postmastectomy radiation in certain groups of patients—those most at risk for local recurrence in the scar after mastectomy, such as the ones with four or more positive nodes, lymphatic vascular invasion, or large tumors (see Chapter 11).

INITIAL CONSULTATION

Most of the time you have a choice of places to receive your radiation. As with surgeons and medical oncologists, you can shop around. Look for a doctor who treats a lot of breast cancer and considers the whole patient and not just the breast. Such a doctor is more likely to work with you to integrate your treatment into your schedule and life. And as always, it's a good idea to bring a recording device to the consultation to make sure you catch everything that is said.

Radiation oncologists (who are always medical doctors) like to see patients soon after the biopsy—ideally while they still have the lump—to get a firsthand sense of the tumor. Sometimes the initial consultation is held in the radiation therapy department. The doctor will want to discuss the usual side effects of the treatment and will also explain plans involving a team approach. Crucial to the team is a specially trained radiation nurse who inquires into your specific needs, taking into account your emotional response to your cancer. The consultation also involves a physical exam.

This first visit to a radiation oncologist doesn't mean you'll necessarily have radiation treatment. The oncologist will talk with you and get your medical history, do an examination, review the X rays and slides from your surgery, and talk with your primary doctor, your surgeon, and, if you have one, your medical oncologist. Together, they will then come up with a recommendation. Make sure you are offered options. Ask what your risk of local recurrence is, with and without radiation therapy. If the choice of radiation seems appropriate to you, you'll be sent for a planning session and whatever X rays are needed after surgery, if any surgery has been done.

There are issues that affect the decision to use or not use radiation. First, if you have large breasts, the available equipment may or may not be able to accommodate them. You then may need to find a center that has the correct equipment. But breast size should *not* be a criterion for excluding radiation.

Second, a bit of the lung gets radiated, which can be dangerous if you have chronic lung disease. So with patients who have conditions like chronic obstructive pulmonary disease, chronic asthma or emphysema, we often have a planning session just to do the measurements—to see how much lung will be affected and whether or not radiation therapy is safe for your lungs. In women who have collagen vascular diseases like lupus or scleroderma, the response to radiation can be less predictable, so it might be a bad idea for them.

Previous radiation to the chest is usually a contraindication to breast radiation. So the radiation oncologist should carefully review your previous treatment records to assess whether it's safe to give you breast radiation.

In any of these cases, when the potential risks of radiation are greater than the potential gains, you should have a mastectomy rather than lumpectomy and radiation.

The Planning Session

A planning session is also called a simulation—sort of a dry run. Usually you'll wait at least two weeks after surgery before this session, to make sure everything's healed and you can get your arm over your head comfortably.

The session takes about an hour. It can be technical and impersonal, unlike your earlier conversation with the radiation oncologist. The goal is to set up, or simulate, the exact position you will be in during your treatment and program this into the computer that delivers the radiation. You put on a hospital gown and lie on a table with your arm lifted and resting on a form above your head. Over you there's a machine similar to the radiation machine, called a simulator (see Figure 16.2). It doesn't actually give the treatment, but it uses X rays for planning. Many radiation oncology facilities these days use CT simulators to do the radiation

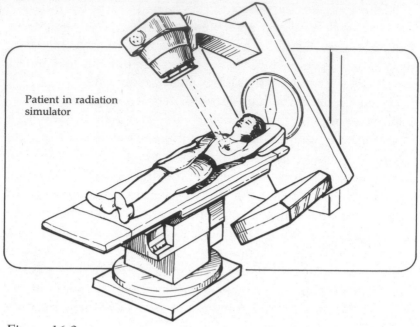

Figure 16.2

planning so the CT information is readily available. In some cases a mold is made to hold your arm, so that you'll be in the same position every day of your treatment. Women with very large breasts are sometimes treated lying on their stomachs or in a special device with the soothing name of breast cradle.

You are imaged in the same position you'll keep for treatments. A lot of measurements and technical X rays are taken to map where your ribs are in relation to your breast tissue, where your heart is in relation to your ribs, and so on, figuring out precisely how that area of your body looks (See Figure 16.1). Depending on what area of your body is going to be radiated, you may also be sent for X rays, a CT scan, or ultrasound to get more information. Then they'll put all the information into a computer that calculates the angles at which the area of your body should be radiated. This also helps protect your heart and lungs.

Before the planning starts, the radiation oncologist or therapist marks out the area of the body that's going to be treated. In most cases, it is only the breast. Sometimes it's the breast and lymph

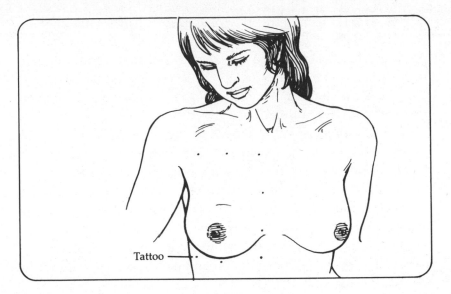

Figure 16.3

nodes. You should be aware that the breast and the lymph node areas will be treated from different angles, thus covering a fairly large area of your chest. Many doctors use tattoos—permanent little blue dots—to outline the area to be radiated (see Figure 16.3). There are a couple of reasons for that. One is to be sure that during the treatment they use the same "landmarks" and position you exactly the same way. The other is to assure that in future any radiation oncologist will know you've had radiation in that area, since you can have it only once on any given spot. For example, if you were to get cancer in the other breast and the area was near the previous cancer, the tattoo mark would tell the radiation oncologist where the field that could be radiated ends. I found tattoos useful because often when I was doing a follow-up exam on a patient whose surgery wasn't extensive, I couldn't remember which breast was treated—it could be a year or so after the last exam. So I looked for the tattoo.

Although the dots may be unattractive, they're not going to turn you into Lydia the Tattooed Lady. They're tiny and, depending on your skin coloring, can be invisible. One radiation nurse I know says, "I've had patients call me up and say, 'I've washed my tattoos off—I can't find them!'" Some doctors use Magic Markers, especially if the patient is adamant about not having tattoos; the problem with this is that the markings will wash off, and you don't have this guidance for the doctors working with you in the future. You can limit the number of tattoos to four if you dislike the thought of several of them.

The tattooing can be somewhat uncomfortable, like pinpricks or bee stings at worst. The other discomfort patients sometimes feel from the planning and tattooing procedure is a stiff arm; especially after recent surgery, it can be awkward to lie with your arm above your head for 20 minutes. Because of this, you may want to practice at home beforehand.

Another useful thing to do before the actual treatments start is to visit the area where the actual treatments will take place ahead of time. This will take the mystery out of the machine, which can look awfully intimidating when you're not familiar with it. Finally you will set up your appointments with the radiation oncologist. During the treatment you will see your radiation oncologist only weekly, but your radiation therapist or technologist and nurse daily.

THE TREATMENTS

Postlumpectomy Radiation

Radiation treatments are scheduled, and they are spaced out, once a day for a given number of weeks. There is always a balance between killing as many cancer cells as possible and avoiding as much injury to the normal tissue as we can. The treatment schedule varies from place to place. Usually it's given in two parts. First, the breast as a whole is radiated, from the collarbone to the ribs and the breastbone to the side, making sure the entire area is treated, including, if necessary, lymph nodes. This is the major part of the treatment and lasts about five weeks, often using about 4,500–5000 rads—also known as centigrays—of radiation (a chest X ray is a fraction of a rad). If there are any microscopic cancer cells in the breast, this should get rid of them. After this, the "boost" (described later) is given. As mentioned in Chapter 12, the value of whole breast radiation therapy has been questioned. Accelerated partial breast radiation (APBI), discussed later in this chapter, is being compared in studies to the standard technique to answer these questions.

How soon after the planning session the treatment begins varies from hospital to hospital, depending on how many radiation patients there are, how much room there is in the radiation department, and how large the staff is. Sometimes the patient waits two weeks to a month. This may cause her to worry that the delay will allow the cancer to spread. It won't, in that amount of time, but waiting can be emotionally hard on the patient.

Radiation may be delayed for other reasons too. Depending on the status of the lymph nodes, you may get chemotherapy right away, and your doctors may not want you to get them both at the same time. With some drugs, such as CMF (see Chapter 17), you can have chemo and radiation together; with others, like doxorubicin (Adriamycin), you usually have the chemo first and then the radiation. Sometimes they're given in a sandwich sequence: chemotherapy, then radiation, then more chemotherapy.

There are important skin care guidelines to follow during your treatment. You should use a mild soap, such as Ivory, Pears, or Neutrogena. During the course of your treatment don't use soaps with fragrance, deodorants, or any kind of metal. All of these can interact with the radiation, and it's important that you avoid them. Don't use deodorant on the side receiving treatment; almost all deodorants contain lots of aluminum. (You can use one of the "natural" ones, such as Tom's, that have no aluminum and often come unscented. If you do this, read the label very carefully. Not all "natural" products are the same.) Through the course of the treatment, you can also use a light dusting of cornstarch as a deodorant; it's pretty effective but varies from person to person.

When you go for your first treatment, you may want to bring someone with you for support. You're facing the unknown, and that's scary. Most patients don't need anyone after the first session. On a more practical level, if you've come by car make sure to request parking accommodations, which most institutions will help you with.

For the treatment itself, you'll change into a hospital gown from the waist up. It's wise to wear something two-piece so you

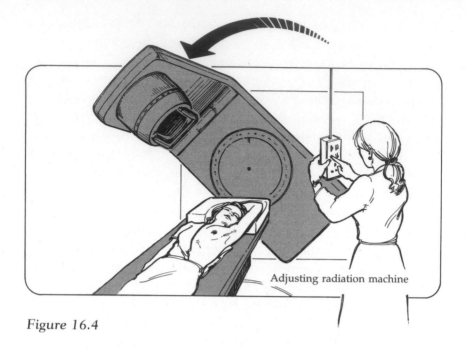

Adjusting radiation machine

Figure 16.4

have to remove only your upper garment. You can wear earrings or bracelets during the treatment, but no neck jewelry. After you've changed, you'll be taken into a waiting room. The wait may be longish and varies from place to place and day to day, so you may want to bring a good book or your iPod player or DVD viewer. Then you're taken into the treatment room. You're there for about 10 minutes, and most of that time is spent with the technologist setting up the machine and getting you ready. There's a table that looks like a regular examining table, and, above it, the radiation machine (Figure 16.4). Just as with your planning session, you lie down on the table, and a special cradle is placed under your head. This has an armrest above your head, which will hold your arm during the treatment. After you're set up, the technician will position you, leave, and turn on the machine for a little less than a minute. The radiation isn't given all at once, but is done a number of times from different angles—twice if only the breast is radiated, more if lymph nodes are also being treated. The technician will then come back in, reposition the machine, and go out again. If you're claustrophobic, you may find lying under the machine a little uncomfortable, but it is open, not like an MRI, and doesn't last long, and the machine never moves toward you.

Radiation therapy units have cameras, so they can see you while you're being treated, and an intercom system so that if you're anxious and need to talk with the technologist, you can. If a friend or family member has come with you, many hospitals allow that person to sit in the room outside the treatment area, watching on the monitor and hearing you through the intercom. If your children are old enough to be curious or are scared at not knowing what's going on, you may permit them to wait outside the treatment room so they can communicate with you if the hospital allows. This can demystify the process and alleviate their fears.

The most important thing for you to do during the treatment is to keep still. You can breathe normally but don't move otherwise. Just close your eyes and think of your favorite place. It will be over before you know it.

Your blood may be drawn during the course of treatment— once at the beginning of the therapy process or maybe once a few weeks later, to make sure there's no drop in your blood count. This usually isn't a problem with breast cancer, since there's not much bone marrow treated. But we prefer to check, especially in patients who have had chemotherapy.

What most people find hardest to deal with is the length of treatment—approximately six weeks, five days a week. If your workplace and home are near the hospital, you may be able to come in before or after work. Otherwise, you may have to cut into the middle of the workday or take time off from your job. Some mothers use baby-sitters; others bring their children to the hospital, along with a friend who stays with them while the mother has her treatment.

The Boost

After a course of radiation to treat your breast, you may be given a boost—extra radiation to the spot where the tumor was. This is usually done by the electron beam. Electrons are a special kind of charged particle; they give off energy that doesn't penetrate very deeply, so it's good if the original tumor wasn't very deep. It doesn't require hospitalization. There is some controversy regarding the need for a boost. It was added in the days when we did not demand clean margins from surgery. With the current practice of removing more breast tissue, the boost may not be as important, but it still seems to add a small degree of local control.

Partial Breast Radiation

As mentioned in Chapter 12, there is increasing interest in confining radiation after lumpectomy to the area of the tumor bed alone. Several different techniques are being studied, all of which attempt to get the same local control in less time. In general, these new techniques reduce the six weeks to four or five days.

The most commonly used form of partial breast radiation in the United States is balloon-delivered intracavitary brachytherapy. It takes advantage of the fact that after a tumor is removed there is a cavity left behind in the breast that fills up with fluid as the area slowly heals. Since the place where tumor cells are most likely to be left behind will be the lining of that cavity, it makes sense to use the cavity to deliver the radiation. In this situation, a week or two after surgery, the doctors will review the pathology to make certain that the margins are clear (see Chapter 11). Once they are satisfied of this, they'll have you make an appointment and go to your breast surgeon's office to have the balloon placed. A small incision is made under local anesthesia and an empty surgical balloon with an attached catheter is inserted into the cavity. A small amount of saltwater and X ray contrast material is then introduced into the balloon, and its position is examined under ultrasound or CT scan. If all looks well—at least 6–8 millimeters between skin and balloon, for example, so that the skin will not be damaged—a radiation oncologist calculates the appropriate dose for the computer to deliver. The treatments themselves consist of hooking the protruding catheter to a computerized delivery device that fills the balloon with the radioactive material. This is done twice a day, six hours apart, for five days. At the end of each treatment the radioactive material is removed and you are detached from the treatment machine and free to go about your business. You are not radioactive.

At present, there are several devices on the market, each with its own benefit. Most commonly used is the Mammosite. It works well unless your tumor is too close to the skin. This happens about 10 percent of the time.[1] Competing devices are Cianna's Savi and Contura Catheters, which can conform the dose to the biopsy cavity. This allows each area around the biopsy cavity to get a different amount of radiation therapy if appropriate, thus potentially sparing the skin and muscle. These can be used with less skin clearance and so may be better if your tumor is superficial. Xoft uses electrons and consequently does not require shielding. These differences are important because there are side effects from this balloon delivery radiation approach as well. The more immediate problems include radiation dermatitis (redness of the skin) and infection. These can be prevented, or at least reduced, by making sure there is adequate clearance from the skin and by taking prophylactic antibiotics. Long-term effects are similar to those of traditional radiation therapy and are described below. We are still in the early days of this approach, and I have no doubt that there will be other variations on this theme over the next several years. If you are interested in using this approach, the key is to find an experienced treatment team and go with the device they are most comfortable with using.

Another form of partial breast radiation is *interstitial brachytherapy*. It's been around for a while; we used to use it as a boost before the days of the electron beam. Now it has a more primary role. The tubes can be placed while you're in the operating room or as an outpatient process (Figure 16.5). Thin plastic tubing is hooked like thread into a needle and drawn through a spot on the breast where the biopsy was done. Then the tubing is left in and the needle withdrawn. The number of tubes varies, and sometimes they are inserted in two layers. Small radioactive pellets called iridium seeds, which give off high energy for a very short distance, are put into the tubes, treating the immediate area of the biopsy. This implant is left in for 36 to 48 hours; the time varies depending on how active the seeds are, how big your breast is, and how big the tumor was.

Since the radioactive material stays in the catheters the whole time, this radiation can be picked up by people around you, although not in large doses. Normally that's no problem, but for

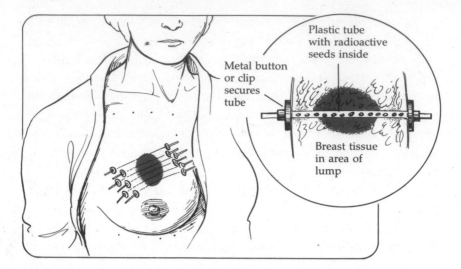

Metal button or clip secures tube

Plastic tube with radioactive seeds inside

Breast tissue in area of lump

Figure 16.5

some people, such as pregnant women, exposure to even that much radiation could be dangerous. You will be kept in the hospital with a sign on the door that reads "Caution: radioactive." After about 36 hours, both the radioactive sources and the tubes are removed, a process that requires no anesthesia. Unless there's some other reason for you to remain hospitalized, you can go home. Initial results from this approach have been comparable to those achieved with conventional radiation therapy.[2] While this approach allows the radiation dose to be given more precisely where it is needed, it is also the most technically difficult way to do partial breast irradiation and so is used less often.

Since the balloon approach requires special equipment to deliver the radiation and the brachytherapy approach is difficult to get right, there was pressure to develop an approach using the linear accelerators that are already in many hospitals to deliver radiation therapy to just the involved area. This third approach uses external beam radiotherapy from a linear accelerator and is called *conformal or intensity-modulated partial breast irradiation.* This treatment also lasts four or five days. A randomized controlled trial of the three techniques compared to traditional radiation therapy is now under way.[3]

Finally there is the single dose intraoperative approach favored in some European centers. A lumpectomy is done and then a barrier is placed between the muscle and the breast tissue to protect the chest wall. A mobile linear accelerator made especially for the operating room is used to aim the radiation therapy directly into the bed of the tumor. In a single treatment the breast tissue receives 21 grays of radiation. The first 101 patients treated were followed for approximately eight months, with good results.[4] A promising large, randomized study was reported in the Spring of 2010 comparing intraoperative radiation therapy to traditional six weeks treatment with similar recurrence rates after four years follow up suggesting that this may well be the wave of the future for breast conservation.[5]

Postmastectomy Radiation

The procedures for postmastectomy radiation are much the same as those used with breast conservation surgery. You will have a planning session, will be given tattoos, and will be treated in the department of radiation therapy. It usually takes about 5–6 weeks. Depending on the clinical situation, it may include radiating the lymph nodes behind the breast bone and above the clavicle as well as any remaining ones under the arm. A boost to the scar may or may not be used depending on the circumstances.

SIDE EFFECTS OF RADIATION

The side effects depend on the part of the body being treated. Those who receive radiation to the breast and have soft bones may have asymptomatic rib fractures: you don't feel them but they show up on X ray. Depending on how your chest is built, a little of the radiation may get to your lung and give you a cough. Your radiation oncologist will tell you about possible side effects before your treatment starts. It's a good idea to ask to talk to someone who has already been treated.

You'll probably have a mild sunburn effect. The severity varies considerably from patient to patient—one person gets a severe skin rash while another is hardly bothered at all. As you may expect, there is a correlation between skin tone and reaction to radiation therapy: the fairer your skin, the worse the reaction you're likely to experience.

The other major symptom experienced by virtually every radiation therapy patient is tiredness. I used to attribute this to the length of treatment, but there's more and more evidence that, like anesthesia (see Chapter 14), radiation itself creates fatigue. The body seems to exhaust its resources coping with the radiation and doesn't have much energy for anything else. This tiredness usually gets worse toward the end of the treatment, and its severity depends on what else is going on in your life. You'll probably want to cut back on your activities to the extent possible. The fatigue may last several weeks after the treatment has finished, or longer if you have already received chemotherapy; it may even begin after the course of treatment is over.

The extent of the fatigue varies greatly. One of my patients, a lawyer, had no problem working a full day but said she "didn't feel like going out for dinner after work." A Facebook friend didn't even have that much trouble: it was "no big deal. I had the radiation over my lunch hour."

For others, the fatigue is a bigger problem. One patient compared hers to the effects of infectious hepatitis, which she'd had years before. "The symptoms sound very nondescript," she says. "But I felt really rotten. I was tired all the time—not the tiredness you feel after a hard day's work, which I've always found fairly pleasant. My body just felt wrong—like I was always coming down with the flu. Some days I couldn't function at all—I had to keep a cot at my job." She also experienced peculiar appetite changes. "My body kept craving lemon, spinach, and roast beef—I ate them constantly, and I couldn't make myself eat anything else."

When the breast is being radiated, it may swell and become more sensitive; if you sleep on your stomach, you may feel uncomfortable. As I explained in Chapter 14, one trick is to hold a pillow between your breasts and sleep on the side that hasn't been treated. This sensitivity, like the other side effects, can take months to disappear, and you may find that breast especially sore or sensitive when you're premenstrual. When the treatments are over, you'll continue to have tenderness and soreness in your breast that will gradually go away. Some continue to experience sharp, shooting pains from time to time; how often varies greatly from woman to woman.

Few of my patients would get depressed during radiation, but many got depressed afterward—possibly because, time-consuming as the treatments are, there is a sense of activity, of doing something to fight the cancer. Once treatment ends, there's a sense of letdown. This really isn't surprising. It occurs in other intense situations, like the classical postpartum depression, or the feelings that occur when any time-consuming structure in your life is over—a job you've worked at, the end of a school term. This may be the time to get involved in a support group, if you haven't already done so. You'll have a little more time since you're not going to the treatments, and the company of others who know how you're feeling may help you get through these emotions.

Often the skin feels a little thicker right after radiation, and sometimes it's darker colored. That will gradually resolve itself over time. The nipple may get crusty, but that too will go away as the skin regenerates. This can take up to six months, and in the meantime you'll look like you've been out sunbathing with one breast exposed.

If you have received a lot of radiation to the lymph node areas, it will compound whatever scarring the surgery caused, and the combination can also increase your risk of lymphedema (see Chapter 19). A rare side effect of radiation to the lymph nodes is problems with the nerves that go from the arm to the hand, causing numbness to the fingertips.

Aside from skin reactions and tiredness, there can be later side effects. Some women get costochondritis, a kind of arthritis that causes inflammation of the space between the breasts where the ribs and breastbone connect (Figure 16.6). The pain can be scary—you wonder if your cancer has spread. It's easy to reassure yourself, though. Push your fingers down right at that junction; if it hurts, it's costochondritis and can be treated with aspirin and antiarthritis medicines. It will go away in a few weeks. Another side effect can occur between three and six months after you've finished your treatment. The muscle that goes above and behind your breast, the pectoralis major muscle, will get extremely sore, and it's worse if you grab it between your fingers. That's because the radiation caused inflammation of the muscle, and as it begins to regenerate, it can get sore and stiff, just as it would if you strained it during strenuous exercise. Most women think it's the

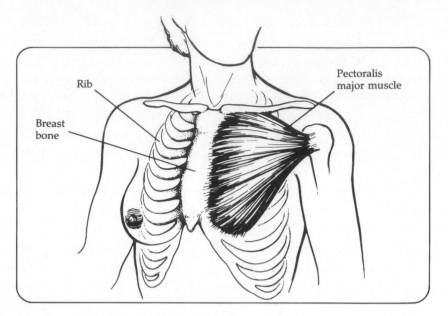

Figure 16.6

cancer spreading—especially since the radiation has been over for months and they're not expecting new side effects from it.

Frequently patients worry that being radioactive can cause them to inadvertently harm other people. They ask, "Can I hug my grandchild? Can I pick up my kids?" Once you leave the treatment room, you can be close to anyone (the implants described earlier are an exception). It's like lying in the sun. Once you're out of it, the effects remain, but the sunlight isn't inside you and can't be transmitted to anyone else.

Rarely, radiation can cause second cancers. This is usually a different kind of cancer, a sarcoma, and doesn't occur for at least five years after radiation therapy. Our best guess is that, for every 1,000 five-year survivors of wide excision and radiation, about two will develop a radiation-induced sarcoma over the next 10 years.[6]

After your treatment is completed, your radiation oncologist and your surgeon may continue to see you. In addition to making certain there are no new tumors, the radiation oncologist is watching for complications from the radiation, and the surgeon for surgical complications. These complications are rare, and radiation remains one of our most valuable tools in the treatment of local breast cancer.

Chapter 17

SYSTEMIC THERAPY

THE HALLMARK OF SYSTEMIC THERAPIES IS THEIR ABILITY TO AFFECT the whole body, not just one area. The systemic treatments used for breast cancer include chemotherapy, hormone therapy, and targeted therapy. When the treatment is given at the time of diagnosis, it is termed "adjuvant therapy" because it started out as an addition to the primary treatment, surgery. If it is given prior to surgery to shrink a tumor, it is called neoadjuvant therapy (because it's still of secondary importance to the surgery, but it's "added" before the primary treatment is used). If it is given to treat known metastatic disease it is just called "systemic therapy," since at this stage it is indeed the most important therapy. That being said, the way it is given and the side effects don't change based on where or why you get it. So this discussion covers all three of its applications.

Chemotherapy has had a lot of bad press, and it's a pity, because it's one of the most powerful weapons against cancer that we have. "Chemotherapy" literally means the use of chemicals to treat disease. As we colloquially use it, however, it usually refers only to the use of chemicals as opposed to hormone therapy or targeted therapy.

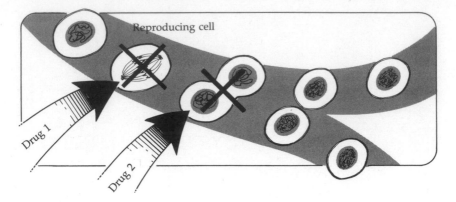

Reproducing cell

Drug 1

Drug 2

Figure 17.1

In the past, chemotherapy was used only to treat metastasis. Oncologists at that time weren't thinking about long-term effects; they hoped to keep the patient living a few years longer than she would without the treatment. If she lived long enough to deal with long-term effects, she and her doctors were happy. Because we now detect micrometastases and use chemotherapy on people whose cancers haven't significantly spread, this has changed. A woman treated with chemotherapy may now live for many years, and the issues surrounding her long-term well-being are more important.

How does chemotherapy work? Cells go through several steps in the process of cell division, or reproduction. Chemotherapy drugs interfere with this process so that the cells can't divide and consequently die. Different drugs are used in this process at different points, and often more than one kind of drug is used at a time (Figure 17.1). Unfortunately this effect on cell division acts on all cells that are rapidly dividing—not just cancer cells but also hair cells and, more importantly, bone marrow cells. Bone marrow produces red blood cells, white blood cells, and platelets continuously (Figure 17.2). This is one of the reasons chemotherapy is given in cycles, with a time lapse between treatments to allow the bone marrow to recover.

Another reason the drugs are given in cycles is that not all the cancer cells are dividing at any one time. The first treatment kills

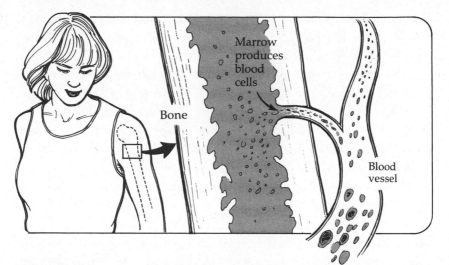

Figure 17.2

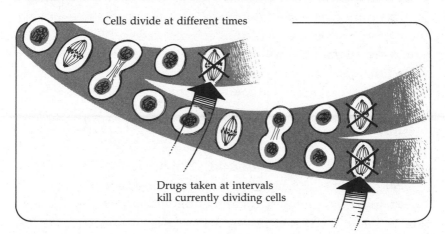

Figure 17.3

one group of cells; three weeks later a new set of cancer cells is starting to divide, and the drugs knock them out too (Figure 17.3). The idea is to decrease the total cancer cells to a number small enough for your immune system to take care of, without wiping out the immune system while we're at it. When we first started giving adjuvant chemotherapy after breast surgery, we gave the treatments over a two-year period. Later studies showed that six months was as good as one year, which was as good as two.[1]

The extra treatment may have actually harmed the immune system without having any additional effect on the cancer. There probably is a certain key dosage or duration beyond which an additional drug is useless, but what it is hasn't been determined yet.

Another kind of systemic therapy is the use of hormones or hormonal manipulations to change the body's own hormonal environment in order to affect the growth of hormonally sensitive tumors. This can include surgical procedures such as oophorectomy (removing the ovaries), radiating the ovaries, using drugs that block hormones, or even using hormones themselves. We don't fully understand all the reasons these hormone treatments work, but there is no question that they do work well in certain patients. Since hormone therapy affects only hormone-sensitive tissues, its side effects are more limited than those of chemotherapy. It doesn't kill other growing cells, such as hair and bone marrow. Hormone therapies can kill or control tumor cells by depriving them of the estrogen they require in order to grow. Without estrogen, some tumor cells will, in effect, commit suicide (apoptosis) while others will go to sleep, in a sort of coma.

Certain systemic therapies are more targeted, such as trastuzumab (Herceptin), which is being used to treat cancers that overexpress Her-2/neu (see Chapter 4), Lapatinib, which blocks tyrosine kinase, an enzyme involved in all the epidermal growth factors, and bevacizumab (Avastin), which is directed against the growth of new blood vessels (angiogenesis). Several more are in the pipeline, including ones that target epidermal growth factor (EGF) and poly(ADP)-ribose polymerase (PARP) (see Chapter 11).

If you need systemic therapy, you'll meet with a medical oncologist who specializes in systemic treatment. After talking with you at length and reviewing your records, the doctor will discuss with you the kind of cancer you have and the systemic options that might be appropriate for you and why (see Chapters 11–12). There are general guidelines for breast cancer treatment, drawn up by a group of nationwide breast cancer specialists. Check the Internet for the latest recommendations. (www.nccn.org has patient guidelines for many cancers). You may also want to become involved in a protocol or clinical trial (see Chapter 10).

There are many well-trained medical oncologists throughout the country, and you can usually find very good treatment close to home. You may, however, want to get a second opinion about chemotherapy or hormone therapy at a cancer center before you start. Doctors at these centers are usually involved in the research into the newest approaches to cancer and may know of exciting clinical trials you could participate in. Sometimes the cancer center and your local medical oncologist can work together in designing and supplementing your treatment, giving you the best of both worlds.

Your doctor or medical team will also discuss with you the role of systemic treatment in your overall treatment, the expected toxicity, and the projected management of your side effects. Before you make a decision and sign a consent form, all these things must be made very clear to you. (See Chapter 10 for how to pick a good doctor or team.)

Sometimes oncologists spend a lot of time explaining chemotherapy but relatively little time telling you about the side effects, risks, and complications of hormone therapy such as tamoxifen. Make sure you understand exactly what drugs you are getting, how you will be getting them, what short- and long-term side effects you can expect, and what can be done to prevent or lessen these side effects. Also ask exactly how much benefit you can expect in your situation from these drugs; they may or may not be worth it to you. Finally, remember to bring a tape recorder so that you don't have to worry about forgetting anything.

In Chapter 12 I explained the decision-making process and options for adjuvant therapy at length. Now we will look at the actual experience of receiving chemotherapy, hormone therapy, and/or targeted therapy.

ADJUVANT CHEMOTHERAPY

Once you have decided with your doctor to receive adjuvant chemotherapy, you'll be scheduled to come in for your treatment. It may be in a clinic, your doctor's office, or, rarely, a hospital. A blood sample is usually taken to check your blood count before your treatment, so that the doctor or nurse can determine whether your body is capable of taking chemotherapy—and as a baseline for comparison later. Your initial dose is determined in part by your body size (height and weight). This is a good (but not perfect) guess at what the optimally safe and effective dose of chemotherapy is for you.

The bone marrow's recovery rate helps the doctor adjust the drug dosage. Sometimes when the blood count is too low, you have to wait for a week before treatment to allow your bone marrow more time to recover. When giving adjuvant chemotherapy, your oncologist should be reluctant to administer anything but the standard dosage. Dose reduction (lowering) should be undertaken only for severe, life-threatening toxicities because it is the standard doses that have been shown to be effective.

Think of the bone marrow as a factory churning out red blood cells, white blood cells, and platelets. Chemotherapy injures a portion of the factory's employees, and the factory doesn't work as well till they have recovered. Recently we've discovered drugs that help accelerate the recovery of the patient's bone marrow—keeping all the workers healthy so the factory can get back on track.

The major drug we have for this is GCSF (granulocyte colony stimulating factor), a substance you normally have in your blood. It stimulates the bone marrow to make more white blood cells in times of stress or infection, when you need to build up your immune system. Now we've found a way to utilize this in chemotherapy treatment.[2] It's a natural product made from bacteria through genetic engineering. (Although this may sound unnatural, it's just a way for bacteria to serve as the production factory.) We have found that when we give it to someone, it whips up her bone marrow, so that instead of having a normal white blood cell count of 10,000, she has 40,000 or 50,000. So now when a woman's white blood cell count becomes too low we give her GCSF in an injection, to hasten the bone marrow's recovery. It's like operating on those injured factory workers and getting them back to work. GCSF is thus able to reduce the time it takes your bone marrow to recover after chemotherapy. Our initial enthusiasm for GCSF has been dampened recently as data have begun coming in which suggest that the use of the drug increases the risk of developing bone marrow abnormalities and even leukemia. These side effects also occur in about 1 percent of women on chemotherapy alone, but the addition of GCSF doubled this risk.[3] This has led to more caution in its use. Women taking a dose-dense schedule of chemotherapy (see Chapter 12) may need GCSF because the abbreviated schedule does not give the bone marrow time to recover on its own. One recent study found that when the GCSF was given with paclitaxel, women complained of severe bone pain. This led doctors to discontinue the GCSF, and they were then pleased to find that most of the women tolerated paclitaxel (Taxol) alone quite well.[4] This has led many oncologists to point out that we probably use too much GCSF. Although in animal tumors we can usually show that higher doses of chemotherapy are more effective, in many cases this has not been demonstrated in women. A good example is Adriamycin and Cytoxan in the adjuvant setting.

If your treatment begins the day the blood count is taken, you'll have to wait 15–45 minutes for tests results before you begin. In any event, you'll probably have to wait while the drugs are being mixed, though again this will depend on the practice in your institution. The wait may be annoying, but it can also be an advantage: often this is an opportunity for women to talk to each other and find support in being together.

Standard chemotherapy treatments are given on a variety of schedules including weekly, 3 weekly, monthly, or 6 weekly. The schedules vary depending on the drugs that are being used. The 3 and 4 weekly schedules may be the most common. This means for example that you'll get them every three weeks, in 21-day cycles or 28-day cycles. If it's a 21-day cycle, you may come in for an infusion every three weeks. On a 28-day cycle, on the other hand, you may come in for treatment on day 1 and day 8, and then go two weeks with no therapy. That's two weeks with therapy and two weeks off or 28 days before you start the cycle again. During this time your treatment may be all intravenous or a combination of intravenous medicine and a pill you take at home. The treatments can last anywhere from 12 weeks to 6 months to a year. Dose-dense scheduling means you receive the drugs every two weeks for four to eight cycles.

Treatment areas vary. In the hospital there may be an entire floor for oncology patients and sometimes just a separate area of a

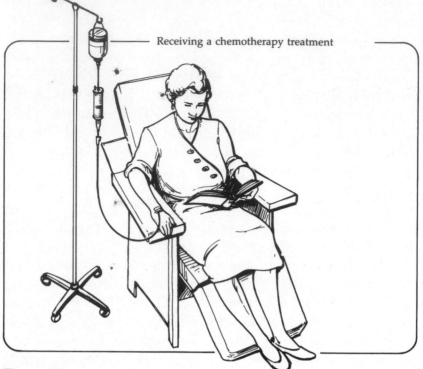

Receiving a chemotherapy treatment

Figure 17.4

larger floor. In a doctor's office or an outpatient clinic there is usually a special area that has been set aside. Chemotherapy can also
be given in a private doctor's office. Everyone is aware of patient
anxiety levels and tries to make the area as comfortable as possible. Since the process doesn't involve machines, the chemo room
doesn't look as intimidating as the radiation area. The room is
comfortably lit and often has television sets or stereos in it. You
may have a room to yourself or may sit among several other patients who are getting their treatment. You'll sit in a comfortable
lounge chair for the procedure (Figure 17.4). Many patients bring
books, tape players, or MP3 players with them for the treatment.
For a very long treatment, you may want to invest in an iPod, handheld TV, or a portable DVD player to catch up on movies. With
easily transportable paperwork or a laptop, you can work while the
treatment is in progress. If you want to have a friend or family

member with you, most hospitals and doctors will permit that. One woman I know would bring her own pillow and blanket from home to help her get through the four hours of her dose-dense treatment while friends came along and kept her entertained. .

The length of time a treatment takes and the intervals at which treatments are given will vary depending on the type of drugs, the institution administering the treatment, and the protocol being used. Several different drug combinations may be used, each requiring its own time length for administration; in addition, you will likely be given extra fluid as well as medications to control nausea and vomiting. Sometimes a treatment will last 10 minutes, sometimes three or four hours.

The treatments are given by your medical oncologist or a specially trained nurse. There's nothing particularly painful about the treatment, which feels like any IV procedure. The chemicals come in different colors; the drugs we use for breast cancer are usually clear, yellow, and red. One woman I counseled told me that she used to have the nurse give the red doxorubicin under the covers because she did not like the color. Never hesitate to ask for something like this if it doesn't inconvenience the staff and helps you get through the treatment.

You usually don't feel the medications go into your body, though some patients feel cold if the fluids are run very fast or if they're cold to begin with, or if their bodies are especially sensitive to cold. Cyclophosphamide can cause a weird feeling of pressure in your sinuses, which stops once the infusion is finished. The doctor or nurse will always be there with you, and they're both highly trained specialists in chemotherapy. Sometimes the drugs irritate veins and cause them to clot off and scar (sclerose) during the course of the treatment. This can make it very hard to get needles into the veins.

Vascular access devices are available that allow for intravenous administration of your medication. They come in a variety of types including Hickman, Groshong, and porta cath. They are all catheter-type devices placed under the skin into a major blood vessel in the upper chest (Figure 17.5). Needles can go in and out of that device and spare the patient the discomfort of having peripheral veins (the ones close to the surface, which are normally

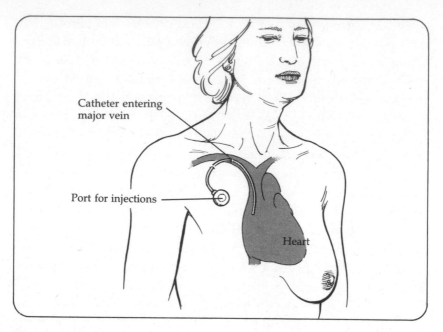

Figure 17.5

used for needles) stuck. The catheter must be inserted in the side of the body away from the affected breast, in case you eventually have a mastectomy or radiation therapy. This involves a surgical procedure, usually done under local anesthetic. It can be a bit uncomfortable but it's a trade-off. Patients like the fact that they don't have to get stuck with a new needle each treatment, but on the other hand having a catheter under your skin can feel strange. The other problem is that the catheter is a foreign body and on rare occasions can cause an infection. It also needs to be flushed occasionally with a blood thinner to prevent a clot. For most women, the decision to use or not use a catheter is reasonable either way, but a catheter is essential for a patient who has trouble with her veins.

Seven drugs are commonly given as adjuvant chemotherapy for breast cancer: cyclophosphamide (Cytoxan) (C), methotrexate (M), 5-fluorouracil (F), doxorubicin (Adriamycin) (A), or epirubicin (E); and paclitaxel (Taxol) or docetaxel (Taxotere) (T). (See Appendix A.) These are usually given in combinations, CMF or AC followed by T or FEC or TAC. In addition, drugs are given to maintain your white blood count based on GCSF. Filgrastim (Neupogen) and sargramostim (Leukine) have to be taken as injections daily over 10–14 days. A new long-acting form called pegfilgrastim (Neulasta), which is injected only once a cycle, may also be used.

Other drugs are used for metastatic disease. Some of the most common are Abraxane and Gemzar, which are given IV, and Xeloda, which can be taken by mouth (see Chapter 20). While the side effects vary somewhat from one drug to another, they are basically similar to those of the adjuvant drugs.

While you are on chemotherapy, your immune system will not be functioning at its best. Although your blood cells may be fairly normal (particularly if you are getting GMCSF support), the immune system is affected in less obvious ways. This doesn't mean you have to hide in your house and avoid all contact with the human race during therapy. Talk with your oncologist or nurse about your daily activities. Are you a teacher, do you have young children in the house, do you own pets? The doctor can give you specific advice about how to minimize your risk of getting an infection. You should make sure you are up to date with your vaccinations (seasonal flu, pneumonia, etc.). You may also want to get a good dental cleaning before starting chemotherapy if there is time (you do not want to do this during chemotherapy, as dental cleanings can introduce bacteria into your bloodstream while your cell counts are low). Practice good hand washing, and consider investing in a small bottle of alcohol-based sanitizer for when you can't get to a sink.

SIDE EFFECTS OF CHEMOTHERAPY

Nausea and Vomiting

Side effects vary according to the drugs used. (See Appendix A for a detailed list of some of the drugs most commonly used against breast cancer and their side effects.) The most immediate potential side effect concerns doxorubicin (Adriamycin), which can leak out of the vein and cause a severe skin burn that could require skin grafting. For this reason, it's generally given in a specific way: avoiding weak veins and running in the IV with lots of fluids, so that it can't cause as much harm if it does leak out.

A common side effect seen with many types of chemotherapy is nausea and vomiting. Overall, about 20 percent of women who get CMF, as well as more of the women who receive AC, complain of nausea and vomiting. These symptoms are more common the younger a woman is and much less so as women age. We've learned that not all chemotherapy-induced nausea is the same. Some drugs are worse than others. Unfortunately the ones commonly used for breast cancer—doxorubicin (Adriamycin) and cyclophosphamide (Cytoxan)—are in the high group. Taxanes (Taxol and Taxotere) tend to have less of a tendency to provoke nausea. Although the drugs themselves cannot be changed, there are many protocols and drugs available to prevent and treat these symptoms, and nobody should have to suffer.

The timing of nausea differs as well. Cyclophosphamide starts about 6–8 hours after treatment and lasts 8–24 hours, while doxorubicin starts in 1–3 hours and lasts 4–24 hours. Acute vomiting, which usually occurs in the first 24 hours after a chemotherapy treatment, seems to be related to serotonin and responds well to serotonin inhibitors like dolasetron (Anzemet), granisetron (Kytril), ondansetron (Zofran), and plaenosetron (Aloxi). Dexamethasone (a steroid related to, but not the same as, those used illegally by athletes) is also helpful for acute vomiting. Delayed nausea and vomiting are caused by something called substance P and occur 1–5 days after therapy, with a peak effect around 48–72 hours, and respond to a drug called aprepitant (Emend). For treatments with high potential for nausea and vomiting, the National Comprehensive Cancer Network (NCCN) currently recommends starting drugs before chemotherapy with apreptitant, dexamethasone, and one of the serotonin inhibitors.[5] Once nausea has set in, it is much harder to control. The NCCN website is worth checking (www.nccn.com). If these approaches are not enough, dopamine antagonists (Metochlopramide, Procholoperazine, domepridone, or Metoprimazine) can be added to the serotonin inhibitors and steroids. Cannabinoid (dronabinol, marijuana) has also been used for both acute and delayed chemotherapy-induced nausea and vomiting, and studies show that it is very effective. (The woman who brought her blanket and pillow to her dose-dense treatments swore by it.) It is also available as a pill (Marinol), which is legal but not as effective. Obviously using marijuana has all the downsides—both legal and physical—that you are aware of. If you are going to try it, do so under an experienced doctor's supervision and prescription. And of course only if it is legal in your area.

The final type of nausea and vomiting is anticipatory and occurs days to hours prior to chemotherapy. This means you have experienced nausea and vomiting in the past, and now just thinking about getting chemotherapy next week makes you nauseated today. This type can be controlled with benzodiazepines starting one or two days prior to treatment or behavioral techniques. These days most oncologists try to prevent nausea and vomiting in the first place. Make sure you discuss this aspect of your care with your doctor and nurse so that you understand which drugs are being given to prevent nausea and why.

Because the thought of chemotherapy can be frightening, it is a good idea to bring someone with you for your first treatment to see how well it goes and drive you home if necessary. Then if the first treatment goes well and you feel all right afterward, you may not need anyone for the following ones. Usually, if you start off feeling all right and your antinausea drugs are effective, you'll get through the rest of the treatments with relative comfort.

In addition to the drugs, some hospitals, like Beth Israel Deaconess in Boston, incorporate such antistress mechanisms as visualization, imagery, and relaxation techniques into their treatment program. These are often very effective. If your hospital or doctor doesn't offer such techniques, you may want to try some of the ones described in Chapter 18. Many of the techniques are simple and easy to learn. In addition, many adult education centers and holistic health institutes in cities and towns all over the country have visualization programs. Acupuncture and Chinese herbs, discussed in Chapter 18, can also bring nausea relief. There are many options, and if what you are receiving from your doctor does not work, you need to ask for something different. There is no reason for anyone to suffer needlessly.

Weight Gain

Although the cause of weight gain with chemotherapy is not clear, one study found that 50 percent of patients gained more than 10 pounds.[6] Twenty-one will gain between 5 and 15 pounds. [7] This was independent of type of chemotherapy, age, and menopausal status, although the women who gained weight did have a decrease in activity. Some data suggest that overweight women have a higher mortality than lean ones.[8] This has stimulated interest in nutritional and exercise programs for survivors (see Chapter 18).

Effects on Appetite and Sense of Smell

Sometimes chemotherapy causes you to lose your appetite (anorexia, which is different from anorexia nervosa). Food may taste different to you, and some chemicals interact badly with certain foods, though both loss of appetite and chemical interaction are less common with breast cancer drugs than with others. The National Cancer Institute publishes a helpful recipe booklet for people whose eating is affected by their chemotherapy. You may also experience peculiar odors. Barbara Kalinowski, who co-facilitated a support group for women with breast cancer in Boston, describes a woman who talked of constantly walking through her house opening windows so she could get rid of an odor that she described as similar to that of a new car.

Premature Menopause

Fifty-seven percent of premenopausal women have hot flashes while on adjuvant chemotherapy. The drugs can create a chemically induced menopause, with hormonal changes, hot flashes, mood swings, and no periods.

An article in the *Journal of Clinical Oncology* suggests that the strongest predictors of whether or not you go through menopause with treatment are age and type of chemotherapy.[9,10] The closer you are to natural menopause, the higher your risk. The average age of menopause is 51. A woman of 45 who receives chemotherapy has an 80 percent likelihood of going into menopause as a result, which is much greater than is the case with tamoxifen (note that tamoxifen works just as well regardless of menopausal status). A thirty-five-year-old woman has a 20 percent chance of becoming postmenopausal. Many women don't know this ahead of time and have to deal with something unexpected in the midst of their treatment.

With CMF given for six months, the risk of premature menopause is approximately 35 percent in women younger than 40 versus 90 percent in women older than 40. In contrast, less than 15 percent of women younger than 40 who receive four cycles of AC (doxorubicin and cyclophosphamide), and 60 percent of those over 40, will become menopausal.[11,12] Overall, it is the cumulative dose of cyclophosphamide that is strongly related to premature menopause. What effect the recent addition of taxanes to AC has on the ovaries is unknown. Although roughly half of the women younger than 40 may regain some menstrual function, the percentage is much lower in older women. There is some evidence in animals that putting the ovaries into reversible menopause with GNRH agonist during chemotherapy may be more protective, but it has not been tested yet in women.[13,14]

If you do experience early menopause, you will of course be infertile. If your period comes back, you can still conceive. Since it's difficult to tell which group you're in, you should use mechanical birth control during treatment if you're heterosexually active. Hormone-based contraception may stimulate the tumor, and the chemotherapy drugs could severely injure a first trimester fetus. (See Chapter 13 for a discussion about fertility options for women who are about to undergo chemotherapy and Chapter 19 for a further discussion of the treatment of menopausal symptoms.)

Hair Loss

Chemotherapy treatments used in breast cancer, as in many other cancers, often cause partial or total hair loss. This is somewhat predictable according to the drugs used and duration of treatment. Women who get doxorubicin as part of their treatment almost always lose their hair, usually within two to four weeks after the onset of treatment. On the other hand, women who receive CMF usually lose their hair, but it is gradual over weeks and months and often it is mild or insufficiently severe to require a wig. You'll wake up one morning and find a large amount of hair on your pillow or in the shower, or you'll be combing your hair and notice a lot in the comb. This is almost always traumatic, so it's probably wise to buy a wig before your treatment starts. You can ask your oncologist to give you a prescription for a "cranial prosthesis" (wig), and often insurance will cover it. It's best to go to a hairdresser or wig salon at the start of treatment, so the hairdresser knows what your hair usually looks like and how you like to wear it—it makes for a better match. Women receiving CMF often end up not using the wig. (You can always donate it to a local breast resource center.) Patients who don't prepare in advance for the hair loss tend to have a difficult time emotionally if it does occur. The Network of Strength, a national support organization, sends wigs to women with hair loss for a nominal fee.

Remember, though, it isn't only the hair on your head that falls out. Pubic hair, eyelashes and eyebrows, leg and arm hair—some or all of the hair on your body will fall out, although in most women the eyelashes and eyebrows only thin a bit. Most of the time that isn't a big problem cosmetically—you can thicken your eyebrows with pencil, for example, and apply false eyelashes— but it can be startling if you're not prepared for it.

It may take a while after the treatments have ended for your hair to grow back. A little down will probably appear even before your treatments have ended, and within six weeks you should have some hair growing in, though the time depends on how fast your hair normally grows. Often it comes back with a different texture—curly if it's been straight. Eventually the curl relaxes and your hair returns to normal after several haircuts. It may come back in a different color, most commonly gray or black.

Sexual Problems

Some women experience sexual problems, often related to the vaginal dryness of menopause. And you may suddenly encounter problems with your diaphragm or an IUD due to dryness. In addition there are the physical and psychological effects of the treatment. It's hard to feel sexy when you are tired and bald. This is an important time to communicate with your partner about each other's feelings and needs and to try and find a comforting compromise. (See Chapter 19 for a discussion of sexual issues and breast cancer.)

"Chemo Brain"

There are many aftereffects of chemotherapy that we're just beginning to acknowledge, either because they're subtle or because
they take longer to materialize. For example, studies show decreased cognitive function (what patients call "chemo brain").
Several studies have been published showing cognitive impairment in women with breast cancer who have undergone adjuvant
chemotherapy.[15,16] All of the studies have been criticized for the
way they were done; for example, they compared the survivors as
a group to healthy controls. Although on the surface this may
seem a good thing to do, in fact it is unlikely to pick up subtle differences. Is this the result of the chemotherapy or of the premature menopause brought on by chemotherapy in younger women?
How does tamoxifen contribute to the changes? Is it because of
depression about having breast cancer in the first place? Or the
hot flashes and night sweats that prevent sleep and result from
the premature menopause?

Research is going on to investigate whether specific groups of
women are more susceptible than others and whether cognitive
retraining can overcome the difficulties.[17] Although most of the
women in these studies are still highly functioning and holding
down jobs, it can be noticeable and distressing to them. For
someone who needs the treatment to survive, it's worth it, but in
cases where chemotherapy offers only a minuscule survival improvement, it may not be. See Chapter 21 for a fuller discussion.

Other Side Effects

Other common side effects include mouth sores, conjunctivitis,
runny eyes and nose, skin, nail changes, diarrhea, and constipa-
tion. You may get headaches, which is often from the antinausea
medication. Any of these can be mild or severe, or anything in
between.

The long-term side effects of chemotherapy include chronic
bone marrow suppression and second cancers, especially
leukemias. The risk of leukemia is small—0.5 percent in the NS-
ABP series—and probably worth the benefit of the treatment, but
you need to be aware that it exists.[18]

Doxorubicin in particular can be toxic to the heart. The likelihood of this is related to the cumulative dose of doxorubicin that you get over a lifetime, and it's rare with four to six cycles. Some people who were treated with doxorubicin many years ago for childhood cancers are now experiencing heart failure and need heart transplants.[19] We're only beginning to consider this now because in the past we used doxorubicin only for metastatic cancers, and those patients usually died of the cancer within a few years. Now that we're using it more frequently for women with negative lymph nodes, the patients may well be alive in 20 or 30 years, and we may see more side effects than we did before. It is important not to assume that a drug or treatment that is relatively safe at the time will be safe over the long haul. We know that doxorubicin causes heart damage by itself, but it also interacts with some other forms of heart disease. Consequently a patient on this drug may have more problems with coronary artery disease years later. Overall, the risk of having a heart problem due to doxorubicin is about 1 in 200 treated women. One of my former patients developed heart disease after being treated with doxorubicin and ended up with a heart transplant.

I'm not suggesting that we abandon doxorubicin for adjuvant treatment; my patient, after all, survived long enough to develop a heart ailment. Doxorubicin is one of the best drugs we have to treat metastatic breast cancer. If it is indicated, it should certainly be used. But we should not use it indiscriminately in women who are not at particularly high risk for metastases. There are several ongoing studies looking to see if we can omit doxorubicin from adjuvant regimens in some women.

Paclitaxel (Taxol) can cause a reversible, dose-dependent, cumulative *neuropathy*. This is a pins-and-needles sensation, often in the hands and feet, which can get worse with each dose but is generally at least partially reversible. Taxol can also cause hand-foot syndrome, an itchy rash on the palms of the hands and the soles of the feet. In about 5–15 percent of women a syndrome of muscle and joint aches and pains can occur, starting about 24–72 hours after the infusion and lasting 2–4 days. It ranges from mild, requiring only occasional nonnarcotic pain relievers, to incapacitating. A woman I counseled through her treatment experienced this and required narcotics to deal with it. The narcotics led to nausea and vomiting. Once you know that you react this way, you can be treated with dexamethasone for several days to prevent the pain. Docetaxel (Taxotere) also causes the neuropathy but is generally milder than paclitaxel. Docetaxel also causes a unique syndrome of swelling and fluid retention; some fluid retention is fairly common but occasionally it can be severe. Fortunately this is reversible but takes a long time. A newer form of paclitaxel, nab-paclitaxel (Abraxane) has been shown to be at least as effective and possibly more effective than paclitaxel and is used for metastatic breast cancer. Although it generally has fewer side effects than paclitaxel, the one side effect that is worse than paclitaxel's is the neuropathy. Though there's no way to know in advance how you'll react to your treatments, your doctor or nurse can tell you how other people treated with the drugs you're on have done in the past.

While it's important to be prepared for possible side effects, it's equally important not to assume you'll have all, or even any, of them. This assumption can intensify and sometimes even create the symptoms. Sometimes people see the side effects as a sign that their illness is getting worse and consequently contribute to their own negative feelings. Bernie Siegel, the doctor who has worked intensively with mental techniques to reduce pain and help heal diseases, reports in his book *Love, Medicine, and Miracles* on a study done in England in which men were given a placebo and told it was a chemotherapy treatment.[20] Thirty percent of the men lost their hair! Positive thinking and—importantly—exercise, as well as keeping up your normal activities, can significantly reduce the side effects of chemotherapy.

Most chemotherapy treatments are given on an outpatient basis. You will soon know whether you are going to feel sick and, if so, on which day the nausea hits and how bad it is. Most women are able to continue their normal lives and maintain their jobs with minor adjustments while receiving treatment. You won't feel great, but you'll be functional. At this point, adjuvant breast cancer chemotherapy should be tolerable and you should be able to function well. If it's not, ask your doctor or nurse for strategies to reduce the side effects. Many options are available.

This may be a good time to take up your friends' offers of help. A ride to your treatment can be wonderful, both for the company and the release from worry about traffic and parking. Child care may give you a breather in a stressful time, as can offers to cook dinner or clean the house. Most friends and family members really do want to help, and this may be the best time to use their support.

Don't expect to feel perfect the minute your last treatment is over. Your body has been under a great stress and needs time to recuperate. It often takes six months or even a year to feel normal again. It will happen, however, so don't despair. (See Chapter 19 for a discussion of rehabilitation after breast cancer.)

Fatigue

An interesting study looked at fatigue during and after chemotherapy. (Anyone who's had chemotherapy knows about such fatigue; now we doctors are catching up to the patients!) The women who had chemotherapy suffered 61 percent more fatigue than the women in the control group.[21] If you are finding this a problem, you should bring it to the attention of your doctor or nurse. There are five factors that are often associated with fatigue: pain, emotional distress, sleep disturbance, anemia, and low thyroid. These are all treatable and so should be checked out. Other possible causes can be infection, electrolyte disorders, and cardiac dysfunction. Moderate to severe fatigue is always worth complaining about.

More tolerable fatigue can be considered the "pooped-out syndrome." Your body has been assaulted by surgery, radiation, and chemotherapy and is still trying to heal. It needs longer to get back to normal than we previously understood. One patient says it takes as long to get back to normal as it took to get the treatment: if you have six months of chemotherapy, you have six months of fatigue.

ADJUVANT HORMONE THERAPY

Tamoxifen

The best-known and most widely used hormone therapy is tamoxifen. In terms of administration, hormone therapies are the simplest of the breast cancer treatments. You don't need to go any-where or have anything done to you—you simply take a pill. The most important thing about tamoxifen is that it treats the cancer you have, and it reduces your chance of getting cancer in the op-posite breast by 50 percent; that is, from 15–20 percent to 7.5–10 percent. So considering all these pros and cons, it is worth taking unless you have had problems with blood clots in the past.

As I explained in Chapter 12, the current data suggest you take tamoxifen for five years and then stop. Much to everyone's surprise, the benefits of decreasing the chance of relapse and of second cancers continue even after you stop taking the drug. Ta-moxifen is therefore likely to kill cancer cells or, more probably, put them into a long-lasting dormant state.

It takes six weeks for tamoxifen to clear from your system after you stop. So if you miss a pill one day, it isn't the end of the world. Just resume taking it the next day.

Hormone therapies generally have fewer side effects than chemotherapy. Because we look at hormones in relation to chemotherapy, we tend to minimize their side effects. And indeed they are milder than those of chemotherapy. But they do exist, and for some women they can be significant, including phlebitis (blood clots), pulmonary embolism, premature menopause, visual problems, depression, nausea (but very rarely vomiting), vaginal discharge, muscular aches and pains, and hot flashes.[22] All of these are rare except for the hot flashes and muscle pains. A lot of women who have these symptoms ask me if they could be caused by their medication. When I say yes, they say, "Thank God. I thought I was going crazy because my doctor said I wouldn't have side effects."

The most common long-term side effect of hormonal therapies is premature menopause and the resulting infertility. I discussed the latter in Chapter 12 and will discuss the former at length in Chapter 19.

The other most common side effects are hot flashes, which oc-cur in about 50 percent of women on tamoxifen. Like all hot flashes, they can be severe or mild. They eventually go away, but "eventually" may mean years. New drugs like venlafaxine (Effexor) or Neurontin can reduce the number and intensity of these hot flashes.[23] Alternative choices are discussed in Chapter 19.

About 30 percent of women on tamoxifen experience major gynecological discomforts—anything from vaginal discharge to severe vaginal dryness. If you are premenopausal on tamoxifen, be aware that new gynecological complaints may be related to it.

There's some evidence that tamoxifen may, in unusual cases, increase thrombophlebitis, a form of phlebitis in the leg in which the vein gets irritated and forms clots.[24] This is rare, about 1 percent, but very dangerous, as the blood clot can travel to the lung, causing pulmonary embolus. It can even be fatal. Let your doctor know right away if you develop leg swelling and pain.

The most serious side effect of tamoxifen is uterine cancer. In the NSABP prevention study (see Chapter 7), researchers found the risk doubled after five years, although the absolute risk is very low.[25] It occurs almost entirely in women over 50. This is reassuring because postmenopausal women now have a safer option with the aromatase inhibitors (see below), and premenopausal women can take this drug without worrying about getting uterine cancer.

Premenopausal women have an increased risk of benign gynecological problems, including uterine polyps, fibroids, endometriosis, and ovarian cysts.[26] (See Chapter 13 on the use of tamoxifen to induce ovulation for IVF.) Because tamoxifen can damage a fetus, it's very important not to get pregnant while you're taking it. A heterosexually active woman undergoing chemotherapy should use some type of effective mechanical contraceptive while receiving treatment.

Some women have elevated liver blood enzymes, which go away once they stop taking tamoxifen. Many women on tamoxifen experience eye problems, including blurry vision and, uncommonly, cataracts.

Nonetheless, there are several benefits with tamoxifen. It raises your high-density lipoproteins and lowers your low-density lipoproteins, which may make you less likely to get heart disease.[27] Tamoxifen often improves osteoporosis in postmenopausal women and sometimes stabilizes it, much like raloxifene.[28]

Other Antiestrogens

Toremifene, a drug that has been approved by the FDA for treatment of metastatic disease, is sometimes used in place of tamoxifen, especially for women who do not tolerate it. Raloxifene is a SERM (see Chapter 7) that has been shown to decrease breast cancer in postmenopausal women with low bone density. One study of 14 women with metastatic breast cancer showed no effect from raloxifene.[29] A second study showed an 18 percent response rate in metastatic disease.[30] At this time it is definitely *not* an alternative to tamoxifen as adjuvant treatment of breast cancer.

Fulvestrant (Faslodex) is a new steroidal antiestrogen. Unlike tamoxifen and raloxifene, it has no estrogenic effects. In the metastatic setting it appears to be as good as anastrozole and causes fewer joint problems (see below). It is given by intramuscular injection once a month rather than by mouth. It is not clear at this time whether it will be used for adjuvant treatment in the future.

Aromatase Inhibitors

Until recently only tamoxifen was given as an adjuvant hormone treatment. As I mentioned in Chapter 12, aromatase inhibitors are now being used just as frequently in postmenopausal women. Like tamoxifen, they are taken in pill form. Three drugs are commonly used: anastrozole, letrozole, and exemestane. The postmenopausal ovary and adrenal glands produce the precursors of estrogen, which are converted in particular organs into estrogen by the enzyme aromatase. These drugs block this conversion, reducing the amount of estrogen in most organs. Since they block estrogen production and have no estrogenic effects, it is not surprising that some of the side effects are similar to those of tamoxifen; others are quite different. In the initial study that compared the aromatase inhibitor (AI) anastrozole to tamoxifen head-to-head, the main differences were the endometrial cancer with tamoxifen and the increased fractures and muscular and joint pain with anastrozole.[31] This was the first adjuvant trial reported, and it is instructive to look at the side effects. Unfortunately the study compares their side effects only to those caused by tamoxifen. Nonetheless the major problems seem to be joint pain, which increased by 32 percent, and fractures, which increased by 50 percent. The fracture problem may not be as bad as we think because tamoxifen tends to reduce fractures; so the difference between the two groups is probably much bigger than if they had compared the aromatase inhibitor to a placebo. When you hear people say that the AIs have fewer side effects than tamoxifen, it is true—but it is also true that we looked only for the side effects that are common with tamoxifen. It will be some time before we know all of women's experiences with these drugs.

When the fourth edition of this book was published, we had just started using these drugs. Now we have several studies investigating the best way to use them. They can be used in a variety of schedules: upfront for five years, switching after two to three years of tamoxifen, or as extended therapy after five years of tamoxifen. Which approach makes most sense for you will depend on your age, how many years it's been since you began menopause, risk of recurrence, bone health, history of blood clots, menopausal symptoms, and sexual activity. Women who are not sure whether they are menopausal, are within a year of their last period, or have chemotherapy-induced menopause are best started on tamoxifen with monitoring of blood hormone levels. If they have no periods for two years and show a menopausal hormone pattern, they can be switched to an AI. As I was writing this fifth edition of the book, a presentation at the San Antonio Breast Meeting showed that premenopausal women can benefit from extended AI therapy once they become menopausal and that the benefit was similar in women who were up to six years after finishing five years of tamoxifen.[32] Why not just use an AI from the beginning? Because it does not work in premenopausal women who are still producing hormones.

When you ask women or oncology nurses what the biggest complaint about the aromatase inhibitors is, they specify bone pain and musculo-skeletal stiffness, but these symptoms may not last. Further follow-up of the ATAC trial mentioned above suggested that in approximately one-third of women, joint symptoms

improved usually within six months while continuing on therapy.[33] Although all three forms of AI cause symptoms, studies
show that switching from one to another will often lessen the
symptoms.[34] Usually these symptoms go away after about three
months, but getting through that time period takes patience and
endurance. Anti-inflammatories (NSAIDs) seem to help some
women, as do warm baths, acupuncture, and massage. Because
many women are also coming off hormone replacement therapy,
it is sometimes difficult to know which of the side effects are
from that and which from the new drugs. A nurse friend of mine
says that bioflavonoids help both bone pain and hot flashes in
some women. Indeed, the ATAC study reported a 20 percent incidence of this. Vaginal dryness and pain on intercourse are also
side effects of the lack of estrogen in some women and can be
managed with lubricants and vaginal moisturizers.

Goserelin (Zoladex)

This drug is one of the GNRH agonists, which block the pituitary's
production of the hormones that stimulate the ovary. The result is
that you are put into a reversible menopause. Goserelin is given by
a monthly injection under the skin of the abdomen. As you might
expect, it has many of the side effects of normal menopause. First,
your periods stop. This is not a contraceptive, however, so you
should be sure to use another means of contraception as well if
you are heterosexually active. Hot flashes, lower sex drive, joint
pain, and weight gain are common side effects. Most of the time
your period will return when you complete your course of treatment, although in some women close to menopause it will not.
Goserelin has been combined with tamoxifen and an aromatase
inhibitor in a randomized controlled trial. After four years the
disease-free survival rates were the same (92 percent), whether
the combination was an AI plus goserelin, or tamoxifen plus
goserelin. This suggests that the benefits of aromatase inhibitors
over tamoxifen seen in postmenopausal women do not hold for
premenopausal women. The side effects, however, are worse—a
quarter of the women have joint pain, as do a third of those who
also took zoledronic acid. Most interesting was the fact that the

women who also received zoledronic acid (Zometa) had 3.2 percent decrease in recurrence (see below). Based on this data three years of goserelin plus tamoxifen and zoledronic acid is probably the best choice for premenopausal women with hormone positive tumors, either after chemotherapy if they are still having periods, or instead of chemotherapy if they are at lower risk.[35]

BONE LOSS AND BISPHOSPHONATES

Women with breast cancer tend to have high bone density. The problem is that chemotherapy (by putting some women into premature menopause) and some of the current hormone therapies accelerate the normal bone loss that occurs with aging. But others, notably tamoxifen and to a lesser extent toremifene, help maintain bone by preventing its loss. They have about the same effect as raloxifene (Evista), improving bone density by 2–3 percent and preventing vertebral fractures. In one study that used goserelin to induce temporary menopause for two years, there was a 5 percent decrease in bone density, which started improving once the therapy was withdrawn.

Women who took tamoxifen while they were on the goserelin showed only a 1.4 percent decrease in bone density.[36] Considering that the study quoted above showed that this combination was the same as using an AI plus goserelin, it is probably preferable.

For women on aromatase inhibitors, the issues are more complicated. At a minimum, women who have had breast cancer should follow the general recommendation from the National Osteoporosis Foundation: first bone density test at 65 or at the latest, when the therapy is finished. It is not clear that the decrease in bone density with treatment will last indefinitely. A study of two years of the aromatase inhibitor exemestane showed that after the drug was stopped, the bone density of the lumbar spine improved and that of the hip stabilized, suggesting that the effects of these drugs are not permanent.[37] A year after the treatments were stopped, there was no difference in bone density in the two groups—a reminder that all women lose some bone. Bone does not change fast and the test itself is not that precise, so the current recommendations are to repeat a bone density test only after a minimum of two years.

In an attempt to prevent the bone loss and subsequent fractures, it has become clinical practice to put women taking AIs on drugs to try and maintain their bones. This usually involves zoledronic acid (Zometa). Interestingly, bone density is maintained[38] but a recent meta-analysis did not show that the number of fractures decreased.[39] This suggests that the effect of AIs on bone may be more than just a reduction in bone density and may affect bone quality in some undefined way.

While one could argue against a need to treat a temporary decrease in bone density, there is another intriguing side effect of the treatment that may well make it worthwhile. The bisphosphonate drugs zoledronic acid (Zometa), palmidronate (Aredia), and alendronate (Fosamax) have been shown in some studies to decrease bone metastases. While this is currently being examined in large studies, it does make the use of one of these drugs more appealing. The one group where it has been shown to be of use is in premenopausal women with early stage estrogen sensitive breast cancer receiving ovarian suppression. Other groups are currently being studied. Meanwhile bisphosphonates have been shown to have the ability to preserve bone density during hormone therapy. Whether this is important is not clear, nor is it clear whether it is better to take them prophylactically or only if there is bone loss. All of these questions should be answered in the next five years.

Most of the time intravenous bisphosphonates have been used in cancer patients. They do not have the gastrointestinal problems seen with oral drugs such as Fosamax but can be associated with flu-like symptoms such as bone pain, transient joint and muscle pain, nausea, and fever. These symptoms usually occur after the first or second infusion and last about 48 hours. They respond well to aspirin and NSAIDs. Since low calcium can be seen with these drugs, women are encouraged to take vitamin D and calcium and are monitored for their calcium blood levels. Kidney toxicity is also possible with these drugs, especially in women who already have diminished renal function. The other side effect is necrosis (tissue death) in the jaw bone. This usually follows dental work and consists of an area of exposed bone that does not heal. For this reason any woman considering taking one of these drugs should have a good dental exam first.

TARGETED THERAPIES

Trastuzumab (Herceptin)

Trastuzumab is Her-2/neu. Although it is pretty safe when given alone, it has shown an increased risk of heart failure in women who also take or have taken Adriamycin. Particularly in women taking it as adjuvant treatment as opposed to treatment of metastatic disease, this possibility is usually monitored. This typically involves a multigated acquisition scan (MUGA) scan or echocardiogram (echo) to evaluate how well your heart is pumping prior to treatment. The test is then checked every three months during Herceptin therapy and every six months for at least two years following the completion of the one-year course. If your heart's ability to pump blood decreases, the drug will be suspended for at least four weeks to see if the situation improves. If there is no improvement in eight weeks, then it is stopped permanently.

Herceptin is given by injection weekly or every three weeks. The side effects are most common with the first treatment and include fever and/or chills in about 40 percent of women. They are easily managed with Tylenol. Other possible but less likely side effects include nausea, vomiting, diarrhea, headaches, difficult breathing, and rashes. These side effects tend to be worse with the first cycle. Trastuzumab is usually given with chemotherapy, at least in the initial cycles, and thus all the usual chemotherapy side effects are present.

Another drug that has an effect in Her-2/neu positive cancers is Lapatinib. It is a tyrosine kinase inhibitor and has been shown to be beneficial in women who are resistant to Herceptin. Though it is often used in metastatic disease, it is not yet used as an adjuvant therapy.

Bevacizumab (Avastin)

The other new targeted drug, currently used only in metastatic disease, is bevacizumab (Avastin). This drug blocks the signal (vascular endothelial growth factor) that the cancer sends out to recruit new blood vessels to grow in and feed it. By doing this it is thought to serve as an embargo around the tumor, leading the cells to die. It is generally used with chemotherapy and has not been used in newly diagnosed women. Its most common side effects (found in 1,032 patients) were weakness, pain, hypertension, diarrhea, and lowered white blood count. Other side effects include nosebleeds, high blood pressure, and protein in the urine. Again the complications from this drug are compounded by whatever chemotherapy is done in conjunction. These drugs are the first of a new wave of long-awaited targeted therapy. The next few years will show us how much promise they really have.

Chapter 18

LIFESTYLE CHANGES AND COMPLEMENTARY TREATMENTS

PATIENTS OFTEN ASKED ME WHAT A WOMAN CAN DO TO ASSIST HER treatment and decrease the chance of recurrence. Frequently, they were thinking about such complementary treatments as acupuncture or meditation. These have their place in healing, but there are other equally important, often better studied complementary tools—lifestyle changes.

Most of the treatments discussed in the previous chapters are aimed at killing breast cancer cells. But as I explained in Chapter 4, we also have other tools to treat this disease. We can change the environment of the body or the neighborhood the cells live in. We are starting to understand what some of the more toxic environments look like, and how they can be changed. This knowledge is beginning to give scientific underpinnings to some of the lifestyle changes and complementary treatments that may have been dismissed in the past. Most lifestyle changes and complementary treatments have few or no side effects, and they often improve the quality of your life and prevent other diseases. I encourage all who have had breast cancer to consider these techniques and try to find ways to incorporate them into their new lives. Usually the lifestyle changes and complementary treatments can be combined with your medical treatments and then continued long after. Complementary medicine is often confused with so-called alternative medicine, but the two are very different. The Office of Cancer Complementary and Alternative Medicine (OCCAM) defines complementary medicine as any medical system, practice, or product not thought of as standard care but *used along with* standard medicine; alternative medicine is a system, practice, or product that is *used in place of* standard treatments.

I think it's very important to be looking at lifestyle changes and complementary (not alternative) treatments if you have breast cancer. For all its limitations, Western medicine is still an important component of any successful effort to cure cancer or put it into significant remission. At the same time, lifestyle changes are gaining more support as we find evidence of their ability to further improve outcomes.

LIFESTYLE CHANGES

There are many theories as to how lifestyle changes may affect breast cancer recurrence. In the past most research focused on hormone levels. Fat has aromatase and can make estrogen, so it was thought to feed many tumors.[1] Thus weight loss can help by decreasing that excess estrogen. While this may well be true, the fact that obesity and physical inactivity also seem to be harmful in nonhormonal cancers like colon cancer suggests that an additional mechanism may be playing a role.

In an effort to find another explanation, Pamela Goodwin from Toronto has been exploring the relationship between insulin resistance and breast cancer. "Insulin resistance syndrome" is the term we use to talk about the condition in which the body makes high levels of insulin in an attempt to overcome the fact that the muscle and fat seem to be less sensitive to it than normal. This syndrome is associated with obesity, hypertension, and type 2 diabetes. In our overweight society it is thought to be present in 20–30 percent of the general population and 60 percent of obese individuals. Goodwin's study is interesting for those of us concerned with breast cancer because it shows that nondiabetic women with high insulin levels (reflecting insulin resistance syndrome) have twice the risk of recurrence and three times the risk of death as women with low levels.[2,3] This may be one factor in the connection between obesity and breast cancer. Goodwin is currently exploring whether this can be modified with an insulin-lowering drug such as Metformin. Of course it can also be modified through weight loss.

The third related area that is attracting attention is chronic inflammation, which is increasingly being seen as a component in the development of many cancers. Note I said inflammation, not infection. Infection is caused by an outside pathogen, while inflammation is a reaction in the body itself against harmful stimuli. This is a reflection of the immune system constantly being in a hyperalert state. It could be considered another factor in the neighborhood, urging the mutated cancer cell on (see Chapter 4). Chronic inflammation has been shown to promote breast cancer cells in a petri dish in the lab. And recently blood markers of inflammation at the time of diagnosis have been found to be associated with reduced survival in breast cancer patients.[4] We are studying whether we can detect evidence of chronic inflammation in ductal fluid before women get cancer.

Okay, I realize that you may not be as interested as I am in the why and want to cut to the chase. What does this mean for you, the individual with breast cancer? What can you do with this information? To start with, there are a lot of observational data suggesting that obesity, low physical activity, and a Western diet may worsen breast cancer prognosis.[5,6,7]

Weight

Weight is a sore topic for most women, and as someone who has struggled all my life to maintain my weight, I am very sensitive to it. However, I have to tell you that the data increasingly indicate that being overweight increases the incidence of postmenopausal cancer, and that women who are obese when diagnosed with breast cancer have a worse prognosis than women of normal weight with comparable cancers and treatments. This difference in prognosis appears to be most important in pre- and perimenopausal women.[8] A recent randomized controlled trial of women with positive nodes receiving chemotherapy showed that obese women had a 5 percent lower overall survival than others. This was true for both pre-menopausal and postmenopausal women.[9] Amazing as it may seem, this difference is similar to the difference we see in many chemotherapy trials, but weight loss has much more tolerable side effects than chemo. Whether this is related to hormone levels (fat can make estrogen after menopause), insulin resistance, or low-grade chronic inflammation is not clear.

Gee, thanks, you say bitterly. But here you are with breast cancer *now*, and unless they've come up with a method of time travel, you can't go back and lose weight before you were diagnosed.

So the question arises, Can weight loss—or gain—*now* make a difference? One study showed that in early stage breast cancer, women who gained about 17 pounds had a higher risk of breast cancer recurrence, breast cancer death, and all causes of early mortality than did women who did not gain weight.[10] A few small studies have shown that increased physical activity and mild calorie restriction can help prevent weight gain during and after breast cancer treatment.[11,12]

"Great," you mutter, unpacified. Like many women, you've already gained weight from your medical treatments. Well, that doesn't have to continue. An ongoing study (prettily named LISA) is investigating an intervention designed to reduce weight through increased physical activity and dietary modification. Once the results are out they will help determine whether losing weight will help prevent recurrence and improve survival. Meanwhile, the very possibility might make giving it a try worthwhile.

Physical Activity

Physical activity has been shown to decrease the risk of developing breast cancer. Now we have several studies which consistently show that a modest increase in physical activity is associated with substantial improvement in survival for patients with early-stage breast cancer. One study lends even more support to this approach, showing that walking three to five hours a week at an average pace, or equivalents of that, reduced the subjects' recurrence risk by 6 percent. In another study[13] an additional five metabolic equivalents (METs) per hour/week resulted in a 15 percent decrease in breast cancer mortality. (Five METs is what you'd get walking at 4 miles per hour for an hour, or ballroom dancing for an hour, among other things). (See Appendix E for a list of activities and their equivalent METs.) Most intervention trials of physical activity have been relatively short, with end points of quality of life, improved fitness, and increased weight loss rather than improved survival. But they have shown that physical activity is certainly feasible during and after breast cancer treatment and is associated with an improved quality of life, including decreased fatigue.[14,15,16]

This area of research is beginning to go beyond just talking about the fact that exercise appears to be good for you and is trying to figure out why. Interesting data are emerging that exercise has an effect on reducing inflammation and insulin resistance, even when it does not cause weight loss. This is another area that is likely to yield new information over the next few years.[17]

There are many ways you can increase your physical activity—and have fun. Make sure you obtain your doctor's approval first, since some chemotherapy drugs, such as doxorubicin, can affect your ability to exercise strenuously. You can start a walking group with friends, or dance, or swim, or roller blade. If there's a sport you've thought of starting, this is a good time to do it. The key is to find something you will do and enjoy (or at the very least can tolerate) to achieve the goal of attaining a longer, healthier life.

You can even combine exercise and activism by participating in walks and other activities to call attention to the need for breast cancer awareness. You can join a dragon boat team and train to participate with other survivors rowing a dragon boat. These are very popular in Canada, and they're catching on in the United States. In Boston there is a yearly swim against breast cancer. Further, increased physical activity has been shown to decrease the symptoms of menopause and improve brain function.[18]

Diet

The effects of diet have been more difficult to prove, but there is some evidence that it can help. Two recently reported randomized clinical trials have explored the effects of dietary change after breast cancer diagnosis. The Women's Intervention Nutrition Study

(WINS)[19] and Women's Healthy Eating and Living (WHEL)[20] study looked at different populations and investigated different dietary patterns, both including the potential role of fat reduction. The WINS results suggest that a lifestyle intervention reducing dietary fat intake and associated with modest weight loss may possibly improve the outcome for breast cancer patients receiving conventional cancer management. The WHEL study, on the other hand, showed that a low-fat diet high in fruits and vegetables but without associated weight loss had no effect on cancer recurrences after 7.3 years.

There are many diets recommended for cancer in general, and some for breast cancer in particular, most of which will come as no surprise, since they have been proven in many areas of health: a diet low in fat, high in fruits and vegetables, low in processed foods, sugar, alcohol, and hormone-treated beef and chicken.

At this point we have the most data on the Mediterranean diet, which encourages an abundance of food from plants, moderate amounts of cheese and yogurt, weekly consumption of small to moderate amounts of fish and poultry, limited sweets and red meat, and low to moderate consumption of wine. This diet will not only help you lose or maintain your weight but has been shown to decrease mortality from many causes, of which breast cancer is only one. There is suggestive observational data that it will also reduce the risk of breast cancer, although no randomized studies directly addressing this have been done.

Whether or not you embrace the Mediterranean regime, look for a serious diet rather than any of the current trendy diet fads out there. A diet high in any fat or sugar—the usual baddies—is never "best for you," no matter how good it tastes. You don't need to give up all the goodies you enjoy, but you do need to limit their place in whatever food plan you embrace.[21,22]

If you decide to include a nutrition approach to your healing, you should work very closely with your nutritionist and your physician to create your particular diet and coordinate it with your other treatments. Certain foods may be better to avoid, or to consume, during specific aspects of your medical treatments.

Overall I think that this is the simplest decision regarding breast cancer treatment. Here are things *you* can do to make a difference that are worthwhile and that lie in your power. Not surprisingly, these recommendations are also suggested to improve the quality of your life and decrease chronic diseases of aging.

Lately I have been speaking out in public forums about the need to increase physical activity. A 2009 Women of Color luncheon in Los Angeles gave me a great boost when an elderly woman who had already been established as a forty-year survivor stood up and testified that after her diagnosis she had gotten off the couch and started walking—and had not stopped yet!

COMPLEMENTARY THERAPIES

Placebo Effect

Many techniques seem to work because of the placebo effect: your mind tells your body that it's getting a certain healing substance, and your body responds as though it were true. As Norman Cousins pointed out years ago in *Anatomy of an Illness,* the effect has worked throughout history—doctors once had some success with such "treatments" as bloodletting and administering powdered unicorn horns. He calls the placebo "the doctor who resides within," who "translates the will to live into a physical reality."[23]

The application of this concept to cancer treatments was recently examined when Gisele Chvetzoff and Ian Tannock reviewed all the studies in oncology that included a placebo arm.[24] They found that placebos sometimes help control symptoms such as pain and appetite but rarely effect positive tumor response.

While most of the following therapies have not been studied or have shown no effect on the survival of women with breast cancer, many have been shown to improve the quality of life. For example, in 1989 David Spiegel from Stanford ran a support group for 86 women with newly diagnosed metastatic breast cancer. For a year, the groups met weekly for 90-minute sessions, focusing on enhancing social support and encouraging the expression of disease-related emotion.[25] Much to everyone's surprise, the study showed an improvement in survival. However, it was a small study, which means that the result could well have been due to chance. Since then a large multicenter randomized study was done that demonstrated no survival benefit, although the distress of many women lessened.[26] This study found that placebos sometimes help with control of symptoms such as pain and appetite that result from medical treatments, but rarely affect tumors. While this was disappointing to those who believe in the mind-body approach, it certainly does not discredit its ability to improve the quality of your life if not lengthen it.

Prayer

For centuries, people of all religions have believed in the power of prayer—and for some of them it seems to have worked. Estelle Disch, a Boston-area therapist who has worked with many cancer patients, says, "If you're praying for health, on some level you're seeing yourself as healthy, and I believe that makes a difference." Faith in a power that can make you well—whether that's God, or your surgeon, or your own will—can help you to get well. I often pray for my patients, hoping to harness whatever forces I can to help them achieve the result that is best for them. As with Spiegel's group, the initial small studies[27,28] suggested a benefit for patients with various conditions, while a larger study of patients undergoing coronary artery bypass surgery in six hospitals found that intercessory prayer had no effect on complication-free recovery.[29] Does this mean those of you who believe in prayer should abandon it? Absolutely not. In a time of crisis such as breast cancer we all reach for familiar approaches that might help. If praying or having someone pray for you gives you comfort and support, you should not let research findings stop you. If you don't find this approach helpful, the research suggests you don't need to start.

Meditation and Visualization

Meditation and visualization have helped survivors deal with stress, pain, and anxiety. But again, they have not been shown to make a difference in survival. Meditation has been an important part of almost every major religion in history. While there are many forms, the ones most commonly used in conjunction with healing work are variants of that very simple one in which the person sits in a comfortable position, eyes closed, focusing on the inhaling and exhaling of breath, and chanting a mantra, a particular word or phrase. The Eastern *om* is fine, but you can also use different language—"peace," for example, or a brief phrase from a prayer.

Herbert Benson, a physician who has extensively studied forms of nonmedical healing, describes this particular form of meditation as the relaxation response, and it is the basis of his work as director of the Mind/Body Medical Institute in Boston. He and his colleagues run a number of groups for people with various diseases. The technique creates physiological responses that contribute to stress reduction.

Most programs that use meditation combine it with visualization or imagery. This too is an ancient technique, based on the belief that if you create strong mental pictures of what you want, while affirming to yourself that you can and will get it, you can make virtually anything happen.

The pioneers of visualization in disease treatment were Carl and Stephanie Simonton, an oncologist and a psychologist. Their book *Getting Well Again* recounts their experiences with "exceptional cancer patients"—those who recover in spite of a negative prognosis—and maintains that their visualization techniques have significantly extended patients' lives.[30] However, no controlled studies have proven this. Studies *have* proven that visualization and meditation combined can reduce pain and the uncomfortable side effects of cancer treatments, which certainly makes them worth trying.[31]

Visualization typically begins with a meditation-relaxation exercise; then you begin to envision your cancer in terms of some concrete image—like gray blobs inside your breast (or whatever area you're dealing with). Next you picture your white blood cells, or your radiation or chemotherapy treatments, as forces countering the cells. You can do visualization with a group or on your own. I've had patients who've used the techniques in both contexts. The Simontons favored violent images—soldiers attacking the cells, or sharks destroying them, but some prefer different images. A friend with metastatic breast cancer felt much better singing her cells a lullaby to put them to sleep.

Affirmations are similar to visualization and often used in conjunction with it. They are statements affirming one's value and intentions, recited aloud if possible, mentally if not. One of my patients had a list of her favorites, which included, "I am now renewing my body's ability to heal itself" and "I now let the light from above heal me with love." Others prefer to frame their affirmations in terms of choice: "I choose health." They should always be used positively rather than negatively—not "I will not stay sick" but "I am growing healthier each day." Affirmations can be repeated regularly and frequently. You can say them while taking your shower, walking to your car, or unloading your groceries. Susan Troyan, one of my surgical colleagues in Boston, has patients bring in positive sayings, which are read during their surgery. She says that whether or not the practice helps healing, it gives women a much needed sense of control.

Laughter

Even simple laughter can be a healing tool. When Norman Cousins set about to cure himself of his neurological illness, he "discovered that ten minutes of genuine belly laughter had an anesthetic effect and would give me at least two hours of pain-free sleep."[32] There appears to be some medical basis for this: laughter can stimulate endorphins—chemicals that act like narcotics in the brain.

One of my patients with inflammatory breast cancer said, "I told people I wanted to laugh. Friends send me funny books, cut out cartoons, call me and say funny things." Though she eventually died from her cancer, her multilevel approach to fighting it gave her the strength she needed to live her life fully to the end—including helping launch the breast cancer political movement.

Giving yourself time not to think about your cancer, just escaping into zany humor, can be emotionally healing. Be sure to pick the things that make you laugh heartily, whether it's a P. G. Wodehouse novel or the Marx Brothers or reruns of *Friends*.

Psychic Healing

Psychic healing is another ancient technique and exists in many forms. Much of charismatic Christian healing involves laying on of hands, a classical psychic healing technique. The relatively recent "therapeutic touch," designed by nurses in the United States, is similar. Sometimes it isn't even done in person—healers and ordinary people "send healing energy."

Regardless of what healing thoughts can do in terms of the disease itself, they can achieve a twofold benefit. For the patient, it is a reminder of all the love and support that's out there for her. And for those who love her, it can alleviate some of the terrible sense of helplessness they feel in the face of a loved one's suffering. Your friends can't operate on you or administer chemotherapy, but they can pray or send healing thoughts.

Some people attribute healing power to crystals and other stones. Many believe these can affect different parts of your physical and emotional health, and that using them to meditate, wearing them as jewelry, or simply keeping them around can help you remain healthy or restore health if you're ill.[33] As far as I know, no scientific studies have been done on healing stones, which is not to say they can't work. Some of my patients have great faith in them, and I like to keep a small collection of amethysts in my office. Like the Catholic rosary or the Jewish hamsa, they can provide a concrete symbol of your belief in your ability to heal. Amethyst is seen as an all-purpose healer, while sugalite and tiger's eye are considered particularly effective with cancer, and moonstone with women's cancers, but any stone you feel drawn to is useful.

Some patients find their stones so soothing they bring them to their treatments. One of my patients had her favorite crystal taped to her hand during surgery. Another carried her sugalite to her chemotherapy treatments, holding it to the parts of her body that the chemicals most negatively affected. Some semiprecious stones are expensive, but you can always find cheaper, less "perfect" stones, and since you're using them for healing, not as a financial investment, they'll probably do just as well.

Vitamins, Herbs

The MD Anderson cancer center did a survey of its multidisciplinary breast clinic as well as its gynecological malignancy clinic and found that 48 percent of the patients were using CAM (complementary-alternative medicine), most frequently herbal products and multivitamins. The increase in the use of these products, which are essentially unregulated by the FDA, has led to concern about safety and interactions with chemotherapy. A 2004 review from the National Cancer Institute listed specific herbal remedies that should be *avoided* during chemotherapy.[34] Most relevant to breast cancer patients were garlic, gingko, echinacea, soy, ginseng, St. John's wort, valerian, kava kava, and grape seed. You can still eat garlic, soy beans, and grapes, but avoid them in supplements while you're on chemotherapy.

Some supplements have been reported to reduce the side effects of chemotherapy. For example, a review from the United Kingdom suggested that CoQ10 provides some protection against heart or liver toxicity for patients taking anthracyclines. However, the results were inconclusive.[35] A preclinical study showed that CoQ10 did not affect the metabolism of doxorubicin.

The best way to stay up to date on this subject is to monitor the website of the National Center for Complementary and Alternative Medicine at the NIH (http://nccam.nih.gov). In addition, many of the large cancer centers such as MD Anderson, Dana Farber, or Sloan Kettering have alternative and complementary clinics that can help you either in person or online. I do think it's important to investigate any substance you take into your body. With prayer, meditation, stone work, and the like, you know that the worst that can happen is that they won't do any good. They can't harm you. Herbs and other substances can.

Acupuncture and Chinese Medicine

Some branches of complementary healing involve treatments, such as the ancient Chinese science of acupuncture, which sees healing in terms of "meridians," energy channels that run through the body. Special needles are inserted into the meridians. Acupuncturists have worked with breast cancer patients, usually in conjunction with Western medical treatments.

Marie Cargill, a Boston-area practitioner of traditional Chinese medicine (TCM), has used acupuncture with breast cancer patients. "What they've been using in China is a combination of Western treatments—surgery, radiation, chemotherapy—and traditional Chinese medicine," she says. Acupuncture, she adds, can strengthen the body when other treatments cause weakening.

Cargill and many other practitioners of TCM like to combine acupuncture with Chinese healing herbs. Both, she says, can help relieve the side effects of radiation and chemotherapy. "Cracking toxin herbs" are used to fight the cancer and supplement the work of the other treatments, while other herbs help build the immune system. There are particular herbs for breast cancer, which are different from herbs used for other cancers. In addition, some herbs are said to work on the depression and anxiety that often accompany life-threatening illness. If it's hard to find Chinese herbs and herbal practitioners, Cargill says that acupuncture alone can work well, if it's used frequently enough.

There have been several good studies on the benefits of Chinese medicinal herbs for the treatment of side effects from chemotherapy in breast cancer patients. The Cochrane Collaboration (a voluntary group that reviews the evidence behind many common treatments and procedures; www.cochrane.org/reviews) found seven randomized studies involving 542 breast cancer patients addressing this question. These studies used six different herbal remedies to treat the side effects of chemotherapy. The studies compared the Chinese medicinal herbs in conjunction with chemotherapy versus chemotherapy alone. The results suggest that using Chinese herbs may improve blood counts, immune system functioning, and the overall quality of life.[36]

Homeopathy

Another area of holistic healing is homeopathy, a method of self-healing stimulated by administering very small doses of drugs that produce symptoms like those of the disease being treated. The drugs are chosen by the patient with the assistance of a homeopathic practitioner, who may or may not also be a medical doctor. The substances are all available over the counter. You can take them on your own, but it's wiser to work with an expert practitioner.

Ted Chapman, a homeopathic M.D. in Boston who has worked with breast cancer patients, emphasizes that homeopathy doesn't cure cancer. "Doctors work on the end product of the disease, and they come in from the outside. We're working from the inside, on what makes you vulnerable to your disease in the first place." Like many other adjunctive therapies, homeopathy is thought to work on the immune system.

Eight controlled trials (seven placebo controlled and one trial comparing homeopathy and an active treatment) with a total of 664 participants were reviewed by the Cochrane Collaboration. Three studies concerned the side effects of chemotherapy, three studied the side effects of radiation therapy, and two focused on menopausal symptoms associated with breast cancer treatment. Of these, two well designed studies have shown that homeopathy can work better than standard therapy for the side effects of radiation or chemotherapy. One involved 254 participants and demonstrated benefits from calendula ointment in the prevention of radiotherapy-induced dermatitis (red, sore skin),[37] while the other, with 32 participants, demonstrated benefits from Traumeel S (a complex homeopathic medicine) over placebo as a mouthwash for chemotherapy-induced mouth soreness (stomatitis).[38] Other studies showed no benefit from the homeopathic remedy. One used Hyland's Menopause or a placebo and showed no difference in the hot flash score between the two.[39] Another hot flash study from Scotland showed no difference between individualized homeopathic remedies and placebo, although both groups saw some relief of symptoms.[40]

Mistletoe (Iscador)

Preparations from European mistletoe are among the most prescribed drugs in cancer patients in several European countries.[41] Proponents claim that mistletoe extracts stimulate the immune system, improve survival, enhance quality of life, and reduce adverse effects of chemo and radiotherapy in cancer patients. The Cochrane Collaboration review did not find enough evidence to reach clear conclusions about the effects on any of these outcomes.

Nevertheless, there is some evidence from two well done studies that mistletoe extracts may offer benefits to quality of life during chemotherapy for breast cancer.

Bioelectromagnetics

Magnets are popular with many people for the treatment of a number of diseases. The theory is that magnetic fields penetrate the body and heal damaged tissues, including cancers. There are no good scientific studies supporting this claim. Many of the magnets are sold in the form of attractive, inexpensive jewelry, so you may enjoy them on two levels, and they don't seem to cause any problems.

ALTERNATIVE TREATMENTS

Some therapies have been proposed to take the place of medical treatments, and several have gained notoriety in popular books. Most of them have not been studied in any scientifically rigorous way and their risks and complications are largely unknown. I mention them to be complete, but I don't endorse their use.

The best known alternative treatment is laetrile. It hasn't been shown to work in any randomized, controlled studies,[42] but it has a fair amount of nonscientific support. It's illegal in the United States and is currently being used by clinics in Mexico. It contains cyanide, and there have been reports of deaths from cyanide poisoning in patients taking laetrile.[43]

Shark cartilage was very popular for a time as a cancer treatment, based on its antiangiogenic properties, but a study showed no benefit.[44]

CanCell is a remedy developed by James Sheridan in 1936, composed of common chemicals and apparently nontoxic. It has not been tested in a clinical trial.[45] Essiac, another popular herbal cancer alternative, is made up of burdock, turkey rhubarb, sorrel, and slippery elm. A retrospective study done in Canada showed no improvement in quality of life or mood in women with breast cancer who took this herbal remedy. Data[46] supporting its anti-cancer effects are lacking, but it is available in health food stores in the United States and Canada. A study in 2004 used Flor-Essence (a variant of Essiac) in a rat model and showed it *promoted* mammary tumor development.[47]

Ongoing studies involve Stanislaw Burzynski's antineoplaston therapy, which is available at his clinic in Houston, Texas. Although there have been anecdotal reports on its efficacy, there is no scientific proof. Chemically antineoplastons consist of phenyl acetate, a metabolite of phenylalanine that is being studied for potential anticancer activity by researchers at the National Cancer Institute and elsewhere. He has been working with the NCI on trials of his drugs for brain tumors that are not treatable by conventional means, and he has had some good results.[48,49,50] It is not clear whether the same results are available for breast cancer cases.

RESEARCH

In researching this chapter, I have been impressed by the many good studies done on complementary and even alternative therapies. With the National Institute of Health's National Center for Complementary and Alternative Medicine up and running, there is financial support as well as interest in exploring these avenues of treatment. Many time-tested herbal and diet-based therapies are being studied for ability to induce or extend remission. For now, however, the absence of government regulation of supplements means that scores of unproved remedies or inadequate dosages of proved ones are on the shelves of pharmacies and grocery stores.

Many people go online for information relating to alternative and complementary healing, as well as to traditional medicine. This can be a good tool, but you need to know how to use it. Check a few things. Is the organization that is giving the information well known? Can you tell who's sponsoring the site, and what their qualifications are? Is it for profit or not for profit? Is the information dated and referenced? Are there data for safety and efficacy, or just anecdotes? Remember that anyone can have a website. The government website http://nccam.nih.gov is a good place to start. On www.dslrf.org we offer links to many of the reliable sites, and will be doing clinical studies of many of these herbs. You can also check your local American Cancer Society division office or quackwatch.com. They keep statements on these treatments that describe exactly what is involved, as well as discussing known risks, side effects, opinion of the medical establishment, and any lawsuits that have been filed. Make sure you are really informed.

Though I am leery of using treatments that lack a medical component, this is a highly personal decision. What risks any of us will take for what reasons depends on who we are and what our values are.

When a particular cancer or stage of cancer has a bad prognosis, refusing traditional treatment isn't really much of a risk. When chemotherapy isn't likely to extend your life for any length of time, the discomfort may not be worth the slight chance of cure, and an alternative treatment may offer both better survival hope and more comfort during the remainder of your life. When Audre Lorde[51] learned her cancer had metastasized to her liver, she decided to forgo chemotherapy. She went to homeopathic doctors in Europe for injections of the mistletoe derivative iscador and did visualization and meditation, determinedly living her life to the fullest. She survived for several years—an impressive achievement with liver metastasis. Maybe it was because she chose a treatment that she believed in and allowed her to remain as active as possible, doing the work to which she was so passionately committed.

One of my patients, a forty-six-year-old woman whose cancer metastasized to her bone marrow, also did remarkably well for a time. A devout Catholic, she cherished the advice of a nun who told her to "work as though everything depended on you, and pray as though everything depended on God." She had surgery and tamoxifen therapy, went on a macrobiotic diet, took a mind-body course at Beth Israel, and continued a regular meditation and visualization program. Whenever a church had a healing service, she went to it. She carried a rosary made of healing stones. She went to Lourdes. Though she ultimately died from her cancer, her health improved for a while. In spite of the cancer in her bones, she went mountain climbing and cross-country skiing—and dancing.

Chapter 19

AFTER TREATMENT

YOU'VE HAD BREAST CANCER AND YOU'VE FINISHED THE TREATMENT; now it's time to get on with your life. But your life has changed, and you have to adjust to your new situation on a number of levels. One of my patients told me that "it's like your life breaks into a million pieces and when you put the pieces back together they don't quite fit exactly the same."

When you go back to your normal activities, you look fine and you expect to feel fine. Everybody's relieved that things are back to normal again—everybody but you. Physical problems that wouldn't have bothered you before now seem ominous. The slight headache that two years ago you would have dismissed as tension—has the cancer metastasized to your brain? And does the bruise on your arm mean you have leukemia? You're now in the "I can't trust my body" stage. Well, why should you trust your body? It betrayed you once, and you know it can do it again. Every time you go for a checkup, every time you get a blood test, you're terrified. In my experience with patients, this stage usually lasts two or three years, until you've had enough innocent headaches and bruises, enough reassuring checkups and blood tests, to feel somewhat trusting of your body again.

But you probably don't feel fine—not the way you used to, anyway. For most women the end of treatment is accompanied by lingering side effects. However, they are usually thrilled to be done with treatment, and so they are all the more surprised by the fears that often rear up at this point. Your support network is there for you, but they too are getting on with life now that your treatment is over, and they aren't as intensely there as they were when your needs were primary parts of their lives. New worries arise: will the cancer come back now that I am no longer being treated? (In this regard, taking tamoxifen or an aromatase inhibitor may be reassuring—you're still in a treatment process for a while.) Who do I call if something comes up? What symptoms should I look for? Who is going to follow my health now? Eventually you begin to get used to this new set of feelings, and your life begins to seem a little like it used to be.

And then, just when you are settling down and starting to forget about it, something pops up in the paper or on the news about a risk factor or new treatment, and it all comes back. You start wondering if it was the alcohol you drank or the birth control pills you took (or whatever happens to be on today's "hit list") that caused your cancer. Or you regret a treatment decision you made, thinking, "If I'd known this back then, I might have done things differently."

But you need to remind yourself that what's past is past. You can't change the way you lived your life in the past based on new information just coming to light today. Accept that you probably got the best treatment that was available at the time you were diagnosed, and that your decision was the right one at the time. If there are improved treatments now, that's wonderful—but you can't waste your energy on what might have been. Read the newspapers and keep informed if you're interested, but don't use it to torture yourself about what might have been. Gradually you will regain your perspective.

Life will never be completely the same as it was before, but most women eventually stop living in terms of their cancer. The fears and memories will come back occasionally—maybe at checkups, maybe on the anniversary of diagnosis, maybe when a friend has a recurrence. But they'll be part of life, not the center of it.

As I was writing this update in 2009, I posted a query on my Facebook page asking for comments about what to expect when you are living with a diagnosis of breast cancer. I expected that women would respond about specific symptoms, but most spoke to the emotional pressures and gave some excellent advice: "Expect the unexpected!" wrote one reader. "Every survivor I have met has such different experiences [that] it's so hard to prepare anybody for what to expect. For me the range of emotions I had surprised me. . . . expect to discover new things about yourself physically and emotionally throughout the journey. Expect to be tired!!! I'm four years out and still tired."

Another wrote wryly, "I'd say expect to do battle at least internally with those dear folks who say things they think are helpful but are actually blaming the survivor for his or her breast cancer. Case in point—'just be positive' or 'just have faith' sound supportive to one who hasn't faced the beast, but to the survivor this says 'If I'm not positive enough, or if I don't have enough faith, I'll fail myself and my loved ones'. Then there's, 'What did you do to yourself?' Implying it's your fault."

THE FOLLOW-UP

A diagnosis of breast cancer means, for one thing, being medically followed for the rest of your life. Therefore the first thing you should do when you complete therapy is to ask your oncologist for a summary of your cancer and treatment to keep for your records. ASCO (American Society of Clinical Oncology) has templates you can use if you want. As fresh as everything is in your mind now, it will soon fade as you become used to life after breast cancer. The care summary plus copies of your pathology report, a summary of your radiation therapy treatment if relevant, and a copy of your operative note should then go into a file and be put in the safe or wherever you keep your important papers. Survivors need to have knowledge about what they were treated with, so they can remind their family doctor or tell any new doctor about it, and have medical records to show them. Further, they can make a big difference to your own peace of mind. If you read that new long-term complications of treatment have been discovered or new research can predict certain outcomes (Did I get that drug? Was my tumor sensitive to estrogen?), you can quickly access the answer and either call your doctor if the answer suggests possible problems or go back to not worrying.

While you are asking your oncologist for your care summary, ask also for a guide to your follow-up (ASCO has templates for this) so you know exactly what is planned in terms of scans and tests over the next years. There is a great website—www.journey forward.org—that helps survivors ask their physicians for a survivorship care plan and has electronic templates (following ASCO content) that can allow the provider to complete the treatment summary and survivorship care plan easily.

Sometimes women think their cancer doctors are following their cholesterol and high blood pressure. This is usually not the case. In our segmented health care system, the oncologists usually focus only on cancer. So don't neglect the rest of your health. Keep getting regular checkups from your primary care physician, so any other health problems that emerge independent of your cancer can be dealt with.

At a minimum, follow-up involves regular monitoring for a recurrence. It also involves addressing chronic treatment-related results of your therapy (e.g., fatigue, sexual dysfunction, "chemo brain," pain syndromes) and monitoring for potential late effects of treatment such as heart disease, lymphedema, and non–breast cancer malignancies. While this may sound depressing, it shouldn't. It means that we now have enough experience with long-term survivors to know what to look for and what to do about it. Surgeons, for example, are looking for lumps in the breast, mastectomy scar, or other breast. They check your neck and the area above the collarbone for lumps that may indicate an affected lymph node, and feel under both arms. In addition, they question you carefully about how you're feeling. They ask if you've had persistent and unusual pain in your legs or back, a persistent dry cough, or any of the other symptoms described at length in Chapter 20.

UCLA and other centers have follow-up programs in which patients are seen every three to six months for the first two to three years and every year after that. The program includes not just exams and mammograms but also physical therapy, nutritional counseling, psychosocial support, and involvement in research. Usually the surgeon and/or other specialists who did your primary treatment will follow your health at regular intervals for a period of time.

And you yourself should be vigilant. If you have a new symptom that doesn't go away in a week or two, tell your doctor about it. Usually that's what most patients do anyway. One study found that a third of recurrences were manifested by the symptoms, a third were detected by physical exam, and a sixth were found by mammogram (for those of you mathematically inclined, the other one-sixth covers everything else).[1]

Patients are often surprised when their doctor doesn't find anything on their follow-up exam; they've been waiting for the cancer to pop up again and tend to be anxious about examinations. Some women start getting nervous days before these visits, and the visits themselves often trigger fears of recurrence. This is normal. However, if worry creeps in weeks before, further evaluation of how you are coping may be useful. You may want to consider seeing a counselor or getting some antianxiety medications. And certainly you should consider sharing your feelings with others in the same boat in a support group, an online chat, or even just casually with a friend who has been through it.

Studies of a large group of breast cancer survivors by my oncologist colleague Patricia Ganz found that the age of the patient when she's followed up and the fact of having received adjuvant chemotherapy (versus other treatments) increased worry about a recurrence.[2] Younger women perceive themselves as having more to lose, and most women consider the use of chemotherapy as a marker of more aggressive disease. Interestingly, the type of surgery did not seem to affect worry. Women who underwent a mastectomy worried no more or less than those who had lumpectomy and radiation. Although this seems counterintuitive, since many women say they have a mastectomy so that they won't worry, it probably occurs because women today have more choice as to which surgery they will get.

Unfortunately the posttreatment worry seldom disappears. While some women worry less as they put their treatment behind them, others experience constant concern. As one woman said, "Worry just comes with the territory." Unless it is disrupting your daily life and plans, this recurrence anxiety need not be treated with psychotherapy or antianxiety medication.

Not all symptoms that you will find over time mean your cancer has spread. Women who have had cancer are as likely as anyone else to get other diseases as they age. Having had cancer does not make anyone immune to arthritis or diabetes, for example. Furthermore, aside from ordinary, nonrelated problems, patients may experience conditions that result from the cancer treatment, such as heart disease, leukemia, and osteoporosis. There are also some physical changes that your body experiences as a direct result of your therapy. It's important to have frequent checkups because a breast that's been radiated undergoes a lot of changes. There will be a lumpy area under the scar and perhaps some skin firmness and/or puckering. By keeping track on a regular basis, the doctor can assure you that the changes you're experiencing are related to the treatment, not the disease itself—and if there's a different, more ominous change, the doctor can distinguish it from the others.

For the same reasons, your surgeon will probably want you to have mammograms every six months for a year or two, and then once a year. In addition to monitoring the treated breast, the doctor will examine your other breast yearly for the possible development of a new cancer, since women with cancer in one breast have an increased risk of getting it in the other. This is particularly important if you are a carrier of the BRCA 1 or 2 gene (see Chapter 6), and you may want to have an MRI as well (see Chapter 8). In non-gene carriers, breast cancer in the other breast is less likely; the risk is about 1 percent per year, or an average of 15 percent over a lifetime.[3] (See Chapter 13 for a discussion of the second primary cancer.) In the latter situation MRI is usually not done. Some types of breast cancer indicate a greater propensity for a second breast cancer to develop. Cancers with a lot of lobular carcinoma in situ (see Chapter 13) have been thought to fit into this category.[4] Even in this situation, however, the increased risk to the second breast is just 2 percent per year, a cumulative lifetime risk of 30 percent. Obviously the younger you are and the longer you live, the greater your chance of developing a second cancer.

In addition to your surgeon, your whole team may follow you; your radiation oncologist and/or your medical oncologist may also want to check on you regularly. Some patients find this overwhelming and don't want to spend all that time trekking back and forth to doctors. More typically, you'll be followed up by one of the members of the team, or even by your local family doctor, if she or he has experience with breast cancer. In a 1996 study, women were randomized to be followed up by either their primary care doctor or a specialist. Interestingly, specialist care did not lead to earlier diagnosis of a recurrence, improved quality of life, or even lower anxiety levels.[5] Your HMO or insurance company may limit which kind of follow-up it will pay for. But basically the choice is yours: don't worry about hurting your doctor's feelings. It's your feelings that matter now. Pick the doctor with whom you have the greatest rapport or in whom you have the greatest confidence. You can even find a new doctor after treatment if you have not been happy with your medical oncologist. You were probably in a hurry to get treatment under way when first diagnosed, but now you are picking someone for a long-term relationship and may want to shop around.

Many doctors still do blood tests every three to six months, including not only your blood count (CBC) but also specific tests (for example, a CEA, CA 15–3, or CA 27.29), as well as liver blood tests with the goal of catching metastatic disease at the earliest point. Both patients and physicians assume that early diagnosis of metastases improves outcomes. Unfortunately we have lots of data indicating that it doesn't work this way, at least as of at the time of this writing. For one thing, these tests don't always succeed. Most are not very sensitive or specific. They go up when there is metastatic disease but they also go up for other conditions. And even when they find metastases, there's no evidence that such early detection gives you an advantage.[6] As you will learn in Chapter 20, we still have no guaranteed way of curing metastatic disease, though we can relieve symptoms and perhaps add a few years to your life.[7,8] In terms of quality of life, knowing sooner that you have a metastasis probably doesn't do you much good. Of course this could change if a treatment emerges that actually works better when started sooner rather than later. Such a treatment would be a huge boon to patients and their doctors. But until such time, these tests can impair the quality of your life without lengthening it. Even if they turn out negative, you still may have a metastasis that is too small to show up on the tests. This also holds true for the routine use of bone scans, chest X rays, and CT scans. These and other data led to follow-up surveillance guidelines issued by ASCO and NCCN (National Comprehensive Cancer Network) that advised only routine discussion of whatever symptoms you may have plus a physical and yearly mammogram.[9,10] ASCO periodically issues updated guidelines for follow-up. The most recent were published in 2006 and recommended careful history taking, physical examination, and regular mammography as appropriate for detection of breast cancer recurrence.[11] If you are taking tamoxifen, you should also have a yearly pelvic exam. The mammogram, unlike the blood tests we've been discussing, can make a difference in longevity, since it can show a local recurrence in the breast or a cancer in the other breast. So unless you're taking part in a protocol that requires regular testing, you may not want to have the other tests.

With breast cancer, unlike some other cancers, we can't be sure that if it hasn't recurred within five years, it won't. However, as I mentioned in Chapter 11, recent studies show that women who have triple negative breast cancers have their peak rate of recurrence at three years while those with estrogen positive tumors have theirs at four years. This means that if you make it to five years you have only a 2–3 percent per year chance of recurrence thereafter. The estrogen receptor positive cancers are usually slow growing, and there are people with such cancers who have had recurrences 10 or even 20 years after the original diagnosis. These later recurrences are likely related to lifestyle changes, or other things that affect the local environment (neighborhood) around dormant cancer cells, causing them to wake up. In some ways this is similar to a chronic disease. You are never quite sure if or when it will come back. Time can affect the likelihood of recurrence—the longer you go without a recurrence, the less likely you are to have one.

So going 10 years without the cancer coming back should give you reason for optimism, if not certainty.

As part of the Army of Women (see the Epilogue), we are planning to do a study of long-term survivors as well as women whose cancer has spread to see if we can figure out what factors determine recurrences.

Since most women are now, thankfully, living a long time after being treated for breast cancer, they need as much information as possible about the long-term side effects of treatment. In the following section I will attempt to address this need.

LONG-TERM SIDE EFFECTS OF SURGERY AND RADIATION

In Chapter 14, I discussed some of the possible long-term effects of surgery such as scarring, cellulitis, and pain. The most serious possible long-term effect of surgery on the lymph nodes is lymphedema.

Lymphedema

Swelling of the arm and sometimes even the breast—lymphedema—can result from lymph node removal (see Chapter 14). It can be so slight that you notice it only because your rings begin to feel too tight on your fingers, or so severe that your arm becomes huge, even elephantine (Figure 19.1). It can be temporary or permanent. It can set in immediately or years after your operation. What causes it? Basically lymphedema—sometimes called milk arm—is a plumbing problem. Normally the lymph fluid is carried through the lymph vessels, passes through the lymph nodes, and is returned to the bloodstream near the heart. The lymph nodes act like a strainer, removing foreign material and bacteria. So if you have surgery in the area and it scars over, some of the holes are blocked and the drainage is affected. The fluid doesn't drain as well as it needs to, and everything backs up and swells. Protein leaks into the tissue and then it scars, causing the condition to become chronic.

This used to be much more common—we'd see it in about 30 percent of cases—because more extensive surgery was done. The

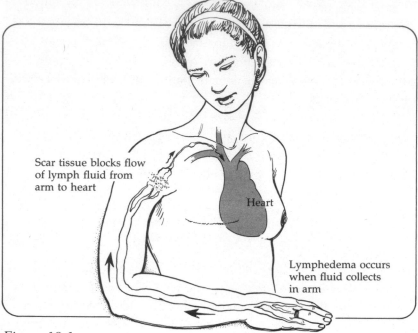

Scar tissue blocks flow
of lymph fluid from
arm to heart

Heart

Lymphedema occurs
when fluid collects
in arm

Figure 19.1

late Dr. Jeanne Petrek reported on 263 women who were alive and symptom free 20 years after their initial treatment for breast cancer. She noted that 13 percent reported severe lymphedema, with 49 percent reporting the sensation of lymphedema. Seventy-seven percent of the women with swelling noted it within three years of their surgery, while the remaining developed swelling at a rate of 1 percent a year.[12]

Though this remains a serious problem for many breast cancer survivors, the current use of sentinel node biopsy promises to decrease women's chances of getting it. Initial studies show that women who underwent sentinel node biopsies had lymphedema 2–6 percent of the time, compared to 17–34 percent for full axillary dissection.[13,14,15]

Most women are cautioned about hand and arm care after surgery so they can prevent lymphedema from happening in the first place. These recommendations are hypothetical and are based on trying to prevent the production of excess lymph and blocked flow. In Dr. Petrek's 20-year study mentioned above, the only factors other than treatment that correlated with lymphedema were weight gain after surgery and arm/hand infection or injury. This is yet another reason to try to avoid weight gain. It's a good idea to watch out for infections in the affected arm and have them treated sooner rather than later. You may also want to consider using a compression bandage when doing vigorous arm exercises. In general, however, common sense should guide you.

One study comparing women who had bilateral mastectomies and axillary dissections to those who had surgery on only one side showed no difference in the incidence of lymphedema.[16] Most of them continued to have blood pressure taken and blood drawn from one of their arms, suggesting that those procedures are not as likely to cause lymphedema as we might have thought.

New studies are being done to determine whether the classical precautions are really necessary. One new study showed that having women lift weights under supervision not only didn't cause increase in lymphedema, but actually resulted in decreased swelling, reduced symptoms, and increased strength.[17] Another study contradicted the common recommendation that all women who have had axillary surgery wear a compression garment in airplanes. In this study 145 of 287 breast cancer survivors without lymphedema were exposed to air travel and there was no difference in the rates of either chronic or temporary lymphedema.[18] This was not a randomized controlled study and contradicts the experience of many women with lymphedema. It remains an understudied area.

Lymphedema proceeds through stages. First is the latency stage; the arm is not swollen but the surgery has caused a reduced capacity for transporting lymph fluid. As long as there are no undue stresses on the system all will be well. Stage 1 is reversible, soft swelling. The skin is normal and you can relieve the swelling by elevating your arm. Stage 2 is no longer spontaneously reversible because there are fibrous changes in the tissues that make your arm feel hard. This stage includes frequent infections, which exacerbate the situation. The final stage is "lymphostatic elephantiasis." This is an extreme increase in volume and changes in the texture of your arm, including deep skin folds. Although there is no cure for lymphedema, we can reduce the swelling and maintain the reduction—in other words, bring lymphedema back to a state of latency.

A treatment devised in Germany, complete decongestive physiotherapy, appears effective in numerous observational studies. It is well-known in Europe and, increasingly, in the United States.[19,20,21] It is usually done by a physical therapist and involves six steps.

1. Skin and nail care, which may include topical and systemic antifungal drugs (making the skin free of infection before treatment)
2. Manual lymph drainage
3. Multilayer short-stretch bandaging
4. Exercise
5. Fitting for compression garments or alternative compression devices
6. Instruction in a home management program

The treatment, which is expensive and time-consuming, is done in two phases. The first attempts to mobilize the accumulated protein-rich fluid and start breaking up the chronic scarring. This phase is intense and can last four weeks; ideally, treatment is given twice a day five days a week. The next phase, which follows immediately, includes compression garments and bandaging at night. A number of recent studies[22,23,24,25] have demonstrated the efficacy of this treatment approach with breast cancer patients. They have shown that the treatment can reduce both the girth of the arm and its volume; one study reported a 41 percent decrease in lymphedema. Most of the studies conclude that effective maintenance therapy following the intensive phase is crucial to preserving the initial reduction.

The best results, not surprisingly, come when the patient is in stage 1. My theory about lymphedema is that we're probably approaching it backward. Patients are advised to go home and elevate the arm if they have a little swelling, to wear an elastic arm stocking for a lot of swelling, and to use an electric pump for an extreme amount of swelling. But by the time they use the pump, their tissues are so stretched out they've lost their normal elasticity. (It's like putting on a pair of panty hose you wore yesterday.)

As soon as they get off the pump, more fluid fills up the loose skin. I think we should act aggressively when we find a small amount of swelling—physical therapy, manual massage, compression—and try to reverse it. We'd probably be able to reverse the process in more people because their skin would still be elastic.

If you think you have swelling, find a lymphedema center or a physical therapist or doctor who has been trained in lymphedema treatment. The National Lymphedema Network (www.lymph-net.org) can help you locate one in your neighborhood.

Physical therapy and exercise can help in early cases. Long support gloves, similar to the stockings used for varicose veins, although unattractive, can reduce the swelling. (Ask for class 2 [30–40 mm Hg] or class 3 [40–50 mg Hg] support.) Although Australian researchers initially reported good results with the group of drugs called benzopyrones[26] such as coumarin, more recent randomized controlled studies have shown them to have no value.[27]

Several operations have been applied to this problem, including liposuction, which is thought to help grow new lymphatics and improve drainage, and lymphatic reconstruction. In both of these situations the women are put into compression garments immediately after surgery. So far there is no randomized data comparing surgery with just compression; nonetheless they report good results.[28,29,30,31]

Lymphedema has been vastly underestimated by the medical profession. Women with lymphedema experience enormous physical and psychological difficulties. Anne Coscarelli, director of the Simms-Mann Center for Integrative Oncology at UCLA's Johnson Cancer Center, feels that the medical profession underestimates the psychological stress of having lymphedema. It is a constant reminder that the ordeal is not over, and that you can't get back to your old life. On top of this, it elicits less support from caregivers and family members because it is not life threatening. Most women with lymphedema benefit greatly from talking to others about the experience, either in a support group or on an Internet bulletin board. In 1995 at UCLA we started what I think was the first lymphedema support group in an attempt to address some of these problems. Lymphedema will end only when axillary dissections are no longer performed.

Other Long-Term Effects

Rarely, radiation can cause second cancers. This is usually a different kind of cancer, a sarcoma, and doesn't occur for at least five years after radiation therapy. Our best guess is that, for every 1,000 five-year survivors of wide excision and radiation, about two will develop a radiation-induced sarcoma over the next 10 years. Another infrequent consequence of radiation is heart disease. Women who have received modern radiation therapy for breast conservation have shown a lower than expected 2.7 percent increase in heart attack or coronary artery disease after ten years.[32] Another study from the University of Pennsylvania showed that 10 percent of women who had received radiation to the right breast developed coronary artery disease by 20 years after treatment. The highest risk was in women with left-sided radiation and hypertension.[33]

A large analysis of all of the randomized studies of surgery and axillary clearance with and without radiation has shown a small increase in mortality in the radiated women. Most of the studies were in women who received postmastectomy radiation that included the nodes under the breastbone. It also was observed mostly in women surviving more than 5–10 years from treatment and particularly women who were treated with less attention to sparing the heart. I am not surprised. My aunt was treated in the 1960s for a left-sided breast cancer with four positive nodes. She had the standard treatment of the day: a mastectomy and cobalt radiation therapy. She suffered acute difficulty in swallowing that I now know was from treating the nodes under the breastbone. Years later she developed significant heart disease requiring bypass surgery and ultimately left-sided lung cancer from which she died in the early 1990s. She was also a smoker, which I am sure contributed: however, I am also sure that these problems stemmed in part from the radiation therapy. The real question is whether we would have had her around for the additional 30 years without it—and that we will never know.

LONG-TERM SIDE EFFECTS OF CHEMOTHERAPY

In the past, chemotherapy was used only to treat metastasis. Oncologists at that time weren't thinking about long-term effects;
they hoped to keep the patient living a few years longer than she
would without the treatment. If she lived long enough to deal
with long-term effects, she and her doctors were happy. Because
we now detect micrometastases and use chemotherapy on people
whose cancers haven't significantly spread, this has changed. A
woman treated with chemotherapy may now live for many years,
and the issues surrounding her long-term well-being are more important. Since the last edition of this book, greater attention has
been paid to these issues, with increased and better research.

"Chemo Brain"

In any group of breast cancer survivors someone is bound to refer
to "chemo brain" to the knowing smiles of her audience. As mentioned in Chapter 17, numerous women have shared this feeling
that their brain just wasn't working the same as it had before their
cancer and ensuing treatments. Their experience was initially dismissed by most oncologists, but it is finally undergoing serious
study. At this point, however, there seem to be more questions
than answers. A recent study looked at women after they'd had
surgery but before they went through chemotherapy or hormone
therapy. They found that a small subgroup performed lower than
expected as compared to healthy controls and patients with noninvasive breast cancer. And, yes, they did also test them for depression, anxiety, and fatigue, finding that these feelings were similar
to those among the cancer patients but not among healthy control
groups.[34] This brought up some interesting hypotheses about associations between low-grade inflammation and DNA repair problems (see Chapter 4), both of which are associated with the
development of cancer and neurocognitive disorders (see Chapter
18). A meta-analysis[35] of all the studies thus far concluded that
cognitive impairment occurs reliably in women who have undergone adjuvant chemotherapy but that the degree of impairment

tends to be mild. These impairments usually occur in attention, concentration, verbal and visual memory, and processing.

In my mind, the best study so far is one by Dr. Valerie Jenkins.[36] She studied women with early breast cancer, representing a combination of those who would get chemotherapy, hormone therapy, or both, and compared them to healthy women who did not have breast cancer. Overall, 128 finished the study (85 who got chemotherapy and 43 who did not). They found little convincing evidence to suggest that there is measurable and meaningful impairment in the vast majority of women who receive standard adjuvant treatments for breast cancer. However, they did find that women who experienced a sudden premature menopause had a higher likelihood of showing a decrease in brain function. This should not come as a surprise to any woman who has gone through menopause or any large hormonal shift. Does anyone's brain work right during puberty or postpartum, much less during perimenopause? Mine certainly didn't! Sudden menopause brings on hot flashes, night sweats, and difficulty in sleeping—all of which can affect your brain. Their summary was that only a small proportion of women receiving adjuvant treatments for breast cancer experience objective measurable change in their concentration and memory, which is reassuring.

Nonetheless, if you still think your brain is not working right, you are probably correct. Remember, these studies are looking for big changes, while you are aware of more subtle differences that may not be captured on neuropyschological tests. But there is hope for you. A study done by MD Anderson in Texas in 2004[37] found that at the 18-month follow-up, approximately 50 percent of the women who had experienced decreases in function showed improvement, whereas 50 percent remained stable. Self-reported ability to work also improved. Although this study is small, the way it was done is important in showing the effects of chemotherapy over time. Approximately 46 percent of the women would not have been classified as experiencing a decline in cognitive function based on their postchemotherapy evaluations alone. In other words, compared to their prechemo functioning they had declined, but they were still above the average for healthy women of their age. This study is consistent with published retrospective postchemotherapy reports that identify a subgroup of patients who experienced cognitive decline that improves over time.[38,39]

The good news is that a group of international researchers focusing on this problem have formed a task force to advance the understanding of the impact that cancer and cancer-related treatment can have on cognitive and behavioral functioning in adults.[40,41] This collaboration will result in a lot more findings for the next edition of this book.

I doubt that most oncologists talk about this potential side effect with women who are considering chemotherapy. If they did, women would probably make a variety of choices, as mentioned earlier. For someone who needs the treatment to survive, it's worth it, but in cases where chemotherapy offers only a minuscule survival improvement, it may not be.

Fatigue

Many cancer survivors identify fatigue as the most frequent and distressing cancer-related symptom.[42] A subset of breast cancer survivors experience moderate to severe symptoms years after cancer treatment has ended.[43] For example, large prospective studies have found that 30–41 percent of breast cancer survivors report fatigue one to five years post diagnosis.[44,45]

This fatigue is related to radiation therapy (see Chapter 16) as well as chemotherapy. Some of the most interesting studies have come out of UCLA, where researchers have found an increase in blood markers of low-grade inflammation.[46] Another study from this group has shown a blunted hormonal stress reaction in survivors with chronic fatigue.[47] It is exciting to finally see biological explanations for the experiences of many survivors. Next will come specific ways to prevent or treat them.

Several studies show that aerobic exercise decreases fatigue.[48] One large prospective study found that women who exercised four or more hours per week had 50 percent less fatigue. This may be hard to enforce—the last thing you feel like doing when you're exhausted is exercise! But it's worth pushing yourself. Exercise is a proven way to decrease all those inflammatory markers and has been shown to decrease recurrence as well. And it can help prevent the next side effect: weight gain.

Weight Gain

Although weight gain resulting from breast cancer treatment is less of a problem with modern therapies than it was in 1978 when first described, it still can be a problem.[49] It is more common in women who receive chemotherapy and are put into menopause. It seems the culprit is not increased eating but rather decreased exercise.[50] Some data suggest that overweight women have a higher mortality than lean ones. However, it is not clear whether gaining weight with treatment increases recurrence of the cancer. The death increase may involve other weight-related problems—stroke, diabetes, and so on. In Chapter 18 we reviewed the growing data on the effects of weight and physical inactivity, whether by increasing diabetes and insulin resistance or provoking a state conducive to low-grade inflammation, or increasing the side effects of treatment and the chance of recurrence. All of this leads me to strongly suggest that maintaining your weight at a healthy level is important after a breast cancer diagnosis.

Bone Loss

Women who have entered menopause prematurely due to chemotherapy or hormone therapy experience some of the bone loss that normally occurs with aging. (See the discussion of bisphosphonates and bone loss in Chapter 17.) Nevertheless, most fractures occur late in life and there is no evidence that treating osteopenia (low bone density short of osteoporosis) reduces your chances of having one. The thinking is that by the time you're 65, we know where your bone density has stabilized and have lots of opportunity to treat you if you indeed have osteoporosis. Although women who have been treated for breast cancer may accelerate this process and fracture at an earlier age, this has certainly not been proven. It doesn't make sense to test bone density before, though it may be good to have a bone density test at the conclusion of therapy to see what you ended with.

Based on this thinking and on the absence of data, I am not sure why many oncologists give bisphosphonates to women who are taking adjuvant hormone therapy or are in premature menopause. These drugs may prevent bone loss, but there is no evidence suggesting that they help prevent fractures in women who do not already have osteoporosis.[51] If you decide to have a bone density test, be careful of falling into the trap of thinking that you should take a bisphosphonate if you have osteopenia; don't confuse bone density with fractures. These drugs are meant to prevent fractures, not treat bone density. The trend is not to give drugs to women to prevent bone loss but to reserve them for those at high risk of fracture (5–10 percent) in the next five to ten years. All women should be taking calcium and vitamin D and getting enough weight-bearing exercise and weight training. Randomized clinical trial evidence supports the use of vitamin D supplements (400–800 U/d) plus calcium to reduce fracture risk in older postmenopausal women and those with low bone mineral density.[52] Although there have been some early data suggesting this vitamin may also be related to lessening breast cancer recurrence, there is still inadequate evidence to support this as a regular practice.

MENOPAUSAL SYMPTOMS

A woman can arrive at menopause in one of three ways: naturally, simply by living long enough; surgically, by having her ovaries removed; and chemically, through chemotherapy. This is as true for the woman with breast cancer as it is for everyone else. The difference is that the options for dealing with her symptoms are dictated in part by her history of breast cancer.

Someone who has had a mastectomy but not chemotherapy or tamoxifen may go into natural menopause right on cue. Or she can be thrown into menopause by a hysterectomy that includes oophorectomy (removal of ovaries) for bleeding or some other problem unrelated to her cancer. In these situations she will have the same symptoms as those who have not had breast cancer (which means they can range from nonexistent to severe). The only difference is that the estrogen question looms larger for her than for someone who is not at any particular risk of breast cancer or recurrence.

A woman who is thrown into menopause by chemotherapy and/or by suddenly discontinuing hormone replacement therapy may find her symptoms doubly hard to sort out. Chemotherapy and tamoxifen add their own symptoms or side effects to the mix. Similarly, a woman may be prescribed goserelin, which creates a state of reversible menopause.

With natural menopause the ovaries continue to produce hormones, albeit at a much lower level than before. Obviously a woman who has gone through surgical menopause—removal of her ovaries—has no ovarian hormone production, although her adrenal glands may produce a very small amount of estrogen, as well as testosterone and androstenedione, which are converted by fat, muscle, and breast tissue into estrogen by aromatase. However, we don't know what happens with women who have chemical menopause. Does the chemotherapy destroy the ovaries so they never produce estrogen again? Or does it simply throw the woman into regular menopause, so she gets postmenopausal levels of hormone production? We do know that women around 30 who receive chemotherapy often go into temporary menopause and then get their periods back (see Chapter 12). This may mean that the chemicals don't totally wipe out the ovaries' capacity to produce hormones. But in a middle-aged woman, the chemicals simply push her in the direction she's already heading. Thus women who are apparently thrown into permanent menopause may still have some ovarian hormone production. Or maybe some of them do and some don't. This is an area we still need to study more.

There are two aspects of menopause that a woman needs to consider. The first is that symptoms can come with a sudden or an erratic change in hormones. These symptoms, as I explained in Chapter 1, are usually transient, lasting for two to three years on average. They need to be treated specifically, and there is a large menu of options.

The second is the way menopause is often portrayed by the media and the pharmaceutical companies—as the cause of diseases that occur in later life, such as dementia and osteoporosis. There are several global approaches to these problems, and there are specific remedies for specific symptoms and prevention of specific diseases. Before I launch into an analysis of the pros and cons of the options, I think it is important to point out that doing nothing is an acceptable choice. You don't have to "treat" or "manage" menopause unless it is interfering with your life.

First let's talk about hormones. As I explained at length in Chapter 5, the data are pretty compelling that taking HRT (hormone replacement therapy) increases the risk of breast cancer. This alone should be enough to cross it off the list as an option for the woman who already has the disease. Recent studies have added further data leading to the conclusion that such women should never use HRT. The HABITS trial began in 1997 to recruit volunteers willing to help investigate whether a two-year HRT treatment for menopausal symptoms was safe in women with a previously treated breast cancer.[53] Women with in situ to stage 2 breast cancer were eligible, whether or not they were on tamoxifen (21 percent), if they had menopausal symptoms for which they felt they needed treatment. A total of 434 women were randomized, and 345 had at least one follow-up. After a mean follow-up of 2.1 years, 26 women in the HRT group and 7 in the non-HRT group had a new breast cancer. Because of this, the researchers stopped the trial and announced that HRT posed an unacceptable risk to women with breast cancer. Of the women with a new cancer in the non-HRT group, two had been taking HRT on their own. (This, by the way, was unfair. If you are part of a study group and decide not to abide by its rules, you should always admit that and leave the study.)

A more recent treatment for menopausal symptoms is bioidentical hormones—hormones identical to the ones your own body makes when it is premenopausal. The studies aren't conclusive yet, but there is no reason to believe that bioidentical hormones are safer than synthetic ones. As we saw in Chapter 5, women with high levels of their own hormones—estrogen and testosterone— are at greater breast cancer risk. A recent abstract by a group at

Northwestern University indirectly implicated the body's own progesterone.[54] Researchers measured salivary levels of progesterone and breast tissue density (a strong risk factor for breast cancer mentioned in Chapter 6) over six months. Only the women on tamoxifen who had an increase in progesterone had an increase in breast density. I should point out that the PEPI study discussed in Chapter 5 also showed increased breast density in the women on natural progesterone.[55] Indeed, the mere fact that women who go through menopause late have a higher risk of breast cancer should suggest that even your own hormones are not all that good for you after a while. So the fact that we don't yet have any data suggesting that bioidentical hormones are dangerous does not mean they are safe. A review of estriol and bioidentical formulations of estrogen (Triest) confirmed that estriol causes endometrial stimulation, just as HRT does, and that it stimulates breast cancers to grow (6 of 24 women).[56] A recent review of bioidentical hormone therapy concluded that hormones specially compounded for a woman may well decrease her symptoms, but there is no evidence that they are safe.[57] It is very likely not the type of hormones that you are taking but the fact that you are taking "replacement" hormones at all that puts you back in premenopausal range. To date there is more hype than science about bioidentical hormones, including over-the-counter natural progesterone creams.[58]

Finally there is tibolone. This is a nonestrogenic drug available only outside of the United States. Studies are investigating its use in breast cancer patients, but the Million Women Study, which looked at women in England on various forms of HRT, found that it too increased risk of breast cancer as well as endometrial cancer.[59,60] A large randomized study of 2004 breast cancer patients reported that although the drug reduced bone loss and hot flashes, it also increased breast cancer recurrence.[61]

TREATMENT FOR SYMPTOMS

If HRT is out, what can you do for menopausal symptoms? Although there are sometimes symptoms during the postmenopausal years, most of the symptoms that cause discomfort come in the transition when your body is experiencing shifts in hormones. So treatments may last for only a few years rather than a lifetime. Treatments vary with symptoms.

Hot Flashes

A behavioral approach can help. For one thing, you can avoid triggers. These vary greatly among individual women, but you can soon figure out what yours are by keeping a daily hot flash diary. Spicy foods, caffeine, stressful situations, and hot drinks are among the more common triggers. Once you've identified them you can avoid them. Sleep in a cool room; carry a hand fan (I keep one in my briefcase); dress in cotton and in layers; do paced respiration exercises (practicing deep, slow abdominal breathing); try acupuncture; eat a serving of soy foods (see later in this chapter) and ground flax seeds daily; walk, swim, dance, or ride a bike every day for at least 30 minutes. If none of this helps, try vitamin E (800 mg) or the herb black cohosh (Remifemin; see later in this chapter). If nothing helps symptoms, you can join or create a support group to help you deal with them.

How well do these treatments work? There are data from randomized controlled studies supporting acupuncture and paced respiration to reduce hot flashes. There are also good data from randomized controlled double-blind studies on black cohosh, using both conjugated estrogen (Premarin) and a placebo as the controls. These studies found that the herb reduces hot flashes and helps vaginal dryness. Many U.S. researchers aren't aware of these studies because they were done in Germany.[62,63]

Soy Protein. A Natural SERM? When I lecture on menopausal hormones or breast cancer, the question I am asked most is about soy. Soy is a food source of isoflavones. Sometimes it is called a phytoestrogen. This is a poor word choice. Although soy acts like estrogen in some organs, it blocks estrogen in others—so it's more like a phyto SERM (selective estrogen receptor modulator; see Chapter 7) than a pure estrogen. In addition, it has many effects besides hormonal ones. It blocks tumor cells in a petri dish, whether or not they're sensitive to estrogen. We are only beginning to study the properties of this natural substance. Data are mixed on its usefulness in treating hot flashes.

Although there has been a lot of concern over the years about whether soy is safe for women to eat,[64] recent data suggest that it probably is. In a study of 5,042 breast cancer survivors from Shanghai researchers found that soy intake actually decreased the risk of death or recurrence.[65] This held through even if the women were estrogen positive and taking tamoxifen.

How should you take soy? Ideally you should consume it as tofu, soybeans, or soy milk. There are many soy cookbooks around. (It also helps prevent prostate cancer and thus is good for the whole family.) If you do not have time to cook, then try one of the soy protein powders such as Healthy Source or Revival. However, I'd advise against taking soy capsules or capsules of isoflavones or genistein. Although these two are ingredients of soy, we do not know which one is more important. Nor do we know whether they work the same way in isolation as they do in food. Also, it is much easier to overdose on soy in capsule form or the soy-based meat substitutes made to resemble burger, franks, or other forms of meat than as tofu. Always remember moderation.

Black Cohosh. Black cohosh (Remifemin) is a natural alternative used to treat menopausal symptoms, but its mechanism is not understood. A group at the Mayo Clinic and two other research groups have studied black cohosh in a randomized controlled trial of hot flashes in women. The studies did not support an effect.[66,67] They also showed no benefit from Vitamin E.[68] Recently a study in mice suggested that black cohosh increased metastatic disease.[69] This reminds me of the studies in animals that suggested soy was dangerous and studies in women that did not. It is always hard to know whether animal studies translate to women. You will have to decide whether you want to try this remedy in the face of conflicting data or not.

Nonhormone Drugs. The same group at the Mayo Clinic did a good study of menopausal symptom relief in women who have had breast cancer, which can also be used by other women.[70] This group, the North Center Cancer Treatment Group (NCCTG), studied more than 650 women with breast cancer and reported a number of findings. First, researchers found that a placebo alone appeared to cause a 20–25 percent reduction of symptoms in four weeks. This may show a psychological component to hot flashes, or it may reflect the nature of hot flashes: they tend to come and go on their own. My own example is fairly common and serves to illustrate the capricious nature of hot flashes. I had ten and a half weeks of horrible hot flashes and no period. "This is it," I thought. "These things will go on for a few years, my periods will stop, and—if I don't end up in an insane asylum first—so will the hot flashes." All of a sudden, on a Sunday while I was at a medical convention in Atlanta, the hot flashes stopped, and I found myself wondering what had happened. I'm sure if I had been started on a new treatment or had been on a placebo in a study, I would have thought happily, "I'm not in the placebo group, and this blessed treatment works!" Since this wasn't the case, I just whispered a prayer of devout gratitude to my guardian angel. Four weeks later, my period was back, and of course that was why the flashes had stopped.

The Mayo Clinic recently published a summary of their studies over the years. Hot flashes are markedly decreased by venlafaxine (antidepressant), mildly to moderately decreased by fluoxetine (antidepressant), mildly decreased by clonidine (antihypertensive). These drugs, other than clonidine, are a mixture of antidepressants.[71] A review of all nonhormonal therapies for hot flashes found data supporting the efficacy of antidepressants (SSRIs and SNRIs), clonidine (antihypertensive), and gabapentin (antiseizure drug) in reducing the frequency and severity of hot flashes. These are all drugs with potential side effects. If hot flashes are a serious problem for you, you should ask your doctor to help you sort through the options to find something that works in your case.

As an occasional flashing woman myself, I think there is one key component to getting through this temporary disruption in life—a sense of humor. If you can laugh at yourself and revel in this change you will, as the saying goes, turn the hot flashes into power surges.

Vaginal Dryness

Vaginal dryness as a result of vaginal atrophy is perhaps the most distressing and least talked about symptom of menopause. It occurs in about 20 percent of women, sometimes transiently and other times permanently. Sexual activity, including masturbation, reduces vaginal atrophy. The problem is that if you're sore from vaginal dryness, you probably don't want to have sex, and if you don't have sex, your vaginal dryness gets worse—a classic catch-22. There are two approaches. Water-based lubricants like KY jelly and Astroglide don't cure the basic condition, but they can help the immediate problem of painful intercourse. Many women find two common, inexpensive, and nonembarrassing products to be the best lubricants: canola oil and Abolene. If you are experiencing pain with intercourse, Abolene (which is sold in drugstores as a facial cleanser) is especially effective. The other approach is to try to increase the vagina's own moisture. Replens, which can be purchased over the counter, causes your vagina to absorb water and become more supple. In one study 61.5 percent of patients preferred Replens, 26.5 preferred a lubricant, and 12 percent had no preference. In fact the use of both a moisturizer and a lubricant may provide the best results.

Both black cohosh and soy have been reported to reduce vaginal dryness. Vitamin E capsules have been used vaginally with some success as well. (You break open the capsule and rub the vitamin E on the lining of your vagina.)

If nothing else works, you may decide to try estrogen to improve the quality of your life. You should use the smallest amount necessary and apply it to where the problem is (interestingly, estrogen by mouth often doesn't relieve vaginal dryness). There's a vaginal ring (Estring) that releases a very small amount of estrogen over a long period of time. In the first 24 hours after you've had it inserted (or inserted it yourself, like a diaphragm), you have a little spurt of estrogen; beyond that it doesn't increase hormone levels because it is low-dose and sustained-release. You keep it in for three months and then change it. Another alternative is the vaginal tablet, which again is slow release over a period of time. These are a great solution for women with breast cancer and vaginal dryness. As a last resort you can try vaginal estrogen creams. If you go that route, however, ignore the instructions on the label, which tell you to use an applicator full. Since estrogen as a cream is well absorbed from the vagina, you'll end up with blood levels that rival what you would get with estrogen pills. All you really need is a little dab on your fingertip. If you apply it every day for two weeks, then two or three times a week, it will solve your problems. (But don't use it as a lubricant at the time of sex; it won't help that way and your male partner may grow breasts—kinky, perhaps, but probably a bit alarming for the poor fellow!)

If you have not had intercourse for a while, you may find that along with dryness your vagina can become tighter as it loses elasticity. A dilator can help with this by stretching things out again. If problems persist despite all of these suggestions, ask your doctor to refer you to a counselor with sex therapy training for further help.

Insomnia, Mood Swings, and Fuzzy Thinking

Although insomnia is often related to night sweats, it is also true that you don't sleep as well when your hormones are awry. Some easy measures can help. Keep your bedroom cool, exercise (but earlier in the day; exercising right before going to bed will keep you awake), avoid caffeine and liquor, take warm baths or showers, increase soy intake, have cereal and milk products at bedtime.

To counter mood swings and anxiety, try using the relaxation response (see Chapter 18), exercising (including yoga), eating a plant- rather than meat-based diet, going to a psychotherapist, and finding creative outlets.

For fuzzy thinking, soy seems to help. Other possibilities are exercise, low-fat diet, nonsteroidal anti-inflammatories (Motrin), and vitamin E. The best thing to do for your brain is use it: for example, work, study, do crossword puzzles, play chess, read, and play card games. Further, a recent study showed that people who stayed socially active had less cognitive decline with age—so hang out with your friends! Remember, menopausal symptoms do not last forever. On average their duration is about two to three years off and on. The best approach to both symptom relief and prevention is to pursue a healthy lifestyle.

Healing the Mind

Emotional healing techniques are more varied and individual than physical ones, and many have proved helpful to my patients and other women with breast cancer.

Psychotherapy can be a tremendous tool at this time, as it is whenever you experience great emotional stress. About a quarter to a third of women have posttreatment symptoms that warrant evaluation. Persistent feelings of sadness, loss of self-esteem, and lack of interest in things that brought you pleasure before you had cancer are not typical and should be followed up.

This may be the time to try a support group, especially if you were too overwhelmed to do it during therapy. Or you can join an online chat group, bulletin board, or mailing list. Check out www.breastcancer.org, Living Beyond Breast Cancer (www.lbbc .org), or Breast Cancer Action Nova Scotia (www.bca.ns.ca). Sometimes brief one-on-one counseling helps, particularly if you are finding it difficult to move on from the aftermath of your illness.

Many women keep a journal of their experiences to refer to later and to help them cope with their feelings. Some take their healing beyond themselves—reaching out to other women who are going through what they've been through. Writers like Audre Lorde, Linda Ellerbee, Katherine Russel Rich, and Carol Dine and performers like singer Melissa Etheridge and skater Peggy Fleming have spoken out or written about the experience. Indeed, much of the success we've had in removing the stigma attached to breast cancer comes from early pioneers such as Shirley Temple Black, Happy Rockefeller, and Rose Kushner, who publicly fought the stigma.

Often, indeed, the need to give back and find a positive side to this experience can be channeled to helping other women with breast cancer. Sometimes this can be done through work. Two of my patients are psychotherapists who now specialize in breast cancer therapy. Another did breast cancer workshops at her corporation. If you're a sales clerk, you may want to work in a store selling prostheses, since you now have a special understanding that may help your customers.

If your profession isn't one that can be adapted to some form of working with breast cancer, or if you don't feel drawn toward spending your work life dealing with the disease, you can still help other women—and thus yourself—on a volunteer basis. For example, you may want to get involved with Reach for Recovery or a similar group that works with breast cancer patients. You know how frightened you were when you were first diagnosed. The presence of someone who's survived the disease can be enormously reassuring to a newly diagnosed woman.

You can also become involved in political action, possibly with the National Breast Cancer Coalition (www.stopbreastcancer.org). You can define the level of your participation according to your own energy, time constraints, and degree of commitment: anything from writing an occasional letter to your congressperson to organizing demonstrations and fund-raising events. Jane Reese Colbourne, a former NBC vice president, found that in her own experience in political activism was "a very good way to channel anger at the fact that you've had this disease. For me, it was the next step after a support group. Talking about it with other women was important, but I wanted to do something about it."

Finally, make sure you don't feel ashamed of what you've been through. Cancer still carries a stigma in our culture, and breast cancer can have especially difficult associations. You need to demystify it to yourself and to others. You don't have to dwell on it, but it's not a good idea to repress it either. You need to have friends you can talk freely to about your disease and your feelings about it; you need to know you can include it in casual conversation, that you don't have to avoid saying, "Oh, yes, that was around the time I was in the hospital for my mastectomy."

One of the newest areas of survivorship research is called "benefit finding." As usual, it takes doctors and researchers awhile to catch up to what patients have known all along—that there are many positive things you can take from this experience. I often hear women say that while they would not wish cancer on anyone, they find themselves living more fully: they "don't sweat the small stuff," they cherish their families, and they truly value each day.

RELATIONSHIPS AND SEX

One of the least discussed subjects about life after breast cancer is sexuality. Your surgeon won't bring it up if you don't; in fact most surgeons will assume that if you're not complaining, everything must be fine. Yet most women find sex hard to talk about—especially when it concerns feelings, perhaps only half recognized, about losing both their sexual attractiveness and their libido when they lose a part of their bodies so strongly associated with sexuality. Doctors need to learn how to open the subject delicately, in a way that doesn't feel intrusive to the woman but communicates that she has a safe place to discuss sexuality concerns. I remember one surgeon who had referred a patient to me on his retirement. He said that after her mastectomy she had surprised everyone with her rapid recovery and exclaimed over how well she had "dealt with it." I took over the case, and in my first conversation with her I found out that, however well adjusted she seemed on the surface, she had not yet looked at her scar—and this was five years after the operation. She had never resumed sex with her husband and even dressed and undressed in the closet so he couldn't see her.

Many women have difficulties with sex and intimacy following a breast cancer diagnosis. Aside from feeling that your body has betrayed you, you may have a sense of invasion from the treatments. All these strangers have been poking and prodding you for weeks; you may almost feel violated, and you forget that your body can provide you with pleasure. It takes awhile to feel good and in control of your body again. You need to communicate these feelings to your partner so he or she can help you in your healing.

Some women find that after surgery, whether mastectomy or lumpectomy, a sexual relationship becomes even more important in helping them regain their sense of worth and wholeness. There may, however, be changes. One patient of mine who had bilateral mastectomies felt that all the erotic sensations she had formerly had in her breasts had "moved south," and that her orgasms were doubly good. Other women miss the stimulation from a lost breast so much that they don't want their other breast touched during sex. Dr. Patricia Ganz, who has both worked with and studied the problems of women with breast cancer, talks about the issues that women who have had lumpectomy and radiation may experience: "Especially with women who had radiation a number of years ago, they often find the breast isn't as soft and beautiful as it was before the radiation." These changes in the conserved breast can carry over into their sexual relationships.

Some of the changes may be more practical than emotional. Your arm or shoulder may not be as strong on the side of your surgery, and this can make certain positions more difficult during intercourse, such as kneeling above your partner. You may feel uncomfortable lying on the side of the surgery for many months. It is important that you communicate with your partner so that together you can explore new ways of lovemaking that you both enjoy.

Chemical menopause can also affect a woman's sexuality. Menopause, like aging itself, often lessens sexual desire, and when that combines with breast cancer issues a woman can find that her libido is abruptly and seriously lessened. Studies are now being done to see whether the libido loss of women with chemically induced menopause is more severe than that of women who have experienced menopause normally.

Dr. Ganz adds that it's difficult to separate out the physiological and emotional aspects of libido loss. "Sex is at least partly in the brain," she says, "and the hormones circulating in the body affect the brain and thus sexual arousal. Psychological distress can affect hormones; we've found in our work that women who have a lot of psychological distress have more sexual dysfunction." This was demonstrated by a recent study from the Mayo Clinic using transdermal testosterone or placebo in breast cancer survivors suffering low libido.[72] Interestingly, both groups, those with the testosterone and those without it, showed equal improvement in all the measures. This suggests a large placebo effect as well as the fact that sexual desire in women is complicated, with many factors involved.[73]

There are no aspects of sexual intimacy that cause cancer or increase the chance of recurrence. Nor can cancer be "caught" by someone sucking on a nipple. Barbara Kalinowski, who once co-led support groups with me at the Faulkner Breast Centre in

Boston, finds that "sometimes women who have had lumpectomy and radiation have a fantasy that the breast still has cancer in it, and don't want it fondled because they fear it will shake things up and send the cancer cells through the rest of the body." Even when your intellect knows such fears are groundless, your emotions may not, and that's bound to affect both partners' sexual pleasure.

Sheila Kitzinger in her book *Woman's Experience of Sex* writes that for some women having a brief affair was an important part of their healing process.[74] They said it was all well and good for a husband of 35 years to still love them without a breast, but they needed confirmation of their sexual attractiveness to feel whole again. That might work for you, though it could also put a severe strain on your marriage. At the very least, however, you'll want to be in touch with whatever feelings you're having about sex and decide which ones to act on and which ones to simply fantasize about.

This brings up another issue. If you are single and dating, should you tell or not? Again, this is an individual decision. Some women will tell a prospective lover way in advance, preferring to have it out in the open before the moment of passion. Others will wait until the last instant when there is no turning back to disclose their secret (never a good idea). For the woman who has had a small lumpectomy or has had mastectomy with a natural-looking reconstruction, the need to tell a casual lover about her situation may or may not arise. However, in a long-term relationship, it's important to be honest. For the woman whose surgery leaves visible alteration, dating can be a matter of concern. Yet it doesn't mean you have to resign yourself to a life of celibacy. Barbara Kalinowski found that several women in her support groups were able to form new romantic relationships shortly after surgery. She recalls one woman who had never married and had a mastectomy with reconstruction in her fifties. "I got a call from her a couple of years ago. She was as giggly and happy as a teenager. 'Guess what!' she told me. 'I'm getting married!' They were planning a honeymoon in Paris and she was ecstatic." Another woman from one of Kalinowski's groups was happily married to a man who was wonderful to her during treatment. Two years later he died of a heart attack. Soon after his death she met a widower and they fell in love. "They decided not to wait," Kalinowski says, "because they both knew how chancy life was. She told me, 'We both learned that we don't want to wait for anything anymore.'"

Many women worry that their partner will be turned off by their condition and new body. There are many horror stories of husbands and significant others who opt out of having sex or even walk out entirely. The impact of cancer can be as devastating to the partner as to the patient herself. Partners may feel angry, ashamed, and vulnerable to illness themselves. Their lives and dreams have been changed, but they typically get little support. They feel guilty complaining when they are not the ones undergoing treatment. Some people have problems dealing with serious illness, and others may use it as an excuse to get out of a relationship they thought was not working anyway. Most important is the quality of the relationship and the level of communication. Work by David Wellisch at UCLA indicates that the husband's involvement in the decision-making process, hospital visitation, early viewing of scars, and early resumption of sexual activity are important for couples to function optimally.[75] Open dialogue is critical in this process, for nonmarried and lesbian couples as well as married ones.

Another study found that patients' and partners' levels of adjustment were significantly related; when one partner was experiencing difficulties in adjustment, the other was also likely to be having problems.[76] Difficulties in communication and sex need to be addressed promptly. Patricia Ganz found that most sexual issues were resolved by one year; if not, they were never resolved.[77] She recently did a randomized controlled trial comparing a six-week psychological education group versus printed material for women who reported moderately severe problems in body image, sexual function, or partner communication. They found that the women randomized to the group had more improvements in relationship adjustment and increased satisfaction with sex than those given only written material.[78]

Counseling or a group—where you can talk about your feelings in a protective environment—can be important in preventing serious problems. Hoping a situation will get better on its own rarely works and usually allows the problem to become chronic. You should request help for such problems as decreased libido and vaginal dryness; you may even consider seeing a sex therapist.

PREGNANCY

If you are still menstruating, a question that nearly always comes up is whether or not you should risk getting pregnant once you've had breast cancer. There are two areas to consider—the ethical implications and the health-related implications.

In the past doctors (usually male) tended to impose their own value judgments on patients and told them not to get pregnant for least five years after having breast cancer. If you survived five years, they reasoned, there was a good chance you'd won your bout with breast cancer; otherwise, they didn't want you bringing a child you couldn't raise into the world.

This is a moral decision for the patient to make, not the doctor, and there are two equally valid ways of looking at it. Some women do not want to have a child they're not reasonably sure they'll be around to raise. Others feel that even if they do die in a few years they'll still be able to give a child the love and care needed in the early years, and they want to pass on their genes before they die. Considerations of a husband's or partner's ability to nurture a child and support from family and friends will weigh on the decision as well.

Having a child is never a decision anyone should make lightly, and a life-threatening illness complicates it further. Think it through carefully and get the thoughts of people whose opinions you respect—and then make your decision.

The other question is medical. Can getting pregnant decrease your chances of surviving breast cancer? I wish I knew. Although there are no randomized studies, cancer centers that have reported on the outcome of women who have had pregnancies following breast cancer have shown no difference in survival (see Chapter 13).[79,80]

We do know that getting pregnant won't cause the cancer to spread; either it has spread or it hasn't before you become pregnant. But if you had a tumor that left microscopic cells in your body, it's possible that pregnancy, with its attendant hormones, could make them grow faster than they would have if you weren't pregnant. This could reduce the time you have left; for example, if you would have died of breast cancer four years from now, you'll die in three years instead.

So the question is, Do you want to take that risk? If you had a lot of positive nodes, a very aggressive tumor, or some other factor that increases the likelihood of micrometastases, you'll want to take that into consideration. It might be worth the risk to you, or it might not. Again, that's a very individual decision.

If you get pregnant, how will your breasts react? If you've had a mastectomy, obviously nothing will happen on the chest area where your breast was, but your other breast will go through all the usual pregnancy changes I described in Chapter 1. If you've had lumpectomy and radiation, the nonradiated breast will probably go through the normal changes. Radiation damages some of the milk-producing parts of the breast, so the radiated breast, while it will grow somewhat larger, won't keep pace with the other breast, and will produce little or no milk. You can nurse on one side only if you want. The problem with that is increased asymmetry; the milk-producing breast will grow and may stay larger after you finish breast-feeding. If you wish, you can have the larger breast reduced later through plastic surgery (see Chapter 2). One of my patients got pregnant shortly after finishing radiation treatments and successfully breast-fed the baby. But one breast ended up twice as large as the other. Knowing she wanted another child, she decided to wait till after her next pregnancy to get the breast reduced.

It's probably a good idea to wait a year or so after your treatment to get pregnant. It's a stressful process and you won't want to add morning sickness to the nausea you're likely to get from the chemicals.

On the other hand, I had a patient who inadvertently got pregnant right after finishing chemotherapy. After talking it over with her husband and her caregivers, she decided to have the baby; last I heard, mother and daughter were both doing fine.

I have been talking about having a child after breast cancer when you are still fertile, of course. In Chapter 13, I discussed

newer research on transplanting ovarian tissue and using tamoxifen and letrozole for in vitro fertilization (IVF). But the fact that
we can do it does not mean it is safe to do. As the numbers of
young women who are breast cancer survivors increase, we need
more studies to answer these questions. (Two good places to research the latest information on this are www.fertilehope.org and
www.youngsurvival.org.)

The decision is up to you. If the stress of dealing with cancer
and its uncertainties is too great, you may not want to have a
child. On the other hand, if you do want to have a child and feel
prepared for it, perhaps creating a new life can help you to cope
with the knowledge of mortality that a life-threatening illness carries with it—a reminder that death isn't the end.

Insurance and Getting a Job

Unfortunately, medical and emotional problems aren't the only
ones you'll have to face. People with cancer often experience
what amounts to discrimination, and there are some precautions
you need to take.

First, you don't want to let your insurance lapse. Your company
can't drop your policy because of your illness, so you're safe on
that score. But many insurance companies won't take on someone
who's had a life-threatening illness, and others will take you on
but exclude coverage in the area of your illness. If you change jobs
and go from one company's coverage to another, you'll probably be
all right (but make certain of this before you accept the new job).
If you quit for a while, make sure you keep up your insurance on
your own. It's costly, but not nearly as costly as having no coverage
if you get a recurrence.

Life insurance and disability insurance are also harder to get if
you've had breast cancer. More and more cancer survivors are
fighting to get this changed, and it should get better in the future.
But for now, be very alert.

One of the hardest questions is whether or not to tell employers and coworkers about your cancer. There are pros and cons either way. Federal law prohibits federal employers, or employers
who get federal grants or federal financial assistance, from dis-

criminating against the handicapped or anyone mistakenly thought to be handicapped. The Americans with Disabilities Act (ADA), which was passed in 1992 and amended in 1994, extends this concept to the private sector. Any employer with 15 or more employees is prohibited from discriminating against qualified applicants and employees because of any disability. Cancer and other diseases are considered disabilities under the terms of this legislation. The employer must also make reasonable accommodations to the disability; for example, if you have trouble reaching a high shelf because of pain from your mastectomy your employer must make material accessible on a lower shelf, or even build you a lower shelf if feasible. A 2004 follow-up study from Canada showed that slightly more survivors than controls were unemployed three years after diagnosis, but among the women still employed no one noted a change in their working conditions because of their cancer diagnosis.[81]

Many women fear employers will find subtle ways to discriminate against them if their cancer is discovered. One of my fellow breast cancer activists tells a great story of how she handled the loss of her job after her mastectomy, before the ADA was passed. Furious, she stormed into her boss's office, reached into her dress, pulled out her prosthesis, and slapped it on his desk. As he gaped at her in horror, she snapped, "Sir, you are confused—I had a mastectomy, not a lobotomy!" Then she calmly walked out, leaving her boss to buzz his secretary and ask her to remove the prosthesis.

The other possibility is that your boss and coworkers will offer you increased support if you are open. More and more attention is being given to cancer survivors in the workplace, and you may find a career counseling center that can give you good advice.

If you are looking for a new job, you may find even more difficulty. Some companies are reluctant to hire a person with cancer. This too is illegal under the ADA, but there is always the fear that an employer will find some excuse not to hire you. You may want to be open about your cancer because you don't want to work for someone with that attitude. On the other hand, you may need the job too much to risk being turned down. But if you don't tell and then end up missing a lot of time for medical appointments or sickness, you could run into problems that might have been avoided if you'd been frank in the beginning. It's a tough dilemma, and there are no easy answers. (A good place for information is the National Coalition for Cancer Survivors, www.canceradvocacy.org.)

To quote one of my Facebook friends: "All I can say is a new door opens and the old one closes. So expect a new perspective on life and living."

Part Six

RECURRENCE

Chapter 20

WHEN CANCER COMES BACK

WHEN BREAST CANCER CELLS REAPPEAR IN THE AREA AROUND THE breast (local or regional recurrence) or in other areas of the body (metastasis), you have a recurrence. For the most part, these are the microscopic cells that presumably got out before your diagnosis and found a niche elsewhere in your body. The cells can get out through the bloodstream or the lymphatic system into other organs, where they can remain dormant for years.

It may be that radiation or chemotherapy kills some cells and injures others, knocking them out. Then after a long while the ones that survived recover and begin doubling again. Another possibility is that the surviving cells were put to sleep by tamoxifen or chemical menopause and are now awakening (Figure 20.1). (If we could figure out what puts these cells to sleep and then what wakes them up, we'd be a long way toward eliminating breast cancer or controlling it for a much longer time—maybe a normal lifetime.) Or perhaps the local environment controlled the cells for a time and then ceased.

Being diagnosed with a recurrence can be devastating. The process of psychosocial adjustment starts all over again; learning to trust your body may take longer when you've been doubly

575

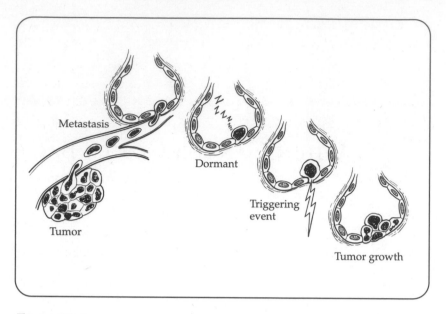

Figure 20.1

betrayed by it. The feelings you experienced the first time around are intensified because now you not only don't trust your body but begin to wonder about your doctors and treatment in general. This is a common feeling. But remember that a recurrence is not your fault; it's the result of factors that we do not understand and cannot control. You should discuss your feelings with your caregivers. In addition, you'll want to get support and help from friends and family, counselors, therapists, and support groups.

The kinds of support groups that are available vary widely, depending on where you are. Even general cancer groups can be very helpful, but most women find breast cancer groups better. In big cities you may want to search out groups for women with recurrences or with metastases. There are advantages to each type of group. Barbara Kalinowski, a clinical nurse specialist, co-led both a first-diagnosis group and a recurrence group that went on for several years. In the recurrence group, the women all faced similar issues for three years, but the dynamics changed as the women with metastases began to worsen. "The women who are sick are very happy for the women who are getting better, and the women who are getting better are very supportive of the women who are sick," Kalinowski says. One of the women who was well had lunch with one of the others whose metastasis was worsening. Jackie Onassis had just died, and the sick woman said she wanted white and pink flowers at her funeral, the way Jackie had. The next week the other woman sent her a gorgeous bouquet of white and pink flowers, with a note saying, "You don't have to wait until you die for your flowers."

In order to better deal with your recurrence, you need to know more about the nature of breast cancer recurrences. In the rest of this chapter we'll examine the types of recurrences, their symptoms, and their treatments. In describing these situations I will use statistics to help you get a sense of how often they occur. As with all statistics in breast cancer (see Chapter 4), it is important to remember that whatever happens to you is happening 100 percent— no matter how often it does or doesn't happen to other people. Statistics are good only for giving you an overall idea of what can happen. They can't tell you what will happen with your particular cancer in your particular body with your particular treatment.

LOCAL AND REGIONAL RECURRENCE

Local recurrence means the cancer has come back in the remaining breast or, in the case of mastectomy, in the scar. Regional recurrence means it has come back in the nodes in the armpit or around the collarbone.

Local and regional recurrences may feel just as devastating to the patient as distant disease, but depending on the circumstances, they may represent a different situation with a somewhat better prognosis. First, it is important that the type of breast cancer that has recurred is identified. If the recurrence is noninvasive cancer (see Chapter 13), it's most likely left over from the original cancer and just needs to be cleaned up with further surgery. On the other hand, if the recurrence is invasive, it may have had a second opportunity to spread. In addition, women with invasive local recurrences generally have more aggressive disease. Scientists have been studying the possibility that there are molecular patterns of the original tumor that can predict local recurrences.

As I am writing this, the first reports have started to come out. While so far there is nothing definitive, I suspect that before long we will be better able to identify which tumors are more likely to recur locally. This will enable us to tailor the local treatment from the beginning, and this section of the book will become unnecessary. At this point, however, we still seek to find out how the recurrences appear and how to treat them. We base our conclusions in part on what the initial therapy was.

Local Recurrence After Breast Conservation

Most local recurrences (6 percent) after breast conservation occur in the area of the original tumor, on average three to four years after the initial therapy.[1] If your initial treatment was a lumpectomy followed by radiation, the first sign of a local recurrence can be a change in how your breast looks or feels. Changes in the physical exam that occur more than one to two years after the completion of radiation therapy should always be looked into immediately. Retrospective studies show that the woman herself detects 76–86 percent of local recurrences, just as she detected the original tumor.[2,3] Less commonly, a mammogram reveals something suspicious. Although MRI has been used to try to distinguish between a local recurrence and scar tissue, only a biopsy can show for certain. Usually a core needle biopsy is sufficient, though sometimes the procedure shows that further surgery is necessary.

Once a local recurrence has been diagnosed, we do tests (see Chapter 11) to see if there are signs of cancer elsewhere in the body. These may include bone scan, chest X ray, CT scan, MRI, or PET scan, and blood tests (some of the latter are looking for tumor markers). If the tests are normal (only 5–10 percent of women with local recurrence have signs of disease elsewhere), then we have to figure out how best to eradicate the tumor from the breast. Usually in these cases we do a mastectomy, since the less drastic surgery and radiation didn't take care of it. After a salvage mastectomy for a local recurrence following partial mastectomy, the prognosis is still pretty good, with a five-year disease-free survival rate of 55–73 percent.[4] Some centers try to preserve the breast with additional limited surgery.[5,6] At this point we do not know whether this approach will work out as well.

Overall, the prognosis is better in women who are older, have smaller lesions, and have gone a long time between the initial treatment and the recurrence. A recent study suggests that local recurrences happening more than five years after initial treatment may have an even better prognosis. The role of systemic therapy after a local recurrence in the breast is still not clear, but it is often considered in high-risk women. If your tumor is sensitive to estrogen and you were on tamoxifen, it is reasonable to switch to an aromatase inhibitor, or vice versa. The role of chemotherapy, especially if you were previously treated with it, is not clear and is still being studied.

There's something else we call a local recurrence that actually isn't a local recurrence at all—it's a new cancer in the breast (often referred to as a new primary). This typically occurs many years after the original cancer and in an entirely different area of the breast. Its pathology is often different—lobular instead of ductal, for example. These second cancers account for only 15–23 percent in the larger series that have followed women after their first diagnosis.[7,8] But they are possible as long as you have your breast. Though they are often counted as recurrences in the statistics for breast conservation, they should be treated as completely new cancers, much as with new cancers in the opposite breast. Most often the local treatment will be a mastectomy, since you can receive radiation therapy only once to any area. However, the newer approaches of partial breast radiation (see Chapter 16) may change this. The addition of chemotherapy and/or tamoxifen will depend on the size and biomarkers of the tumor (see Chapter 11).

Local Recurrence After Mastectomy

You can also get a local recurrence in the scar or chest wall after a mastectomy (risk is about 6 percent). Actually the term "chest wall" is inaccurate here because it implies that the cancer is in the muscle or bone. But usually such a recurrence appears in the skin and fat sitting where the breast was before; only rarely does it include the muscle (see Figure 20.2). In fact 40–60 percent of local

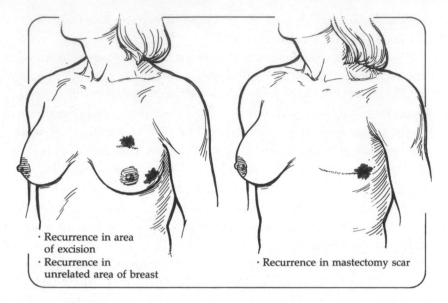

· Recurrence in area
  of excision
· Recurrence in
  unrelated area of breast

· Recurrence in mastectomy scar

Figure 20.2

recurrences occur where the breast was before, and the risk of this
happening is about 10 percent. Ninety percent of these recurrences happen within the first five years after the mastectomy. Approximately 20–30 percent of women with local recurrences after
mastectomy have already been diagnosed with metastatic disease
and another 20–30 percent will develop it within a few months of
diagnosis. Therefore, just as with local recurrences after breast
conservation, tests should be done to look for distant disease.

Local recurrence after mastectomy usually shows up as one or
more pea-size nodules on or under the skin near the scar or on it.[9]
After reconstruction a recurrence can appear at the suture line of
the flap or in front of the implant. When it's in the skin itself, it is
red and raised. It's usually so subtle the surgeon is likely to think
at first that it's just a stitch that got left in after the operation.
Then it gets bigger and needs to be biopsied. That can be done
under local anesthesia, since the area is numb. Reconstruction
rarely if ever hides a recurrence. With implants, the recurrences
are in front of the implant. With a flap the recurrences are not in
the flap itself (tissue from the abdomen) but along the edge of the
old breast skin.[10]

The treatments for a local recurrence are also local. Most commonly the lesion is removed surgically and followed by radiation to the chest wall if the woman has not previously had radiation. Occasionally larger areas are surgically removed, including sections of rib and breastbone. Although this approach has not been shown to increase survival, it can improve the quality of life by preventing further local spread, which can be difficult to manage.

Despite aggressive local treatment, 80–85 percent of women with an isolated local recurrence following mastectomy eventually develop distant metastases. This is higher than the prognosis for a local recurrence after breast conservation treated with a mastectomy, probably because local recurrences after lumpectomy are often leftover disease and can be "salvaged" with a mastectomy. However, local recurrences in the scar after mastectomy are more likely to be blood-borne metastases from elsewhere in the body and are harbingers of a more serious situation. Studies, both randomized and nonrandomized, have suggested, however, that removing the recurrence and giving radiation, with the addition of systemic therapy such as tamoxifen or chemotherapy, can lead to five-year remissions in 36–52 percent of such women.[11,12] The current recommendation is similar to that for a breast recurrence, described above. The biggest predictor of overall survival is the length of time between the original therapy and the recurrence—that is, the disease-free interval.[13] The later the recurrence, the better. It's a good idea to look for a clinical trial you can participate in to help us answer the questions about chemotherapy.

Rarely a woman has extensive local recurrence after mastectomy, with many nodules in the skin. They merge and act almost like a coat of armor across the chest and even into the back and the other breast. At this point we call it *en cuirasse*, a French-origin word meaning "in casing." This is because the tumor, which can be fairly limited, may block lymph vessels in this area and these, in turn, become scarred. Some women have large tumor masses on the chest wall that weep and bleed. Both of these situations are rare, but they're very distressing because you are watching the cancer grow on the outside. We believe there must be a different genetic mutation for this type of local recurrence than for distant metastasis because these women usually do not have extensive disease in the rest of their body for a long time. Unfortunately we lack a good therapy for it. Surgery cannot cut out enough tissue to clear it, and radiation therapy is limited in extent as well. Some have tried hyperthermia (very high heat) in an attempt to burn off the tumor, but its effect has also been limited. Sometimes chemotherapy gives some relief, but not always. There are reports of success using heat and chemotherapy, especially Doxil, a form of doxorubicin (Adriamycin) that tends to concentrate in skin. These cases are very upsetting for the doctor and patient, and we are still searching for the right treatment approach.

Regional Recurrence

A regional recurrence is one in the lymph nodes under the arm or above the collarbone. Now that we are taking out fewer lymph nodes from the axilla (see Chapter 14), a cancerous node can be left behind. This is rare, occurring in only about 2 percent of breast cancers. Further treatment to this area with either surgery or radiation often takes care of the problem, although systemic therapy may also be used. My cousin had a mastectomy in 1985 with a local recurrence in 1988 and another recurrence under her arm in 1994. She was already taking tamoxifen and so had the lump removed, with clean margins, followed by radiation for three weeks. She has been disease-free since. This disease is full of surprises; please don't ever write yourself off!

Regional recurrence in lymph nodes elsewhere, such as in the neck or above the collarbone, is more likely to reflect spread of the tumor through the bloodstream. Akin to local recurrence following mastectomy, it usually warrants a more aggressive approach.[14]

As physicians, we tend to downplay local and regional recurrences because they are not as life threatening as metastatic disease can be. Nonetheless, for the patient they can be devastating. When a woman gets a local recurrence, she finds it much harder than she did the first time not to think of herself as doomed. She gave it her best shot and it didn't work—how can she trust any treatment again? This became obvious to me when we first set up our support group for women with metastatic disease at the Faulkner Breast Centre in Massachusetts. I wanted to exclude women with local recurrence because I thought their situation wasn't serious enough for this group. My coworkers and patients convinced me that this was not true, and they turned out to be right. The desperate feelings are the same. Barbara Kalinowski, one of the oncology nurses there, describes the difficulties women with recurrences have, even around other women with breast cancer. "They find themselves being 'polite' in mixed groups. One woman was talking about having just had her sixth chemotherapy treatment, and the woman next to her said, 'Oh, good, you're almost through!' And she didn't have the heart to tell her this was her second time around." A woman who has gone through the tough round of surgery, radiation, and chemotherapy and thinks she has put it behind her can feel overwhelmed to find out that she has to go through it all over again. (I discuss ways to cope with this situation later in this chapter.)

DISTANT RECURRENCE (METASTATIC DISEASE)

When a cancer spreads to a different organ, it's known as a distant recurrence, or a metastasis. If a metastasis is detectable at the time of first diagnosis, the patient is described as being in stage 4 (see Chapter 11).

As hard as it is to face a local recurrence, metastatic disease can be even more devastating. It causes the same feelings that go with any recurrence, compounded by the knowledge that the chance of cure is slim. Here you need to face the fact that you are not immortal and create the best quality of life for yourself in the time you have, while maintaining hope. Contrary to common belief, metastatic breast cancer is rarely an immediate death sentence, and with good treatment women with metastasis often live for a number of years, with reasonable quality of life. Cushman Haagensen, a famous breast surgeon of the 1970s, described a few patients who lived 20 to 30 years after finding their first distant metastases. To quote Andrew Seidman, a medical oncologist from Memorial Sloan-Kettering Cancer Center in New York, you need to remember that "metastatic breast cancer often behaves biologically . . . like a novel with many chapters, fortunately, rather than a short story."[15]

Like other cancers, breast cancer can spread anywhere, but it's most likely to show up in the bones, lungs, liver, and occasionally brain. Why this is we don't know. Researchers are studying it and perhaps one day will give us a better understanding of it. The cancer cell may be making some sort of "homing" receptor for a particular organ, or perhaps the environment of certain organs is more conducive to growth for this type of cancer cell. Bone is overwhelmingly the most common organ that hormone positive breast cancer cells go to, and some physicians speculate that all breast cancer spreads to the bone before going to any other organ. This may be why bisphosphonates seem to improve the survival of breast cancer patients, even those with disease in organs such as the liver (see Chapter 17). Researchers are studying this question and perhaps one day will give us a better understanding of it.

As I mentioned in Chapter 11, when breast cancer shows up in your lungs, liver, or bones, it's still breast cancer—not lung or liver or bone cancer. We can usually tell which it is by looking at it under the microscope. We have always known that some types of breast cancers, the hormonal ones, like to spread to the bones and skin while the hormone negative ones are more likely to go to the lungs, liver, and brain. It may also be true that the estrogen negative ones also go to bone first but show up first in other organs so we discount the bone, focusing on the more life-threatening disease in the liver, lungs, and brain. More recently we have been able to refine that further with the subtypes of breast cancer discussed at length in Chapter 11. The research in the basic biology of metastatic disease has blossomed. For example, there are data in mice suggesting that the local neighborhood of the tumor can determine where the metastatic cells will be able to survive. These data also show that bisphosphonates (see Chapter 17) prevent bone metastases by changing the receptiveness of the bone to the cancer cells.

At the time I'm writing this book, nothing we know of can offer a cure for metastatic breast cancer. However, as new therapies are continuously being developed, we have reason to hope that, as with AIDS, we can one day convert metastatic breast cancer into a chronic disease. Recent studies suggest that in certain situations where the recurrence is limited and the woman can be rendered disease free with multidisciplinary treatments, 3–30 percent of women with metastatic breast cancer can be put into remission for over 20 years.[16] Is that a cure? I suspect it doesn't matter to those women what you call it—what matters is that they are alive and well.

Remember that these numbers are averages. There will always be women who are "above average." There are cases in the medical literature like that of the woman who had metastases throughout her bones, had hormone treatment, and was well 24 years later.[17] I wish we could take credit for such rare and wonderful occurrences, but we have no idea what causes the cure in any of them. Possibly these patients have cancers that remain extraordinarily sensitive to the available therapies, while most metastatic cancers have so many genetic changes that they develop resistance fairly quickly. Alternatively, occasional long survival may occur because the cancer is just very slow growing and has little or nothing to do with the therapy. Some people may think of it as a miracle—and until or unless we can prove otherwise, it's as good an explanation as any.

On a hopeful note, one population study from British Columbia, Canada, looked at survival after breast cancer recurrence and documented a steady increase in two-year survival from 34 percent in 1991 and 1992 to 45 percent in 1999 and 2001. The median survival increased from 435 days to 661 days, or 22 months, which suggests that our improved therapy is at least increasing the length of time women live with metastatic disease, if not the cure rate.[18] This trend has been confirmed by the group at MD Anderson who appear so often in this book.[19]

Many factors can help predict who will live a long time, but they're not absolute. One is the length of time between the original diagnosis and metastasis. If the metastasis shows up six months after the diagnosis, it suggests that the cancer is much more aggressive than if it's six years after the diagnosis. However, patients with metastases at the time of initial diagnosis often do quite well. This is probably because their cancer has been growing slowly below the surface for some time, unlike the woman whose cancer reappears six months after a thorough look has found no distant metastases.

Still another factor is whether or not the tumor was sensitive to hormones. We also look at how many places it's metastasized to—if there's only one or if multiple organs are involved. Where it recurs is also a consideration. Metastasis to the bone or the skin is less serious than metastasis to the lung or liver.

This is all just so many statistics, however, and as noted above, what happens to an individual woman may or may not fall within the norm. I've had patients with metastatic disease outlive the most optimistic prognosis. One patient developed lung metastasis while she was getting her adjuvant chemotherapy. So she had hardly any disease-free interval, and the cancer seemed resistant to chemotherapy. Statistically, she should have been dead within a year or two. She was treated with hormones and the cancer disappeared for two years. It came back, and another treatment made it disappear for another two years. When it came back that time, we gave another hormone. Ten years after her initial diagnosis, she died of breast cancer. When she was diagnosed she had an eight-year-old son, and she was able to raise him almost into adulthood. So we can't accurately predict the course of any individual's illness. This is true of initial disease, and metastatic disease is even more unpredictable.

Usually I find that women who have just finished breast cancer treatments don't want to think about the possibility of spread. They're busy dealing with the healing process, and a metastasis is too painful to think about. But of course it's always somewhere in the back of a woman's mind. Usually about a year after initial treatments a patient would start asking me about symptoms of metastasis. (This is an observation, not a guideline. If you want to know right away or two months later, talk to your doctor. There's nothing particularly brave about toughing it out when you're worried. Every woman's pace is different.)

In medical school, we were taught that we shouldn't tell people who had been treated for cancer what to look for if they were worried about recurrences, because they'd start imagining that they had every symptom we told them about. I've never liked that idea. It doesn't soothe people at all; it just means they'll be afraid of everything, instead of a few specific things. When you've had cancer, you're acutely aware of your body, and any symptom that's new—or that you never noticed before—can take on terrifying significance for you. Anything unexpected in your body has you petrified. Inevitably this will mean a lot of fear over symptoms that turn out to be harmless.

But if you know that the symptoms of breast cancer metastasis are usually bone pain, shortness of breath, lack of appetite, and weight loss, and neurological symptoms like pain or weakness or headaches, there are at least limits to your fear. You'll probably be frightened when anything resembling those symptoms comes up, even if it turns out to be nothing but a tension headache or a mild flu. But at least you won't be terrified by a sore spot on your big toe or an unexpected weight gain. Knowing what symptoms to look for reduces fear; it doesn't increase it. Dr. Daniel Hayes, the clinical director of the breast cancer oncology program at the University of Michigan and an old friend of mine, puts it this way: "I tell patients it is common sense: if you stub your toe and it hurts just like it did before your diagnosis of breast cancer, it is normal. If you have a new symptom that is particularly unusual, severe, and lasts longer than you expect, then you should see your caregiver. And be sure he or she remembers you had breast cancer, even 10 or 20 years ago. (I frequently see late metastases that get missed because doctors forget the patient had breast cancer once a long time ago.)"

Most women whose breast cancer has metastasized don't show any symptoms until the disease is quite extensive. It doesn't involve years and years of terrible suffering, the way TV melodrama likes to show it.

As I pointed out earlier, most recurrences are diagnosed because of symptoms noticed by the woman. Diagnosing metastatic disease early on a scan or blood test does not make the treatment easier or more effective. This means you do not have to kick yourself for not complaining sooner. If you have a symptom that feels abnormal, get it checked out but don't feel it is an emergency.

Symptoms

Symptoms appear differently in different areas of the body. So now we'll consider some of the most common sites of metastasis.

Bone. Bone, as I mentioned earlier, is the most common site of metastases in women with breast cancer. This is true partly because it's more common there than in other places, and partly because it creates definite symptoms. Even if it first appears elsewhere, as the disease progresses it usually reaches the bone at some stage.

Metastasis to the bone is generally diagnosed when the patient experiences pain. Sometimes it's hard to know if the pain is ordinary low back pain or some other condition, like arthritis. Usually the pain you get with breast cancer in the bones is fairly constant and doesn't improve over time, but it may wax and wane and it may move around. With arthritis, you wake up in the morning and feel stiff but get better as you move around during the day. Also the location is important. Pain in the feet, ankle, and hands is usually caused by arthritis or even by your treatment; tamoxifen and especially the aromatase inhibitors can cause muscle and joint pain. With some muscular problems that cause bone pain, the more you do the worse the pain gets. But the pain from cancer is steady and usually persists during the night, when you're not doing anything. Sometimes, however, it is more erratic. Oncologist Craig Henderson tells me he has been "impressed with how often the cancer pain would decrease substantially or even disappear for weeks or months on end and then reappear without any treatment at all. I think bone pain is sometimes overlooked as bone mets because it is not steady." The pain is probably caused by the cancer taking up room in the bone and pressing on it, and it can be worse in different positions and under different conditions. If you have pain that lasts for more than a week or two with no sign that it's going away, and it isn't like whatever pains have become familiar to you, you should get it checked out.

We usually check bone pain by doing a bone scan. This is a radioactive test I described in Chapter 11. It's not very specific because it can be positive for a lot of different conditions, but it's quite accurate for showing when a cancer may be present.

If the bone scan is suspicious, the next step is an X ray. If there's metastasis, this will show one of two things: either lytic lesions (holes where the cancer has eaten away the bones) or blastic lesions (an increase of bone where the growth factor of the cancer has caused the bone to get more dense). CT scans and MRI, described in Chapters 8 and 11, can be used to confirm a diagnosis of cancer in specific bones.[20] PET scanning is also being done more, although its accuracy is unproven. However, there may be a lag in time between the first evidence of cancer on a bone scan and the appearance of metastases on an X ray or even a CT scan.

A woman I know told me her experience with discovering bone metastasis. She felt generalized pain around her rib cage and groin and called her internist. He was out of town and so she was seen by a nurse practitioner, who attributed the pain to tendonitis and ordered an anti-inflammatory drug, which relieved the pain. Later when she saw her surgeon, he suggested it could be bone metastases and ordered a PET scan (a bone scan would have been as good or better). But she was feeling better and did not follow through until four weeks later, when she was hiking and experienced severe pain. She was found to have bone metastases and was started on a hormonal therapy and an intravenous bisphosphonate. She has been feeling well since but now wishes that she had followed up on the scan sooner. The result would not have been different, but she would have had pain relief earlier.

When women have cancer in their bones, we worry about the possibility of fractures. If the cancer eats away enough bone, it will no longer be strong enough to hold you up. Then you can get what's called a "pathological fracture," which is caused by something wrong in the bone itself, not by a blow from outside (Figure 20.3). It's similar to osteoporosis in that it doesn't take much to cause this fracture because the bone is so weakened. A slight pressure that usually wouldn't even cause a bruise triggers the fracture. (It's different from osteoporosis, however, in that it doesn't affect all your bones.)

Luckily the use of intravenous bisphosphonates, pamidronate (Aredia) and zolendronic (Zometa), has dramatically lowered the risk of bone fractures.[21] The exact frequency of giving these drugs is still being determined, but many oncologists are backing off on monthly treatment because of the risk of complications such as the osteonecrosis of the jaw described in Chapter 19.

We try to make sure that the key bones are not at risk. The ones to worry most about are the ones that hold you up—your leg or hip

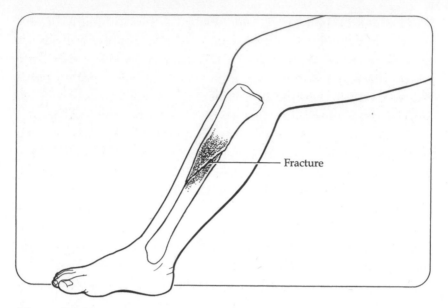

Fracture

Figure 20.3

bones. The upper arm can also fracture, but it's less likely because you don't put as much constant pressure on it. You can also get a fracture in your spine. If X rays show that a bone in a critical place has metastatic disease that puts it at risk for a fracture, we can do surgery ahead of time to pin the hip or stabilize the bone. Again, the idea is to keep you stabilized and functional, with the highest quality of life possible for the longest time possible. Bone metastases are often treated with radiation, especially if they are in a place that is likely to fracture or there are just one or two metastases that appear long after your original diagnosis. More often the patient has both radiotherapy and systemic therapy (chemotherapy or hormone therapy.) However, these therapies may kill the tumor in the bone without relieving the pain, leading you to think that the therapy hasn't worked. In these cases there may be residual fractures that haven't healed and can't be managed with radiotherapy or systemic therapy alone. Some sort of brace or, in some cases, surgical insertion of a pin or rod may be necessary to stabilize the fracture so you don't keep refracturing that area.

Lung. We also see breast cancer metastasis fairly often in the lungs. Usually the symptoms are shortness of breath and/or a chronic cough. Among patients who die of breast cancer, 60–70 percent have it in their lungs. The lungs are the only obvious site of metastasis in about 21 percent of cases. There are a couple of different ways it can form. One is in nodules—usually several—that show up on a chest X ray. If it shows only one nodule, we can't tell if it's lung cancer or breast cancer that has spread. So we do a needle biopsy or a full biopsy to find out. (Lung cancer usually starts in just one spot, but a cancer that has spread to the lung through the bloodstream or lymphatic channels is likely to hit multiple spots in the lung.)

If your breast cancer has spread to your lungs, you may experience shortness of breath on less exertion than normal. It can be fairly subtle. It comes on slowly, since the cancer has to use up a lot of your lungs before it compromises your breathing.

Another form of metastasis in the lung is called lymphangitic spread. Here the cancer spreads along the lymphatics. Instead of forming nodules it occurs in a fine pattern throughout the lung. This isn't all cancer since, like the en cuirasse of the skin described above, some of the changes in the lung are due to back-of-lymphatic drainage and fibrosis of these lymph channels. It's subtler and harder to detect on a chest X ray. It ultimately causes shortness of breath, since it takes up room and scars the lungs, making them less able to expand and contract and bring oxygen into your bloodstream.

The third way it can show is through fluid in the pleura, the lining of the lung. (The pleura is a sac with a smooth lining around it; the lung sits in it so that it can move without sticking to the chest wall.) This usually indicates that the spread is in there rather than in the lung itself. The cancer creates fluid around the lung (effusion), and the fluid causes the lung to collapse partially (see Figure 20.4). Here again, you'll experience shortness of breath. Usually breast cancer in the lungs doesn't cause pain.

If we think your cancer may have metastasized to your lung and the chest X ray doesn't show nodules, fluid, or any of the other signs, we can still do a CT scan.

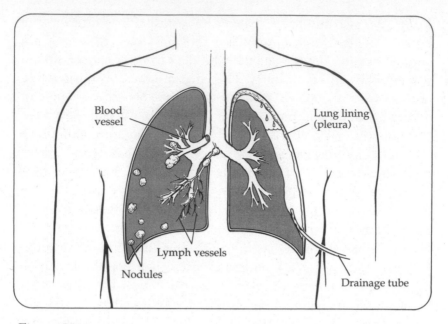

Figure 20.4

For lung metastases the treatment is usually systemic; fluid in pleura can also be treated by sticking a needle into the chest and draining the fluid. This works immediately, but frequently for only a short time. Often the fluid comes back right away. In order to prevent the reaccumulation, we fasten the pleura to the lung itself. When I was in medical school we used to open up the chest, take a piece of gauze, and rub it against the lung to irritate the spot. That got it red and raw and so it stuck together and created a scar, leaving no room for fluid. A less invasive approach is to drain the fluid through a tube and then put in material that will scar up the lining of the sac. Talc powder irritates the pleural surfaces and causes them to scar together so that fluid can't accumulate between them. However, often an effective hormonal therapy or chemotherapy will keep the fluid in the lung from reaccumulating, at least for a while. Eventually many women with recurrent pleural effusions do receive the scarring procedure with talc and chest tube drainage. Occasionally women with recurring fluid will have a catheter left in so that they can be drained as needed.

However, many women with such fluid in the pleura will get permanent relief by a combination of local drainage, scarring of the pleura (using any one of the methods just described), and a systemic therapy.

Liver. The liver is the third most common site for metastases. Again, this can be subtle. The symptoms occur because the cancer takes up a lot of room in the liver, and that takes some time to happen. About two-thirds of women who die of breast cancer have it in their liver, and about a quarter have it there initially. The symptoms are common—weight loss, anorexia (loss of appetite), nausea, gastrointestinal symptoms, and pain or discomfort under the right rib cage. You may have some pain in the right upper quadrant of your liver, which occurs when the liver's covering tissue is stretched out.

A diagnosis of liver metastasis is often suspected from blood tests and confirmed by CT, MRI, PET scanning or, on occasion, ultrasound. The major treatment for extensive liver disease is chemotherapy, especially if your liver function blood tests are elevated. Hormone therapy can work well on hormone receptor positive and slower-growing liver metastases, and the decision to use it usually depends on the extent of damage present in the liver. In certain kinds of cancer, like colon cancer, liver metastasis can be a single lesion or just a few, and thus on rare occasions can be cut out. But with breast cancer there is usually more than one spot involved and surgery becomes impossible. In the uncommon exceptions when there is only one spot, we can surgically remove part of the liver to relieve symptoms or use X ray therapy, but this is a last resort when the patient has a large, painful liver that is not responding to chemotherapy.

There are also new techniques for a small number of liver metastases that involve putting hot (hyperthermia) or cold (cryosurgery) probes into the tumors and burning or freezing them. This can help the obvious spots but must be followed with systemic therapy to control the rest of the micrometastatic liver disease.

Sometimes when patients have a lot of pain, we radiate the liver to shrink it. But we do this only for particularly severe symptoms that are not responding to systemic therapy or for the rare case of a woman whose only apparent disease is in the liver. Sometimes we put chemotherapy directly into the liver through a catheter in the artery leading into the organ, to achieve a more direct treatment of the metastases if we can't get a good a response with less drastic and more comfortable forms of chemotherapy. Liver transplants do not work in this situation because the disease is usually more extensive, not just in the liver.

Brain and Spinal Cord. Neurological metastases are less common but very serious. Breast cancer can spread to the brain and the spinal cord. It's still fairly uncommon—about 10 percent. However, women with triple negative and HER-2 positive cancers have a very high incidence of brain recurrence, between 33 and 45 percent or so. Adjuvant chemotherapy does not get into the brain as effectively as it does into the rest of the body. Because of this, we are seeing brain metastases with somewhat greater frequency as systemic adjuvant therapies have become better at eradicating disease outside the brain. This is particularly true in women with Her-2/neu overexpressing breast cancers, whose disease outside the brain is well controlled with Herceptin. The most common symptoms are headache, visual changes, and/or persistent nausea. I almost hate to say that, since most people get a lot of headaches during their lives, and I'm afraid any reader with breast cancer who gets a tension headache or the flu will be terrified. But if the headache doesn't go away in a reasonable time, check it out. In some patients it's the kind of headache that occurs with a brain tumor. It begins early in the morning before you get out of bed, improves as the day goes on, but then gets worse and worse over time.

Behavior or mental changes are sometimes, though rarely, caused by the tumor. You can have weakness or unsteadiness in walking or seizures. It can resemble a stroke: you suddenly can't talk, part of your body is abruptly very weak, or you can't see out of one eye. Those kinds of symptoms occur when a portion of your brain is blocked, which the cancer growth can cause. The best way to diagnosis it is through CT scan or MRI. About half of patients have one lesion; the rest have several.

Another kind of brain metastasis you can get is a form of meningitis called *carcinomatosis meningitis*. This affects the lining of the brain rather than the brain itself. It causes weakness in the eye and mouth muscles, headaches, stiff neck, and sometimes confusion, the way any form of meningitis does.

For brain metastases the treatment is usually radiation, which shrinks the metastasis. If there's only one or a few lesions, surgery or radiosurgery is indicated, followed by whole brain radiation therapy; this has been shown effective in improving survival[22] in a randomized controlled trial. Unfortunately this is useful only for a single or a few lesions. Radiosurgery is a technique for removing a lesion; it permits a higher radiation dose delivered to a very specific area where the tumor is, sparing surrounding tissue, but has not yet been proven to make a difference in overall survival.

You'll also probably be put on steroids—dexamethasone—right away to reduce the brain swelling, although when brain metasteses are very small, detected on screening by MRI—something increasingly done on high-risk metasteses patients—there may be no brain swelling or other symptoms and steroids may not be needed. Since the skull in which the brain sits is a hard, bony shell, there isn't much room for swelling before important structures are injured. If you're having seizures, you'll also be put on antiseizure medication. Unfortunately chemotherapy and hormone therapies don't work well on brain metastasis, although responses can occur with both.

Metastasis to the spinal cord is also very serious. This is the one area where early detection makes a big difference. The tumor can push on the cord and cause paralysis. Sometimes this happens because the bone metastasis is in the vertebrae and pushes against the spinal cord as it grows out of the bone into the spinal canal (Figure 20.5). Sometimes the tumor grows directly in the spinal cord itself. Before the paralysis, however, there are earlier symptoms—pain, weakness, sensory loss, and bowel or bladder disturbances. Pain is the most common—85–90 percent of patients with spinal cord metastasis have pain. It may be the only symptom for months. The problem is that if you have cancer only in the bones and the back, you'll also have pain. So we have to be able to differentiate, or at least be extremely alert, to be certain

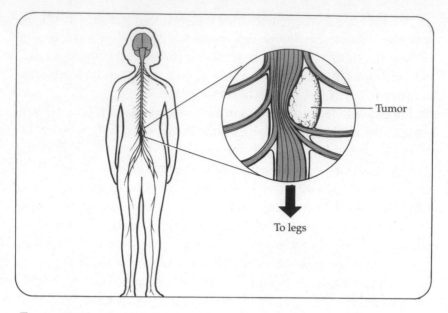

Figure 20.5

that the patient with bone metastasis in her back isn't on the verge of spinal cord compression.

Most of the pain is aching and continuous. Its onset is gradual and it gets worse over time; it often becomes severe as it pushes on the spinal cord. And it's very localized: you feel it exactly on the spot where the tumor is. There is another kind of pain that goes downward the way sciatica does, when a disk compresses the nerves and goes down your leg, getting worse if you cough or sneeze. You may also feel pain in your shoulder or back from spinal cord compression. Seventy-five percent of patients with metastasis to the spinal cord have weakness in their muscles from the tumor pushing against the nerves, and about 5 percent have spots of numbness. Anyone with metastatic breast cancer who has unrelenting pain in one spot, as well as any neurological symptoms, should be concerned. If you have no other signs of metastasis, it probably isn't spinal cord compression, since that's rarely the first sign of metastatic disease, although it can be. We diagnose it with CT scan or MRI. The treatment is generally emergency surgery if there is any evidence of nerve damage, muscle weakness, or a large tumor pressing on the spinal cord. If it's one spot, we may be able to remove the tumor and decompress the spinal cord. Surgery, if performed, is then followed by radiation therapy. Alternatively, the treatment can be emergency radiation alone; it is one of the few instances in which radiation is used as an emergency treatment. The radiation shrinks the tumor and steroids prevent the spinal cord from swelling.

Breast cancer can also metastasize to the eye, though again it's rarely the first place such spread occurs. The initial symptoms are double or blurred vision. It's diagnosed by CT scan or MRI. It's also treated with radiation, which can often prevent loss of vision.

Another area is bone marrow. The main symptom is anemia, caused by a decrease in the number of red blood cells, and the white blood cells and platelets can also decrease. Though it sounds grim, metastasis to bone marrow often responds very well to treatment, either with hormones or with chemotherapy. This remission can last for several years.

Breast cancer in all its manifestations is an unpredictable disease. These are general descriptions. As I write this, many women come to mind whose cancer didn't follow the rules. Use this information to help understand your own situation and ask questions, not as a blueprint for what will happen to you. Your situation will be unique to you no matter what happens.

Chapter 21

LIVING WITH RECURRENCE

THE TREATMENT APPROACHES TO METASTATIC DISEASE DIFFER FROM the approaches to primary breast cancer. As I have already noted, metastatic cancer is not considered curable, so our goal is twofold.

First, we want to prolong your survival by keeping the cancer well under control. Hormone therapy, immunotherapy, and chemotherapy can induce remissions that last about one year on average but, rarely, can last as long as 10 years. Some of the newer treatments for metastatic breast cancer are being shown to improve the time before the cancer begins to progress better than some of the older chemotherapy and hormone options. Remember, however, that increased time to progression does not necessarily mean increased survival. It may simply mean that you have more symptom-free time before the cancer recurs. In this case, you would live comfortably for a longer time and spend less time actually ill.

Trastuzumab (Herceptin) and the taxanes paclitaxel (Taxol), docetaxel (Taxotere), and nab-paclitaxel (Abraxane) have also been shown to substantially help some patients live longer than do the older chemotherapy regimens.[1] As the final draft of this edition was being written, a new targeted therapy for metastatic breast cancer in women with triple negative disease showed great promise.[2] This is an important first step—one we hope is the beginning of a new era in the treatment of metastatic disease.

No one knows how long someone with metastatic breast cancer will live. Therefore our second, main achievable goal is called palliation—keeping you feeling as good as you can for as long as you can. Palliation is achieved by choosing the therapies with the best chance of working and the fewest side effects. What the term "working" means depends on the situation. If the metastases significantly involve a major organ such as the liver or lungs and are compromising its function (major organ dysfunction), then you will need something that shrinks the tumor and stabilizes the situation. If your disease is stable, keeping the tumor from spreading further is the best achievable outcome of treatment.

Dr. Daniel Hayes, clinical director of the breast cancer oncology program at the University of Michigan, tells his patients that "there is bad news and good news. The bad news is you have metastatic breast cancer, meaning that it is unlikely that you will be cured with any therapy, no matter how aggressive." He stresses that both the doctor and the patient must understand this, or the patient can become disillusioned and distrustful. It is too easy for someone with a frightening disease to hear what she'd prefer to hear, and for a caring doctor to allow her to. Indeed, the reluctance to abandon high-dose chemotherapy and stem cell transplant (see Chapter 10), even with little data to support it, grew out of a lack of acceptance of the fact that we don't have a cure. "But," Dr. Hayes continues, "the good news is you have metastatic breast cancer." He explains that there are numerous therapies available to achieve palliation and they are growing yearly. They include local treatments such as surgery, radiation, cryotherapy, radiofrequency knife, chemoembolization and phototherapy. Systemic therapies include at least 18 chemotherapy drugs (both IV and oral) as well as at least 12 hormonal therapies and now four biologic or targeted therapies (see www.advancedbc.org/content/treatments-common-use-metastatic-breast-cancer for an up-to-date list). It is important to recognize that treatment for women with metastatic breast cancer continues throughout life, with short breaks. The goal is to stay ahead of the cancer, which becomes resistant to one treatment but will often respond to another.

In addition there are new supportive therapies such as bisphosphonates (which treat bone metastasis), erythropoietin (which combats anemia), antinausea drugs, white blood cell growth factors (which prevent infection), and better pain medications. "The challenge," says Dr. Hayes, "is judicious application in sequence of these treatments, which will optimize the patient's feeling as good as she can for as long as she can."

Once you are diagnosed with metastatic disease, a major source of stress is having no clear idea of what to expect—how long you will live and how much you may suffer from pain and other problems. There are two important considerations here. One is dealing with your own emotions, through counseling, a support group, religion—whatever works best for you. The other is to get as much information as your doctor has about the probable progress of your illness and what it entails. Sometimes doctors deal with a patient's fear by using every kind of therapy as rapidly and in as great a dose as possible, in an attempt to ward off the inevitable. Often the patient also goes along with this approach. But it's as dangerous as the opposite extreme of shying away from any treatment at all. In the rest of this chapter I'll explain treatments for metastatic disease, and what you can reasonably expect from them.

HORMONE (ENDOCRINE) TREATMENTS

We've known for a long time that breast cancer in women is often an endocrine disease—the endocrine glands are the ones that make hormones. We can test the cancer when the tumor is first removed and tell if it's sensitive to hormones by doing the estrogen receptor test described in Chapter 11.

In women who have metastatic disease and a tumor that's sensitive to hormones, using endocrine treatments first often makes more sense than chemotherapy, at least in the beginning, while the tumor is still sensitive to this approach. When a patient has responded to one hormone therapy, we know she's likely to respond to a second and possibly a third one—and occasionally more—so we use them in sequence.

The first hormone treatment was used in premenopausal women and consisted of oophorectomy—surgically removing the ovaries. Now we can either do this surgically or use drugs (ablation). In menstruating women whose tumors are estrogen receptor positive, the response to oophorectomy is 35 percent. This means their obvious disease will temporarily disappear. An additional 25 percent will have improved symptoms and a prolonged period of stable disease.

Removing your ovaries puts you into menopause right away, complete with mood swings and hot flashes (see Chapter 19). But it also can relieve your metastatic breast cancer symptoms almost immediately, often by the time you leave the hospital. In fact, patients with painful bone metastasis have been reported to wake up from the anesthesia post-oophorectomy pain free.

This approach went out of fashion with the introduction of chemotherapy, but it has resumed an important place in the treatment of metastatic disease with the introduction of several new drugs that can turn off the ovaries' ability to make estrogen. Such an approach can be just the right treatment for a woman with bone metastasis and an estrogen receptor positive tumor. Whether we remove the ovaries or inactivate them with drugs, the treatment is effective. Reversible menopause can be induced by using GnRH agonists such as goserelin (Zoladex) or leuprolide (Lupron) (see Chapter 17), which block FSH and LH and stop your periods.

Another way to treat breast cancer is to use drugs that can change the local hormonal milieu. This is the way antiestrogens such as tamoxifen and toremifene (Fareston) work. They can be used in both premenopausal and postmenopausal women whose tumors are sensitive to estrogen. If you were on tamoxifen in the past and then stopped, it's worth trying it again to treat your metastatic disease. On the other hand, if the metastasis became apparent while you were on tamoxifen, your tumor is probably resistant and you should try something else. Note that toremifene (Fareston) and raloxifene (Evista) work the same way tamoxifen does. Consequently if you are on one of these and your cancer comes back or grows, it is useless to switch to the other one.

In women who are postmenopausal (whether by chemotherapy or naturally) estrogen is principally made by the enzyme aromatase, which converts testosterone and androstenedione to estrogen. This enzyme is found in the adrenal glands, fat, muscle, and breast tissue. The first aromatase inhibitor used was aminoglutethimide, but it isn't very potent. In addition, it causes other symptoms by blocking the adrenal glands' production of other hormones. The most recent aromatase inhibitors—anastrozole (Arimidex), letrozole (Femara), and exemestane (Aromasin)—are more potent and specific blockers of aromatase; they are therefore much less toxic than aminoglutethimide and have very good response rates. They are currently the drugs of choice once a tumor becomes resistant to tamoxifen or even if a patient has never received tamoxifen or stopped it years ago. The aromatase inhibitors have been shown to improve women's overall survival better than the standard hormone therapy, such as tamoxifen or megestrol acetate (Megace), discussed below. The common side effects are hot flashes (30 percent) and weight gain (20 percent), as with tamoxifen, musculoskeletal pain (40 percent), and gastrointestinal complaints (5 percent). But the aromatase inhibitors work only in postmenopausal women. For premenopausal women they are ineffectual and potentially dangerous.

Fulvestrant (Faslodex) is a newer estrogen receptor blocker that does not have the estrogenic effects of tamoxifen. It benefits 20–30 percent of women when used after an aromatase inhibitor. Its effects are equivalent to tamoxifen and anastrozole.[3,4,5] It will often work in patients with tumors that have become resistant to tamoxifen and other forms of endocrine therapy. It is usually given as an intramuscular injection once monthly.

Another interesting choice for women resistant to aromatase inhibitors is estrogen, surprising though that might be.[6] One hypothesis is that cancer cells subjected to the estrogen deprivation of aromatase inhibitors become more sensitive and are responsive to low dose estrogen therapy. It seems we have to keep the cancer cells guessing.

Megestrol acetate (Megace) is a kind of progestin. Its biggest side effect is increased appetite, which leads to weight gain. This occurs in about half of patients, and they gain between 10 and 20 pounds. Twelve percent of women gain more than 30 pounds. (In fact, megestrol acetate is so likely to cause weight gain that physicians often use it to treat people with AIDS and other wasting diseases.) It has been used in women with metastatic breast cancer who have loss of appetite. Megestrol acetate works for about

20–30 percent of women and is used after the aromatase inhibitors, tamoxifen, and fulvestrant. For the rare patient who has responded to more than three lines of hormonal therapy, there is also Halotestin (fluoxymesteron).

You might think that if all these hormones work separately they'd work even better together. However, as I mentioned in Chapter 12, the ATAC study did not show a synergistic effect between tamoxifen and anastrozole in the adjuvant setting. Several studies of combination hormone therapy versus single agents have shown increased likelihood of response but no increase in overall survival, except perhaps in premenopausal women, for whom the combination of ovarian ablation and tamoxifen may be beneficial. A current trial is studying anastrozole versus anastrozole plus fulvestrant. But sequential use is a different situation: patients who respond to one therapy are more likely to respond to the next one when the first treatment fails.

Similarly, combinations of hormones and chemotherapy have no long-term advantage over either therapy alone. Patients whose tumors are ER positive but only marginally sensitive to hormones are more likely to have a response, but for those who respond to hormone therapy alone, the response from adding chemotherapy will not be longer and there will be no better survival. Moreover, the combination of hormones and chemotherapy will be much more toxic than hormone therapy alone. If a woman's tumor is ER positive, it is better for her doctors to wait to give chemotherapy if she does not respond to hormones or after she has had a response (or series of responses) and then stops responding. At that point she is very likely to benefit from the chemotherapy alone.

Some women experience a phenomenon called "flare" with hormone treatment of metastatic breast cancer (and this can sometimes occur with chemotherapy too): within the first month of therapy there is an exacerbation of the patient's disease. It actually indicates a good prognosis. Typically it occurs with someone who has bone metastasis and is put on tamoxifen. Suddenly her pain is worse than ever. But then she's back to normal soon after. We think this happens because tamoxifen actually works initially as a weak estrogen in some women, stimulating their cancer, before it starts to function as an antiestrogen. But you need to be aware of this because a flare can be very scary. We also can see a flare in the tumor markers. This is important to know because your doctor, seeing a rise in the markers, may assume that the treatment is not working, instead of recognizing the flare as a sign that it is working. Even if you don't have a flare, markers such as CEA or CA 15–3 may rise for a while before they begin to fall and you may continue to have symptoms such as bone pain (see Chapter 20 regarding microfractures or compression fractures), so be sure to give any therapy—hormones or chemotherapy—a chance to work before changing treatment. Generally you want to stay on any treatment for at least three months unless there is un-equivocal evidence that your disease is growing rapidly in spite of the treatment.

Overall, the hormone treatments work about 40 percent of the time. But it doesn't work out equally for all women. If your tumor is strongly estrogen and progesterone receptor positive, you'll have a 60 percent chance of responding. That means in over half such cases symptoms are alleviated for a significant period of time. Women with lower levels of estrogen (ER) and progesterone (PR) have a lower response rate, but it is still significant. Of the women whose breast cancers are truly ER and PR negative by modern tumor-staining techniques, only 5 percent have a chance of bene-fiting from hormone therapy. It is reasonable to try a hormone therapy in a patient who has no symptoms and whose disease is slow growing.

Usually the effects of endocrine treatments last for 12–18 months, but many women stay in remission (with their disease under control) for 2–5 years, and some are free of disease for as long as 10 years. The 24-year survivor mentioned earlier was treated with hormone therapies only. A widely held belief among medical oncologists is that chemotherapy works faster than hor-mone therapy in reversing symptoms. One reason for this belief may be that chemotherapy often results in faster tumor shrinkage, as seen on X rays. Another reason may be that patients who re-spond to endocrine therapy are usually those with the more slowly growing disease. There is probably a relationship between the rate at which the disease grows and the rate at which it disap-pears. When the tumor does show up again, especially if the patient is on tamoxifen, sometimes just stopping the drug can give a secondary response. We think this is because the antiestrogen tamoxifen can, after long periods of treatment, sometimes become estrogenic and eventually stimulate tumor growth; therefore, stopping tamoxifen can halt the growth of the tumor cells again. This "withdrawal" therapy has not been reported for the aromatase inhibitors or fulvestrant, and it is rarely used anymore because there are so many effective, low-toxicity agents to use after stopping tamoxifen.

To sum up, for the premenopausal woman, we usually start by trying ovarian ablation, by either surgical or chemical means. If she has a response, we stay with it until the symptoms recur and then go on to one of the other hormone agents not used the first time (tamoxifen or an aromatase inhibitor, depending on whether she is still menstruating). Then, if she has had her ovaries removed, we may try fulvestrant, then megestrol acetate or one of the other hormone treatments. With postmenopausal women we start with an aromatase inhibitor (since ablating the ovaries of a postmenopausal woman doesn't change much). In 25–30 percent of cases, when one kind of aromatase inhibitor fails (steroidal or nonsteroidal), changing to the other type can produce a further response.

When the tumor seems resistant to the aromatase inhibitors, estradiol may be tried before moving down the list, which includes fulvestrant (an estrogen blocker) or tamoxifen, megestrol acetate, fluoxymesterone. If a woman was on tamoxifen adjuvant therapy at the time of her metastasis we would start with anastrozole for postmenopausal women and goserelin (Zoladex) or oophorectomy for premenopausal women. Only when a woman stops responding to hormones do we go on to chemotherapy. It is important to remember that this may not be a matter of extending life but of maintaining the best quality of life for the longest time. Sometimes oncologists, especially if there is tumor in the liver or lungs, may lead off with combination chemotherapy for a number of cycles to get a quick response, before backing off to hormonal treatment to maintain it. As hormonal options are increasing rapidly, we suggest you check the practice guidelines of the NCCN for up-to-date information (www.nccn.org).

The woman with metastatic breast cancer whose tumor is sensitive to hormones is comparatively lucky, since she has more avenues of treatment that are less toxic than does the woman whose tumor is resistant to hormonal influence. As I noted earlier, however, even a woman with hormone receptor negative tumors occasionally responds to hormone therapy. This may be because the older methods of measuring ER and PR were somewhat inaccurate and women whose cancer was called negative were actually low positive. Most oncologists feel that a woman with any degree of ER or PR positivity, however small, should be given treatment with hormone therapy at some time during the course of her metastatic disease. All women with metastasis should question their medical oncologist about the possibility of hormone treatment. It may not occur to them to try a hormone maneuver first (or at all) unless you bring it up. The best quality of life is associated with less toxic but successful hormone treatments. It is always a discussion worth having, although chemotherapy is probably the better choice if you have moderate to severe symptoms or life-threatening organ dysfunction.

CHEMOTHERAPY

Chemotherapy is the best choice for women whose tumors are not responsive to hormone therapy and those whose estrogen receptor positive tumors are or have become resistant to hormone treatment. It is usually used in women with ER and PR negative tumors, and women who need a rapid response because the metastases are causing organ dysfunction. Between 20 and 59 percent of patients respond at least partially to the commonly used single-drug chemotherapy treatments, and about 10–15 percent have a complete response: their tumors vanish on X ray examination for 6–12 months. The average time to respond is around 2–3 months, which means that only half of all patients who eventually go on to respond will have evidence of it within 2–3 months. This is important because both patients and doctors often get impatient and don't give the treatment enough time. In addition, the scans and markers are not that accurate. Sometimes a 25 percent increase in the size of a lesion (within the error margins of the test) will prompt a shift in treatment. Craig Henderson points out that in the original Herceptin trial, "the earliest that any patient was evaluated was 11 weeks (the protocol called for 12 weeks), and I think it is one reason why we found the 11.3 percent responders that we did find—in someone else's hands the drug would have been abandoned."

Symptoms generally improve within a few weeks, and the average duration of the response is 5–13 months on the drug, but individual patients' responses can last longer. The maximum duration that we've so far found is over 180 months—that is over 15 years and thus could be called a cure. (Unfortunately this length of survival is very rare.) The average survival of the responders is 15–42 months. So chemotherapy, like hormone therapy, can help you live with symptom improvement for anywhere between one and four years, and there's a small chance it can give you 10 or more years of quality life.

More than 80 cytotoxic drugs—drugs that kill cells—have been tested. Thirteen are used commonly in breast cancer treatment. Interestingly, breast cancer creates the kind of tumor that is responsive to the greatest array of drugs. Most other cancers don't respond to as many chemicals (hence Dr. Hayes's "good news" observation cited above). The standard drugs are the same ones I discussed in Chapter 17 in terms of adjuvant treatment: cyclophosphamide (Cytoxan) (C), methotrexate (M), 5-fluorouracil (F), doxorubicin (Adriamycin) (A), epirubicin (E), and paclitaxel (T) or docetaxel (D). These drugs have the highest antitumor activity among all the patients studied, and only limited cross-resistance.

What is used depends on what was used at the time metastatic disease was diagnosed. If you already had CMF, then doxorubicin (or pegylated liposomal doxorubicin) (Doxil) may be tried. If you had doxorubicin when you were diagnosed, paclitaxel or docetaxel or nab paclitaxel may be the next choice. Fortunately there are other drugs as well. These include capecitabine (Xeloda), mitoxantrone (Novantrone), vinorelbine (Navelbine), gemcitabine (Gemzar), and less commonly irinotecan (Captosar), cisplatin or carboplatin, and mitomycin C, all of which have documented antitumor activity in breast cancer. They are usually given alone rather than in the combinations we use for adjuvant therapy (see Chapter 17) because possible single agent therapy simplifies treatment planning, has less toxicity, and does not appear to compromise length of survival.

Each drug has limitations. With doxorubicin, we can give only a certain dosage, and then it becomes toxic to the heart. Once you reach that point you can't ever use it again. Some of the other drugs you can take indefinitely.

Many chemotherapy drugs produce the standard side effects (vomiting, bone marrow suppression, etc.), and when the drugs are combined they tend to be worse. For this reason, giving one chemotherapy drug at a time can significantly reduce side effects. At this point a sensible approach may be to use a sequential single agent in situations where there is no organ dysfunction and mild to moderate symptoms, saving the combinations for cases with organ dysfunction and severe symptoms. As I mentioned in Chapter 17, there are now terrific antinausea drugs that have almost eliminated this problem.

Most chemotherapy drugs involve some hair loss. Several have a very low potential to cause leukemia down the road. Since you're dealing with metastatic breast cancer, though, that's not a reason to eliminate them. Most will decrease your white cell count. Attempts have been made to test the tumor cells against a variety of drugs in a test tube to predict the right drug or combination of drugs. Although it sounds like a great idea, it hasn't worked in practice as well as we would like.

While cancer cells can build resistance to a particular drug, they don't always do so. Sometimes we treat metastatic cancer with a drug and get a response; then the disease recurs and we are able to use the same drug again, and again it works. I am always amazed at how often we find a drug that doesn't work for the majority of patients but turns out to be exactly what one particular person needs. I had a patient with horrible lumps all over her chest. We treated her with just about everything, including experimental drugs, and nothing seemed to work. Then we went back and tried straight 5-fluorouracil, which usually works only modestly in breast cancer—and everything disappeared. So we sometimes can't predict what the right drug is for a particular person, and if you have metastatic disease, you need to keep that in mind. You may feel discouraged if particular drugs don't seem to be working, especially if they're the standard breast cancer drugs. But you never know when we'll hit on the one that will alleviate your symptoms.

Once we've found a drug that works, we generally continue it for a long time. How long is something on which doctors disagree. There are two philosophies. One is that we'll get as much response as we're going to get in about six months, so we should give the chemo for six months and then stop. The other philosophy is to give it continuously until the patient becomes resistant to it, and then move on to something else. There are arguments for both schools. Most of the studies suggest improved quality of life and better symptom control with continuous therapy, but again this may not be best for every woman. It's something you should discuss with your doctor and be clear about before you start treatments.

Dr. Hayes tells his patients that four things can happen with treatment for metastatic disease:

1. Terrible toxicity; it is the wrong drug and should be stopped and something else tried
2. Obvious disease progression; it is the wrong drug or the cancer has become resistant and it is time to stop that drug and try something else
3. A stable situation; it is not clear whether the drug is holding the disease in check or not; continue the drug with monitoring of disease and side effects
4. Improvement with little toxicity; it is the right drug and should be continued

It is not hard to figure out which of the four categories you are in—you know how you feel, what your physical exam reveals, and the data from X rays and markers. Often women have symptoms that are not really associated with their disease but frighten them nonetheless, leading them to assume their disease is getting worse when it is not. Oncologists too tend to assume that everything that happens is due to cancer. Both need to be sure that the tumor really is getting worse before changing drugs. For this reason many oncologists monitor the relevant X rays every three to four cycles of chemotherapy with the same tests you had in the beginning—comparing apples to apples. In addition they do routine blood tests for liver function and tumor markers (CA 15–3, 27, 29, and CEA) every three months. More recent studies have shown that we can measure specific tumor cells known as circulating tumor cells (CTC) in the blood of women with metastatic disease. If there is an increase in circulating tumor cells, you probably are on the wrong drug and should switch. A new study now taking place will examine whether this strategy actually improves survival.

It might seem that combining chemotherapy and hormone therapy would work better than either one alone. But it doesn't. In women with hormone-sensitive tumors, adding chemotherapy to hormones doesn't increase the disease-free or overall survival and they get unpleasant side effects. However, chemotherapy works just as well later after hormone therapy has been used.

Any woman with metastatic disease needs to investigate the available clinical trials. New drugs and/or new combinations of drugs and biologic agents are being tested continuously and may be the best choice for someone with metastatic disease. It's important to talk with your doctor and get clear, precise information about what drugs are best for you, how long and in what sequence you can take them, and what their side effects are.

For a while it was popular to use high-dose chemotherapy with stem cell rescue (also referred to, incorrectly, as a bone marrow transplant) to treat metastatic disease. We now have six randomized controlled studies examining its use in women with metastasis and none have shown a benefit over standard chemotherapy.[7] Although there's always a temptation to go for what appears to be the most aggressive therapy, in this case the benefit isn't worth the increased side effects for most women.

TARGETED THERAPY

We have always dreamed of finding something distinctive about the cancer cell and developing a therapy specific to it. We would then give the antibody, kill or control all of the cancer cells, and do little or no harm to the rest of the body. Recently several drugs have been developed to target other molecules that might be specific to or overexpressed by the cancer cells. Two of these are monoclonal antibodies that target Her-2 (trastuzumab) or new blood vessels that are necessary for the cancer to grow (bevacizumab). About 20 percent of women with breast cancer have too many copies of the Her-2/neu oncogene. This particular oncogene tells the cell to grow: harder, stronger, and longer. Trastuzumab is an antibody to that oncogene, which blocks it in its tracks.

There are now several trials suggesting that trastuzumab, either by itself or with chemotherapy, is very effective in Her-2/neu overexpressing breast cancer. In one larger randomized controlled trial,[8] women who received chemotherapy plus trastuzumab not only had an increased time without the cancer growing but also had an increased time in survival while they were involved in the study. However, trastuzumab can cause heart failure. This is uncommon (less than 5 percent of cases) when it is used alone or with nonanthracycline therapy, but when it was given with doxorubicin the rate of congestive heart failure rose to about 28 percent. Thus it should not be given with doxorubicin or other anthracyclines. So all women with Her-2/neu-overexpressing metastatic breast cancer should receive trastuzumab either alone or with chemotherapy unless they have preexisting heart failure. When or if breast cancer progresses on trastuzumab, it is not clear that this antibody should be continued. This has been examined in a small German study, which suggested that continuing trastuzumab after the disease grows is still worthwhile. Another option is to add a different approach to blocking Her-2/neu, such as Lapatinab. This is being used in combination with trastuzumab, or for women who are become resistant to trastuzumab in place of it.

In 2004 the second monoclonal antibody to be used for metastatic breast cancer was reported. The antiangiogenesis drug bevacizumab (Avastin) is an antibody to VEGF, a growth factor responsible for inducing new blood vessels to grow and feed the tumor. Angiogenesis is the cancer's attempt to develop new blood vessels to support its growth. With drugs that block this function, the cancer theoretically will not be able to get enough nourishment from its inadequate blood vessels and will die. In a review of the five studies that have been done there was a greater benefit when bevacizumab was added to chemotherapy than in chemotherapy alone.[9] This is big news on two levels. As with trastuzumab, the next step will be to see if it has any benefit in women who are newly diagnosed.

Other forms of immunotherapy such as vaccines are also being tested. Although we commonly think of a vaccine as prevention, such as the ones used for polio or measles, it can also be used in treatment. These vaccines are made by training immune cells to hone in on a certain target found on breast cancer cells. It sounds great, but problems have prevented it from being effective so far. For one thing, not every cancer cell is the same. This means that a vaccine against one element such as Her-2 will kill only the cells that express it, leaving the others behind. Vaccines for metastatic breast cancer are being tested in clinical trials and may be useful in the near future.

BISPHOSPHONATES

Most of the treatments we have considered involve killing or controlling the cancer cell. The other approach is to alter the tissue that the cancer is trying to grow in. A bisphosphonate is a drug that blocks the resorption (breakdown) of bone, as previously discussed. It has been shown to be very effective in treating bone metastasis. When there is cancer in the bone, the bone is resorbed—one of the reasons the bone gets weaker and often fractures. Several studies have shown that women who take pamidronate (Aredia) or zolendronic acid (Zometa) every four weeks will have a decrease not only in the resorption of the bone but also in the number of new bone metastases that develop and the incidence of bone fractures and bone pain.[10,11] One study also suggested that it decreased other sites of metastatic disease, although this has not been confirmed yet by other studies. It certainly is worth taking if you have bone metastasis. However, there may be complications in the jaw as described in Chapter 17, and many oncologists are deferring IV bisphosphonate use or using it only every three months.

OTHER TREATMENTS

I've been discussing systemic therapies so far, but sometimes local treatment is called for. Certain kinds of metastatic disease respond best to local treatments because they're local problems.

Radiation, for example, works best if the cancer has spread to your eye. Spinal cord involvement with impending bone fracture (in which your bone is so weakened that it is about to break) also lends itself well to radiation, since it too is a local problem and there is only one spot to be treated. For impending bone fractures following spinal cord compression, surgical treatment is often needed to stabilize the bone before radiation.

Radiation for metastatic cancer is the same as for initial breast cancer, but its purpose is different—to alleviate pain or other symptoms. A couple of weeks usually pass before the pain noticeably lessens. After any treatment of any organ, and especially bone, healing of damage from the cancer must occur before fully normal function returns. Thus, just as it takes months after you break a bone for normal tensile strength to return, it takes months after the treatment with radiotherapy to have normal bone strength again. During this time it is easy to fracture the bone, and in some cases you'll never regain full strength because the therapy (especially radiotherapy) may reduce the bone's capacity to heal fully.

The timing is somewhat different too. There are usually 10–15 treatments, spread over two and a half to four weeks. A smaller dose of radiation is used. While a primary radiation treatment to your breast might use 6,000 centigrays of radiation over six and a half weeks, with 180 centigrays per treatment, the treatment for someone with, for example, bone metastasis in the hip might use 3,000 centigrays over 10 treatments of 300 centigrays each.

Surgery, as I mentioned earlier, is best if there is one spot in the lung or brain, for example, in a woman who has had a reasonably long interval between primary diagnosis and development of metastatic disease. If the cancer has recurred in several places, however, systemic treatment is best.

Pain Control

In terms of palliation—getting rid of symptoms so you feel better—treatments of the cancer itself aren't the only options. We've come an enormous way in pain control. If, for example, you're in severe pain because of bone metastasis, we now have ways of putting a catheter in the space along the spinal cord and dripping continuous low-dose morphine to get rid of all the pain. Administered this way, it won't affect your mind the way it would if administered systemically. This won't cure you, but in your last three or four months of life, when systemic therapy is no longer working, it can give you quality time and reduce or eliminate suffering. There's now a whole specialty of pain management that includes psychiatrists, anesthesiologists, and internists. Since a thorough discussion of all the options lies outside the scope of this book, suffice it to say that we have acquired a lot of knowledge about chronic pain and how to deal with it. Anybody who has chronic pain because of metastatic cancer and isn't getting relief should ask to be referred to a pain unit. Sometimes oncologists and people who work on cancer are so focused on treating and curing the disease that they forget about these ancillary things that can make an enormous difference in a patient's life. So ask to see a pain specialist; even if it means having to travel to the local medical school, it can make a big difference to you.

And beware of uninformed medical personnel who still worry about addiction to narcotics in terminally ill patients. They are not going to "abuse" the drugs; they are simply going to suffer less. Nor should drug abuse in the larger population be an excuse for withholding pain relief from patients who need it. Effective pain drugs like Oxycontin have even been dropped from pharmacies in New England for fear of theft. While drug abuse is a serious problem, not treating people's pain is also a form of abuse.

Experimental Treatments

This is a perfect time for women to participate in phase 3 clinical trials (see Chapter 10)—trials of drugs or treatments that have been tested in earlier phases and shown not to harm the patient. There is a trickier area to consider with metastatic cancer too—

phase 1 or phase 2 trials. These are earlier stages in the testing of a drug, designed to determine first the toxicity of a possibly useful drug and then whether it works.

Since you know that traditional treatments, which were so helpful with your first diagnosis, offer only a slim chance of cure, an experimental treatment may be worth considering. Generally there is no harm in trying an innovative new therapy and postponing treatment with other standard therapies.

When is the best time to join an experimental trial? Classically, people do it when nothing else has helped and they've run out of options. However, by the time you run out of options you're least likely to be able to respond to the new treatment: you have no resources left. So the best time may be when you have been diagnosed with metastatic disease but are feeling well. You have a chest X ray or bone scan that shows a lesion but you have modest symptoms. At this stage, there's no rush to use chemotherapy or hormone therapy since, as I noted before, there's no evidence that treating with chemo earlier will give you better survival odds than waiting until you have symptoms. If you now try something experimental, you have an opportunity to see if it works; if it doesn't you can still get the usual chemotherapy if symptoms worsen.

Only a doctor who is working on the particular experiments is likely to offer such treatments routinely. The best way to find out about them is to go to your local cancer center and see what they're involved in. You can also go to www.clinicaltrials.gov and obtain a list of every clinical trial you're eligible for, either in your own geographical area or in the whole United States if you're willing and able to travel. You can also register at www.breastcancer trials.org to be notified regarding trials you may be eligible for.

I think this is really worthwhile. It's a gamble, but sometimes the gamble pays off. For example, some of the women who first participated in the tests for docetaxel or trastuzumab had a remarkable response that lasted between 18 and 24 months. Another good example is one of the patients on the first trastuzumab (Herceptin) trial. When this trial started, it was not clear that this drug would cause tumors to shrink, but we did know that patients whose tumors overexpressed Her-2 did not respond well to conventional chemotherapy or hormone therapies. When the trial was complete, only 5 out of 43 patients in the study had evidence of tumor shrinkage. One of those patients had experienced a recurrence in the chest wall shortly after receiving doxorubicin. We knew from both her Her-2 status and the rapidity of the disease recurrence that her prognosis wasn't good. After the trial, the disease in the chest wall disappeared completely, and the last I heard she was still tumor free more than a decade after going on the study. This dramatic, long-lasting response doesn't happen too often in phase 1 and phase 2 trials, but every so often it does, and this is what makes it worthwhile for the individual patient to participate in these studies.

Exciting new experiments are going on for metastatic disease. One example is the PARP inhibitors that are showing great promise in triple negative and BRCA-positive disease—a form of breast cancer that does not respond well to conventional treatments. Clinical trials are going on with this category of drugs.

While they may help you, these trials can involve side effects as well. But only you can decide what price in toxicity you are willing to pay. Some women want to try everything new and others don't. Don't let yourself be pushed by your doctor or family. Decide in your own heart what the best approach is for you.

During and after your treatment for metastatic disease you'll be followed with staging tests—bone scan, chest X ray, and blood tests—as well as a few other tests such as CT scans, PET scans, or MRI. These can help determine if you're indeed responding to treatment, although your symptoms are the best test of effectiveness.

TAKING CARE OF YOURSELF EMOTIONALLY

Women with metastatic disease often feel very isolated. Other survivors, finding their stories too scary, may not want to listen to them, and family and friends may not be able to deal with the seriousness of the situation. Luckily there are many women living with breast cancer recurrences and metastatic disease who are willing to help you at the click of a mouse. Advocate Musa Mayer participates in a listserv for women with metastatic disease (http://bcmets.org), and she maintains the websites www .advancedbreastcancer.org and www.brainmetsbc.org. These sites have a wealth of information regarding the latest treatments as well as reports of women's experiences with them, like the message from Cindi on their home page about how she has been in treatment for metastatic breast cancer for nine years and is still working as a zookeeper! I strongly recommend them.

David Spiegel tells the story of a woman who had always wanted to write poetry and started after her diagnosis of metastatic disease. She had a book of poems published before her death. One of my own patients, Susan Shapiro, was very distressed with the lack of analysis of breast cancer from a feminist political perspective. She wrote an article in the local feminist paper and called a meeting. From this she started the Women's Community Cancer Project in Boston a few months before she died. I'm certain she would be happy to know her work sparked a national movement that continues today.

A diagnosis of recurrence or metastasis will remind you that you do not have control over your body. But you certainly do have control over your mind, emotions, and spirit. This is a good time to revisit some of the complementary treatments such as visualization, self-hypnosis, and imagery (see Chapter 18). And find a doctor you can talk to and who will listen to you. Shop around if you have to. If you are in a small town and/or have an insurance plan with limited choice, then schedule an appointment with your oncologist so that you can talk about what you need, as well as what she or he expects from you. (See Appendix C for the patient's and doctor's rights.) You need to know as accurately as possible what to expect from your condition and your treatments so that you can plan. Ask for the information you need and tell your doctor if there are things you would rather not know. As in any relationship, frank communication about your needs will go far toward having them met.

There are two main fears that accompany a diagnosis of recurrent breast cancer: pain and death. As I discussed earlier in this chapter, pain is certainly not inevitable. Pain control has finally gone mainstream in the United States. There are pain centers, and many methods have been developed to deal with pain without clouding your mind and ruining your life.

Not everyone dies from a recurrence or metastatic breast cancer, but it is certainly a possibility. Spiegel's book *Living Beyond Limits* is invaluable in addressing the needs of the heart and soul in confronting terminal illness.[12] You may not be able to avoid death, but you can control how you want to handle it. One of my patients was a great denier. From the first moment of her diagnosis she refused to let her cancer interfere with her life. When she developed metastatic disease, this pattern continued. She continued to hurl herself through life: sailing, traveling, and enjoying herself. My first reaction was to be a little critical of her inability to face the reality of the situation, until I realized that she *had* faced it. She knew exactly what she was doing and was determined to take control of whatever time she had left. She slipped into a coma on her sailboat among friends and died as she wanted, where she wanted, in control to the end.

WHEN TO STOP TREATMENT

When a patient would ask me, "How long do I have to live?" I'd never answer—not because I wanted to withhold information but because I simply didn't know. There are statistical likelihoods, but they do not tell what will happen to each individual. There are patients who, according to the statistics, should die in four months but live four years; there are others who should last four years but die in four months. I'm always amazed at the variations. One of my patients had a small cancer and negative nodes with what should have been a good prognosis, but when she finished her radiation we discovered the cancer had metastasized to her lungs, and she died in three months. Another patient, a Chinese woman who spoke no English, had a cancer that was very bad, and I privately thought she wouldn't live very long. I had to talk to her through her sons, who kept trying to get me to say how long she had. I wouldn't tell them. It's a good thing, because she was still alive seven years later. Sometimes I think she lived so long because she didn't know she was supposed to die.

At the same time, it's important for your doctor to be honest with you. I think it's sensible to say to a patient who has asked for a frank response, "This is serious, but we don't know how long you'll live until we see how you respond to treatment. You'll probably eventually die of breast cancer, and you probably won't live another 40 years, so you may want to plan your life with that in mind." If you insist on more specific predictions, a doctor may quote statistics—but you should always be reminded that there are exceptions to statistics. If 99 out of 100 patients in your condition die within a year, 1 out of 100 doesn't—and there's no reason to assume you won't be that one. You should know that this is a hard task for your doctor, who really wants to "get it right" for you, neither denying you a chance of extra life in which you might accomplish things you want to get done or putting you through needless treatment that only makes the last days more miserable. This is something the doctor can learn only by experience. They don't teach it in medical school, and this is a situation where a doctor who has been through this many times before may have an advantage.

Eventually, however, there comes the hardest part. We've tried all the available treatments, and we know that you don't have much longer. Even then, we don't know if it's days or weeks, and there is still the possibility of a miracle. But there's a point at which you're clearly dying, and you have a right to know that. The prevailing belief used to be that it was better not to tell patients they were dying. But this sets up an unhealthy climate of denial. It's likely you'll sense it yourself, but since no one wants to talk about it you pretend it's okay in order to spare them, and they pretend it's okay in order to spare you. Such denial can keep you from finishing your business—clearing up relationships, saying good-bye, saying the things you won't get another chance to say to the people you love, giving them the chance to say those things to you. I think doctors make a great error in denying death: we tend to look at it too much as a defeat and get caught up in our own wishful thinking, at the patient's expense.

While you're still feeling fairly well, you may want to talk with your doctor, and with your family members or friends, about how you want to die when the time comes. Do you want to be kept alive at all costs, or not? Do you want to die at home, or in the hospital?

Often people die in a hospital or a nursing home, and many think of that as an inevitability. But it isn't, and it's important to consider whether it might be better for you to die in your own home or in the home of a loved one. For many people this is the best option, particularly if a loved one is able to stay with you full-time. Dying at home offers more control over your surroundings and a greater likelihood that you will die with loved ones around you. If this is an option you want to explore, there are many hospice programs that can help you. They are experienced in caring for both the patient and the family in a way that can make all the difference. I had firsthand experience when my cousin was dying of bile duct cancer, and I cannot say enough about how terrific they are.

For some women and their families, this is not possible. If it makes more sense for you to die in a hospital, there is much you and your loved ones can do to ensure that the environment is as comfortable as possible. Many hospitals have hospice rooms for dying patients, and even those that don't can make a regular room more homelike. You will want to discuss your wishes with the caregivers there, to be sure they are willing and prepared to follow them.

There are other issues you'll want to look into—perhaps even before you have decided that it's time to stop fighting your illness. When the time comes—whether in months or years—do you want to be heavily medicated or as alert as possible? No way is universally better, but one way might be better for you. If your wishes are clearly known—especially if they can be documented in a living will—you might be able to prevent those tragic situations in which doctors and family members are fighting over whether to keep you on a life-support system.

A living will is only part of an advance directive—a set of written instructions that also include a health care proxy. The living will spells out what medical treatment you do and don't want if the time arrives when you are unable to verbalize your own decisions. A health care proxy specifies a particular person you authorize to make decisions about your care when you no longer can.

Living wills vary from state to state, and in some cases you may need to add information to yours. As Dr. Daniel Tobin writes in *Peaceful Dying*, the language of the typical living will may not be specific enough.[13] If the document merely says you don't want life-prolonging measures if you have an "incurable or irreversible condition," your doctor may define such a condition differently than you do. So you might want to add a specific "do not resuscitate" to your living will, and other additions concerning artificial nutrition and hydration. You need to spend some time thinking about what you do want when the time comes. Do you want to be tube-fed? Do you want to be given antibiotics to fight infections? Or do you prefer to die from the infection rather than continue for a short time and die of your cancer? These things may not be fun to think about, but they're important.

Betsy Carpenter, a speaker and activist around issues of advance directives, emphatically agrees. You may or may not want life-extending treatment at some point, and you have a right to decide. It's important to make those decisions before you reach the point where you can no longer speak for yourself. Like Dr. Tobin, Carpenter stresses the importance of talking with your family and friends in advance, discussing the options open to you and how you feel about them, and listening respectfully to the feelings of your loved ones. Your illness and your ultimate death will affect those who love you deeply, and it's important to involve them in your decision-making process. Understanding your feelings and sharing theirs with you will make it far less likely that they'll go against your wishes when the time comes.

In deciding what you do and don't want, Carpenter advises, think about four areas in particular. What are your fears? Most people fear pain, loss of control, inappropriate prolongation of life, and becoming a burden to loved ones. Each of these fears should be explored fully, in terms of what is reasonable to think may happen and in terms of your own emotions.

Pick out your health care proxy carefully, she says, and spell out who you don't want involved in making health care decisions for you as well. "This doesn't have to be hostile," she says. "You can write, 'although I dearly love my son Jim, I don't wish him to have any part in decision making around my care.'" The agent you choose should be someone you love and fully trust to honor your wishes, who knows you well enough to make decisions that you haven't spelled out, in ways that you would want. "For example," she says, "my husband is my proxy agent, and he knows that I wouldn't want my life artificially prolonged. But suppose my daughter, who lives in London, wasn't here when I went into a coma. He might be certain that it was important for her to see me living and breathing one last time. So he might decide to keep me on life support for 24 hours until she could get back home. And he would know that, loving her, I would also want this for her." Because of such contingencies, she adds, while your living will should be specific, it shouldn't be too specific to preclude your agent from making judgments in such unforeseen circumstances. You may want to write out a declaration of precedence: "If a conflict arises between my list and my agent's decision, I give precedent to my agent over my own written word."

If there is someone you don't want visiting you when you're dying, this too should be spelled out, says Carpenter, in a priority of visitation statement. Such documents are important even for those not facing imminent death, she says. Healthy people are sometimes injured in accidents and lose the ability to verbalize their wishes.

And remember that there is no universally right choice. You may want to be allowed to die if, for example, you're in a reversible coma. On the other hand, you may decide that no one can know absolutely if a coma is irreversible and you want to have whatever chance there is to go on living, even if that chance is minute. A woman I know tells of walking with a friend and passing an old-age home, where a very elderly, frail man in a wheelchair sat staring in front of him, seemingly unaware of his surroundings. Her friend shuddered and said, "I wouldn't want to live if it had to be like that." My friend shook her head. "Maybe he's looking at the trees and feeling the breeze on his face, and maybe that's worth living for." Neither woman was right or wrong.

These scenarios are important for every one of us to consider, since none of us is immortal, and death can come for anyone anytime. Of course, you may live another 10 or 20 years, but you lose nothing by having those discussions, and you might even gain some peace of mind.

Epilogue

ERADICATING BREAST CANCER: POLITICS AND RESEARCH

THE POLITICS OF BREAST CANCER

Breast cancer has certainly come out of the closet in the past several years. There are three-day walks, mountain climbs, races for cure, bike rides, art exhibits, lobby days, gala fund-raisers, and pink ribbons. Few women are embarrassed to admit they have breast cancer, and all are aware of the advances we have made. With all this publicity and public support, it's easy to forget that this awareness is a relatively new phenomenon. The first edition of this book made no mention of the politics of the disease: there were none. The second edition chronicled its birth. And someday soon we will be able to rest on our laurels because politics will not be necessary. Until that day I think it is very important that we continue to remember and record our recent history. For those of you who have been a part of it—read with pride. For those who are just joining the sisterhood—know that you stand with many strong women before you.

The politics of breast cancer had its forerunners more than 50 years ago. In 1952 the American Cancer Society started the Reach to Recovery program. This was a group of breast cancer survivors who were helping newly diagnosed women. Members of Reach to Recovery, all of whom had undergone mastectomies, would visit the patient in the hospital and reassure her that there was life after surgery. They were, as they continue to be, a wonderful resource for women with breast cancer.

From there, support groups for women with breast cancer evolved. Women sat together and talked about their experiences and their feelings. It was tremendously helpful for these people to learn they were not alone. Others shared their feelings about their disease, which was shrouded in so much mystery and fear.

All this underlined the fact that there was little psychological support from the medical profession; you had to get it from somewhere else. And since breast cancer continued to be hidden from public view, there remained an aura of something shameful and disreputable about it.

The next big step came in the 1970s, when famous women such as onetime child actor Shirley Temple Black, first lady Betty Ford, and Happy Rockefeller, the wife of the then-governor of New York, told the world they had breast cancer. Their openness began to create an environment in which breast cancer could be looked at as a dangerous disease that needed to be addressed by public institutions, rather than a private and shameful secret. There was a dramatic increase in the number of women in America who got mammograms, and in the number of breast cancers diagnosed.

Those were the days of the one-step procedure. You'd go in for the biopsy; it would be done under general anesthetic; and, if the lump was positive, your breast would be immediately removed.

1n 1977 Rose Kushner, a writer who had breast cancer, wrote a groundbreaking book entitled *Why Me?* It ushered in the two-step procedure. Kushner saw no reason for a woman to have to decide whether to have a mastectomy before she even knew whether she had breast cancer. She argued passionately that it was important for the woman to have her biopsy, learn if she had cancer, and then, if she did, decide what avenue to pursue. Doctors were still working on the erroneous assumption that time was everything: if they didn't get the cancer out the instant they found it, it would spread and kill the patient. Kushner had done enough research to realize that a few weeks between diagnosis and treatment wouldn't do any medical harm, and would do a great deal of emotional good. She pushed for the two-step procedure, and her book influenced large numbers of women to demand it for themselves.

Another force on the horizon at that time was Nancy Brinker. Brinker's sister, Susan G. Komen, was diagnosed with breast cancer in 1977 and died in 1980. In 1983 Brinker founded the Susan G. Komen Breast Cancer Foundation, now called Susan G. Komen for the Cure, which is based in Dallas, Texas. Ironically, Brinker herself was diagnosed with breast cancer soon afterward. Since the mid-1980s the foundation has been working to raise money for research and for making mammograms available to more women. They organized the yearly Race for the Cure, which takes place in a number of cities.

By the 1980s the second wave of feminism had emerged, demanding redress for all of the inequities against women. Participants adopted the old Marxist expression "the personal is political" and began to define many social realities in a larger context: rape, battered wives, the need for child care. A large component of the movement worked on health issues, promoting the need for women to take control of their own health and learn all they could about their own bodies. Doctors would no longer be seen as omniscient father figures, and would become medical specialists who worked with their patients to help them determine individually what was best for them in any health situation.

Then in the late 1980s, almost spontaneously in different parts of the country, a number of political women's cancer groups sprang up. One, whom I spoke of earlier, was in the Boston area, started by a patient of mine, feminist writer Susan Shapiro. When she was diagnosed with breast cancer, she began to search for anyone working on the political issues around women and cancer. She didn't find anything but remained passionately convinced that there were political implications to cancer. She wrote an article entitled "Cancer as a Feminist Issue" for the feminist newspaper *Sojourner*, in which she announced a meeting at the Cambridge Women's Center. A lot of women who had been as frustrated as she by the lack of political response to their disease showed up. They formed the Women's Community Cancer Project. Their scope was fairly broad. It included all cancers that women got as well as women's role as caregivers for children, spouses, and parents with cancer. Inevitably, much of the focus was on breast cancer. Shapiro died in January 1990, but the project continues to exist.

Around the time the Women's Community Cancer Project was beginning, the Women's Cancer Resource Center in Oakland, California, Breast Cancer Action in the Bay Area, and the Mary-Helen Mautner Projects for Lesbians with Cancer in Washington, D.C., got under way. All of these groups were aware of the work the AIDS movement had been doing when for the first time we were seeing people with a killer disease aggressively demanding more money for research, changes in insurance bias, and job protection. Women with breast cancer took note of that, particularly feminists. Like gay activists with AIDS, they were aware of ways in which social systems contributed to disease and to the medical responses around them. They understood that this needed to be confronted politically.

At the time these groups were emerging, I was finishing the first edition of this book. As I went on my book tour, talking with women, I began to realize how deep women's anger was, and how ready they were to do something. The key moment for me was in Salt Lake City in June 1990, when I gave a talk to 600 women. It was a weekday afternoon, and the audience was mostly older women. It was a pretty long talk, and at the end I said, "We don't know the answers, and I don't know what we have to do to make President [HW] Bush wake up and do something about breast cancer. Maybe we should march topless to the White House." I was making a wisecrack, hoping to end a somber talk with a little lightness.

I got a great response, and afterward women came up to me asking when the march was, how they could sign up for it, and what they could do to organize it. I realized that this issue touched all kinds of women throughout the country, and that they were all fed up with the fact that this virtual epidemic was being ignored. I saw that it wasn't just in the big centers like San Francisco and Boston and Washington, D.C., where I'd have expected to see political movements springing up. It was everywhere. Women were ready to fight for attention to breast cancer.

I felt that we needed a national organization to give these women the hook they needed to begin organizing. I spoke to Susan Hester of the Mautner Project, Amy Langer of NABCO (the National Coalition of Breast Cancer Organizations), and Nancy Brinker of the Komen Foundation about the idea. We were all enthusiastic, and the result was a planning meeting. The initial groups involved included Breast Cancer Network of Strength (formerly Y-ME), the Women's Community Cancer Project, Breast Cancer Action, Cancer Care, and Canact from New York. Then we called an open meeting to be held in Washington and wrote to every women's group we knew of.

We had no idea who'd show up. On the day of the meeting the room was packed. There were representatives from all kinds of groups; the American Cancer Society and the American Jewish Congress were there. So was the Human Rights Campaign Fund, a big gay and lesbian group. There were members of breast cancer support groups from all around the country, such as Arm in Arm from Baltimore, the Linda Creed group from Philadelphia, and Share from New York. Overall there were about 100 or so individuals representing 75 organizations. We were overwhelmed, and we started the National Breast Cancer Coalition on the spot. Out of that meeting came the first coalition board.

Amy Langer of NABCO chaired the initial meetings until the bylaws and officers could be chosen. A year later Fran Visco, a lawyer from Philadelphia who had breast cancer in her late thirties, became the first elected president, and remains the president today. Our first action, in the fall of 1991, was a project we called Do the Write Thing. We wanted to collect and deliver to Washington 175,000 letters, representing the 175,000 women who would be diagnosed with breast cancer that year, and we wanted the number of letters from each state to match the number of women there who would get breast cancer. We managed to identify groups in each state who could work with us. In October we ended up with 600,000 letters—it was an enormous response. On the day we delivered the letters to the White House, the guards just stood there; nobody would help us lift the boxes. So all these women who'd had mastectomies were lifting heavy boxes of letters onto the conveyer belt.

We were all certain that the letters would be dumped into the shredder—that our first action had been a flop. But in reality, we had succeeded on a number of levels. For one thing, we had organized in such a way that we had a group in every state. That meant a large and potentially powerful organization. For another, even if the White House ignored us, the members of Congress didn't. When we started lobbying for increased research money, they granted us $43 million more, raising the 1993 appropriation to $132 million. That was a small triumph.

We held hearings to determine how much research money was really needed, and it was one of the first times scientists and activists interested in breast cancer had met together. This created an interesting coalition. As a result of the hearings we decided we needed $433 million for breast cancer research. The total budget was $93 million, so we started lobbying for $300 million more, armed with our report based on scientists' testimony.

At first the reaction was overwhelmingly negative. Everybody in Congress kept saying there was no money and it would be impossible to come up with anything like another $300 million. But we kept at it, and when the politicians told us there wasn't anymore money, we said, "Well, you found money for the savings and loan bailout. You found money for the [first] Gulf War. We think you can find this money too, if you really decide it's important that women are dying." We testified in the Senate and the House. We lobbied, we sent faxes, and we called. But despite support from many Congress members we couldn't figure out how to get enough money.

Then Senator Tom Harkin noticed that, amazingly, in the past there had been some money for breast cancer in the Defense Department—$25 million spent on mammogram machines for the army. At our urging he decided to try and increase that to $210 million. Added to an increase in the NIH funding, that would bring the total to $300 million.

At that point, the Defense Department people were so worried that the firewall between the domestic budget and the defense budget might be breached that they agreed to have a breast cancer research program within the DOD!

So there was $210 million in the Defense budget and the extra $100 million in the NCI budget. That was $10 million over the $300 million we had gone after. Against all odds, we had succeeded. Part of it was being in the right place at the right time. But most of it was the enormous amount of work all the women in the coalition and around the country had put in. Overnight we gained an enormous amount of clout and became recognized as a force to be reckoned with.

We were ready to move on to our next step: we wanted to have a say in how the money we had raised was spent. We wanted women with breast cancer to be involved in the decision-making panels on review boards for grants, on the National Cancer Advisory Board, and in all the decision making. We started lobbying, and our next major project was to deliver 2.6 million signatures to the White House in October 1993 to represent the 2.6 million women living with breast cancer at the time—1.6 million who knew they had breast cancer and 1 million who were yet to be diagnosed. We mobilized around the country collecting signatures, and we delivered our 2.6 million signatures to President Clinton on October 18. As a measure of how far we'd come from October 1991, this time we were welcomed in the East Room, where Fran Visco and I shared the stage with Hillary and Bill Clinton, along with Donna Shalala, secretary of Health and Human Services. The room was filled with 200 of our people. It was an awesome moment.

And President Clinton followed up. In December we had a meeting of activists, politicians, scientists, doctors, laypeople, and businesspeople to set national strategy, and we came up with a national action plan. Each of the subgroups working on this plan included one of our activist members. We were all at that table and we were changing the policy of business as usual around breast cancer.

Being with the scientists, talking and working with them, the activists learned that the answers aren't always easy, that scientists have to work months and years to come up with one useful discovery. The scientists saw that the activists weren't shrill, uninformed troublemakers but intelligent, concerned people fighting to save their own and others' lives.

One of the reasons we wanted the money from the Department of Defense was to attract new people, to get researchers working on new aspects of breast cancer. And it worked. When the $210 million was made available by the Department of Defense, they got 2,400 grant applications. Many of these were from people who had never done breast cancer research before. The DOD program has thrived over these years, although we still have to fight for the money each year in Congress. The National Breast Cancer Coalition also continues to do the difficult work of challenging the status quo and representing real change. One big win was the enactment of the Breast and Cervical Cancer Treatment Act. After four years of an intense and aggressive grassroots lobbying campaign this legislation was signed into law, guaranteeing treatment to low-income uninsured women screened and diagnosed with breast and cervical cancer through the CDC National Breast and Cervical Cancer Early Detection Program. Before the law went into effect, poor women could be diagnosed but there was no money for treatment. Other work passed two Medicare bills—one to make sure that breast cancer drugs were covered by Medicare and one requiring Medicare to cover the cost of routine patient care associated with clinical trials.

Through Project LEAD, a program that brings scientists together for a weekend to teach advocates the basics if breast cancer research, we are currently training activists to be effective advocates and to contribute when they get a seat at the table. The yearly Advocacy Conference in the spring in Washington puts it all to good effect, as advocates meet with Congress to lobby for our cause. And we are fighting for research into the causes of breast cancer, how to prevent it and how to cure it. The increase in environmental research as well as in basic research is in part in response to our efforts. We want to attract more basic research, rather than focus all our energy on how to treat existing disease.

I've learned through this that you really can affect how the government acts. A small group of committed people can do a lot. So few people let their feelings be known that the people who do it, and who do it vociferously, get an undue amount of power. We didn't have any money, but we were organized.

Our movement continues to grow. Many of the women in the coalition have never been involved in political action before. Now they find themselves working side by side with the baby boomers who marched in the 1960s and learned the value of political protest and who now are confronting breast cancer, realizing that, like civil rights and war resistance and the early women's movement issues, breast cancer research needs to be fought for.

The current breast cancer political movement is becoming international. The National Breast Cancer Coalition has held two international conferences in Brussels and is helping nascent politic groups get started in Eastern Europe and Africa. The Komen Foundation has held the Race for the Cure in Italy, Germany, and Argentina, and is spreading its message of empowerment. Women all over the world are learning that this is more than a personal issue.

The issues that are being addressed have broadened as well. The NBCC is involved with setting the standards for quality breast care, and the Komen Foundation has funded a large project with the American Society for Clinical Oncology to identify the level of care that is currently being delivered. All of the political groups have taken up the cause of clinical enrollment and are helping to educate women about the benefits of participating in trials. Breast cancer politics have matured beyond pink ribbons and shower cards.

PUSHING THE ENVELOPE: THE DR. SUSAN LOVE RESEARCH FOUNDATION

While documenting the changes in the diagnosis and treatment of breast cancer, the *Breast Book* through its five editions has also chronicled over 20 years of my career, from clinical practice and the birth of advocacy, through academics and work on the multidisciplinary delivery of breast cancer to research in my own foundation on what causes the breast to get cancer in the first place.

Throughout this book I have told you about what the studies show and what has not been studied. I am amazed as I do the

fifth edition of this book every five years at how our new understanding of the biology of the disease has led to new targeted
treatments and better outcomes. At the same time, I have become
increasingly frustrated that we have not made equal progress in
finding the cause of breast cancer. I keep thinking about cancer of
the cervix. When I was in training as a surgeon in the late 1970s,
an abnormal Pap smear meant you had a total hysterectomy.
Many young women lost their fertility because we really did not
know what else to do. Then over time we figured out that local
therapies worked as well as hysterectomy, and were much less invasive. If this concept sounds familiar to you, it's because we later
applied it to breast cancer: in most cases, lumpectomy does as
well as mastectomy when it's combined with radiation, and it pre-
serves the breast itself.

The parallels, however, stop at that level. Research on cervical
cancer uncovered the fact that it was sexually transmitted and
then that it was caused by the human papilloma virus (HPV).
Now we have a vaccine against cervical cancer. One of my
cousins had a hysterectomy many years ago for an abnormal Pap
smear, and more recently my sister had a hysterectomy for HPV.
But my daughter doesn't have to worry about that—she's been
vaccinated. All of this happened within thirty years—and with
much less money and no pink ribbons or walks or art exhibits. So
why we have we been able to do this with cancer of the cervix and
not with cancer of the breast? Why have we not learned the
cause(s) of breast cancer or how to prevent it? Ironically, one reason may be that less money was raised for cervical cancer. Are we
victims of our own success? Lots of money makes it possible to
study interesting molecular biology without addressing the human disease. In addition, cancer of the cervix, until recently, did
not have an animal model that could be used for research. This
meant the studies had to be done on women. Although we have
learned a lot from rats and mice, it doesn't always translate to humans in any clinically useful way.

I went to some basic scientists and asked them why they did
not do breast cancer research on women. The response floored
me: "Women are too messy! I can control rats and mice from their
genes to their every activity, leading to nice pretty science!" one of

them said to me. "And besides," he added, lamely, "I don't know where to find the women." Well, that was something I could solve.

With a generous grant from the Avon Foundation for Women, the Dr. Susan Love Research Foundation launched the Love/Avon Army of Women in October 2008. The goal is to recruit a million women and a few good men (the women can be good or not) who are willing to participate in research. It is not a matching service or a study, but rather an email list of women willing to consider participating in research to find the cause of breast cancer and prevent it. It's a bit like an online dating service; you don't have to date everyone, or anyone, you are matched with. In the Army of Women you reply to our program only if you fit a study *and* you want to. And if you don't fit the specific study, or you don't feel comfortable with it, you can pass the information on to a friend who may be. The studies we find women for are not usually clinical trials or drug research, but rather a variety of studies examining women's experiences with cancer or looking for the as yet unknown causes of the disease.

You can sign up online at www.armyofwomen.org. In the first year over 320,000 women joined, 80 percent of whom neither had breast cancer nor were at high risk. Our members come from every state and range in age from 18 to 100. Researchers from all around the United States and potentially the world submit their studies for our review. If a study is approved, we eblast a description out to everyone in the army. The ones who fit the study and are interested RSVP, while the others do not. We then screen them again and if they still fit, pass their name on to the scientist. In the first year we launched 15 studies, and 13,000 women participated in the research process. Many studies were closed within 24 to 48 hours, having recruited all the women they needed and saving years of work and lots of money. So researchers were able to bring their lab findings into the real world far sooner than they would have without our volunteers.

Our biggest problem with the army is not with the women: they get it right away! The problem is with the scientists who take longer to try a new way of doing things. This, plus my frustration that there is little original research on finding the cause of breast cancer, is now leading us to start the first large online cohort study, the Health of Women Study (HOW).

As you may know, a cohort study is a group of people who answer questionnaires about their health and are followed over a long period of time so that correlations can be found between factors in their lives and later disease development. The Nurse's Health Study from Boston and the California Teacher's Study are examples of cohort studies that have shown the links between hormone replacement therapy and breast cancer, as well as the effects of physical activity in its prevention. The difference with our study is that we are doing it completely online. This means that we can have many more women in the cohort, 1 million, giving us power to detect less common factors in the disease or factors that relate only to certain populations. In addition, because we are doing it all online we don't have to develop a whole questionnaire before we can start. We can be more flexible, sending the participants a short online survey on different topics every few months. We can easily add timely questions and simultaneously address some of the issues that our readers want to know—such as the potential environmental factors involved in the development of breast cancer.

I am writing this as the study is being launched in a partnership with two epidemiologists at City of Hope, Katie Henderson and Leslie Bernstein, as well as with the help of the CaBIG at the National Cancer Institute. It is very exciting and provides a perfect opportunity for every woman to become involved in finding the cause of this disease once and for all. If we can find a vaccine for cancer of the cervix, we certainly can find something similar for cancer of the breast.

As I continue to speak around the country, I always finish my talks with an anecdote about my daughter, Katie. Although she is no longer four years old and her future aspirations have changed, this story has become a symbol to many women of what this movement is all about.

In 1993, at the Los Angeles Breast Cancer Coalition "War Mammorial" created by artist Melanie Winter, 1,300 white plastic casts of women's torsos were set on a hill. From a distance they looked like graves, but up close they showed the variety of

women's bodies: large breasts, small breasts, some with mastectomies, and some with implants. Katie was walking around trying
to figure out which breasts she wanted when she grew up. Then
she turned serious.

"Are these the graves of women with breast cancer?" she
asked.

"No, these women are all alive," I told her. "But some women
do die from breast cancer."

"Well, you're trying to stop that aren't you, Mommy?"

"Yes, Katie, I would like to stop breast cancer before you
grow up."

She thought about that a minute. "What if you die first?" she
asked.

"I'd like to stop breast cancer before I die," I replied.

She thought again, then turned to me and said, "If there is
breast cancer left after you die it's a big problem. Because I'm not
going to be a breast surgeon. I'm going to be a ballerina."

Well, Katie is now 21 and neither a breast surgeon nor a ballerina. But I still have great hopes that neither she nor her future
children or any others will be haunted, as so many of us are now,
by the fear of getting breast cancer. As long as we keep fighting,
the discoveries we're making, buttressed by the political activism
that lets the scientists and the government know we won't let up
until we've ended breast cancer, will bring about her wish. And
maybe her daughters won't even have to ask that question. That's
what keeps me going.

APPENDIXES

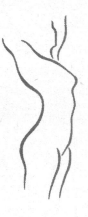

Drugs Used for Systemic Treatment of Breast Cancer

This list of drugs is not meant to be exhaustive. Check with your oncologist about your specific drugs. Unusual signs and symptoms should be reported to your doctor immediately.

I. CHEMOTHERAPY

capecitabine (Xeloda) oral
Use: for metastatic disease resistant to anthracyclines and paclitaxel
Method of action: converted to 5-FU in body; prevents DNA and RNA synthesis
Adverse effects: nausea, diarrhea, tingling hands and feet, fatigue, anemia, reduced immunity

cyclophosphamide (Cytoxan) IV or oral
Use: primary therapy and metastatic disease
Method of action: interferes with tumor cell growth
Adverse effects: temporary or permanent infertility, hair loss, cystitis, immune suppression

docetaxel (Taxotere) IV
Use: locally advanced or metastatic disease after failure of first treatment
Method of action: inhibits cell division
Adverse effects: fluid retention, suppressed immunity, hair loss, loss of feeling in hands and feet

doxorubicin (Adriamycin, Rubex) IV
Use: primary therapy and metastatic disease
Method of action: inhibits DNA synthesis
Adverse effects: nausea, hair loss, immune suppression, may cause heart
    damage, increased risk of leukemia

epirubicin (Ellence) IV
Use: primary therapy and metastatic disease
Method of action: inhibits DNA synthesis
Adverse effects: nausea, hair loss, immune suppression, may be less toxic to
    heart than doxorubicin, increased risk of leukemia

etoposide (VePesid) oral
Use: metastatic disease
Method of action: stops cell division
Adverse effects: immune suppression, nausea, diarrhea

5-fluorouracil (5-FU) IV
Use: primary and metastatic disease
Method of action: prevents DNA and RNA synthesis
Adverse effects: nausea, diarrhea, tingling hands and feet, fatigue, anemia,
    reduced immunity, less hair loss than other drugs

methotrexate IV
Use: primary and metastatic disease
Method of action: interferes with DNA synthesis and repair
Adverse effects: immune suppression, nausea, gastrointestinal distress,
    flu-like symptoms

mitomycin C (Mutamycin) IV
Use: metastatic disease
Method of action: inhibits DNA synthesis
Adverse effects: nausea, hair loss, immune suppression, may cause heart
    damage, increased risk of leukemia

mitoxantrone (Novantrone) IV
Use: metastatic disease; may be less effective than doxorubicin and
    epirubicin
Method of action: inhibits DNA synthesis
Adverse effects: nausea, hair loss, immune suppression, may cause heart
    damage, increased risk of leukemia

paclitaxel (Taxol) IV
Use: metastatic disease
Method of action: inhibits cell division
Adverse effects: fluid retention, suppressed immunity, hair loss, loss of feel-
    ing in hands and feet

vinblastine (Velban) IV
Use: metastatic disease
Method of action: inhibits cell division
Adverse effects: nausea, diarrhea, tingling hands and feet, fatigue, anemia, reduced immunity

vinorelbine (Navelbine) IV
Use: metastatic disease
Method of action: inhibits cell division
Adverse effects: Nausea, diarrhea, tingling hands and feet, fatigue, anemia, reduced immunity

II. BIOLOGIC

bevacizumab (Avastin) IV
Use: metastatic disease with chemotherapy
Method of action: blocks VEGF and new blood vessels to feed tumor
Adverse effects: gastrointestinal perforations, problems with wound healing, bleeding

trastuzumab (Herceptin) IV
Use: metastatic disease in patients who overexpress Her-2/neu
Method of action: blocks Her-2, a growth factor receptor, to inhibit tumor cell growth
Adverse effects: anemia, immune suppression, flu-like symptoms

III. HORMONE THERAPY

anastrozole (Arimidex) oral
Use: for treatment of primary and metastatic disease in postmenopausal women
Method of action: inhibits production of aromatase—an enzyme that converts precursor hormones to estrogen in the breast
Adverse effects: fractures, muscular and joint pain, hot flashes

exemestane (Aromasin) oral
Use: for treatment of primary and metastatic disease in postmenopausal women
Method of action: inactivates aromatase
Adverse effects: fractures, muscular and joint pain, hot flashes

fulvestrant (Faslodex) IV
Use: in postmenopausal women to treat metastatic breast cancer
Method of action: blocks estrogen
Adverse effects: headaches, hot flashes, gastrointestinal distress

goserelin (Zoladex) IV
Use: advanced breast cancer, primarily in premenopausal women
Method of action: blocks release of luteinizing hormone and follicle-stimulating hormone to shut down ovaries
Adverse effects: hot flashes, vaginal dryness

letrozole (Femara) oral
Use: for treatment of primary and metastatic disease in postmenopausal women
Method of action: nonsteroidal aromatase inhibitor that blocks production of estrogen
Adverse effects: fractures, muscular and joint pain, hot flashes

megestrol acetate (Megace) oral
Use: Advanced breast cancer in women whose disease has progressed after tamoxifen treatment
Method of action: uncertain; may prevent estrogen from reaching tumor
Schedule: 40 mg tablet, 4 times a day
Adverse effects: weight gain, PMS-like effects, increased risk of blood clots

tamoxifen (Nolvadex) oral
Use: breast cancer prevention and treatment of primary and metastatic disease
Method of action: selective estrogen receptor modulator (SERM) that blocks estrogen in breast but not in uterus
Adverse effects: hot flashes, vaginal dryness, increased risk of blood clots, endometrial cancer

toremifene citrate (Fareston) oral
Use: metastatic disease in postmenopausal women with ER positive tumors
Method of action: selective estrogen receptor modulator (SERM) that blocks estrogen in breast
Adverse effects: hot flashes, vaginal dryness, increased risk of blood clots; risk of endometrial cancer still unknown

Appendix B

Resources

In past editions we have listed resources, references, and books that may be of help. Because the Internet is so much more extensive and up-to-date than anything we can present here, we are limiting our recommendations to what we feel are the best websites for you to use. For those of you not adept at searching the Web, remember that your local library will be happy to help.

Websites

www.drsusanloveresearchfoundation.org (Dr. Susan Love Research Foundation). Obviously we feel this is your best resource. We keep it up-to-date as new research data come along.

www.cancer.gov (National Cancer Institute). This is a very comprehensive site, with data for both doctors and patients. It lists clinical trials and is a good source of accurate, unbiased information.

www.cancer.org (American Cancer Society). This is also a good resource for the general public.

www.nccn.com (National Comprehensive Cancer Network). Here is where you can find the practice guidelines quoted throughout this book.

www.y-me.org (Y-ME). A national organization that is focused on support. It maintains a 24-hour hotline (800/221–2141 in English and 800/986–9505 in Spanish) to help answer and provide direction for clinical questions.

www.adjuvantonline.com (Adjuvant!). This is where your doctor can find a program that will calculate the benefit of various treatments in your individual case.

www.breastcancer.org (Living with Breast Cancer). This site is another good overall resource. It was created by Dr. Marisa Weiss, a radiation oncologist.

www.youngsurvival.org (Young Survival Coalition). Focuses on young women diagnosed and living beyond their breast cancer treatment.

www.stopbreastcancer.org (National Breast Cancer Coalition). The best national organization focused on political and policies issues.

www.facingourrisk.org (FORCE). Website for women at high risk to provide support and information.

www.nccam.nih.gov (National Center for Complementary and Alternative Medicine). Good starting place for scientific information regarding complementary and alternative therapies.

www.ibcsupport.org. Inflammatory breast cancer site that provides accurate and helpful information for patients with IBC.

www.fertilehope.org. Focuses on fertility issues in women with breast cancer.

www.lymphnet.org (National Lymphedema Network). Support for all kinds of lymphedema, including that caused by breast cancer.

http://bcmets.org. A list serv for women with breast cancer metastisis.

www.brainmetsbc.org. Understanding brain metastases, available treatments, and emerging research.

www.nho.org (Hospice Resources). National Hospice Organization. Provides a directory of hospice programs by state.

www.armyofwomen.org. Home of my effort to find the cause of breast cancer.

cancercenters.cancer.gov. Lists the NCI-designated cancer centers by state and includes a map.

The Wellness Community
Physician/Patient Statement

In 1990, six prominent Los Angeles oncologists met with the staff of the Wellness Community over a period of six months to answer the question, What can cancer patients expect from their oncologists? The question was considered important since they believed that the relationship between the patient and the physician could affect the course of the illness. After many meetings they arrived at *The Wellness Community Patient/Oncologist Statement.* They then tested the statement with their patients and found that a great majority had confidence in their physician and considered their relationship "excellent." However, there was agreement among patients that the issues considered in the statement were important to a continuation of excellent relationships. The statement reproduced below was then published in the UCLA Jonsson Comprehensive Cancer Center Bulletin and is given by physicians to their patients.

The effective treatment of serious illness requires a considerable effort by both the patient and the physician. A clear understanding by both of us as to what each of us can realistically and reasonably expect of the other will do much to enhance the outlook. I am giving this "statement" to you as one step in making our relationship as effective and productive as possible. It might be helpful if you would read this statement and, if you think it appropriate, discuss it with me.

As your physician, I will make every effort to:

1. Provide you with the care most likely to be beneficial to you.
2. Inform and educate you about your situation, and the various treatment alternatives. How detailed an explanation is given will be dependent upon your specific desires.
3. Encourage you to ask questions about your illness and its treatment and to answer your questions as clearly as possible. I will also attempt

to answer the questions asked by your family; however, my primary responsibility is to you, and I will discuss your medical situation only with those people authorized by you.

4. Remain aware that all major decisions about the course of your care shall be made by you. However, I will accept the responsibility for making certain decisions if you want me to.

5. Assist you to obtain other professional opinions if you desire, or if I believe it to be in your best interests.

6. Relate to you as one competent adult to another, always attempting to consider your emotional, social and psychological needs as well as your physical needs.

7. Spend a reasonable amount of time with you on each return visit unless required by something urgent to do otherwise, and give you my undivided attention during that time.

8. Honor all appointment times unless required by something urgent to do otherwise.

9. Return phone calls as promptly as possible, especially those you indicate are urgent.

10. Make available test results promptly if you desire such reports and I will indicate to you, at the time the test is given, when you can expect the results and who you should call to get them.

11. Provide you with any information you request concerning my professional training, experience, philosophy, and fees.

12. Respect your desire to try treatment that might not be conventionally accepted. However, I will give you my honest opinion about such unconventional treatments.

13. Maintain my active support and attention throughout the course of the illness.

I hope that you as the patient will make every effort to:

1. Comply with our agreed-upon treatment plan.

2. Be as candid as possible with me about what you need and expect from me.

3. Inform me if you desire another professional opinion.

4. Inform me of all forms of therapy you are involved with.

5. Honor all appointment times unless required by something urgent to do otherwise.

6. Be as considerate as possible of my need to adhere to a schedule to see other patients.

7. Attempt to make all phone calls to me during the working hours. Call on nights and weekends only when absolutely necessary.

8. Attempt to coordinate the requests of your family and confidantes, so that I do not have to answer the same questions about you to several different persons.

Pathology Checklist

Your name _____

Your age _____

Your menopausal status

    Premenopausal _____

    Postmenopausal_____

Your hospital number _____

Your hospital _____

Your doctors

    Primary care_____

    Surgeon _____

    Medical oncologist _____

    Radiation oncologist _____

Date of biopsy/surgery_____

Place of biopsy/surgery _____

Name of doctor doing procedure _____

Place of pathological reading _____

Name of pathologist _____

Pathology reference number_____

Specimen type

  Biopsy

    Core (needle)_____

    Surgical _____

    Lumpectomy _____

    Mastectomy_____

Lymph node sampling
    Axillary node dissection_____
    Sentinel node biopsy _____
Specimen size (for excisions less than total mastectomy)
    Greatest dimension (cm) _____
    Additional dimensions _____
Side of tumor
    Right _____
    Left _____
Tumor site
    Upper outer quadrant _____
    Lower outer quadrant _____
    Upper inner quadrant _____
    Lower inner quadrant _____
    Central _____

MICROSCOPIC

Invasive or in situ
In situ
    Ductal carcinoma in situ (DCIS) _____
    Lobular carcinoma in situ (LCIS) _____
    Ductal and lobular in situ _____
    Paget's disease in the nipple _____
    Invasive/infiltrating
    Ductal _____
    Tubular _____
    Mucinous _____
    Adenoid cystic _____
    Inflammatory _____
    Secretory _____
    Medullary _____
    Papillary _____
    Undifferentiated _____
    Not otherwise specified (NOS) _____
    Lobular _____
Size of invasive tumor in greatest dimension
    Less than 2 cm _____
    Less than 0.1 cm (microinvasion) _____

Between 0.1 cm–0.5 cm _____
Between 0.5 cm–1 cm _____
Between 1 cm–2 cm _____
Between 2 cm–5 cm _____
Greater than 5 cm _____
Any size with direct extension to
Chest wall _____
Edema (swelling) _____
Both chest wall and edema _____
Inflammatory carcinoma _____

Histology
Grade of tumor
Low _____
Moderate _____
High _____

Differentiation
Low _____
Moderate _____
High _____

Mitosis
Low _____
High _____

Lympho/vascular invasion
Positive _____
Negative _____
Extent of DCIS associated with the tumor (EIC) _____

Margins
Negative
No tumor within 1 cm or no residual tumor _____
No tumor within 1 mm of margin _____
Tumor focally (at one spot) next to a margin _____
Positive
Invasive tumor involving the inked margin _____
In situ tumor involving inked margin _____

Markers

Hormones

    Estrogen receptor positive/progesterone receptor positive _____

    Estrogen receptor positive/progesterone receptor negative _____

    Estrogen receptor negative/progesterone receptor positive _____

    Estrogen receptor negative/progesterone receptor negative _____

Her-2/neu

    Negative _____

    Positive _____

    By IHC _____

        By FISH _____

Others

    P 53 positive _____

    Ki-67 _____

    S phase _____

Axillary lymph nodes

        No lymph nodes _____

Lymph nodes negative

    Negative on histology but positive on IHC _____

    Negative on histology but positive on RTPCR _____

Lymph nodes positive

    1–3 nodes positive _____

    4–9 nodes positive _____

    10 or more positive _____

General Physical Activities Defined by Level of Intensity

The following is in accordance with CDC and ACSM guidelines.

MODERATE ACTIVITY[+] 3.0 to 6.0 METs* (3.5 to 7 kcal/min)	VIGOROUS ACTIVITY[+] Greater than 6.0 METs* (more than 7 kcal/min)
Walking at a moderate or brisk pace of 3 to 4.5 mph on a level surface inside or outside, such as • Walking to class, work, or the store; • Walking for pleasure; • Walking the dog; or • Walking as a break from work. Walking downstairs or down a hill Racewalking—less than 5 mph Using crutches Hiking Roller skating or in-line skating at a leisurely pace	Racewalking and aerobic walking—5 mph or faster Jogging or running Wheeling your wheelchair Walking and climbing briskly up a hill Backpacking Mountain climbing, rock climbing, rapelling Roller skating or in-line skating at a brisk pace
Bicycling 5 to 9 mph, level terrain, or with few hills Stationary bicycling—using moderate effort	Bicycling more than 10 mph or bicycling on steep uphill terrain Stationary bicycling—using vigorous effort

Moderate activity[+] 3.0 to 6.0 METs* (3.5 to 7 kcal/min)	Vigorous activity[+] Greater than 6.0 METs* (more than 7 kcal/min)
Aerobic dancing—high impact Water aerobics	Aerobic dancing—high impact Step aerobics Water jogging Teaching an aerobic dance class
Calisthenics—light Yoga Gymnastics General home exercises, light or moderate effort, getting up and down from the floor Jumping on a trampoline Using a stair climber machine at a light-to-moderate pace Using a rowing machine—with moderate effort	Calisthenics—push-ups, pull-ups, vigorous effort Karate, judo, tae kwon do, jujitsu Jumping rope Performing jumping jacks Using a stair climber machine at a fast pace Using a rowing machine—with vigorous effort Using an arm cycling machine—with vigorous effort
Weight training and bodybuilding using free weights, Nautilus- or Universal-type weights	Circuit weight training
Boxing—punching bag	Boxing—in the ring, sparring Wrestling—competitive
Ballroom dancing Line dancing Square dancing Folk dancing Modern dancing, disco Ballet	Professional ballroom dancing—energetically Square dancing—energetically Folk dancing—energetically Clogging
Table tennis—competitive Tennis—doubles	Tennis—singles Wheelchair tennis
Golf, wheeling or carrying clubs	———
Softball—fast pitch or slow pitch Basketball—shooting baskets Coaching children's or adults' sports	Most competitive sports Football game Basketball game Wheelchair basketball Soccer

Moderate activity[+] 3.0 to 6.0 METs* (3.5 to 7 kcal/min)	Vigorous activity[+] Greater than 6.0 METs* (more than 7 kcal/min)
	Rugby Kickball Field or rollerblade hockey Lacrosse
Volleyball—competitive Playing Frisbee Juggling Curling Cricket—batting and bowling Badminton Archery (nonhunting) Fencing	Beach volleyball—on sand court Handball—general or team Racquetball Squash
Downhill skiing—with light effort Ice skating at a leisurely pace (9 mph or less) Snowmobiling Ice sailing	Downhill skiing—racing or with vigorous effort Ice-skating—fast pace or speed-skating Cross-country skiing Sledding Tobogganing Playing ice hockey
Swimming—recreational Treading water—slowly, moderate effort Diving—springboard or platform Aquatic aerobics Waterskiing Snorkeling Surfing, board or body	Swimming—steady paced laps Synchronized swimming Treading water—fast, vigorous effort Water jogging Water polo Water basketball Scuba diving
Canoeing or rowing a boat at less than 4 mph Rafting—whitewater Sailing—recreational or competition Paddle boating Kayaking—on a lake, calm water Washing or waxing a powerboat or the hull of a sailboat	Canoeing or rowing—4 or more mph Kayaking in whitewater rapids

Moderate activity[+] 3.0 to 6.0 METs* (3.5 to 7 kcal/min)	Vigorous activity[+] Greater than 6.0 METs* (more than 7 kcal/min)
Fishing while walking along a river-bank or while wading in a stream—wearing waders ——	——
Hunting deer, large or small game Pheasant and grouse hunting Hunting with a bow and arrow or crossbow—walking	——
Horseback riding—general Saddling or grooming a horse	Horseback riding—trotting, gallop-ing, jumping, or in competition Playing polo
Playing on school playground equipment, moving about, swinging, or climbing Playing hopscotch, 4-square, dodgeball, T-ball, or tetherball Skateboarding Roller-skating or in-line skating—leisurely pace	Running Skipping Jumping rope Performing jumping jacks Roller-skating or in-line skating—fast pace
Playing instruments while actively moving; playing in a marching band; playing guitar or drums in a rock band Twirling a baton in a marching band Singing while actively moving about—as on stage or in church	Playing a heavy musical instrument while actively running in a marching band
Gardening and yard work: raking the lawn, bagging grass or leaves, dig-ging, hoeing, light shoveling (less than 10 lbs per minute), or weed-ing while standing or bending Planting trees, trimming shrubs and trees, hauling branches, stacking wood Pushing a power lawn mower or tiller	Gardening and yard work: heavy or rapid shoveling (more than 10 lbs per minute), digging ditches, or carrying heavy loads Felling trees, carrying large logs, swinging an ax, hand-splitting logs, or climbing and trimming trees Pushing a nonmotorized lawn mower

Moderate activity[+] 3.0 to 6.0 METs* (3.5 to 7 kcal/min)	Vigorous activity[+] Greater than 6.0 METs* (more than 7 kcal/min)
Shoveling light snow	Shoveling heavy snow
Moderate housework: scrubbing the floor or bathtub while on hands and knees, hanging laundry on a clothesline, sweeping an outdoor area, cleaning out the garage, washing windows, moving light furniture, packing or unpacking boxes, walking and putting household items away, carrying out heavy bags of trash or recyclables (e.g., glass, newspapers, and plastics), or carrying water or firewood General household tasks requiring considerable effort	Heavy housework: moving or pushing heavy furniture (75 lbs or more), carrying household items weighing 25 lbs or more up a flight of stairs, or shoveling coal into a stove Standing, walking, or walking down a flight of stairs while carrying objects weighing 50 lbs or more
Putting groceries away—walking and carrying especially large or heavy items less than 50 lbs	Carrying several heavy bags (25 lbs or more) of groceries at one time up a flight of stairs Grocery shopping while carrying young children *and* pushing a full grocery cart, or pushing two full grocery carts at once
Actively playing with children— walking, running, or climbing while playing with children Walking while carrying a child weighing less than 50 lbs Walking while pushing or pulling a child in a stroller or an adult in a wheelchair Carrying a child weighing less than 25 lbs up a flight of stairs Child care: handling uncooperative young children (e.g., chasing, dressing, lifting into car seat), or handling several young children at one time Bathing and dressing an adult	Vigorously playing with children— running longer distances or playing strenuous games with children Racewalking or jogging while pushing a stroller designed for sport use Carrying an adult or a child weighing 25 lbs or more up a flight of stairs Standing or walking while carrying an adult or a child weighing 50 lbs or more

Moderate activity[+] 3.0 to 6.0 METs* (3.5 to 7 kcal/min)	Vigorous activity[+] Greater than 6.0 METs* (more than 7 kcal/min)
Animal care: shoveling grain, feeding farm animals, or grooming animals Playing with or training animals Manually milking cows or hooking cows up to milking machines	Animal care: forking bales of hay or straw, cleaning a barn or stables, or carrying animals weighing over 50 lbs Handling or carrying heavy animal-related equipment or tack
Home repair: cleaning gutters, caulking, refinishing furniture, sanding floors with a power sander, or laying or removing carpet or tiles General home construction work: roofing, painting inside or outside of the house, wall papering, scraping, plastering, or remodeling Outdoor carpentry, sawing wood with a power saw	Home repair or construction: very hard physical labor, standing or walking while carrying heavy loads of 50 lbs or more, taking loads of 25 lbs or more up a flight of stairs or ladder (e.g., carrying roofing materials onto the roof), or concrete or masonry work Hand-sawing hardwoods
Automobile bodywork Hand washing and waxing a car	Pushing a disabled car
Occupations that require extended periods of walking, pushing or pulling objects weighing les than 75 lbs, standing while lifting objects weighing less than 50 lbs, or carrying objects of less than 25 lbs up a flight of stairs Tasks frequently requiring moderate effort and considerable use of arms, legs, or occasional total body movements. For example: • Briskly walking on a level surface while carrying a suitcase or load weighing up to 50 lbs • Maid service or cleaning services • Waiting tables or institutional dishwashing	Occupations that require extensive periods of running, rapid movement, pushing or pulling objects weighing 75 lbs or more, standing while lifting heavy objects of 50 lbs or more, walking while carrying heavy objects of 25 lbs or more Tasks frequently requiring strenuous effort and extensive total body movements. For example: • Running up a flight of stairs while carrying a suitcase or load weighing 25 lbs or more • Teaching a class or skill requiring active and strenuous participation, such as aerobics or physical education instructor

MODERATE ACTIVITY[+] 3.0 to 6.0 METs* (3.5 to 7 kcal/min)	VIGOROUS ACTIVITY[+] Greater than 6.0 METs* (more than 7 kcal/min)
• Driving or maneuvering heavy vehicles (e.g., semi-truck, school bus, tractor, or harvester)—not fully automated and requiring extensive use of arms and legs • Operating heavy power tools (e.g., drills and jackhammers) • Many homebuilding tasks (e.g. electrical work, plumbing, carpentry, dry wall, and painting) • Farming—feeding and grooming animals, milking cows, shoveling grain; picking fruit from trees, or picking vegetables • Packing boxes for shipping or moving • Assembly-line work—tasks requiring movement of the entire body, arms or legs with moderate effort • Mail carriers—walking while carrying a mailbag • Patient care—bathing, dressing, and moving patients or physical therapy	• Firefighting • Masonry and heavy construction work • Coal mining • Manually shoveling or digging ditches • Using heavy nonpowered tools • Most forestry work • Farming—forking straw, baling hay, cleaning barn, or poultry work • Moving items professionally • Loading and unloading a truck

Source: U.S. Department of Health and Human Services, Public Health Service, Centers for Disease Control and Prevention, National Center for Chronic Disease Prevention and Health Promotion, Division of Nutrition and Physical Activity. *Promoting physical activity: a guide for community action.* Champaign, IL: Human Kinetics, 1999. (Table adapted from Ainsworth BE, Haskell WL, Leon AS, et al. Compendium of physical activities: classification of energy costs of human physical activities. *Medicine and Science in Sports and Exercise* 1993;25(1):71–80. Adapted with technical assistance from Dr. Barbara Ainsworth.)

* The ratio of exercise metabolic rate. One MET is defined as the energy expenditure for sitting quietly, which, for the average adult, approximates 3.5 ml of oxygen uptake per kilogram of body weight per minute (1.2 kcal/min for a 70-kg individual). For example, a 2-MET activity requires two times the metabolic energy expenditure of sitting quietly.

+ For an average person, defined here as 70 kilograms or 154 pounds. The activity intensity levels portrayed in this chart are most applicable to men aged 30 to 50 years and women aged 20 to 40 years. For older individuals, the classification of activity intensity might be higher. For example, what is moderate intensity to a 40-year-old man might be vigorous for a man in his 70s. Intensity is a subjective classification.

Data for this chart were available only for adults. Therefore, when children's games are listed, the estimated intensity level is for adults participating in children's activities.

To compute the amount of time needed to accumulate 150 kcal, do the following calculation: 150 kcal divided by the MET level of the activity equals the minutes needed to expend 150 kcal. For example: $150 \div 3$ METS = 50 minutes of participation. Generally, activities in the moderate-intensity range require 25–50 minutes to expend a moderate amount of activity, and activities in the vigorous-intensity range would require less than 25 minutes to achieve a moderate amount of activity. Each activity listed is categorized as light, moderate, or vigorous on the basis of current knowledge of the overall level of intensity required for the average person to engage in it, taking into account brief periods when the level of intensity required for the activity might increase or decrease considerably.

Persons with disabilities, including motor function limitations (e.g., quadriplegia) may wish to consult with an exercise physiologist or physical therapist to properly classify the types of physical activities in which they might participate, including assisted exercise. Certain activities classified in this listing as moderate might be vigorous for persons who must overcome physical challenges or disabilities.

~Note: Almost every occupation requires some mix of light, moderate, or vigorous activities, depending on the task at hand. To categorize the activity level of your own position, ask yourself: How many minutes each working day do I spend doing the types of activities described as light, moderate, or vigorous? To arrive at a total workday caloric expenditure, multiply the minutes spent doing activities within each intensity level by the kilocalories corresponding to each level of intensity. Then, add together the total kilocalories spent doing light, moderate, and vigorous activities to arrive at your total energy expenditure in a typical day.

abscess: Infection that has formed a pocket of pus.

adenine: A nucleotide base that pairs with thymine in forming DNA.

adenocarcinoma: Cancer arising in gland-forming tissue. Breast cancer is a type of adenocarcinoma.

adjuvant chemotherapy: Anticancer drugs used in combination with surgery and/or radiation as an initial treatment before there is detectable spread, to prevent or delay recurrence.

adrenal gland: Small gland found above each kidney that secretes cortisone, adrenalin, aldosterone, and many other important hormones.

alopecia: Hair loss, a common side effect of chemotherapy.

amenorrhea: Absence or stoppage of menstrual period.

amino acid: The building block of proteins.

androgen: Hormone that produces male characteristics.

angiogenesis (angiogenic): Stimulates new blood vessels to be formed.

anorexia: Loss of appetite.

apoptosis: Cell suicide.

areola: Pigmented area around the nipple.

aromatase inhibitors: A class of drugs that block an enzyme called aromatase, thereby reducing estrogen levels in the breast tissue.

aspiration: Putting a hypodermic needle into a tissue and drawing back on the syringe to obtain fluid or cells.

asymmetrical: Not matching.

ataxia telangectasia: Disease of the nervous system; carriers of the gene are more sensitive to radiation and have a higher risk of cancer.

atypical cell: Mild to moderately abnormal cell.

atypical hyperplasia: Cells that are not only abnormal but increased in number.

augmented: Added to, such as an augmented breast: one that has had a silicone implant added to it.

autologous: From the same person. An autologous blood transfusion is blood removed and then transfused back to the same person at a later date.

axilla: Armpit.

axillary lymph nodes: Lymph nodes found in the armpit area.

axillary lymph node dissection: Surgical removal of lymph nodes found in the armpit region.

basal type: triple negatives or ER negative PR negative and Her-2/neu negative.

base pairs: Two nucleic acids that bind together in DNA and RNA.

benign: Not cancerous.

bilateral: Involving both sides, such as both breasts.

biological response modifier: Usually natural substances such as colony stimulating factor that stimulates the bone marrow to make blood cells, that alter the body's natural response.

biomarker: A measurable biological property that can be used to identify women at risk.

biopsy: Removal of tissue. This term does not indicate how *much* tissue will be removed.

bone marrow: The soft inner part of large bones that produces blood cells.

bone scan: Test to determine if there is any sign of cancer in the bones.

brachial plexus: A bundle of nerves in the armpit that go on to supply the arm.

breast reconstruction: Creation of an artificial breast after mastectomy by a plastic surgeon.

bromocriptine: Drug used to block the hormone prolactin.

calcifications: Small calcium deposits in the breast tissue that can be seen by mammography.

carcinoembryonic antigen (CEA): Nonspecific (not specific to cancer) blood test used to follow women with metastatic breast cancer to help determine if the treatment is working.

carcinogen: Substance that can cause cancer.

carcinoma: Cancer arising in the epithelial tissue (skin, glands, and lining of internal organs). Most cancers are carcinomas.

cell cycle: The steps a cell goes through in order to reproduce itself.

cellulitis: Infection of the soft tissues.

centigray: Measurement of radiation absorbed dose, same as a *rad*.

checkpoint: Point in the cell cycle where the cell's DNA is checked for mutations before it is allowed to move forward.

chemotherapy: Treatment of disease with certain chemicals. The term usually refers to *cytotoxic* drugs given for cancer treatment.

chromosome: Genes are strung together in a chromosome.

cohort study: Study of a group of people who have something in common when they are first assembled and who are then observed for a period of time to see what happens to them.

colostrum: Liquid produced by the breast before the milk comes in: premilk.

comedo: Type of DCIS where the cells filling the duct are more aggressive looking.

comedo: Whitehead (closed comedo) or blackhead (open) pimple.

contracture: Formation of a thick scar tissue; in the breast a contracture can form around an implant.

core biopsy: Type of needle biopsy where a small core of tissue is removed from a lump without surgery.

corpus luteum: Ovarian follicle after ovulation.

cortisol: Hormone produced by the adrenal gland.

costochondritis: Inflammation of the connection between ribs and breast bone, a type of arthritis.

cribriform: Type of DCIS where the cells filling the duct have punched out areas.

cyclical: In a cycle like the menstrual period, which is every 28 days, or chemotherapy treatment, which is periodic.

cyst: Fluid filled sac.

cystosarcoma phylloides: Unusual type of breast tumor.

cytologist: One who specializes in studying cells.

cytology: Study of cells.

cytosine: A nucleotide base that pairs with guanine in DNA.

cytotoxic: Causing the death of cells. The term usually refers to drugs used in chemotherapy.

Danazol (danocrine): Drug used to block hormones from the pituitary gland, used in endometriosis and rarely in breast pain.

diethylstilbesterol (DES): Synthetic estrogen once used to prevent miscarriages, now shown to cause vaginal cancer in the daughters of the women who took it. DES is sometimes used to treat metastatic breast cancer.

DNA: Deoxyriboneucleic acid, the genetic code.

DNA microarray analysis: A way of analyzing the many mutations in many tumors at the same time.

dose dense: chemotherapy where the interval between two courses is shortened while the dose of each course may be increased, decreased or made equivalent to a standard dose so that the dose per unit of time is higher.

double helix: The structure of DNA that allows it to be easily replicated.

doubling time: Time it takes the cell population to double in number.

ductal carcinoma in situ (DCIS): Ductal cancer cells that have not grown outside of their site of origin, sometimes referred to as precancer.

ductoscope: A tiny endoscope that is threaded through the nipple into a duct.

eczema: Skin irritation characterized by redness and open weeping.

edema: Swelling caused by a collection of fluid in the soft tissues.

electrocautery: Instrument used in surgery to cut, coagulate, or destroy tissue by heating it with an electric current.

embolus: Plug or clot of tumor cells within a blood vessel.

engorgement: Swelling with fluid, as in a breast engorged with milk.

epigenetic: Changes in DNA that can be reversible as opposed to permanent mutations. Similar to taping the light switch so that it cannot be turned off rather than permanently damaging it.

erb-B2: Another name for the Her-2/neu oncogene.

esophagus (esophageal): Organ carrying food from the mouth and the stomach.

estrogen: Female sex hormones produced by the ovaries, adrenal glands, placenta, and fat.

estrogen receptor: Protein found on some cells to which estrogen molecules will attach. If a tumor is positive for estrogen receptors, it is sensitive to hormones.

excisional biopsy: Process of taking the whole lump out.

extracellular matrix: The material that surrounds the cells.

fat necrosis: Area of dead fat usually following some form of trauma or surgery, a cause of lumps.

fibroadenoma: Benign fibrous tumor of the breast most common in young women.

fibrocystic disease: Much misused term for any benign condition of the breast.

fibroid: Benign fibrous tumor of the uterus (not in the breast).

flow cytometry: Test that measures DNA content in tumors.

fluoroscopy: Use of an X ray machine to examine parts of the body directly rather than taking a picture and developing it, as in conventional X rays. Fluoroscopy uses more radiation than a single X ray.

follicle-stimulating hormone (FSH): Hormone from the pituitary gland that stimulates the ovary.

follicles: In the ovaries, eggs encased in their developmental sacs.

frozen section: Freezing and slicing tissue to make a slide immediately for diagnosis.

frozen shoulder: Stiffness of the shoulder, which is painful and makes it hard to lift the arm over your head.

galactocele: Milk cyst sometimes found in a nursing mother's breast.

GCSF (granulocyte stimulating factor): A drug that stimulates the bone marrow to recover faster from chemotherapy.

gene: A linear sequence of DNA that is required to produce a protein.

genetic: Relating to genes or inherited characteristics.

genome: All of the chromosomes that together form the genetic map.

germ line: Cells that are involved in reproduction, i.e., sperm and eggs.

ghostectomy: Removal of breast tissue in the area where there was a previous lump.

GNRH agonist: A drug that blocks the pituitary production of hormones that stimulate the ovaries.

guanine: One of the base pairs that form DNA; pairs with cytosine.

gynecomastia: Swollen breast tissue in a man or boy.

hemangioma: A birth mark consisting of overgrowth of blood vessels.

hematoma: Collection of blood in the tissues. Hematomas may occur in the breast after surgery.

hemorrhage: Bleeding.

Her-2/neu: An oncogene that, when overexpressed, leads to more cell growth.

heterogeneous: Composed of many different elements. In relation to breast cancer, heterogeneous refers to the fact that there are many different types of breast cancer cells within one tumor.

homeopathy: System of therapy using very small doses of drugs, which can produce in healthy people symptoms similar to those of the disease being treated. These are believed to stimulate the immune system.

hormone: Chemical substance produced by glands in the body which enters the bloodstream and causes effects in other tissues.

hot flashes: Sudden sensations of heat and swelling associated with menopause.

HRT: Hormone replacement therapy.

human choriogonadotropin (HCG): Hormone produced by the corpus luteum.

hyperplasia: Excessive growth of cells.

hypothalamus: Area at the base of the brain that controls various functions including hormone production in the pituitary.

hysterectomy: Removal of the uterus. Hysterectomy does not necessarily mean the removal of ovaries (oophorectomy).

immune system: Complex system by which the body is able to protect itself from foreign invaders.

immunocytochemistry: Study of the chemistry of cells using techniques that employ immune mechanisms.

incisional biopsy: Taking a piece of the lump out.

infiltrating cancer: Cancer that can grow beyond its site of origin into neighboring tissue. Infiltrating does not imply that the cancer has already spread outside the breast. Infiltrating has the same meaning as invasive.

informed consent: Process in which the patient is fully informed of all risks and complications of a planned procedure and agrees to proceed.

in situ: In the site of. In regard to cancer, in situ refers to tumors that haven't grown beyond their site of origin and invaded neighboring tissue.

interstitial brachytherapy: Partial breast irradiation through tubes loaded with radioactive seeds.

intracavitary brachytherapy: Partial breast irradiation through a balloon filling the biopsy cavity.

intraductal: Within the duct. Intraductal can describe a benign or malignant process.

intraductal papilloma: Benign tumor that projects like a finger from the lining of the duct.

intraoperative limited radiation therapy: Irradiation applied in the operating room to the bed of the tumor.

invasive cancer: Cancers that are capable of growing beyond their site of origin and invading neighboring tissue. Invasive does not imply that the cancer is aggressive or has already spread.

lactation: Production of milk from the breast.

latissimus flap: Flap of skin and muscle taken from the back used for reconstruction after mastectomy or partial mastectomy.

lidocaine: Drug most commonly used for local anesthesia.

lobules: Parts of the breast capable of making milk.

lobular carcinoma in situ: Abnormal cells within the lobule that don't form lumps. They can serve as a marker of future cancer risk.

lobular: Having to do with the lobules of the breast.

local treatment of cancer: Treatment of the tumor only.

lumpectomy: Surgery to remove lump with small rim of normal tissue around it.

luteinizing hormone: Hormone produced by the pituitary, which helps control the menstrual cycle.

lymph nodes: Glands found throughout the body that help defend against foreign invaders such as bacteria. Lymph nodes can be a location of cancer spread.

lymphatic vessels: Vessels that carry lymph (tissue fluid) to and from lymph nodes.

lymphedema: Milk arm. This swelling of the arm can follow surgery to the lymph nodes under the arm. It can be temporary or permanent, and occur immediately, or any time later.

macrophages: Blood cells that are part of the immune system.

malignant: Cancerous.

mastalgia: Pain in the breast.

mastitis: Infection of the breast. Mastitis is sometimes used loosely to refer to any benign process in the breast.

mastodynia: Pain in the breast.

mastopexy: Uplift of the breast through plastic surgery.

menarche: First menstrual period.

metastasis: Spread of cancer to another organ, usually through the blood stream.

metastasizing: Spreading to a distant site.

methylation: Process that occurs when a methyl group (three carbons and a hydrogen) attaches to a gene and results in silencing it

methylxanthine: Chemical group to which caffeine belongs.

microcalcification: Tiny calcifications in the breast tissue usually seen only on a mammogram. When clustered can be a sign of ductal carcinoma in situ.

micrometastasis: Microscopic and as yet undetectable but presumed spread of tumor cells to other organs.

micropapillary: Type of DCIS in which the cells filling the duct take the form of finger-like projections into the center.

mitosis: Cell division.

mutation: An alteration of the genetic code.

myocutaneous flap: Flap of skin and muscle and fat taken from one part of the body to fill in an empty space.

myoepithelial cells: The cells that surround the ductal lining cells and may serve to contain the cells.

necrosis: Dead tissue.

nodular: Forming little nodules.

nuclear magnetic resonance (NMR or MRI): Imaging technique using a magnet and electrical coil to transmit radio waves through the body.

nucleotide: One of the base pairs forming DNA.

observational study: A study in which a factor is observed in a group of people.

oncogene: Tumor genes present in the body. These can be activated by carcinogens and cause cell to grow uncontrollably.

oncogenes: Altered DNA that can lead to cancerous growth.

oncology: Study of cancer.

oophorectomy: Removal of the ovaries.

osteoporosis: Softening of the bones, and bone loss, that occurs with age in some people.

oxytocin: Hormone produced by the pituitary gland, involved in lactation.

p53: A tumor suppressor gene.

palliation: Act of relieving a symptom without curing the cause.

partial breast irradiation: Radiation just to the bed of the tumor rather than to the whole breast.

pathologist: Doctor who specializes in examining tissue and diagnosing disease.

pectoralis major: Muscle that lies under the breast.

phlebitis: Irritation of a vein.

pituitary gland: A gland located in the brain that secretes many hormones to regulate other glands in the body: the master gland.

Poland's syndrome: A congenital condition in which there is no breast development on one side of the chest.

polychemotherapy: Chemotherapy with more than one drug at a time.

polygenic: Relating to more than one gene.

polymastia: Literally many breasts. Existence of an extra breast or breasts.

postmenopausal: After the menopause has occurred.

Premarin (conjugated estrogen): Estrogen from pregnant horses' urine that is sometimes given to women after the menopause.

progesterone: Hormone produced by the ovary involved in the normal menstrual cycle.

prognosis: Expected or probable outcome.

prolactin: Hormone produced by the pituitary that stimulates progesterone production by the ovaries and lactation.

prophylactic subcutaneous mastectomies: Removal of all breast tissue beneath the skin and nipple, to lessen future breast cancer risk.

prosthesis: Artificial substitute for an absent part of the body, as in breast prosthesis.

protein: The building block of life, formed from amino acids.

protocol: Research designed to answer a hypothesis. Protocols often involve testing a specific new treatment under controlled conditions.

proto-oncogene: Normal gene controlling cell growth or turnover.

Provera (medroxyprogesterone acetate): Progesterone that is sometimes given to women in combination with Premarin after menopause.

pseudolump: Breast tissue that feels like a lump but when removed proves to be normal.

ptosis: Drooping, as in breasts that hang down.

punch biopsy: A biopsy of skin done that just punches a small hole out of the skin.

quadrantectomy: Removal of a quarter of the breast.

rad: Radiation absorbed dose, same as centigray. One chest X ray equals one-tenth of a rad.

radial scar: A benign lesion where glands are trapped in fibrous tissue often difficult to distinguish from cancer.

randomized: Chosen at random. In regard to a research study it means choosing the subjects to be given a particular treatment by means of a computer programmed to choose names at random.

randomized controlled study: A study in which the participants are randomized to one treatment or another.

recurrence: Return of cancer after its apparent complete disappearance.

recurrence score: Score developing from analyzing different mutations and predicting the risk of recurrence with tamoxifen or chemotherapy.

remission: Disappearance of detectable disease.

repair endonucleases: Enzymes that can repair mutations.

RNA: Ribonucleic acid; carries the message from the DNA into the cell to make proteins.

sarcoma: Cancer arising in the connective tissue.

scleroderma: An autoimmune disease that involves thickening of the skin and difficulty swallowing, among other symptoms.

scoliosis: Deformity of the backbone that causes a person to bend to one side or the other.

sebaceous material: Oily, cheesy material secreted by glands in the skin.

selenium: Metallic element found in food.

SERM: Selective estrogen receptor modulator: a compound that is estrogenic in some organs and antiestrogenic in others.

seroma: Collection of tissue fluid.

side effect: Unintentional or undesirable secondary effect of treatment.

silicone: Synthetic material used in breast implants because of its flexibility, resilience, and durability.

somatic cell: A cell that forms the organs of the body but is not involved in reproduction.

S phase fraction: A measure of how many cells are dividing at a time; if it is high it is thought to indicate an aggressive tumor.

stem cell: A primitive cell that is self renewing as well as capable of giving rise to daughter cells.

stroma: Tissue and cells forming the support structure of an organ or gland. May include fat cells, fibrous cells, white blood cells, blood vessels, and nerves.

subareolar abscess: Infection of the glands under the nipple.

subcutaneous tissue: The tissue under the skin.

systemic treatment: Treatment involving the whole body, usually using drugs.

tamoxifen: Estrogen blocker used in treating breast cancer.

targeted therapy: An antibody directed to a specific molecular target, for example, Herceptin.

telomerase: An enzyme that reattaches the end of a chromosome when it divides.

telomere: The end of a chromosome, a bit of which is clipped off every time a cell divides.

thoracic: Concerning the chest (thorax).

thoracic nerves: Nerves in the chest area.

thoracoepigastric vein: Vein that starts under the arm and passes along the side of the breast and then down into the abdomen.

thymine: A nucleotide base that pairs with adenine in DNA formation.

titration: Systems of balancing. In chemotherapy, titration means using the largest amount of a drug possible while keeping the side effects from becoming intolerable.

trauma: Wound or injury.

triglyceride: Form in which fat is stored in the body, consisting of glycerol and three fatty acids.

tru-cut biopsy: Type of core needle biopsy in which a small core of tissue is removed from a lump without surgery.

tumor: Abnormal mass of tissue. Strictly speaking a tumor can be benign or malignant.

tumor dormancy: Tumors that are present in a stable state.

tumor suppressor gene: A gene that prevents cells from growing if they have a mutation.

vegf: Vascular epidermal growth factor; a protein that stimulates new blood vessels to grow.

virginal hypertrophy: Extremely large breasts in a young woman.

xeroradiography: Type of mammogram taken on a Xerox plate rather than X ray film.

Notes

Chapter 1

1. Love SM, Barksy SH. Anatomy of the nipple and breast ducts revisited. *Cancer* 2004; 101:1947–1957.

2. Cooper A. *On the Anatomy of the Breast*. London: Orme, Green, Brown & Longmans, 1840.

3. Teboul M, Halliwell M. *Atlas of Ultrasound and Ductal Echography of the Breast*. Oxford: Blackwell Science, 1995.

4. Ramsay DT et al. Anatomy of the lactating human breast refined with ultrasound imaging. *Journal of Anatomy* 2005; 206(6):545–534.

5. Going JJ, Moffat DF. Escaping from flatland: Clinical and biological aspects of human mammary duct anatomy in three dimensions. *Journal of Pathology* 2004; 203:538–544.

6. Rusby JE et al. Microscopic anatomy within the nipple: Implications for nipple-sparing mastectomy. *American Journal of Surgery* 2007; 194(4):433–437.

7. Nelson CM, Bissell MJ. Of extracellular matrix, scaffolds, and signaling: Tissue architecture regulates development, homeostasis, and cancer. *Annual Review of Cell and Developmental Biology* 2006; 22:287–309.

8. Al-Hajj M et al. Prospective identification of tumorigenic breast cancer cells. *Proceedings of the National Academy of Science* 2003; 100(7):3983–3988.

9. Going JJ, Moffat DF. Escaping from flatland.

10. New England Research Institute. *Women and Their Health in Massachusetts. Final Report 1991*. Watertown, MA, 1991.

11. Sluijmer AV et al. Endocrine activity of the postmenopausal ovary: The effects of pituitary down-regulation and oophorectomy. *Journal of Clinical Endocrinology and Metabolism* 1995; 80:2163–2167.

12. Ushiroyama T, Sugimoto O. Endocrine function of the peri- and postmenopausal ovary. *Hormone Research* 1995; 44:64–68.

13. Hreshchyshyn MM et al. Effects of natural menopause, hysterectomy, and oophorectomy on lumbar spine and femoral neck bone densities. *Obstetrics and Gynecology* 1988; 72:631.

14. Parker WH et al. Ovarian conservation at the time of hysterestomey and long-term health outcomes in the Nurse's Health Study. *Obstetrics & Gynecology* 2009; 113(5):1027–1037.

15. Tice JA et al. Using clinical factors and mammographic breast density to estimate breast cancer risk: Development and validation of a new predictive model. *Annals of Internal Medicine* 2008; 148(5):337–347.

16. Ayalah, D, and IJ. Weinstock. *Breasts:Women Speak About Their Breasts and Their Lives.* New York: Summit,1979.

Chapter 2

1. Heuston JT. Unilateral agenesis and hypoplasia: Difficulties and suggestions. In Goldwyn R, ed. *Plastic and Reconstructive Surgery of the Breast,* 361. Boston: Little, Brown, 1976.

2. Gifford S. Emotional attitudes toward cosmetic breast surgery: Loss and restitution of the "ideal" self. In Goldwyn R, ed., *Plastic and Reconstructive Surgery,* 117.

3. Letterman G, Schurter MA. A history of mammoplasty with emphasis on correction of ptosis and macromastia. In Goldwyn R, ed., *Plastic and Reconstructive Surgery,* 361.

4. Silverman BS et al. A critical assessment of the relationship between silicone implants and connective tissue diseases (a review). *Regul Toxicology Pharmacology* 1996; 23(1 Pt 1):74–85.

5. Deapen DM, Brody GS. Augmentation mammoplasty and breast cancer: A 5-year update of the Los Angeles study. *Plastic Reconstructive Surgery* 1992; 89(4):660–665.

6. Berkel H, Birdsell DC, Jenkins H. Breast augmentation: A risk factor for breast cancer? *New England Journal of Medicine* 1992; 326(25):1649–1653.

Chapter 3

1. Herrman JB. Mammary cancer subsequent to aspiration of cysts in the breast. *Annals of Surgery* 1971; 173:40.

2. Greenberg R, Skornick Y, Kaplan O. Management of breast fibroadenomas. *Journal of General Internal Medicine* 1998 Sept 13; 640–645.

3. Kaufman CS et al. Office-based cryoablation of breast fibroadenomas with long-term follow-up. *Breast Journal* 2005; 11:344–350.

4. Ader DN, Shriver CD, Browne MW. Cyclical mastalgia: Premenstrual syndrome or recurrent pain disorder? *Journal of Psychosomatic Obstetrics & Gynecology* 1999; 20(4):198–202.

5. Preece PE et al. Clinical syndromes of mastalgia. *Lancet* 1976; 2:670.

6. Mansel RE. Breast pain. *British Medical Journal* 1994; 309:866–868.

7. Wren BG. The breast and the menopause. *Bailliere's Clinical Obstetrics and Gynaecology* 1996; 10(3):433–447.

8. Barros AC et al. Reassurance in the treatment of mastalgia. *Breast Journal* 1999; 5(3):162–165.

9. Page JK, Mansel RE, Hughes SE. Clinical experience of drug treatments for mastalgia. *Lancet* 1985; 2:373.

10. Steinbrunn BS, Zera RT, Rodriguez JL. Mastalgia: Tailoring treatment to type of breast pain. *Postgraduate Medicine* 1997; 102(5):183–198.

11. Greenblatt RB et al. Clinical studies with an antigonadotropin—Danazol. *Fertility and Sterility* 1971; 22:102.

12. Mansel RE, Dogliotti L. European multicentre trial of bromocriptine in cyclical mastalgia. *Lancet* 1990; 335:190.

13. Fentiman IS et al. Double-blind controlled trial of tamoxifen therapy for mastalgia. *Lancet* 1986; 1:287.

14. Steinbrunn BS, Zera RT, Rodriguez JL. Mastalgia: Tailoring treatment to type of breast pain. *Postgraduate Medicine* 1997; 102(5):183–198.

15. Boyd N et al. Effect of low-fat high carbohydrate diet on symptoms of cyclical mastopathy. *Lancet* 1988; 2(8603):128.

16. LeBan MM, Meerscharet JR, Taylor RS. Breast pain: A symptom of cervical radiculopathy. *Archives of Physical Medicine and Rehabilitation* 1979; 60:315.

17. Pye JK, Mansel RE, Hughes LE et al. Clinical experience of drug treatments for mastalgia. *Lancet* 1985; 2:373.

18. Maddox PR et al. Non-cyclical mastalgia: An improved classification and treatment. *British Journal of Surgery* 1989; 76(9):901–904.

19. Thomsen AC, Espersen MD, Maigaard S. Course and treatment of milk stasis, noninfectious inflammation of the breast, and infectious mastitis in nursing women. *American Journal of Obstetrics and Gynecology* 1984; 149:492.

20. Meguid MM et al. Pathogenesis-based treatment of recurring subareolar breast abscesses. *Surgery* 1995; 118:775–782.

21. Maier WP, Berger A, Derrick BM. Periareolar abscess in the nonlactating breast. *American Journal of Obstetrics and Gynecology* 1982; 149:492.

22. Sartorius O. Personal communication.

23. Watt-Boolsen S, Ryegaard R, Blichert-Toft M. Primary periareolar abscess in the nonlactating breast: Risk of recurrence. *American Journal of Surgery* 1987; 153:571.

24. Livingstone V, Stringer LJ. The treatment of Staphylococcus aureus infected sore nipples: A randomized comparative study (letter). *Journal of Human Lactation* 2001; 17:116–117.

25. Love SM et al. Benign breast diseases. In Harris JR et al., eds. *Breast Diseases,* 22. Philadelphia: Lippincott, 1987.

26. Elzer MH et al. Significance of age in patients with nipple discharge. *Surgical Gynecology and Obstetrics* 1970; 131:519.

27. Pritt B et al. Diagnostic value of nipple cytology: Study of 466 cases. *Cancer* 2004; 102(4):233–238.

28. Cabioglu N et al. Surgical decision making and factors determining a diagnosis of breast carcinoma in women presenting with nipple discharge. *Journal of the American College of Surgeons* 2003; 3:354–364.

29. Pereira B, Mokbel K. Mammary ductoscopy: Past, present, and future. *International Journal of Clinical Oncology* 2005 Apr 10; 2:112–116.

Chapter 4

1. Hanahan D, Weinberg RA. The hallmarks of cancer cells. *Cell* 2000 Jan 7; 100(1):57–70.

2. Nelson CM, Bissell MJ. Of extracellular matrix, scaffolds, and signaling: Tissue architecture regulates development, homeostasis, and cancer. *Annual Review of Cell and Developmental Biology* 2006; 22:287–309.

3. Hoagland M, Dodson B. *The Way Life Works.* New York: Times Books, 1998.

4. Ashworth A. A synthetic lethal therapeutic approach: Poly (ADP) ribose polymerase inhibitors for the treatment of cancers deficient in DNA double-strand break repair. *Journal of Clinical Oncology* 2008; 26:3785–3790.

5. Al-Hajj M et al. Prospective identification of tumourigenic breast cancer cells. *Proceedings of the National Academy of Science USA* 2003; 100:3983–3988.

6. Holst CR et al. Methylation of p16(INK4a) promoters occurs in vivo in histologically normal human mammary epithelia. *Cancer Research* 2003 Apr 1; 63(7):1596–1601.

7. Weaver VM et al. Reversion of the malignant phenotype of human breast cells in three-dimensional culture and in vivo by integrin-blocking antibodies. *Journal of Cell Biology* 1997; 137(1):231–245.

8. Kupperwasser C et al. Reconstruction of functionally normal and laignant human breast tissues in mice. *Proceedings of the National Academy of Science* 2004; 101(14):4966–4971.

9. Kolata G. Forty years war: Old ideas spur new approaches in cancer fight. *New York Times* 2009 Dec 29.

10. Newell GR, Vogel VG. Personal risk factors: What do they mean? *Cancer* 1988; 62:1695.

11. Cuzick J. Women at high risk of breast cancer. *Reviews on Endocrine-Related Cancer* 1987; 25:5.

12. Miller AB. Epidemiology and prevention. In Harris JR et al., eds. *Breast Diseases*. Philadelphia: Lippincott, 1987.

13. Seidman H, Stellman SD, Mushinski MH. A different perspective on breast cancer risk factors: Some implications of the nonattributable risk. *CA: A Cancer Journal for Clinicians* 1982; 32:301.

14. Willett WC et al. Moderate alcohol consumption and the risk of breast cancer. *New England Journal of Medicine* 1980; 316:1174.

Chapter 5

1. Yue W et al. Genotoxic metabolites of estrodiol in breast: Potential mechanism of estrodiol-induced carcinogenesis. *Journal of Steroid Biochemistry and Molecular Biology* 2003; 86(3–5):477–486.

2. Yang L et al. Estimates of cancer incidence in China for 2000 and projections for 2005. *Cancer Epidemiology Biomarkers and Prevention* 2005; 14(1): 243–249.

3. Althuis MD et al. Global trends in breast cancer incidence and mortality 1973–1997. *International Journal of Epidemiology* 2005; 34(2):405–412.

4. Parkin DM et al. Global Cancer Statistics, 2002. *CA: A Cancer Journal for Clinicians* 2005; 55:74–108.

5. Bray F, McCarron P, Parkin DM. The changing global patterns of female breast cancer incidence and mortality. *Breast Cancer Research* 2004; 6:229–239.

6. Brody JG, Rudel RA. Environmental pollutants and breast cancer: The evidence from animal and human studies. *Breast Diseases: A Year Book Quarterly* 2008; 19(1): 17–19.

7. Newell GR, Vogel VG. Personal risk factors: What do they mean? *Cancer* 1988; 62:1695.

8. Morris CR, Wright WE, Schrag RD. The risk of developing breast cancer within the next 5, 10, or 20 years of a woman's life. *American Journal of Preventative Medicine* 2001; 20(3):214–218.

9. Cheblowski RT et al. Ethnicity and breast cancer: Factors influencing differences in incidence and outcome. *Journal of the National Cancer Institute* 2005; 97:439–448.

10. Kelsey JL, Berkowowitz GS. Breast Cancer epidemiology. *Cancer Research* 1988; 48:5615.

11. Okunaga M et al. Breast cancer among atomic bomb survivors. In Boice JD, Jr., Fraumeni JF, Jr., eds. *Radiation Carcinogenesis Epidemiology and Biological Significance,* 45:65. New York: Raven, 1984.

12. Tokuoka S et al. Incidence of female breast cancer among atomic bomb survivors, 1950–1985. *Radiation Research* 1994; 138:209–223.

13. Land C. Epidemiology of radiation-induced breast cancer. *NAPBC Breast Cancer Etiology Working Group Workshop on Medical Ionizing of Radiation and Human Breast Cancer* 1997.

14. Miller AB et al. Mortality from breast cancer after irradiation during fluoroscopic examinations in patients being treated for tuberculosis. *New England Journal of Medicine* 1989; 321:1285.

15. Mettler FA et al. Breast neoplasm in women treated with X rays for acute postpartum mastitis: A pilot study. *Journal of the National Cancer Institute* 1969; 43:803.

16. Hoffman DA et al. Breast cancer in women with scoliosis exposed to multiple diagnostic X rays. *Journal of the National Cancer Institute* 1989; 81:1307.

17. Simon N. Breast cancer induced by radiation: Relation to mammography and treatment of acne. *Journal of the American Medical Association* 1977; 237(8):789.

18. Hildreth NG, Shore RE, Dvoretsky PM. The risk of breast cancer after irradiation of the thymus in infancy. *New England Journal of Medicine* 1989; 321:1281.

19. Wang J, Inskip PD, Bioce JDJ. Cancer incidence among medical diagnostic X ray workers in China, 1950 to 1985. *International Journal of Cancer* 1990; 45:889–895.

20. Vaughan TL, Lee JA, Strader CH. Breast cancer incidence of a nuclear facility: Demonstration of a morbidity surveillance system. *Health Phys* 1993; 64:349–354.

21. Pukkala E, Auvinen A, Wahberg G. Incidence of cancer among Finnish airline attendants. *British Medical Journal* 1995; 311:649–952.

22. Boice JDJ, Mandel JS, Doody MM. Breast cancer among radiologic technologists. *Journal of the American Medical Association* 1995; 274:394–401.55.

23. Boice JD et al. Second cancer following radiation treatment for cervical cancer: An international collaboration among cancer registries. *Journal of the National Cancer Institute* 1985; 74:974. Li FP.

24. Travis LB, Curtis RE, Boice JD, Jr. Late effects of treatment for childhood Hodgkin's disease. *New England Journal of Medicine* 1996; 335:352–353.

25. Rudel, RA et al. Chemicals causing mammary gland tumors in animals signal new directions for epidemiology, chemicals testing, and risk assessment for breast cancer prevention. *Cancer* 2007; 109(S12):2635–2666.

26. Gammon MD et al. Electric blanket use and breast cancer among young women. *Am J Epidemiology* 1998; 148:556–563.

27. Laden F et al. Electric blanket use and breast cancer in the Nurses' Health Study. *Am J Epidemiology* 2000; 152:41–49.

28. Kabat GC et al. Electric blanket use and breast cancer on Long Island. *Epidemiology* 2003; 14:514–520.

29. Brody JG, Rudel RA. Environmental pollutants and breast cancer: The evidence from animal and human studies. *Breast Diseases: A Year Book Quarterly,* 2008; 19(1): 17–19.

30. Soto AM et al. The E-SCREEN assay as a tool to identify estrogens: An update on estrogenic environmental pollutants. *Environmental Health Perspectives* 1995; 103:113–122.

31. Shu XO et al. Soy food intake and breast cancer survival. *JAMA* 2009; 302(22):2437–2443.

32. Horwitz KB, Sartorius CA. Progestins in hormone replacement therapies reactivate cancer stem cells in women with preexisting breast cancers: A Hypothesis. *Journal of Clinical Endocrinology & Metabolism* 2008; 93:3295–3298.

33. Hunter DJ et al. Plasma organochlorine levels and the risk of breast cancer. *New England Journal of Medicine* 1997; 337:1253–1258.

34. Van't Veer P et al. DDT and postmenopausal breast cancer in Europe: Case control study. *British Medical Journal* 1997; 315:81–85.

35. Lopez-Carillo L et al. Dicholorodiphenyltrichloroethane serum levels and breast cancer risk: A case control study from Mexico. *Cancer Research* 1997; 57:3728–3732.

36. Snedeker SM. Pesticides and breast cancer risk: A review of DDT, DDE, and dieldrin. *Environmental Health Perspectives* 2001; 109 Suppl 1:35–47.

37. Cohn BA et al. DDT and breast cancer in young women: New data on the significance of age at exposure. *Environmental Health Perspectives* TK; 115:1406–1414.

38. Gammon MD et al. Environmental toxins and breast cancer on Long Island: Polycyclic aromatic hydrocarbon DNA adducts. *Cancer Epidemiology Biomarkers Prev* 2002; 11: 77–685.

39. Mok MT et al. Mouse mammary tumor virus-like env sequences in human breast cancer. *International Journal of Cancer* 2008 Jun 15; 122(12):2864–2870.

40. Amarante MK et al. Plasma malondialdehyde levels and CXCR4 expression in peripheral blood cells of breast cancer patients. *Journal of Cancer Research and Clinical Oncology* 2009; 135(8): 997–1004.

41. Tworoger SS, Hankinson SE. Prolactin and breast cancer etiology: An epidemiologic perspective. *J Mammary Gland Biol Neoplasia* 2008 Mar; 13(1):41–53.

42. Sasano H et al. In situ estrogen production and its regulation in human breast carcinoma: From endocrinology to intracrinology. *Patholo Int* 2009 Nov; 59(11):777–789.

43. Miller WR et al. Regulation of aromatase activity within the breast. *Journal of Steroid Biochem and Molecular Biology* 1997; 61(3–6):193–202.

44. Murray TJ et al. *Reprod Toxicol* 2007; 23(3):383–390.

45. Palmer JR et al. Risk of breast cancer in women exposed to diethylstilbestrol in utero: Preliminary results (United States). *Cancer Causes Control* 2002; 13:753–758.

46. Michels KB et al. Birthweight as a risk factor for breast cancer. *Lancet* 1996; 348:1542–1546.

47. Potischman N, Troisi R. In utero and early life exposures in relation to risk of breast cancer. *Cancer Causes Control* 1999; 10:561–573.

48. Okasha M et al. Exposures in childhood, adolescence, and early adulthood and breast cancer risk: A systematic review of the literature. *Breast Cancer Research and Treatment* 2003; 78:223–276.

49. Trichopoulos D. Hypothesis: Does breast cancer originate in utero? *Lancet* 1990; 335:939–940.

50. MacMahon B, Cole P, Brown J. Etiology of human breast cancer: A review. *Journal of the National Cancer Institute* 1973; 50:21.

51. Parker WH et al. Ovarian conservation at the time of hysterectomy and long-term health outcomes in the Nurses' Health Study. *Obstet Gynecol* 2009 May; 113(5):1027–1037.

52. Pike MC et al. "Hormonal" risk factors, "breast tissue age," and the age-incidence of breast cancer. *Nature* 1983; 303:767–770.

53. Rosner B, Colditz GA, Willett WC. Reproductive risk factors in a prospective study of breast cancer: The Nurses' Health Study. *American Journal of Epidemiology* 1994; 139:819–835.

54. Lyons TR, Schedin PJ, Borges VF. Pregnancy and breast cancer: When they collide. *J Mammary Gland Biol Neoplasia* 2009 Jun; 14(2):87–98.

55. Melbye M, Wohlfahrt J, Olsen J. Induced abortion and the risk of breast cancer. *New England Journal of Medicine* 1997; 336:81–85.

56. Ye Z et al. Breast cancer in relation to induced abortions in a cohort of Chinese women. *British Journal of Cancer* 2002; 87:977–981.

57. Beral V et al. Breast cancer and abortion: Collaborative reanalysis of data of 53 epidemiological studies, including 83,000 women with breast cancer from 16 countries. *Lancet* 2004; 363:1007–1016.

58. Collaborative Group on Hormonal Factors in Breast Cancer. Breast cancer and breastfeeding: Collaborative reanalysis of individual data from 47 epidemiological studies in 30 countries, including 50,302 women with breast cancer and 96,973 women without the disease. *Lancet* 2002; 360:187–195.

59. Grimbizis GF, Tarlatzis BC. The use of hormonal contraception and its protective role against endometrial and ovarian cancer. *Best Pract Res Clin Obstet Gynaecol* 2009 Oct 29.

60. Marchbanks PA et al. Oral contraceptives and the risk of breast cancer. *New England Journal of Medicine* 2002; 346:2025–2032.

61. Pasanisi P et al. Oral contraceptive use and BRCA penetrance: A case-only study. *Cancer Epidemiol Biomarkers Prev* 2009 Jul; 18(7):2107–2113.

62. Fowke JH et al. Oral contraceptive use and breast cancer risk: Modification by NAD(P)H:Quinone Oxoreductase (NQ01) Genetic Polymorphisms. *Cancer Epidemiological Biomarkers & Prevention* 2004; 13(8):1308–1315.

63. Stone L. *The Family, Sex, and Marriage.* New York: Harper & Row, 1979.

64. Hale JR. *Renaissance Europe.* Berkeley: University of California Press, 1971.

65. Fraser A. *The Weaker Vessel.* New York: Vintage, 1984.

66. Fogle RH et al. Ovarian androgen production in postmenopausal women. *J Clin Endocrinol Metab* 2007; 92:3040–3043.

67. Fournier A et al. Estrogen-progestavgen menopausal hormone therapy and breast cancer: Does delay from menopause onset to treatment initiation influence risks? *J Clin Oncol* 2009.

68. Bernstein L. Combined hormone therapy at menopause and breast cancer: A warning—Short-term use increases risk. *Journal of Clinical Oncology* 2009; 27(31): 5116–5119.

69. Chlebowski RT et al. Influence of estrogen plus progestin on breast cancer and mammography in healthy postmenopausal women: The Women's Health Initiative randomized trial. *Journal of the American Medical Association* 2003; 289:3243–3253.

70. Kumle M. Declining breast cancer incidence and decreased HRT use. *Lancet* 2008; 372 (9639):608–610.

71. Kerlikowske, personal communication.

72. Resnick SM et al. Women's Health Initiative Study of cognitive aging investigators. Effects of conjugated equine estrogen in postmenopausal women with hysterectomy: The Women's Health Initiative randomized controlled trial. *Journal of the American Medical Association* 2004; 291:1701–1712.

73. Calle EE et al. Postmenopausal hormone use and breast cancer associations differ by hormone regimen and histologic subtype. *Cancer* 2009 Mar 1; 115(5):936–945.

74. Ross RK et al. Effect of hormone replacement therapy on breast cancer risk: Estrogen versus estrogen plus progestin. *Journal of the National Cancer Institute* 2000.

75. Vachon CM et al. Case-control study of increased mammographic breast density response to hormone replacement therapy. *Cancer Epidemiology Biomarkers and Prevention* 2002; 11:1382–1388.

76. Ettinger B et al. Reduced mortality associated with long-term postmenopausal estrogen therapy. *Obstetrics and Gynecology* 1996; 87(1):6–12

77. Fournier A, Berrino F, Clavel-Chapelon F. Unequal risks for breast cancer associated with different hormone replacement therapies: Results from the E3N cohort study. *Breast Cancer Res Treat* 2008 January; 107(1):103–111.

78. Chen CL et al. Hormone replacement therapy in relation to breast cancer. *Journal of the American Medical Association* 2002; 287:734–741.

79. Newcomer LM et al. Postmenopausal hormone use and risk of breast cancer by histologic type. *American Journal of Epidemiology* 1999; 149:S79.

80. Li CI et al. Hormone replacement therapy in relation to risk of lobular and ductal breast carcinoma in middle-aged women. *Cancer* 2000; 88:2570–2577.

81. Newcomb PA et al. Postmenopausal estrogen and progestin use in relation to breast cancer risk. *Cancer Epidemiology, Biomarkers & Prevention* 2002; 11:593–600.

82. Eliassen AH, Hankinson SE. Endogenous hormone levels and risk of breast, endometrial, and ovarian cancers: Prospective studies. *Adv Exp Med Biol* 2008; 630:148–165.

83. Tamimi RM et al. Combined estrogen and testosterone use and risk of breast cancer in postmenopausal women. *Arch Intern Med* 2006; 166 (14):1483–1489.

84. Orgeas CC et al. Breast cancer incidence after hormonal infertility treatment in Sweden: A cohort study. *Am J Obstet Gynecol* 2009 Jan; 200(1):72.

85. Lemer-Geva L et al. Infertility, ovulation induction treatments, and the incidence of breast cancer: A historical prospective cohort of Israeli women. *Breast Cancer Res Treat* 2006; 100(2):201–212.

86. Pappo I et al. The possible association between IVF and breast cancer incidence. *Ann Surg Oncol* 2008 Apr; 15(4):1048–1055.

87. Papadopoulos FC et al. Age at onset of anorexia nervosa and breast cancer risk. *Eur J Cancer Prev* 2009; Jun 18(3):207–211.

88. Holmes MD et al. Association of dietary intake of fat and fatty acids with risk of breast cancer. *Journal of the American Medical Association* 1999; 281(10):914–920.

89. Prentice RL et al. Low-fat dietary pattern and risk of invasive breast cancer: The Women's Health Initiative randomized controlled dietary modification trial. *JAMA* 2006 Feb 8; 295(6):629–642.

90. Pierce JP et al. Influence of a diet very high in vegetables, fruit, and fiber and low in fat on prognosis following treatment for breast cancer: The Women's Healthy Eating and Living (WHEL) randomized trial. *JAMA* 2007 Jul 18; 298(3):289–298.

91. Cummings SR et al. Prevention of breast cancer in postmenopausal women: Approaches to estimating and reducing risk. *J Natl Cancer Inst* 2009 Mar 18; 101(6):384 396. Key J et al. Meta-analysis of studies of alcohol and breast cancer with consideration of the methodological issues. *J Natl Cancer Inst* 2006; 17(6):759–770. Zhang S et al. A prospective study of folate intake and the risk of breast cancer. *Journal of the American Medical Association* 1999; 281:1632–1637.

92. Key J et al. Meta-analysis of studies of alcohol and breast cancer with consideration of the methodological issues. *J Natl Cancer Inst* 2006; 17(6):759–770. Sellers TA et al. Dietary folate intake, alcohol, and risk of breast cancer in a prospective study of postmenopausal women. *Epidemiology* 2001; 12:420–428.

93. Zhang SM et al. Plasma folate, vitamin B6, vitamin B12 and homocysteine and risk of breast cancer. *Journal of the National Cancer Institute* 2003; 95:373–380. Sellers TA et al. Dietary folate intake, alcohol, and risk of breast cancer in a prospective study of postmenopausal women. *Epidemiology* 2001; 12:420–428.

94. Zhang SM et al. Plasma folate, vitamin B6, vitamin B12, and homocysteine and risk of breast cancer. *Journal of the National Cancer Institute* 2003; 95:373–380.

95. Rohan TE et al. Dietary folate consumption and breast cancer risk. *Journal of the National Cancer Institute* 2000; 92:266–269.

Chapter 6

1. The Collaborative Group on Hormonal Factors in Breast Cancer. Familial breast cancer: Collaborative reanalysis of individual data from 52 epidemiological studies including 58,209 women with breast cancer and 101,986 women without the disease. *Lancet* 2001; 358:1389–1399.

2. Easton DF et al. Genetic linkage analysis in familial breast and ovarian cancer: Results from 214 families. *American Journal of Human Genetics* 1993; 52:678.

3. Shattuck-Eidens D at al. BRCA 1 sequence analysis in women at high risk for susceptibility mutations: Risk factor analysis and implications for genetic testing. *Journal of the American Medical Association* 1997; 278:1242.

4. Liede A, Karlan BY, Narod SA. Cancer risks for male carriers of germline mutations in BRCA 1 or BRCA 2: A Review of the literature. *Journal of Clinical Oncology* 2004; 22:735–742.

5. Narod, SA. Modifiers of risk of hereditary breast cancer. *Oncogene* 2006; 25:5832–5836.

6. Narod SA, Foulkes WD. BRCA 1 and BRCA 2: 1994 and beyond. *Nature Reviews Cancer* 2004; 4:665–676.

7. Olopade OI, Artioli G. Efficacy of risk-reducing salpingo-oophorectomy in women with BRCA 1/2 mutations. *Breast Journal* 2004; 10(Suppl 1):S5–S9.

8. Bergthorsson JT et al. Chromosome imbalance at the 3pl4 region in human breast tumors: High frequency in patients with inherited predisposition due to BRCA 2. *European Journal of Cancer* 1998; 34(1):1544.

9. Dorum A et al. A BRCA 1 founder mutation, identified with haplotype analysis, allowing genotype/phenotype determination and predictive testing. *European Journal of Cancer* 1997; 33:2390.

10. Weitzel JN et al. Prevalence of BRCA mutations and founder effect in high-risk Hispanic families. *Cancer Epidemiol Biomarkers Prev* 2005 Jul; 14(7):1666–1671.

11. John EM et al. Prevalence of pathogenic BRCA 1 mutation carriers in 5 US racial/ethnic groups. *JAMA* 2007 Dec 26; 298(24):2869–2876.

12. Iglehart JD et al. Overestimation of hereditary breast cancer risk. *Annals of Surgery* 1998; 228(3):375–384.

13. White DB et al. Too many referrals of low-risk women for BRCA 1/2 genetic services by family physicians. *Cancer Epidemiolo Biomarkers Prev* 2008 Nov; 17(11):2980–2986.

14. Newman B et al. Frequency of breast cancer attributable to BRCA 1 in a population-based series of American women. *Journal of the American Medical Association* 1998; 279:915–921.

15. Peto J et al. Prevalence of BRCA 1 and BRCA 2 gene mutations in patients with early-onset breast cancer. *Journal of the National Cancer Institute* 1999; 91(11):943–949.

16. Metcalfe KA et al. Breast cancer risks in women with a family history of breast or ovarian cancer who have tested negative for a BRCA 1 or BRCA 2 mutation. *British Journal of Cancer* 2009; 100:421–425.

17. Frank TS et al. Clinical characteristics of individuals with germline mutations in BRCA 1 and BRCA 2: Analysis of 10,000 individuals. *J Clin Oncol* 2002; 20:1480–1490.

18. Nanda R et al. Genetic testing in an ethnically diverse cohort of high-risk women: A comparative analysis of BRCA 1 and BRCA 2 mutations in American families of European and African ancestry. *JAMA* 2005; 294:1925–1933.

19. Weitzel JN et al. Prevalence of BRCA mutations and founder effect in high-risk Hispanic families. *Cancer Epidemiol Biomarkers Prev* 2005; 14:1666–1671.

20. Domchek S, Weber BL. Genetic variants of uncertain significance: Flies in the ointment. *Journal of Clinical Oncology* 2008; 26 (1):16–17.

21. Isaacs C, Peshkin BN, Schwartz M. Genetic testing and management of patients with hereditary breast cancer. In *Diseases of the Breast,* 231. 4th ed. Philadelphia: Lippincott Williams & Wilkins, 2010.

22. Frank TS et al. Sequence analysis of BRCA 1/2: Correlation of mutations with family history and ovarian cancer risk. *Journal of Clinical Oncology* 1998; 16:2417.

23. Meijers-Heijboer H et al. Breast cancer after prophylactic mastectomy in women with a BRCA 1 or BRCA 2 mutation. *New England Journal of Medicine* 2001; 345:159–164.

24. Brekelmans CTM et al. Effectiveness of breast cancer surveillance in BRCA 1/2 gene mutation carriers and women with high familial risk. *Journal of Clinical Oncology* 2001; 19:924–930.

25. Komenaka IK et al. The development of interval breast malignancies in patients with BRCA mutations. *Cancer* 2004; 100:2079–2083.

26. Kriege M et al. Efficacy of MRI and mammography for breast cancer screening in women with a familial or genetic predisposition. *New England Journal of Medicine* 2004; 351:427–437.

27. Walsh T et al. Spectrumo f mutations in BRCA 1BrCA 2 CHEK2 and TP53 in families at high risk of breast cancer. *JAMA* 2006; 295(12):1379–1388.

28. Offit K. Breast cancer single-nucleotide polymorphisms: Statistical significance and clinical utility. *Journal of the National Cancer Institute* 2009; 101(14):973–975.

29. Hartmann LC et al. Benign breast disease and the risk of breast cancer. *New England Journal of Medicine* 2005; 353:229–237.

30. Gayet A et al. Does hormone replacement therapy increase the frequency of breast atypical hyperplasia in postmenopausal women? Results from the Bouches du Rhone district screening campaign. *Eur J Cancer* 2003; 39 (12):1738–1745.

31. Dupont WD, Page DL. Risk factors for breast cancer in women with proliferative breast disease. *New England Journal of Medicine* 1985; 312:146–151.

32. Rubin E et al. Proliferative disease and atypia in biopsies performed for non-palpable lesions detected mammographically. *Cancer* 1988; 61:2077–2082.

33. Davis HH, Simons M, Davis JB. Cystic disease of the breast relationship to cancer. *Cancer* 1974; 17:957.

34. Marshall LM et al. Risk of breast cancer associated with atypical hyperplasia of lobular and ductal types. *Cancer Epidemiology, Biomarkers, and Prevention* 1997; 6:297–301.

35. Page DL et al. Atypical hyperplastic lesions of the female breast: A long-term follow-up study. *Cancer* 1985; 55:2698–2708.

36. Simpson JF. Update on atypical epithelial hyperplasia and ductal carcinoma in situ. *Pathology* 2009; 41(1): 36–39.

37. Page DL et al. Atypical lobular hyperplasia as a unilateral predictor of breast cancer risk: A retrospective cohort study. *Lancet* 2003; 361:125–129.

38. Arpino G et al. Lobular neoplasia on core-needle biopsy: Clinical significance. *Cancer* 2004; 101:242–250.

39. Fisher B et al. Tamoxifen for prevention of breast cancer: Report of the National Surgical Adjuvant Breast and Bowel Project P-1 study. *Journal of the National Cancer Institute* 1998; 90(18):1371–1388.

40. Radisky DC, Hartmann LC. Mammary involution and breast cancer risk: Transgenic models and clinical studies. *J Mammary Gland Biol Neoplasia* 2009 Jun; 14(2):181–191.

41. Leborgne R. Intraductal biopsy of certain pathologic processes of the breast. *Surgery* 1946; 19:47–54.

42. Papanicolaou GN. Exfoliative cytology of the human mammary gland and its value in the diagnosis of cancer and other diseases of the breast. *Cancer* 1958; II(2):377–409.

43. Buehring GC. Screening for breast atypias using exfoliative cytology. *Cancer* 1979; 43(5):1788–1799.

44. Sartorius OW et al. Cytologic evaluation of breast fluid in the detection of breast disease. *Journal of the National Cancer Institute* 1977; 67:277–284.

45. Wrensch MR et al. Breast cancer incidence in women with abnormal cytology in nipple aspirates of breast fluid. *American Journal of Epidemiology* 1992; 135:130–141.

46. Buehring GC et al. Presence of epithelial cells in nipple aspirate fluid is associated with subsequent breast cancer: A 25-year prospective study. *Breast Cancer Res Treat* 2007 Mar; 102(1):125–127.

47. Baltzell KA et al. Epithelial cells in nipple aspirate fluid and subsequent breast cancer risk: A historic prospective study. *BMC Cancer* 2008 Mar 19; 8:75.

48. Sauter E et al. Nipple aspirate fluid: A promising non-invasive method to identify cellular markers of breast cancer risk. *British Journal of Cancer* 1997; 76(4):494–501.

49. Dooley WC et al. Ductal lavage for detection of cellular atypia in women at high risk for breast cancer. *Journal of the National Cancer Institute* 2001; 93:1624–1632.

50. King BL et al. Immunocytochemical analysis of breast cells obtained by ductal lavage. *Cancer Cytopathol* 2002; 96.

51. Yamamoto D, Tanaka K. A review of mammary ductoscopy in breast cancer. *Breast Journal* 2004; 10(4):295–297.

52. Fabian C et al. Correlation of breast tissue biomarkers with hyperplasia and dysplasia in fine-needle aspirates (FNAs) of women at high and low risk for breast cancer. *Proceedings of Annual Meeting of American Association of Cancer Researchers* 1994; 35(A1703).

53. Gail MH et al. Projecting individualized absolute invasive breast cancer risk in African American women. *J Natl Cancer Inst* 2007 Dec 5; 99(23):1782–1792.

54. Tice JA et al. Using clinical factors and mammographic breast density to estimate breast cancer risk: Development and validation of a new predictive model. *Ann Intern Med* 2008 Mar 4; 148(5):337–347. Summary for patients in *Ann Intern Med* 2008 Mar 4; 148(5):I34.

55. Tyrer J, Duffy SW, Cuzick J. A breast cancer prediction model incorporating familial and personal risk factors. *Stat Med* 2004 Apr 15; 23(7):1111–1130. Erratum in *Stat Med* 2005 Jan 15; 24(1):156.

Chapter 7

1. Stuebe AM. Lactation and incidence of premenopausal breast cancer: Longitudinal study. *Arch Intern Med* 2009 Aug 10; 169(15):1364–1371.

2. Van Gils CH et al. Consumption of vegetables and fruits and risk of breast cancer. *Journal of the American Medical Association* 2005; 293:183–193.

3. Prentice RL et al. Low-fat dietary pattern and risk of invasive breast cancer: The Women's Health Initiative randomized controlled dietary modification trial. *JAMA* 2006 Feb 8; 295(6):629–642.

4. Wu AH et al. Adolescent and adult soy intake and risk of breast cancer in Asian Americans. *Carcinogenesis* 2002; 23(9):1491–1496.

5. Lee SA et al. Adolescent and adult soy food intake and breast cancer risk: Results from the Shanghai Women's Health Study. *Am J Clin Nutr* 2009 Jun; 89(6):1920–1926.

6. Messina M, Wu AH. Perspectives on the soy-breast cancer relations. *Am J Clin Nutr* 2009 May; 89(5):1673S–1679S.

7. Korde LA et al. Childhood soy intake and breast cancer risk in Asian American women. *Cancer Epidemiol Biomarkers Prev.* 2009 Apr; 18(4):1050–1059.

8. Rosolowich V et al. Mastalgia. *J Obstet Gynaecol Can* 2006; 28(1):49–71.

9. Goss PE et al. Effects of dietary flaxseed in women with cyclical mastalgia. *Breast Cancer Res Treat* 2000; 64:49.

10. Thompson LU et al. Dietary flaxseed alters tumor biological markers in post-menopausal breast cancer. *Clin Cancer Res* 2005; 11(10):3828–3835.

11. Fabian CF et al. Evaluation of Ki-67 measured in benign breast tissue acquired from premenopausal women treated with a flaxseed derivative. *J Clin Oncol* 2009; 27:15.

12. Wu AH et al. Green tea, soy, and mammographic density in Singapore Chinese women. *Cancer Epidemiolo Biomarkers Prev* 2008 Dec; 17(12):3358–3365.

13. Druesne-Pecollo N et al. Beta-carotene supplementation and cancer risk: A systematic review and meta-analysis of randomized controlled trials. *J Cancer* 2009 Oct 28.

14. Lappe JM et al. Vitamin D and calcium supplementation reduces cancer risk: Results of a randomized trial. *Am J Clin Nutr* 2007; 85:1586–1591.

15. Chlebowski R et al. Calcium plus vitamin D supplementation and the risk of breast cancer. *J Natl Cancer Inst* 2008; 100:1581–1591.

16. Garland CF et al. Vitamin D and prevention of breast cancer: Pooled analysis. *J Steroid Biochem Mol Biol* 2007; 103:708–711.

17. Chlebowski RT et al. Calcium plus vitamin D supplementation and the risk of breast cancer. *J Natl Cancer Inst* 2008 Nov 19; 100(22):1581–1591.

18. Holick MF. Vitamin D deficiency. *N Engl J Med* 2007; 357:266–281.

19. Holmes MD, Willet WC. Does diet affect breast cancer risk? *Breast Cancer Research* 2004; 6:170–178.

20. Toniolo P et al. Serum carotenoids and breast cancer. *American Journal of Epidemiology* 2001; 153:1142–1147.

21. Sato R et al. Prospective study of carotenoids, tocopherols, and retinoid concentrations and the risk of breast cancer. *Cancer Epidemiology Biomarkers Prevention* 2002; 11:451–457.

22. Kline K et al. Vitamin E and breast cancer prevention: Current status and future potential. *Journal of Mammary Gland Biology and Neoplasia* 2003; 8(1).

23. Neuhouser et al. Multivitamin use and risk of cancer and cardiovascular disease in the Women's Health Initiative cohorts. *Arch Intern Med* 2009.

24. Bernstein L et al. Physical exercise activity and reduced risk of breast cancer in young women. *Journal of the National Cancer Institute* 1994; 86:1403.

25. Dallal CM et al. Long-term recreational physical activity and risk of invasive and in situ breast cancer. *Arch Intern Med* 2007; 167:408–415.

26. Bernstein L et al. The effects of moderate physical activity on menstrual cycle patterns in adolescence: Implications for breast cancer prevention. *British Journal of Cancer* 1987; 55:681.

27. Frisch RE et al. Lower lifetime occurrence of breast cancer and cancer of the reproductive system among former college athletes. *American Journal of Clinical Nutrition* 1987; 45:328.

28. Spicer DV et al. Pilot trial of a gonadotropin hormone agonist with replacement hormones as a prototype contraceptive to prevent breast cancer. *Contraception* 1993; 47:427.

29. Spicer D et al. Changes in mammographic densities induced by a hormonal contraceptive designed to reduce breast cancer risk. *Journal of the National Cancer Institute* 1994; 86(6):431.

30. Bernstein L et al. Treatment with human chorionic gonadotropin (hCG) and risk of breast cancer. *Cancer Epidemiol Biomark Prev* 1995; 4:437–440.

31. Fisher B et al. Tamoxifen for prevention of breast cancer: Report of the National Surgical Adjuvant Breast and Bowel Project P-1 study. *Journal of the National Cancer Institute* 1998; 90(18):1371–1388.

32. Gail MH et al. Projecting individualized probabilities of developing breast cancer for white females who are examined annually. *Journal of the National Cancer Institute* 1989; 81(24):1879–1886.

33. Cuzick J et al. Overview of the main outcomes in breast cancer prevention trials. *Lancet* 2003; 361:296–300.

34. Powles TJ. Twenty-year follow-up of the Royal Marsden randomized double blinded tamoxifen breast cancer prevention trial. *JNCI* 2007; 99:283–290.

35. Veronesi U et al. Tamoxifen for the prevention of breast cancer: Late results of the Italian randomized tamoxifen prevention trial among women with hysterectomy. *JNCI* 2007; 99:727–737.

36. Cuzick J et al. Long-term results of tamoxifen prophylaxis for breast cancer: 96-month follow-up of the randomized IBIS-I trial. *J Natl Cancer Inst* 2007 Feb 21; 99(4):272–282.

37. Gail M et al. Weighing the risks and benefits of tamoxifen treatment for preventing breast cancer. *Journal of the National Cancer Institute* 1999; 91:1829–1846.

38. Bernstein L et al. Tamoxifen therapy for breast cancer and endometrial cancer risk. *J Natl Cancer Inst* 1999 Oct 6; 91(19):1654–1562.

39. Vogel VG et al. Update of the National Surgical Adjuvant Breast and Bowel Project Study of Tamoxifen and Raloxifene (STAR) P-2 Trial: Preventing breast cancer cancer. *Prev Res* 2010; 3(6); OF1–11.

40. Temple W et al. Technical considerations for prophylactic mastectomy in patients at high risk for breast cancer. *American Journal of Surgery* 1991; 161(4):413.

41. Katipamula R et al. Trends in mastectomy rates at the Mayo Clinic, Rochester: Effect of surgical year and preoperative magnetic resonance. *J Clin Oncol* 2009 Sept; 27(25):4082–4088.

42. Parker WH et al. Ovarian conservation at the time of hysterectomy and long-term health outcomes in the Nurses' Health Study. *Obstet Gynecol* 2009 May; 113(5):1027–1037.

43. Rebbeck TB et al. Bilateral prophylactic mastectomy reduces breast cancer risk in BRCA 1 and BRCA 2 mutation carriers: The PROSE Study group. *J Clin Oncol* 2004; 22:1055–1062.

44. Heemskerk-Gerritsen BA et al. Prophylactic mastectomy in BRCA 1/2 mutation carriers and women at risk of hereditary breast cancer: Long-term experiences at the Rotterdam Family Cancer Clinic. *Ann Surg Oncol* 2007; 14:3335–3344.

45. Olopade OI, Artioli G. Efficacy of risk-reducing salpingo-oophorectomy in women with BRCA-1 and BRCA-2 mutations. *Breast J*. 2004 Jan-Feb; 10 Suppl 1:S5–9.

46. Piver MS et al. Primary peritoneal carcinoma after prophylactic oophorectomy in women with a family history of ovarian cancer. *Cancer* 1993; 71:2751–2755.

47. Rebbeck TR et al. Prophylactic oophorectomy in carriers of BRCA 1 or BRCA 2 mutations. *New England Journal of Medicine* 2002; 346:1616–1622.

48. Kurian AW, Sigal BM, Plevritis SK. Survival analysis of cancer risk reduction strategies for BRCA 1/2 mutation carriers. *J Clin Oncol* 2009; 28:222–231.

49. Narod SA. Modifiers of risk of hereditary breast cancer. *Oncogene* 2006; 25:5832–5836.

50. Murata S et al. Ductal access for prevention and therapy of mammary tumors. *Cancer Res* 2006 Jan 15; 66(2):638–645.

51. Jaini R, Kesaraju P, Johnson J et al An autoimmune-mediated strategy for prophylactic breast cancer vacation Nature Medicine published online at http://www.naturemedicine/ and downloaded June 9, 2010.

Chapter 8

1. Roubidoux MA. Invasive cancers detected after breast cancer screening yielded a negative result: Relationship of mammographic density to tumor prognostic factors. *Radiology* 2004 Jan; 230(1):42–48.

2. Sadowski N. Personal communication, 1988.

3. Kornguth P et al. Impact of patient-controlled compression on the mammography experience. *Radiology* 1993; 186(1):99.

4. Lewin JM et al. Comparison of full-field digital mammography with screen-film mammography for cancer detection: Results of 4,945 paired examinations. *Radiology* 2001; 218(3):873–880.

5. Lewin JM et al. Clinical comparison of full-field digital mammography and screen-film mammography for detection of breast cancer. *American Journal of Roentgenology* 2002; 179(3):671–677.

6. Gur D et al. Changes in breast cancer detection and mammography recall rates after the introduction of a computer aided detection system. *Journal of the National Cancer Institute* 2004; 96:185–190.

7. Elmore JG, Carney P. Computer-aided detection of breast cancer: Has promise outstripped performance? *Journal of the National Cancer Institute* 2004; 96:162–163.

8. Homer MJ. Nonpalpable breast microcalcifications: Frequency, management, and results of incisional biopsy. *Radiology* 1992; 185:411.

9. Berend ME et al. The natural history of mammographic calcifications subjected to interval follow-up. *Archives of Surgery* 1992; 127:1309.

10. Stomper P et al. Is mammography painful? A multicenter patient survey. *Archives of Internal Medicine* 1988; 148(3):521.

11. Kolb TM, Lichy J, Newhouse JH. Comparison of the performance of screening, mammography, physical examination, and breast US and evaluation of factors that influence them: An analysis of 27,825 patient evaluations. *Radiology* 2002; 225:165–175.

12. Kolb TM et al. Occult cancer in women with dense breasts: Detection with screening US-diagnostic yields and tumor characteristics. *Radiology* 1998; 207:191–199.

13. Parker SH et al. Stereotactic breast biopsy with a biopsy gun. *Radiology* 1990; 176:741.

14. Delille JP et al. Physiologic changes in breast magnetic resonance imaging during the menstrual cycle: Perfusion imaging, signal enhancement, and influence of the T1 relaxation time of breast tissue. *Breast Journal* 2006; 11:236–241.

15. Warner E et al. Comparison of breast magnetic resonance imaging mammography, and ultrasound for surveillance of women at high risk for hereditary breast cancer. *Journal of Clinical Oncology* 2001; 19:3524–3531.

16. Van der Hoeven JJM et al. 18F-2-Fluoro-2-Deoxy-D-Glucose positron emission tomography in staging of locally advanced breast cancer. *Journal of Clinical Oncology* 2004; 22:1253–1259.

17. Martelli G et al. Diagnostic efficacy of physical examination, mammography, fine needle aspiration, cytology (triple-test) in solid breast lumps: An analysis of 1708 cases. *Tumori* 1990; 76:476.

18. Pass HA. Stereotactic biopsy of breast cancer. *PPO (Principles & Practice of Oncology)* Updates 1998; 12(12):1–7.

19. Martelli et al. Diagnostic efficacy.

Chapter 9

1. Thomas DB et al. Randomized trial of breast self-examination in Shanghai: Methodology and preliminary results. *Journal of the National Cancer Institute* 1997; 89:355–365.

2. U.S. Preventive Services Task Force Guidelines Screening for Breast Cancer. U.S. Preventive Services Task Force Recommendation Statement. *Ann Intern Med* 2009; 151:716–726.

3. Miller A et al. Canadian National Breast Screening Study: 2. Breast cancer detection and death rates among women aged 50–59 years. *Canadian Medical Association Journal* 1992; 147(10):1477.

4. Goodson WH III et al. Optimization of clinical breast examination. *Am J Med* 2010; 123: 329–334.

5. Vainio H, Biacnchini F, eds. *Breast Cancer Screening.* International Agency for Research on Cancer Handbook on Cancer Prevention, Report no. 7. Lyon, France: International Agency for Research on Cancer, 2002.

6. Hofvind S et al. Comparing screening mammography for early breast cancer detection in Vermont and Norway. *J Natl Cancer Inst* 2008; 100:1082–1091.

7. Mandelblatt JS et al. Effects of mammography screening under different screening schedules: Model estimates of potential benefits and harms. *Annals of Internal Medicine* 2009; 151:738–7478.

8. Nelson HD et al. *Screening for Breast Cancer: An Update for the U.S. Preventive Services Task Force.* AHRQ Publication no. 10–05142-EF-5, November 2009. Agency for Healthcare Research and Quality, Rockville, MD. www.ahrq.gov/clinic/uspstf09/breastcancer/brcanup.htm.

9. Berrington de Gonzalez A, Reeves G. Mammographic screening before age 50 years in the UK: Comparison of the radiation risks with the mortality benefits. *British journal of cancer* 2005; 93:590–596.

10. Moss SM et al. Trial management effect of mammographic screening from age 40 years on breast cancer mortality at 10 years' follow-up: A randomized controlled trial. *Lancet* 2006; 368:2053–2060.

11. Armstrong K et al. Screening mammography in women 40–49 years of age: A Systematic review for the American College of Physicians. *Annals of Internal Medicine* 2007; 146(7):516–526.

12. Gotzsche PC, Nielsen M. Screening for breast cancer with mammography. *Cochrane Database Syst Rev* 2009; 7(4):CD0018777.

13. Jorgensen KJ, Gotzsche PC. Overdiagnosis in publicly organized mammography screening programs: Systematic review of incidence trends. *BMJ* 2009 Jul; 9:339.

14. Kriege M et al. Efficacy of MRI and mammography for breast cancer screening in women with a familial or genetic predisposition. *N Engl J Med* 2004; 351:427–437.

15. Hamilton LJ et al. Will MRI screening deliver the expected survival advantage in BRCA 1 carriers. *Clinical Radiology* 2009; 64(11):1045–1047.

16. Berg WA et al. Reasons women at elevated risk of breast cancer refuse breast MR imaging screening: ACRIN 6666. *Radiology.* 2010 Jan; 254(1):79–87.

17. Berg WA et al. Combined screening with ultrasound and mammography vs. mammography alone in women at elevated risk of breast cancer. *JAMA* 2008; 299(18):2151–2163.

18. Jones EA et al. Breast-specific gamma-imaging: Molecular imaging of the breast using 99mTcsestamibi and a small-field-of-view gamma-camera. *J Nuc Med Technol* 2009 Dec; 37(4):201–205.

19. Caprio MG et al. Dual-time-point [(18)F]-FDG PET/CT in the diagnostic evaluation of suspicious breast lesions. *Radiol Med* 2009 Dec 16.

20. Stojadinovic A et al. Electrical impedance scanning for the early detection of breast cancer in young women: preliminary results of a multicenter prospective clinical trial. *Journal of Clinical Oncology* 2005; 2023(12):2703–2701.

21. Arora N et al. Effectiveness of a noninvasive digital infrared thermal imaging system in the detection of breast cancer. *Am J Surg* 2008; 196(4):523–526.

Chapter 10

1. Rollin B. First, *You Cry.* New York: New American Library, 1976.

2. Kushner R. *Alternatives.* Cambridge, MA: Kensington, 1984.

3. Peters-Golden H. Breast cancer: Varied perceptions of social support in the illness experience. *Social Science Medicine* 1982; 16:483.

4. Kaspar A. Telephone interview.

5. Taylor SE, Lichtman RR, Wood JV. Attributions, beliefs about control, and adjustment to breast cancer. *Journal of Perspectives on Sociology and Psychology* 1984; 46:489.

6. Wellisch DK et al. Psychological functioning of daughters of breast cancer patients. Part II: Characterizing the distressed daughter of the breast cancer patient. *Psychosomatics* 1992; 33(2):171.

7. Lichtman RR et al. Relations with children after breast cancer: The mother-daughter relationship at risk. *Journal of Psychosociology and Oncology* 1984; 2:1.

8. Veronesi U. Randomized trials comparing conservative techniques with conventional surgery: An overview. In Tobias JS, Peckham MJ, eds. *Primary Management of Breast Cancer: Alternatives to Mastectomy Management of Malignant Disease Series.* London: E. Arnold; 1985.

9. Peters WP et al. High-dose chemotherapy and autologous bone marrow support as consolidation after standard-dose adjuvant therapy for high-risk primary breast cancer. *Journal of Clinical Oncology* 1993; 11:1132–1143.

10. Tallman MS et al. Conventional adjuvant chemotherapy with or without high-dose chemotherapy and autologous stem cell transplantation in high-risk breast cancer. *New England Journal of Medicine* 2003; 349:17–26.

11. Garcia-Carbonero R et al. Patient selection in high-dose chemotherapy trials: Relevance in high-risk breast cancer. *Journal of Clinical Oncology* 1997; 15:3178–3184.

12. Early Breast Cancer Trialists' Cooperative Group. Effects of chemotherapy and hormonal therapy for early breast cancer on recurrence and 15-year survival: An overview of the randomized trials. *Lancet* 2005; 1687–1717.

13. Lorde A. *A Burst of Light*. New York: Firebrand; 1988.

Chapter 11

1. Dixon JM et al. Infiltrating lobular carcinoma of the breast: An evaluation of the incidence and consequence of bilateral disease. *British Journal of Surgery* 1983; 70:513.

2. Mansi JL et al. Outcome of primary breast cancer patients with micrometastases: A long-term follow-up study. *Lancet* 1999; 354:197–202.

3. Gotteland M et al. Estrogen receptors (ER) in human breast cancer. *Cancer* 1994; 74(3):864.

4. Slamon D et al. Studies of the Her-2/neu proto-oncogene in human breast and ovarian cancer. *Science* 1989; 244(4905):707.

5. Dybdal B et al. Determination of HER2 gene amplification by fluorescence in situ hybridization and concordance with the clinical trials immunohistochemical assay in women with metastatic breast cancer evaluated for treatment with trstuzumab. *Breast Cancer Res Treat* 2005; 93(1):3–11.

6. Allred DC et al. Overexpression of HER-2/neu and its relationship with other prognostic factors change during the progression of in situ to invasive breast cancer. *Hum Pathol* 1992; 23: 974–979.

7. Ewers SV et al. Prognostic significance of flow cytometric DNA analysis and estrogen receptor content in breast carcinomas: A 10-year survival study. *Breast Cancer Research and Treatment* 1992; 24:115.

8. Gazic B et al. S-phase fraction determined on fine needle aspirates is an independent prognostic factor in breast cancer-a multivariate study of 770 patients. *Cytopathology* 2008; 19(5):294–302.

9. Edge SB et al. *Cancer Staging Manual*, chap. 32. 7th ed. New York: Springer, 2010.

10. Diehl IJ et al. Detection of tumor cells in bone marrow of patients with primary breast cancer: A prognostic factor for distant metastasis. *Journal of Clinical Oncology* 1992; 10:1534–1539.

11. Braun S et al. A pooled analysis of bone marrow micrometastasis in breast cancer. *NEJM* 2005; 353:793–802.

12. Ginestier C et al. ALDH1 as a marker of normal and malignant human mammary stem cells and a predictor of poor clinical outcome. *Cell Stem Cell* 2007; 1:555–567.

13. Haagensen C. *Diseases of the Breast*. Philadelphia: Saunders, 1971.

14. Perou CM et al. Molecular portraits of human breast tumors. *Nature* 2000; 406:747–752.

15. Chen WY et al. Risk factors and hormone-receptor status: Epidemiology risk-prediction models and treatment implications for breast cancer. *Nat Clin Pract Oncol* 2007:415–423.

16. Fan C et al. Concordance among gene-expression-based predictors for breast cancer. *N Engl J Med* 2006 Aug 10; 355(6):560–569.

17. Rouzier et al. Breast cancer molecular subtypes respond differently to preoperative chemotherapy. *Clin Cancer Res* 2005; 11:5678–5685.

18. Chen WY et al. Risk factors and hormone-receptor status: Epidemiology risk-prediction models and treatment implications for breast cancer. *Nat Clin Pract Oncol* 2007; 415–423.

19. Paik S et al. A multigene assay to predict recurrence of tamoxifen-treated, node-negative breast cancer. *New England Journal of Medicine* 2004; 351(27):2817–2865.

20. Paik S et al. Expression of the 21 genes in the recurrence score assay and prediction of clinical benefit from tamoxifen in NSABP study B 14 and chemotherapy in NSABP study B 20. *Proceedings of San Antonio Breast Cancer Symposium* 2004; 24.

21. Albain KS, Paik S, van't Veer L. Prediction of adjuvant chemotherapy benefit in endocrine responsive early breast cancer using multigene assays. *Breast* 2009 Oct; suppl 3:S141–145.

22. Albain K et al. Prognostic and predictive value of the 21 gene recurrence score assay in postmenopausal node-positive breast cancer. *Breast Cancer Research and Treatment* 2007; 106(S1):A10.

23. Cardoso F et al. The MINDACT trial: The first prospective clinical validation of a genomic tool. *Mol Oncol* 2007 Dec; 30:246–251.

24. Berry DA et al. Effects of improvements in chemotherapy on disease-free and overall survival of estrogen-receptor negative, node positive breast cancer: 20 year experience of the CALGB and US Breast Intergroup. *Breast Cancer Research and Treatment* 2004; 88(S1):Abstract no. 29.

Chapter 12

1. Nimeus-Malmstrom et al. Gene-expression profiling in primary breast cancer distinguishes patients developing local recurrence after breast-conservation surgery, with or without postoperative radiotherapy. *Breast Cancer Research*. 2008; 10(2):R34.

2. Early Breast Cancer Clinical Trialists' Collaborative Group. Effects of adjuvant tamoxifen and of cytotoxic therapy on mortality in early breast cancer: An overview of 61 randomized trials among 28,896 women. *Lancet* 2005; 365(9472):1687–1717.

3. Fisher B et al. Twenty-year follow-up of a randomized trial comparing total mastectomy, lumpectomy, and lumpectomy plus irradiation for the treatment of breast cancer. *New England Journal of Medicine* 2002; 347:1233–1241.

4. Veronesi U et al. Twenty-year follow-up of a randomized study comparing breast-conserving surgery with radical mastectomy for early breast cancer. *New England Journal of Medicine* 2002; 347:1227–1232.

5. Tuttle TM et al. Increasing use of contralateral prophylactic mastectomy for breast cancer patients: A trend toward more aggressive surgical treatment. *J Clin Oncol* 2007; 25:5203–5209.

6. Holland R et al. Histological multifocality of Tis, T1–2 breast carcinomas: Implications for clinical trials of breast-conserving treatment. *Cancer* 1985; 56:979.

7. Fisher B et al. Twenty-year follow-up.

8. Tillman GF et al. Effect of breast magnetic resonance imaging on the clinical management of women with early-stage breast carcinoma. *Journal of Clinical Oncology* 2002; 20:3413.

9. Houssami N, Hayes DF. Review of preoperative magnetic resonance imaging (MRI) in breast cancer: Should MRI be performed on all women with newly diagnosed, early stage breast cancer? *CA Cancer J Clin* 2009 Sep-Oct; 59(5):290–302.

10. Turnbull LW et al. Multicentre randomized controlled trial examining the cost-effectiveness of contrast-enhanced high yield magnetic resonance imaging in women with primary breast cancer scheduled for wide local excision (COMICE). *Health Technol Assess* 2010 Jan; 14(1):1–182.

11. Solin LJ et al. Relationship of breast magnetic resonance imaging to outcome after breast conservation treatment with radiation for women with early-stage invasive breast carcinoma or ductal carcinoma in situ. *J Clin Oncol* 2008 Jan 20; 26(3):386–391.

12. Bleicher RJ et al. Association of routine pretreatment magnetic resonance imaging with time to surgery, mastectomy rate, and margin status. *J Am Coll Surg* 2009 Aug; 209(2):180–187.

13. Schnitt SJ et al. The relationship between microscopic margins of resection and the risk of local recurrence in patients with breast cancer treated with breast conserving surgery and radiotherapy. *Cancer* 1994; 74:1746.

14. Harris J, Morrow M. Local management of invasive cancer: Breast. In Harris JR et al., eds. *Diseases of the Breast*, 731. 3rd ed. Philadelphia: Lippincott/Williams & Wilkins 2004.

15. Okumura SO et al. Feasibility of breast-conserving therapy for macroscopically multiple ipsilateral breast cancer. *International Journal of Radiation Oncology, Biology, and Physics* 2004; 59(1):146–151.

16. Kroll SS et al. Breast reconstruction with myocutaneous flaps in previously irradiated patients. *Plast Reconstru Surg* 1994 Mar; 93(3):460–469.

17. Early Breast Cancer Trialists' Collaborative Group. Effects of chemotherapy and hormonal therapy for early breast cancer on recurrence and 15 year survival: An overview of the randomized trials. *Lancet* 2005:366:2087–2106.

18. Giordano SH et al. Risk of cardiac death after adjuvant radiotherapy for breast cancer. *Journal of the National Cancer Institute* 2005; 97(6):416–424.

19. Deutsch M et al. The incidence of lung carcinoma after surgery for breast carcinoma with and without postoperative radiotherapy: Results of National Surgical Adjuvant Breast and Bowel Project (NSABP) Clinical Trials B–04 and B–06. *Cancer* 2003; 98:1362–1368.

20. Zablotska LB, Neugut AI. Lung carcinoma after radiation therapy in women treated with lumpectomy or mastectomy for primary breast carcinoma. *Cancer* 2003; 97:1404–1411.

21. Harris JR et al. Consensus statement on post-mastectomy radiation therapy. *International Journal of Radiation Oncology, Biology, and Physics* 1999; 44:989–990.

22. Recht A et al. Post-mastectomy radiotherapy: Clinical practice guidelines of the American Society of Clinical Oncology. *Journal of Clinical Oncology* 2001; 19:1539–1569.

23. National Comprehensive Cancer Network. Clinical Practice Guidelines in Oncology. www.nccn.org.

24. Chung CS, Harris JR. Post-mastectomy radiation therapy: Translating local benefits into improved survival. *Breast* 2007 Dec; 16 Suppl 2:78–83.

25. Smith BD et al. Accelerated partial breast irradiation consensus statement from the American Society of Radiation Oncology (ASTRO). *Radiation Oncology, Biology, and Physics* 2009; 74(4):987–1001.

26. Vaidya JS, Joseph DJ, Tobias JS, et al Targeted intraoperative radiotherapy versus whole breast radiotherapy for breast cancer (TARGIT-A-trial): an international prospective, randomized, non-inferiority phase 3 trial. Published online the Lancet.com June 5 2010 DOI:10.1016/S0140–6736(10)60837–9

27. Nimeus-Malmstrom et al. Gene-expression profiling in primary breast cancer distinguishes patients developing local recurrence after breast-conservation surgery, with or without postoperative radiotherapy. *Breast Cancer Research* 2008; 10(2):R34.

28. Orr RK. The impact of prophylactic axillary node dissection on breast cancer survival: A Bayesian meta-analysis. *Annals of Surgical Oncology* 1999; 6:109–116.

29. Louis-sylvestre C et al. Axillary treatment in conservative management of operable breast cancer: Dissection or radiotherapy? Results of a randomized study with 15 years of follow-up. *Journal of Clinical Oncology* 2004; 22:97–101.

30. Guiliano AE et al. Sentinel lymphadenectomy in breast cancer. *Journal of Clinical Oncology* 1997; 5:2345–2350.

31. Van la Parra RF et al. Validation of a nomogram to predict the risk of nonsentinel lymph node metastases in breast cancer patients with a positive sentinel node biopsy: Validation of the MSKCC breast nomogram. *Ann Surg Oncol* 2009 May; 16(5):1128 1135.

32. Reed J, Rosman M, Verbanac KM. Prognostic implications of isolated tumor cells and micrometastases in sentinel nodes of patients with invasive breast cancer: 10 year analysis of patients enrolled in the prospective East Carolina University/Anne Arundel Medical Center Sentinel Node Multicenter Study. *J Am Coll Surg* 2009 Mar; 208(3):333–340.

33. Pugliese MS et al. Predictors of completion axillary lymph node dissection in patients with immunohistochemical metastases to the sentinel lymph node in breast cancer. *Ann Surg Oncol* 2009 Dec 22.

34. Spanheimer PM et al. Measurement of uterine radiation exposure from lymphoscintigraphy indicates safety of sentinel lymph node biopsy during pregnancy. *Ann Surg Oncol* 2009 May; 16(5):1143–1147.

35. Noguchi M. Axillary reverse mapping for breast cancer. *Breast Cancer Res Treat* 2010 Feb; 119(3):529–535.

36. Love SM, McGuigan KA, Chap L. The Revlon/UCLA Breast Center practice guidelines for the treatment of breast disease. *Cancer Journal from Scientific American* 1996; 2(1):2–15.

37. Rosen P et al. Contralateral breast carcinoma: An assessment of risk and prognosis in stage I (TIN0M0) and stage II (T1N1M0) patients with 20 year follow up. *Surgery* 1989; 106(5):904–910.

38. Hislop T et al. Second primary cancers of the breast: Incidence and risk factors. *British Journal of Cancer* 1984; 49:79–85.

39. Herrington LJ et al. Efficacy of prophylactic mastectomy in women with unilateral breast cancer: A Cancer Research Network Project. *Journal of Clinical Oncology* 2005 July 1; 23(19).

40. Early Breast Cancer Collaborative Trialists' Group, Polychemotherapy for early breast cancer: An overview of the randomized trials. *Lancet* 1998 Sept 19; 352:930–942.

41. Osborne CK, Ravdin PM. Adjuvant systemic therapy of primary breast cancer. In Harris JR et al., eds. *Diseases of the Breast*, 625.

42. Rajagopal S, Goodman PJ, Tannock IF. Adjuvant chemotherapy for breast cancer: Discordance between physicians' perception of benefit and the results of clinical trials. *Journal of Clinical Oncology* 1994; 12(6):1296.

43. Crew KD. Prevalence of joint symptoms in postmenopausal women taking aromatase inhibitors for early-stage breast cancer. *J Clin Oncology* 2007; 25(25):3877–3883.

44. Zander AR et al. High-dose chemotherapy with autologous hematopoietic stem-cell support compared with standard-dose chemotherapy in breast cancer patients with 10 or more positive lymph nodes: First results of a randomized trial. *Journal of Clinical Oncology* 2004; 22:2273–2283.

45. Citron ML et al. Randomized trial of dose-dense versus conventionally scheduled and sequential versus concurrent combination chemotherapy as postoperative adjuvant treatment of node positive primary breast cancer: First report of Intergroup Trial C9741/Cancer and Leukemia Group B Trial 9741. *Journal of Clinical Oncology* 2003; 21:1431–1439.

46. Fisher B et al. Effect of preoperative chemotherapy on local-regional disease in women with operable breast cancer: Findings from National Surgical Adjuvant Breast and Bowel Project B-18. *Journal of Clinical Oncology* 1997; 15:2483.

47. Early Breast Cancer Collaborative Trialists' Group, Effects of adjuvant tamoxifen and of cytotoxic therapy on mortality in early breast cancer: An overview of 61 randomized trials among 28,896 women. *New England Journal of Medicine* 1988; 319:1681.

48. Early Breast Cancer Trialists' Cooperative Group, Effects of chemotherapy and hormonal therapy for early breast cancer on recurrence and 15-year survival; an overview of the randomized trials. *Lancet* 2005; 1687–1717.

49. Parker WH et al. Ovarian conservation at the time of hysterectomy and long-term health outcomes in the Nurses' Health Study. *Obstet Gynecol* 2009 May; 113(5):1027–1037.

50. Taylor CW et al. Multicenter randomized clinical trial of goserelin versus surgical ovariectomy in premenopausal patients with receptor-positive metastatic breast cancer an intergroup study. *Journal of Clinical Oncology* 1998 March 16; (3):994–999.

51. Kaufmann M et al. Survival analyses from the ZEBRA study: Goserelin (Zoladex) versus CMF in premenopausal women with node-positive breast cancer. *European Journal of Cancer* 2003; 39:1711–1717.

52. Jakesz R et al. Randomized adjuvant trial of tamoxifen and goserelin versus cyclophosphamide methotrexate and fluorouracil: Evidence for the superiority of treatment with endocrine blockade in premenopausal patients with hormone-responsive breast cancer. Austrian Breast and Colorectal Cancer Study Group Trial 5. *Journal of Clinical Oncology* 2002; 20:4621–4627.

53. Santner SJ et al. Aromatase activity and expression in breast cancer and benign breast tissue stromal cells. *Journal of Clinical Endocrinology Metabolism* 1997; 82:200.

54. Gnant M et al. Endocrine therapy plus zoledronic acid in premenopausal breast cancer. *N Engl J Med* 2009 Feb 12; 360(7):679–691.

55. Cobleigh MA et al. Multinational study of the efficacy and safety of humanized anti-HER2 monoclonal antibody in women who have HER2-overexpressing metastatic breast cancer. *Journal of Clinical Oncology* 1999; 17:2639–26486.

56. Vogel CL et al. Efficacy and safety of trastuzumab as a single agent in first-line treatment of HER2-overexpressing metastatic breast cancer. *Journal of Clinical Oncology* 2002; 20:719–772.

57. Baselga J et al. Adjuvant trastuzumab: A milestone in the treatment of Her 2 positive early breast cancer. *Oncologist* 2006; 11 Suppl 1:4–12.

58. Gonzalez-Angulo AM et al. High risk of recurrence for patients with breast cancer who have human epidermal growth factor receptor 2-positive, node negative tumors 1 cm or smaller. *J Clin Oncol* 2009 Dec 1; 27(34):5700–5706.

59. Brufsky AM et al. Zoledronic acid effectively prevents aromatase inhibitor-associated bone loss in postmenopausal women with early breast cancer receiving adjuvant letrozole: Z-FAST study 36-month follow results. *Clin Breast Cancer* 2009 May; 9(2):77–85.

60. Brufsky AM et al. Zoledronic acid effectively prevents aromatase inhibitor-associated bone loss in postmenopausal women with early breast cancer receiving adjuvant letrozole: Z-FAST study 36-month follow results. *Clin Breast Cancer* 2009 May; 9(2):77–85.

61. Bundred NJ et al. Effective inhibition of aromatase inhibitor-associated bone loss by zoledronic acid in postmenopausal women with early breast cancer receiving adjuvant letrozole: ZO-FAST Study results. *Cancer* 2008 1; 112(5):1001–1010.

62. Majed B et al. Is obesity an independent prognosis factor in woman breast cancer? *Breast Cancer Res Treat* 2008 Sep; 111(2):329–342.

63. Clarke M et al. Adjuvant chemotherapy in oestrogen-receptor poor breast cancer: Patient-level meta-analysis of randomized trials. *Lancet* 2008; 371(9606):29–40.

Chapter 13

1. Tamimi RM et al. Comparison of molecular phenotypes of ductal carcinoma in situ and invasive breast cancer. *Breast Cancer Research* 2008; 10:R67.

2. Allred DC et al. Ductal carcinoma in situ and the emergence of diversity during breast cancer evolution. *Clin Cancer Res.* 2008 Jan 15; 14(2):370–378.

3. Fisher ER et al. Pathological findings from the National Surgical Adjuvant Breast and Bowel Project: Twelve-year observations concerning lobular carcinoma in situ. *Cancer* 2004; 100:238–244.

4. Hwang ES et al. Clonality of lobular carcinoma in situ and synchronous invasive lobular carcinoma. *Cancer* 2004; 100:2562–2572.

5. Raju U et al. Molecular classification of breast carcinoma in situ. *Curr Genomics* 2006; 7(8):523–532.

6. Akashi-Tanaka S et al. Treatment of non-invasive carcinoma: Fifteen year results at the National Cancer Center Hospital in Tokyo. *Breast Cancer* 2000; 7:341–344.

7. Ottesen GL et al. Carcinoma in situ of the female breast: 10-year follow-up results of a prospective nationwide study. *Breast Cancer Research & Treatment* 2000; 62:197–210.

8. Goldstein NS, Kestin LL, Vicini FA. Clinical pathologic implications of E-cadherin reactivity in patients with lobular carcinoma in situ of the breast. *Cancer* 2001; 92:738–747.

9. Moran M, Haffty BG. Lobular carcinoma in situ as a component of breast cancer the long-term outcome in patients treated with breast conservation therapy. *International Journal of Radiation Oncology, Biology, and Physics* 1998; 40:353–358.

10. Abner AL et al. The relation between the presence and extent of lobular carcinoma in situ and the risk of local recurrence for patients with infiltrating carcinoma of the breast treated with conservative surgery and radiation therapy. *Cancer* 2000; 88:1072–1077.

11. Sasson AR et al. Lobular carcinoma in situ increases the risk of local recurrence in selected patients with stages I and II breast carcinoma treated with conservative surgery and radiation. *Cancer* 2001; 91:1862–1869.

12. Carolin KA, Tekyi-Mensah S, Pass HA. Lobular carcinoma in situ and invasive cancer: The contralateral breast controversy. *Breast Journal* 2002; 8:263–268.

13. Alpers CE, Wellings SR. The prevalence of carcinoma in situ in normal and cancer-associated breasts. *Human Pathology* 1985; 16:796.

14. Nielsen M, Jensen J, Andersen J. Noninvasive cancerous and cancerous breast lesions during lifetime and at autopsy. *Cancer* 1984; 54:612.

15. Betsill WL et al. Intraductal carcinoma: Long-term follow-up after treatment by biopsy alone. *Journal of the American Medical Association* 1978; 239:1863.

16. Page DL, Dupont WD. Intraductal carcinoma of the breast. *Cancer* 1982; 49:751.

17. Tot T. The theory of the sick breast lobe and the possible consequences. *Int J Surg Pathol* 2007; 15(4):369–375.

18. Morrow M, Bucci C, Rademaker A. Medical contraindications are not a major factor in the underutilization of breast conserving therapy. *J Am Coll Surg* 1998 Mar; 186(3):269–274.

19. Solin LJ et al. Relationship of breast magnetic resonance imaging to outcome after breast conservation treatment with radiation for women with early-stage invasive breast carcinoma or ductal carcinoma in situ. *J Clin Oncol* 2008 Jan 20; 26(3):386–391.

20. Kumar AS et al. Biologic significance of false-positive magnetic resonance imaging enhancement in the setting of ductal carcinoma in situ. *Am J Surg* 2006 Oct; 192(4):520–524.

21. Bijker N et al. Breast-conserving treatment with or without radiotherapy in ductal carcinoma-in-situ: Ten-year results of European Organization for Research and Treatment of Cancer randomized phase III trial 10853—a study by the EORTC

Breast Cancer Cooperative Group and EORTC Radiotherapy Group. *J Clin Oncol* 2006 Jul 20; 24(21):3381–3387.

22. Emdin SO et al. DCIS: Radiotherapy after sector resection for ductal carcinoma in situ of the breast. Results of a randomised trial in a population offered mammography screening. *Acta Oncol* 2006; 45(5):536–543.

23. Fisher B et al. Prevention of invasive breast cancer in women with ductal carcinoma in situ: An update of the National Surgical Adjuvant Breast and Bowel Project experience. *Semin Oncol* 2001; 28(4):400–418.

24. Houghton J et al. Radiotherapy and tamoxifen in women with completely excised ductal carcinoma in situ of the breast in the UK, Australia, and New Zealand: Randomized controlled trial. *Lancet* 2003; 362(9378):95–102.

25. Silverstein M et al. Intraductal carcinoma of the breast (208 cases): Clinical factors influencing treatment choice. *Cancer* 1990; 66(1):102.

26. Finkelstein SD, Sayegh R, Thompson WR. Late recurrence of ductal carcinoma in situ at the cutaneous end of surgical drainage following total mastectomy. *American Surgeon* 1993 July; 59:410.

27. Fisher DE et al. Chest wall recurrence of ductal carcinoma in situ of the breast after mastectomy. *Cancer* 1993; 71(10):3025.

28. Kerlikowske K et al. Biomarker expression and risk of subsequent tumors after initial ductal carcinoma in situ diagnosis. *J Natl Cancer Inst* 2010; 102:627–637.

29. Budzar AU et al. Combined modality treatment of stage III and inflammatory breast cancer: MD Anderson Cancer Center experience. *Surg Clin North America* 1995; 4(4):715–734.

30. Mehra R, Burtness B. Antibody therapy for early-stage breast cancer: Trastuzumab adjuvant and neoadjuvant trials. *Biol Ther* 2006; 6(9):951–962.

31. Liedtke C et al. Genomic grade index is associated with response to chemotherapy in patients with breast cancer. *J Clin Oncol* 2009; 27(19):3185–3191.

32. Chen AM et al. Breast conservation after neoadjuvant chemotherapy. *Cancer* 2005; 103(4):689–695.

33. Merajver SD et al. Breast conservation and prolonged chemotherapy for locally advanced breast cancer: The University of Michigan experience. *J Clin Oncol* 1997; 15(8):2873–2881.

34. Liauw SL et al. Inflammatory breast carcinoma: Outcomes with trimodality therapy for nonmetastatic disease. *Cancer* 2004; 1000(5):920–928.

35. Fourquet A, Meunier M, Campana M. Occult primary cancer with axillary metastases. In Harris JR et al., eds. *Diseases of the Breast*, 1048.

36. Ellerbrock N et al. Treatment of patients with isolated axillary nodal metastases from an occult primary carcinoma consistent with breast origin. *Cancer* 1990; 66:1461.

37. Van Ooijen B et al. Axillary nodal metastases from an occult primary consistent with breast carcinoma. *British Journal of Surgery* 1993; 80(10):1299.

38. Graham H. *The Story of Surgery.* New York: Doubleday, Doran, 1939.

39. Wood WS, Hegedus C. Mammary Paget's disease and intraductal carcinoma: Histologic, histochemical, and immunocytochemical comparison. *American Journal of Dermapathology* 1988; 10:183–188.

40. Fu W, Mittel VK, Young SC. Paget disease of the breast: Analysis of 41 patients. *American Journal of Clinical Oncology* 2001; 24:397–400.

41. Kaelin C. Paget's disease. In Harris JR et al., eds. *Diseases of the Breast*, 1008.

42. Marshall JK et al. Conservative management of Paget's disease of the breast with radiotherapy: 10–15 year results. *Cancer* 2003; 97:2142–2149.

43. Lagios MD et al. Paget's disease of the nipple. *Cancer* 1984; 54:545.

44. Kister SJ, Haagensen CD. Paget's disease of the breast. *American Journal of Surgery* 1970; 119:606.

45. Malak G, Tapolcsanyi L. Characteristics of Paget's carcinoma of the nipple and problems of its negligence. *Oncology* 1974; 30:278.

46. Guerrero MA, Ballard BR, Grau AM. Malignant phylloides tumor of the breast: Review of the literature and case report of stromal overgrowth. *Surgical Oncology* 2003; 12:27–37.

47. Chaney AW et al. Primary treatment of cystosarcoma phyllodes of the breast. *Cancer* 2000; 89(7):1502–1511.

48. Intra M et al. Clinicopathologic characteristics of 143 patients with synchronous bilateral invasive breast carcinomas treated in a single institution. *Cancer* 2004; 101:905–912.

49. Anders CK et al. Breast cancer before age 40 years. *Semin Oncol* 2009 Jun; 36(3):237–249.

50. Henderson IC, Patek AJ. Are breast cancers in young women qualitatively distinct? *Lancet* 1997; 349:1488–1489.

51. McCormick B. Selection criteria for breast conservation: The impact of young and old age and collagen vascular disease. *Cancer* 1994; 74:430.

52. Bartelink H et al. Impact of higher radiation dose on local control and survival in breast conserving therapy of early breast cancer: 10 year result of the randomized boost versus no boost EORTC 22881–10882 trial. *J Clin Oncol* 2007; 25:3259–3265.

53. Aebi S et al. Is chemotherapy alone adequate for young women with estrogen-receptor-positive breast cancer? *Lancet* 2000; 355(9218):1869–1874.

54. Goldhirsch A, Gelber RD, Castiglione M. The magnitude of endocrine effects of adjuvant chemotherapy for premenopausal breast cancer patients. The International Breast Cancer Study Group. *Ann Oncol* 1990; 1(3):183–188.

55. Pagani O et al. Prognostic impact of amenorrhea after adjuvant chemotherapy in premenopausal breast cancer patients with axillary node involvement: Results of the International Breast Cancer Study Group (IBCSG) Trial VI. *Eur J Cancer* 1998; 34(5):632–640.

56. Walshe JNM, Denduluri N, Swain SM. Amenorrhea in premenopausal women after adjuvant chemotherapy for breast cancer. *J Clin Oncol* 2006; 24(36):5769–5779.

57. Castiglione-Gertsch M et al. Adjuvant chemotherapy followed by goserelin versus either modality alone for premenopausal lymph node negative breast cancer: A randomized trial. *J Natl Cancer Inst* 2003; 95(240):1833–1846.

58. Oktay K et al. Embryo development after heterotopic transplantation of cryopreserved ovarian tissue. *Lancet* 2004; 363:837–840.

59. Oktay K et al. Fertility preservation in breast cancer patients: IVF and embryo cryopreservation after ovarian stimulation with tamoxifen. *Human Reproduction* 2003; 8(1):90–95.

60. Guinee VF et al. Effect of pregnancy on prognosis for young women with breast cancer. *Lancet* 1994; 343:1587.

61. Petrek JA. Childbearing issues in breast carcinoma survivors. *Cancer* 1997; 79(7):1271–1278.

62. Blakely LJ et al. Effects of pregnancy after treatment for breast carcinoma on survival and risk of recurrence. *Cancer* 2004; 100:465–469.

63. Gelber S et al. Effect of pregnancy on overall survival after the diagnosis of early-stage breast cancer. *Journal of Clinical Oncology* 2001; 19:1671–1675.

64. Mueller BA et al. Childbearing and survival after breast carcinoma in young women. *Cancer* 2003; 98:1131–1140.

65. Silliman RA et al. Breast cancer care in old age: What we know, don't know, and do. *Journal of the National Cancer Institute* 1993; 85(3):190.

66. Hughes KS et al. Lumpectomy plus tamoxifen with or without irradiation in women 70 years of age or older with early breast cancer. *New England Journal of Medicine* 2004; 351:971–977.

67. Deapen MD et al. The relationship between breast cancer and augmentation mammoplasty: An epidemiologic study. *Plastic and Reconstructive Surgery* 1986; 77:361.

68. Jacobson GM et al. Breast irradiation following silicone gel implants. *International Journal of Radiation Oncology, Biology, and Physics* 1986; 12(5):835.

69. Schwartz RM et al. A study of familial male breast carcinoma and a second report. *Cancer* 1980; 46:2629.

70. Jackson AW et al. Carcinoma of the male breast in association with the Klinefelter syndrome. *British Medical Journal* 1965; 1:223.

71. Ikeda RE, Preston DL, Tokuoka S. Male breast cancer incidence among atomic bomb survivors. *Journal of the National Cancer Institute* 2005; 97(8):603–605.

72. Sorensen HT et al. The intrauterine origin of male breast cancer: A birth order study in Denmark. *European Journal of Cancer Prevention* 2005; 14(2):185–186.

73. Campbell JH, Cummins SD. Metastases simulating mammary cancer in prostatic carcinoma under estrogenic therapy. *Cancer* 1951; 4:303.

74. Port ER et al. Sentinel lymph node biopsy in patients with male breast carcinoma. *Cancer* 2001; 91(2):319–323.

75. Chakravarthy A, Kim CR. Post-mastectomy radiation in male breast cancer. *Radiotherapy Oncology* 2002; 65(2):99–103.

76. Zabolotny BP, Zalai CV, Meterissian SH. Successful use of letrozole in male breast cancer: A case report and review of hormonal therapy for male breast cancer. *Journal of Surgical Oncology* 2005; 90(1):26–30.

77. Giordano SH et al. Efficacy of anastrozole in male breast cancer. *American Journal of Clinical Oncology* 25(3):235–237.

78. Hittmair AP, Lininger RA, Tavassoli FA. Ductal carcinoma in situ (DCIS) in the male breast. *Cancer* 1998; 83(10):2139–2149.

Chapter 14

1. Raul CP et al. Incidence of anaphylactoid reactions to isosulfan blue dye during breast carcinoma lymphatic mapping in patients treated with preoperative prophylaxis: Results of a surgical prospective clinical practice protocol. *Cancer* 2005 Aug 15; 104(4):692–699.

2. Boneti C et al. Scientific Impact Award: Axillary reverse mapping (ARM) to identify and protect lymphatics draining the arm during axllary lymphadenectomy. *Am J Surg* 2009 Oct; 1 98(4):482–487.

3. Kell MR et al. Outcome of axillary staging in early breast cancer: A meta analysis. *Breast Cancer Res Treat* 2010 Jan 9.

4. Moskovitz AH et al. Axillary web syndrome after axillary dissection. *Am J Surg* 2001; 181(5):434–439.

5. Baron RH et al. Eighteen sensations after breast cancer surgery: A 5 year comparison of sentinel lymph node biopsy and axillary lymph node dissection. *Ann Surg Oncol* 2007 May; 14(5):1653–1661.

6. Sener SF et al. Lymphedema after sentinel lymphadenectomy for breast carcinoma. *Cancer* 2001; 92(4):748–752.

7. Thompson M et al. Hematoma-directed ultrasound-guided (HUG) breast lumpectomy. *Ann Surg Oncol* 2007; 1:148–156.

8. Jakub JW et al. Current status of radioactive seed for localization of nonpalpable breast lesions. *Am J Surg* 2009 Nov 30.

9. Anderson BO, Masetti R, Silverstien MJ. Oncoplastic approaches to partial mastectomy: An overview of volume-displacement techniques. *Lancet Oncology* 2005; 6(3):145–157.

10. Paepke S et al. Subcutaneous mastectomy with conservation of the nipple-areola skin: Broadening the indications. *Ann Surg* 2009 Aug; 250(2):288–292.

11. Lorde A. *The Cancer Journals.* New York: Spinsters, 1980.

12. Tasmuth T et al. Treatment-related factors predisposing to chronic pain in patients with breast cancer: A multivariate approach. *Acta Oncology* 1997; 36(6):625–630.

13. Wallace MS, Wallace AM, Kobke MK. Pain after breast surgery: A survey of 282 women. *Pain* 1996 Aug; 66:2–3.

14. Tasmuth T, Blomqvist C, Kalso E. Chronic post-treatment symptoms in patients with breast cancer operated in different surgical units. *European Journal of Surgical Oncology* 1999; 25(1).

15. Crawford JS, Simpson J, Crawford P. Myofascial release provides symptomatic relief from chest wall tenderness occasionally seen following lumpectomy and radiation in breast cancer patients [letter]. *International Journal of Radiation Oncology, Biology, and Physics* 1996; 34(5): 1188–1189.

16. Eija K, Tiina T, Pertti NJ. Amitriptyline effectively relieves neuropathic pain following treatment of breast cancer. *Pain* 1996; 64(2):293–302.

Chapter 15

1. Bajaj AK et al. Aesthetic outcomes in patients undergoing breast conservation therapy for the treatment of localized breast cancer. *Plast Reconstru Surg* 2004; 114:1442.

2. Kronowitz SJ et al. A management algorithm and practical oncoplastic surgical techniques for repairing partial mastectomy defects. *Plast Reconstru Surg* 2008; 122:1631.

3. Kushner R. *Why Me?* Cambridge, MA: Kensington, 1982.

4. Fernancez-Frias AM et al. Immediate reconstruction after mastectomy for breast cancer: Which factors affect its course and final outcome? *J Am Coll Surg* 2009 Jan; 208(1):126–133.

5. Pockaj BA et al. Quality of life after breast cancer surgery: What have we learned and where should we go next? *J Surg Oncol* 2009; 99:447–455.

6. Frost MH et al. Satisfaction after contralateral prophylactic mastectomy: The significance of mastectomy type, reconstructive complications, and body appearance. *J Clin Oncol* 2005; 23:7849–7856.

7. El-Tamer MB et al. Morbidity and mortality following breast cancer surgery in women: National benchmarks for standards of care. *Ann Surg* 2007; 245:665–671.

8. Metzger D. "The Woman Who Slept with Men to Take the War Out of Them," in *Tree*. Oakland, CA: Wingbow, 1983.

9. Sutton T. *Boston Globe,* May 3, 2009.

Chapter 16

1. Whelan T et al. Randomized trial of breast irradiation schedules after lumpectomy for women with lymph node-negative breast cancer. *Journal of the National Cancer Institute* 2002; 94:1143–1150.

2. Dirbas FM, Jeffrey SS, Goffinet DR. The evolution of accelerated, partial breast irradiation as a potential treatment option for women with newly diagnosed breast cancer considering breast conservation. *Cancer Biotherapy and Radiopharmaceuticals* 2004; 19(6):673–705.

3. Vicini FA et al. Accelerated treatment of breast cancer. *Journal of Clinical Oncology* 2001; 19:1993–2001.

4. Veronesi U et al. A preliminary report of interoperative radiotherapy (IORT) in limited stage breast cancers that are conservatively treated. *European Journal of Cancer* 2001; 37:2178–2183.

5. Vaidya JS, Joseph DJ, Tobias JS, et al Targeted intraoperative radiotherapy versus whole breast radiotherapy for breast cancer (TARGIT-A-trial): an international prostpective, randomized, non-inferiority phase 3 trial. Published online the Lancet.com June 5 2010 DOI:10.1016/S0140–6736(10)60837–9

6. Kurtz JM et al. Contralateral breast cancer and other second malignancies in patients treated by breast-conserving therapy with radiation. *International Journal of Radiation, Oncology, Biology, and Physics* 1987; 15:277.

Chapter 17

1. Bonadonna G et al. Ten-year experience with CMF-based adjuvant chemotherapy in resectable breast cancer. *Breast Cancer Research and Treatment* 1985; 5:95.

2. ASCO. American Society of Clinical Oncology recommendations for the use of hematopoetic colony stimulating factors: Evidence-based clinical practice guidelines. *Journal of Clinical Oncology* 1994; 12:247.

3. Hershman D et al. Acute myeloid leukemia or myelodysplastic syndrome following use of granulocyte colony-stimulating factors during breast cancer adjuvant chemotherapy. *JNCI* 2007; 99:196–205.

4. Arnedos M et al. Routine prophylactic granulocyte colony stimulating factor (GCSF) is not necessary with accelerated (dose dense) paclitaxel for early breast cancer. *Breast Cancer Research and Treatment* 2008 Nov; 112(1):1–4.

5. NCCN Practice Guidelines in Oncology 2004; v.1. High emetic risk chemotherapy: Emesis prevention.

6. Huntington M. Weight gain in patients receiving adjuvant chemotherapy for carcinoma of the breast. *Cancer* 1985; 65:572.

7. Denmark-Wahnefried W, Winer EP, Rimer BK. Why women gain weight with adjuvant chemotherapy for breast cancer. *Journal of Clinical Oncology* 1993; 11(7):1418.

8. Herbert JR et al. The effect of dietary exposure on recurrence and mortality in early stage breast cancer. *Breast Cancer Research and Treatment* 1998; 51:17.

9. Goodwin PJ et al. Risk of menopause during the first year after breast cancer diagnosis. *Journal of Clinical Oncology* 1999; 17(8):2365–2370.

10. Bines J, Oleske DM, Cobleigh MA. Ovarian function in premenopausal women treated with adjuvant chemotherapy for breast cancer. *Journal of Clinical Oncology* 1996; 14(5):1718–1729.

11. Cobleigh MA et al. Amenorrhea following adjuvant chemotherapy for breast cancer. *Proceedings of the American Society of Clinical Oncology* 1995; 14:115.

12. Bryce CJ et al. Menstrual disruption in premenopausal breast cancer patients receiving CMF (V) vs AC adjuvant chemotherapy. *Breast Cancer Research and Treatment* 1998; 50:284.

13. Montz FJ, Wolff A, Cambone JC. Gonadal protection and fecundity rates in cyclophosphamide-treated rats. *Cancer Research* 1991; 51:2124.

14. Ataya K et al. Luteinizing hormone releasing hormone agonist inhibits cyclophosphamide induced ovarian follicular depletion in rhesus monkeys. *Biology of Reproduction* 1995; 52:365.

15. Wieneke MH, Dienst ER. Neuropsychological assessment of cognitive functioning following chemotherapy for breast cancer. *Psychooncology* 1995; 4:61–66.

16. Schagen SB et al. Cognitive deficits after postoperative adjuvant chemotherapy for breast carcinoma. *Cancer* 1999; 85:640–650.

17. Tannock IF et al. Cognitive impairment associated with chemotherapy for cancer: Report of a workshop. *Journal of Clinical Oncology* 2004; 22(1): 2233–2239.

18. Fisher B et al. Leukemia in breast cancer patients following adjuvant chemotherapy or postoperative radiation: The NSABP experience. *Journal of Clinical Oncology* 1985; 3:1640.

19. Klewer SE et al. Dobutamine stress echocardiography: A sensitive indicator of diminished myocardial function in asymptomatic doxirubin-treated long-term survivors of childhood cancer. *Journal of the American College of Cardiologists* 1992; 19(2):394.

20. Siegel BS. *Love, Medicine, and Miracles*. New York: Harper & Row, 1986.

21. Irvine D et al. The prevalence and correlates of fatigue in patients receiving treatment with chemotherapy and radiotherapy: Comparison with the fatigue experienced by healthy individuals. *Cancer Nursing* 1994; 17(5):367–378.

22. Fisher B et al. Tamoxifen for the prevention of breast cancer: Report of the National Surgical Adjuvant Breast and Bowel Project P-1 Study. *Journal of the National Cancer Institute* 1998; 90:1371–1388.

23. Loprinski CL et al. Venlafaxine alleviates hot flashes: An NCCTG Trial. Abstract 4, Proceedings of ASCO, vol. 19, 2000.

24. Saphner T, Tormey DC, Gray R. Venous and arterial thrombosis in patients who received adjuvant therapy for breast cancer. *Journal of Clinical Oncology* 1991; 9(2):286.

25. Fisher B et al. Tamoxifen for the prevention of breast cancer.

26. Chalas E et al. Benign gynecological conditions among participants in the Breast Cancer Prevention Trial. *American Journal of Obstetrics and Gynecology* 2005; 192(4):1230–1237.

27. Caleffi M et al. Effect of tamoxifen on oestrogen binding, lipid and lipoprotein concentrations, and blood clotting parameters in premenopausal women with breast pain. *Journal of Endocrinology* 1988; 119(2):335.

28. Kristensen B et al. Tamoxifen and bone metabolism in postmenopausal low-risk breast cancer patients: A randomized study. *Journal of Clinical Oncology* 1994; 12(5):992.

29. Budzar AU et al. Phase II evaluation of Ly156758 in metastatic breast cancer. *Oncology* 1988; 45(5):344–345.

30. Gradishar WJ et al. Raloxifene HCl: A new endocrine agent is active in estrogen receptor positive metastatic breast cancer. *Breast Cancer Research and Treatment* 1997; 46(53) (Abstract no. 209).

31. ATAC Trialists' Group Results of the ATAC (Arimidex, tamoxifen, alone or in combination) trial after completion of 5 years' adjuvant treatment for breast cancer. *Lancet* 2005; 365:60–62.

32. Goss P et al. Extended adjuvant endocrine therapy in premenopausal early stage breast cancer: An analysis of younger women from NCIC CTG MA 17. *San Antonio Breast Cancer Symposium* 2009 Dec 10. Abstract 13.

33. Buzdar AU et al. Clinical features of joint symptoms observed in the Arimidex, tamoxifen, alone or in combination (ATAC) trial. *J Clin Oncol* 2006; 24:15S.

34. Briot K et al. Effects of switching aromatase inhibitors on arthralgia: The ATOLL study. Presented at the 31st Annual San Antonio Breast Cancer Symposium, 2008 Dec 10–14, Abstract 1142.

35. Gnant M et al. Endocrine therapy plus zoledronic acid in premenopausal breast cancer. *N Engl J Med* 2009; 360:679.

36. Sverrisdottir A et al. Bone mineral density among premenopausal women with early breast cancer in a randomized trial of adjuvant endocrine therapy. *Journal of Clinical Oncology* 2004; 22:3694–3699.

37. Geisler LE et al. Changes in bone and lipid metabolism in postmenopausal women with early breast cancer after terminating 2 year treatment with exemestane: A randomized, placebo-controlled study. *Eur J Cancer* 2006 Nov; 42(17):2968–2975.

38. Hines S et al. Zoledronic acid for treatment of osteopenia and osteoporosis in women with primary breast cancer undergoing adjuvant aromatase inhibitor therapy. *Breast* 2010; DOI: http://dx.doi.org/10.1016/j.breast.2009.12.001.

39. Valachis A et al. Lack of evidence for fracture prevention in early breast cancer bisphosphonate trials: A meta-analysis. *Gynecol Oncol* 2009; DOI: 10.1016/j.ygyno.2009.12.001.

Chapter 18

1. Lorincz AM, Sukumar S. Molecular links between obesity and breast cancer. *Endocr Relat Cancer* 2006; 13(2):279–292.

2. Goodwin PJ et al. High insulin levels in newly diagnosed breast cancer patients reflect underlying insulin resistance and are associated with components of the insulin resistance syndrome. *Breast Cancer Res Treat.* 2009; 114(3):517–725.

3. Goodwin PJ et al. Fasting insulin and outcome in early-stage breast cancer: Results of a prospective cohort study. *J Clin Oncol* 2001; 20:42–51.

4. Pierce BI et al. Elevated biomarkers of inflammation are associated with reduced survival among breast cancer patients. *J Clin Oncol* 2009; 27:3437–3444.

5. Chlebowski RT et al. Weight loss in breast cancer patient management. *J Clin Oncol* 2002 Feb 15; 20(4):1128–1143.

6. Kushi LH et al. Lifestyle factors and survival in women with breast cancer. *J Nutr* 2007; 137:236S–242S.

7. Holmes MD et al. Physical activity and survival after breast cancer diagnosis. *JAMA* 2005; 293(20):2479–2486.

8. Berclaz G et al. Body mass index as a prognostic feature in operable breast cancer: The International Breast Cancer Study Group experience. *Ann Oncol* 2004 Jun; 15(6):875–884.

9. De Azambuja E et al. The effect of body mass index on overall and disease-free survival in node-positive breast cancer patients treated with docetaxel and doxorubicin-containing adjuvant chemotherapy: The experience of the BIG 02–98 trial. *Breast Cancer Res Treat* 2010; 119:145–153.

10. Kroenke CH et al. Weight, weight gain, and survival after breast cancer diagnosis. *J Clin Oncol* 2005; 23(7):1370–1378.

11. Goodwin P et al. Multidisciplinary weight management in locoregional breast cancer: Results of a phase II study. *Breast Cancer Res Treat* 1998 Mar; 48(1):53–64.

12. Dujuric Z et al. Combining weight-loss counseling with the Weight Watchers plan for obese breast cancer survivors. *Obes Res* 2002 Jul; 10(7):657–665.

13. Holick CN et al. Physical activity and survival after diagnosis of invasive breast cancer. *Cancer Epidemiology and Biomarkers Prev* 2008 Feb; 17(2):379–386.

14. Segal R et al. Structured exercise improves physical functioning in women with stages I and II breast cancer results of a randomized controlled trial. *J Clin Oncol* 2001 Feb 1; 19(3):657–665.

15. Mock V, Frangakis C, Davidson NE. Exercise manages fatigue during breast cancer treatment: A randomized controlled trial. *Psychooncology* 2005 Jun; 14(6):464–477.

16. McNeely ML et al. Effects of exercise on breast cancer patients and survivors: A systematic review and meta-analysis. *CMAJ* 2006 Jul 4; 175(1):34–41.

17. Pedersen BK. The diseasome of physical inactivity and the role of myokines in muscle-fat cross talk. *J Physiol* 2009; 587(23): 5559–5568.

18. Weuve J et al. Physical activity, including walking, and cognitive function in older women. *Journal of the American Medicine Association* 2004; 292:1454–1461.

19. Blackburn GL, Wang KA. Dietary fat reduction and breast cancer outcome: Results from the Women's Intervention Nutrition Study (WINS). *Am J Clin Nutr* 2007 Sep; 86(3):s878–881.

20. Pierce JP et al. Influence of a diet very high in vegetables fruit and fiber and low in fat on prognosis following treatment for breast cancer. Women's Healthy Eating and Living (WHEL) Randomized Trial. *JAMA* 2007; 98:289–298.

21. Knoops KT et al. Mediterranean diet lifestyle factors and 10-year mortality in elderly European men and women. *Journal of the American Medical Association* 2004; 292:1433–1439.

22. Stampfer MJ et al. Primary prevention of coronary heart disease in women through diet and lifestyle. *New England Journal of Medicine* 2000; 343:16–22.

23. Cousins N. *Anatomy of an Illness.* New York: Bantam, 1979.

24. Chvetzoff G, Tannoci IF. Placebo effects in oncology. *Journal of the National Cancer Institute* 2003; 95:19–29.

25. Spiegel D. Effects of psychotherapy on cancer survival. *Nature Reviews: Cancer* 2002; 2:383–388.

26. Goodwin PJ, Lezcz ML, Ennis M. The effect of group psychosocial support on survival in metastatic breast cancer. *NEJM* 2001; 345:1719–1726.

27. Duckro P, Magaletta PR. The effect of prayer on physical health: Experimental evidence. *International Journal of Health and Religion* 1994; 33(3):211–219.

28. Dossey L. *Healing Words: The Healing Power of Prayer.* San Francisco: Harper, 1993.

29. Benson H et al. Study of the Therapeutic Effects of intercessory Prayer (STEP) in cardiac bypass patients: A multicenter randomized trial of uncertainty and certainty of receiving intercessory prayer. *Am Heart J* 2006; 151(4):934–942.

30. Simonton OC, Matthews S, Creighton JL. *Getting Well Again.* New York: Bantam, 1992.

31. Ott MJ, Norris RL, Bauer-Wu SM. Mindfulness meditation for oncology patients: A discussion and critical review. *Imtegr Cancer Ther* 2006 Jun 5; 2:98–108.

32. Cousins N. *Anatomy of an Illness.* New York: Bantam, 1979.

33. Mella DL. *The Legendary and Practical Use of Gems and Stones.* Albuquerque, NM: Domel, 1979.

34. Navo MA et al. An assessment of the utilization of complementary and alternative medication in women with gynecologic or breast malignancies. *J Clin Oncol* 2004; 22:671–677.

35. Sparreboom A et al. Herbal remedies in the United States: Potential adverse interactions with anticancer agents. *J Clin Oncol* 2004; 22:2489–2503.

36. Zhang M et al. Chinese medicinal herbs to treat the side-effects of chemotherapy in breast cancer patients. *Cochrane Database Syst Rev* 2007 Apr 18; (2):CD004921.

37. Pommier P et al. Phase III randomized trial of Calendula officinalis compared with trolamine for the prevention of acute dermatitis during irradiation for breast cancer. *J Clin Oncol* 2004 Apr 15; 22(8):1447–1453.

38. Oberbaum M. A randomized controlled clinical trial of the homeopathic medication TRAUMEEL S in the treatment of chemotherapy-induced stomatitis in children undergoing stem cell transplantation. *Cancer* 2001 Aug 1; 92(3):664–690.

39. Jacobs J et al. Homeopathy for menopausal symptoms in breast cancer survivors: A preliminary randomized controlled trial. *J Altern Complement Med* 2005 Feb; 11(1):21–27.

40. Thompson EA, Reilly D. The homeopathic approach to the treatment of symptoms of oestrogen withdrawal in breast cancer patients: A prospective observational study. *Homeopathy* 2003 Jul; 92(3):131–134.

41. Horneber MA et al. Mistletoe therapy in oncology. *Cochrane Database Syst Rev.* 2008 Apr 16; (2):CD003297.

42. Milazzo S, Lejeune S, Ernst E. Laetrile for cancer: A systematic review of the clinical evidence. *Support Care Cancer* 2007 Jun; 15(6):583–595.

43. Kennedy D. Food and Drug Administration's warning on laetrile. TK

44. Miller DR et al. Phase I/II trial of the safety and efficacy of shark cartilage in the treatment of advanced cancer. *Journal of Clinical Oncology* 1998; 16:3649–3655.

45. Trull L. *The CanCell Controversy: Why Is a Possible Cure for Cancer Being Suppressed?* Norfolk, VA: Hampton Roads, 1993.

46. Zick SM et al. Trial of Essiac to ascertain its effect in women with breast cancer (TEA-BC). *Journal of Alternative and Complementary Medicine* 2006; 12(10): 971–980.

47. Bennett LM et al. Flor-Essence herbal tonic does not inhibit mammary tumor development in Sprague Dawley rats. *Breast Cancer Research and Treatment* 2004.

48. Burzynski SR, Kubove E. Initial clinical study with antineoplaston A2 injections in cancer patients with five years' follow-up. *Drugs Exper Clinical Research* 1987; 13:1–11.

49. Green S. Antineoplastons: An unproven cancer therapy. *Journal of the American Medical Association* 1992; 267:2924–2928.

50. Burzynski SR. The present state of antineoplaston research. *Integr Cancer Ther* 2004; 4788:87–93.

51. Lorde A. *A Burst of Light.* New York: Firebrand, 1988.

Chapter 19

1. Joseph E et al. Evaluation of an intensive strategy for follow-up and surveillance of primary breast cancer. *Annals of Surgical Oncology* 1998; 5:552–528.

2. Ganz PA et al. Quality of life in long-term, disease-free survivors of breast cancer: A follow-up study. *Journal of the National Cancer Institute* 2002; 94:39–49.

3. Robbins GF, Berg JW. Bilateral primary breast cancers: A prospective clinical pathological study. *Cancer* 1964; 17:1501.

4. Haagensen CD, Lane N, Bodian C. Coexisting lobular neoplasia and carcinoma of the breast. *Cancer* 1983; 51:1468.

5. Grunfeld E et al. Routine follow-up of breast cancer in primary care: Randomised trial. *British Medical Journal* 1996; 313:665–669.

6. Insa A et al. Prognostic factors predicting survival from first recurrence in patients with metastatic breast cancer: Analysis of 439 patients. *Breast Cancer Research and Treatment* 1999; 56(1):67–78.

7. Chang J et al. Survival of patients with metastatic breast carcinoma: Importance of prognostic markers of the primary tumor. *Cancer* 2003; 97(3):545–553.

8. Stierer M, Rosen HR. Influence of early diagnosis on prognosis of recurrent breast cancer. *Cancer* 1989; 64:1128.

9. Smith TJ et al. American Society of Clinical Oncology 1998 update of recommended breast surveillance guidelines. *Journal of Clinical Oncology* 1999; 17:1080–1082.

10. Carlson RW et al. Clinical Practice Guidelines in Oncology, Breast Cancer v 1.04. National Comprehensive Cancer Network, 2004. www.nccn.org.

11. Khatcheressian JL et al. American Society of Clinical Oncology 2006 update of the breast cancer follow-up and management guidelines in the adjuvant setting. *Journal of Clinical Oncology* 2006; 24:5091–5097.

12. Petrek JA et al. Lymphedema in a cohort of breast carcinoma survivors 20 years after diagnosis. *Cancer* 2001; 92:1368–1377.

13. Blanchard DK et al. Relapse and morbidity in patents undergoing sentinel lymph node biopsy alone or with axillary dissection for breast cancer. *Archives of Surgery* 2003; 138:482.

14. Martin GM, Dowlatshahi K. Sentinel lymph node biopsy lowers the rate of lymphedema when compared with standard axillary lymph node dissection. *Annals of Surgery* 2003; 69:209.

15. Sener SF et al. Lymphedema after sentinel lymphadectomy for breast carcinoma. *Cancer* 2001; 92:748.

16. Petrek JA, Heelan MC. Incidence of breast carcinoma-related lymphedema. Cancer 1998; 83:2776.

17. Schmitz KH et al. Weight lifting in women with breast cancer-related lymphedema. *New England Journal of Medicine.* 2009; 361:664–673.

18. Graham PH. Compression prophylaxis may increase the potential for flight-associated lymphoedema after breast cancer treatment. *The Breast* 2002; 11(1):66–71.

19. Kasseroller RG. The Vodder School: The Vodder method. *Cancer* 1998; 83:2840.

20. Foldi E. The treatment of lymphedema. *Cancer* 1998; 83:2883.

21. Bernas M et al. Massage therapy in the treatment of lymphedema: Rationale, results, and applications. *IEEE Engineering in Medicine and Biology Magazine* 2005; 24(2):58–68.

22. Mondry TE, Riffenburgh RH, Johnstone PA. Prospective trial of complete decongestive therapy for upper extremity lymphedema after breast cancer therapy. Cancer J 2004 Jan-Feb; 10(1):42–48.

23. Vignes S et al. Long-term management of breast cancer-related lymphedema after intensive decongestive physiotherapy. *Breast Cancer Research and Treatment* 2007; 101(3):285–290.

24. Koul R et al. Efficacy of complete decongestive therapy and manual lymphatic drainage on treatment-related lymphedema in breast cancer. *International Journal of Radiation, Oncology, Biology, and Physics* 2007 Mar; 67(3):841–846.

25. Hamner JB, Fleming MD. Lymphedema therapy reduces the volume of edema and pain in patients with breast cancer. *Annals of Surgical Onocology* 2007 Jun; 14(6):1904–1908.

26. Casley-Smith JR, Morgan RG, Piller NB. Treatment of lymphedema of the arms and legs with 5,6-Benso(alpha)-pyrone. *New England Journal of Medicine* 1993; 329:1158.

27. Loprinzi CL et al. Lack of effect of coumarin in women with lymphedema after treatment for breast cancer. *New England Journal of Medicine* 1999; 340(5):346–350.

28. Brorson H. Liposuction in arm lymphedema treatment. *Scand J Surg* 2003; 92(4):287–295.

29. Campisi C et al. Long-term results after lymphatic venous anastomoses for the treatment of obstructive lymphedema. *Microsurgery* 2001; 21(4):135–139.

30. Baumeister RG, Siuda S. Treatment of lymphedemas by microsurgical lymphatic grafting: What is proved? *Plast Reconstr Surg* 1990; 85(1):64–74.

31. Becker C et al. Postmastectomy lymphedema: Long-term results following microsurgical lymph node transplantation. *Ann Surg* 2006; 243(3):313–315.

32. Jagsi R et al. Rates of myocardial infarction and coronary artery disease and risk factors in patients treated with radiation therapy for early stage breast cancer. *Cancer* 2007; 109:650–657.

33. Vallis KA et al. Assessment of coronary heart disease morbidity and mortality after radiation therapy for early breast cancer. *Journal of Clinical Oncology* 2002; 20:1036–1042.

34. Ahles TA et al. Cognitive function in breast cancer patients prior to adjuvant treatment. *Breast Cancer Research and Treatment* 2008; 110:143–152.

35. Falleti MG et al. The nature and severity of cognitive impairment associated with adjuvant chemotherapy in women with breast cancer: A meta-analysis of the current literature. *Brain and Cognition* 2005; 59:60–70.

36. Jenkins V et al. A 3 year prospective study of the effects of adjuvant treatments on cognition in women with early stage breast cancer. *British Journal of Cancer* 2006; 94:828–834.

37. Wefel JS et al. The cognitive sequel of standard-dose adjuvant chemotherapy in women with breast carcinoma: Results of a prospective randomized longitudinal trail. *Cancer* 2004; 100:2292–2299.

38. Schagen SB et al. Late effects of adjuvant chemotherapy on cognitive function: A follow-up study in breast cancer patients. *Annals of Oncology* 2002; 13:387–1397.

39. Ahles TA et al. Neuropsychological impact of standard-dose systemic chemotherapy in long-term survivors of breast cancer and lymphoma. *Journal of Clinical Oncology* 2002; 20:485–493.

40. Vardy J et al. Cancer and cancer-therapy related cognitive dysfunction: An international perspective from the Venice cognitive workshop. *Ann Oncol* 2008; 19:623–629.

41. Vardy J et al. The fog hasn't lifted on "chemobrain" yet: Ongoing uncertainty regarding the effects of chemotherapy and breast cancer on cognition. *Breast Cancer Research and Treatment* 2010.

42. Curt GA et al. Impact of cancer-related fatigue on the lives of patients: New findings from the fatigue coalition. *Oncologist* 2000; 5:353–360.

43. Bower JE et al. Fatigue in breast cancer survivors: Occurrence correlates and impact on quality of life. *Journal of Clinical Oncology* 2000; 18:743–753.

44. Nail LM. Fatigue in patients with cancer. *Oncology Nursing Forum* 2002; 29:537–544.

45. Meeske K et al. Fatigue in breast cancer survivors two to five years post diagnosis a HEAL study report. *Quality of Life Research* 2007; 16:947–960.

46. Bower JE et al. Inflammatory biomarkers and fatigue during radiation therapy for breast and prostate cancer. *Clinical Cancer Research* 2009; 15(17):5534–5540.

47. Bower JE et al. Inflammatory responses to psychological stress in fatigued breast cancer survivors: Relationship to glucocorticoids. *Brain, Behavior, and Immunity* 2007; 3:251–858.

48. Spence RR, Heesch KC, Brown WJ. Exercise and cancer rehabilitation: A systematic review. *Cancer Treatment Reviews* 2009 Dec 3.

49. Dixon JK, Moritz DA, Baker FL. Breast cancer and weight gain: An unexpected finding. *Oncology Nursing Forum* 1978; 5:5–7.

50. Goodwin PJ. Weight gain in early-stage breast cancer: Where do we go from here? *Journal of Clinical Oncology* 2001; 19:2367–2369.

51. Cummings SR et al. Effect of alendronate on risk of fracture in women with low bone density but without vertebral fractures: Results from the Fracture Intervention Trial. *Journal of the American Medical Association* 1998; 280:2077–2082.

52. Goodwin PJ et al. Prognostic effects of 25-hydroxyvitamin D levels in early breast cancer. *Journal of Clinical Oncology* 2009; 27:3757–3763.

53. Holmberg L et al. HABITS (hormonal replacement therapy after breast cancer): Is it safe? A randomized comparison: Trial stopped. *Lancet* 2004; 363:453–455.

54. Morrow M et al. A prospective study of variability in mammographic density during the menstrual cycle. *Breast Cancer Res Treat* 2009 DOI 10.1007/s10549-009-0496-9.

55. Writing Group for the PEPI Trial. Effects of estrogen or estrogen/progestin regimens on heart disease risk factors in postmenopausal women: The postmenopausal estrogen/progestin interventions (PEPI) trial. *Journal of the American Medical Association* 1995; 273(3):199.

56. Cialli AR, Fugh-Berman A. Is estriol safe? *Alternative Therapies in Women's Health* 2002; 14(10):73–74.

57. Boothby LA, Doering PL, Kipersztok S. Bioidentical hormone therapy: A review. *Menopause* 2004; 11(3):356–367.

58. Wren BG. Progesterone creams: Do they work? *Climacteric* 2003; 6:184–187.

59. Million Women Study Coordinators. Breast cancer and hormone replacement therapy in the Million Women Study. *Lancet* 2003; 362:419–427.

60. Million Women Study Collaborators. Endometrial cancer and hormone-replacement therapy in the Million Women Study. *Lancet* 2005; 365:1543–1545.

61. Kenemans P. Safety and efficacy of tibolone in breast-cancer patients with vasomotor symptoms: A double blind, randomized, non-inferiority trial. *Lancet Oncol* 2009 10(2):135–146.

62. Lieberman S. A review of the effectiveness of cimicifuga racemosa (black cohosh) for the symptoms of menopause. *Journal of Women's Health* 1998; 7(5):525–529.

63. Anon. meeting summary. American Society for Clinical Oncology 1998.

64. Messina MJ, Loprinzi CL. Soy for breast cancer survivors: A critical review of the literature. *Journal of Nutrition* 2001; 131:3095S–3108S.

65. Shu XO et al. Soy food intake and breast cancer survival. *Journal of the American Medical Association* 2009; 302(22):2437–2443.

66. Pockaj BA et al. Phase III double-blind, randomized, placebo-controlled crossover trial of black cohosh in the management of hot flashes: NCCTG Trial N01CC1. *Journal of Clinical Oncology* 2006; 24:2836–2841.

67. Jacobson JS et al. Randomized trial of black cohosh for the treatment of hot flashes among women with a history of breast cancer. *Journal of Clinical Oncology* 2001; 19:2739–2745.

68. Barton DL et al. Prospective evaluation of vitamin E for hot flashes in breast cancer survivors. *Journal of Clinical Oncology* 1998; 16:495–500.

69. Davis VL et al. Black cohosh increases metastatic mammary cancer in transgenic mice expressing c-erb B2. *Cancer Research* 2008; 68(20):8377–8383.

70. Loprinzi CL et al. Mayo Clinic and North Central Cancer Treatment Group hot flash studies: A 20-year experience. *Menopause* 2008; 15:655–660.

71. Nelson HD et al. Nonhormonal therapies for menopausal hot flashes: Systematic review and meta-analysis. *Journal of the American Medical Association* 2006; 295:2057–2071.

72. Barton DL et al. Randomized controlled trial to evaluate transdermal testosterone in female cancer survivors with decreased libido: North Central Cancer Treatment Group Protocol N02C3. *Journal of the National Cancer Institute* 2007; 99:672–679.

73. Ganz PA, Greendale GA. Female sexual desire: Beyond testosterone. *Journal of the National Cancer Institute* 2007; 99(9):659–661.

74. Kitzinger S. *Woman's Experience of Sex*. New York: Putnam's, 1983.

75. Wellisch DK, Jamison KR, Pasnau RO. Psychosocial aspects of mastectomy. II. The man's perspective. *American Journal of Psychiatry* 1978; 135:543.

76. Baider L, Kaplan-DeNour A. Couples' reactions and adjustments to mastectomy: A preliminary report. *International Journal of Psychiatry and Medicine* 1984; 14:265.

77. Ganz PA et al. Life after breast cancer: Understanding women's health related quality of life and sexual functioning. *Journal of Clinical Oncology* 1998; 16:501.

78. Rowland JH et al. Addressing intimacy and partner communication after breast cancer: A randomized controlled group intervention. *Breast Cancer Research and Treatment* 2009; 118(1):99–111.

79. Mignot L et al. Breast cancer and subsequent pregnancy. *American Society of Clinical Oncology Proceedings* 1986; 5:57.

80. Peters M. The effect of pregnancy in breast cancer. *Prognostic Factors in Breast Cancer* 1968; 65.

81. Maunsell E et al. Work situation after breast cancer: Results from a population-based study. *Journal of the National Cancer Institute* 2004; 96:1813–1822.

Chapter 20

1. Solin LJ, Harris EER, Weinstein SP. Local-regional recurrence after breast conservation treatment or mastectomy. In Harris JR et al., eds. *Diseases of the Breast*, 840. 4th ed. Philadelphia: Lippincott, Williams & Wilkins, 2004.

2. Rutgers E, Van Slooten E, Kluck H. Follow-up after treatment of primary breast cancer. *British Journal of Surgery* 1989; 76:187–190.

3. Kurtz J et al. The prognostic significance of late local recurrence after breast conserving therapy. *International Journal of Radiation Oncology, Biology, and Physics* 1990; 18:87–93.

4. Solin LJ et al. Local-regional recurrence after breast conservation treatment of mastectomy. In Harris JR et al., eds. *Diseases of the Breast*, 844.

5. Chada M et al. The feasibility of a second lumpectomy and breast brachytherapy for localized cancer in a breast previously treated with lumpectomy and radiation therapy of breast cancer. *Brachytherapy* 2008; 7(1):22–28.

6. Kuerer HM, Arthur DW, Haffty BG. Repeat breast-conserving surgery for in-breast local breast carcinoma recurrence: The potential role of partial breast irradiation. *Cancer* 2004; 100:2269–2280.

7. Voogd AC et al. Local recurrence after breast conservation therapy for early stage breast carcinoma: Detection, treatment, and outcome in 266 patients. *Cancer* 1999 Jan 15; 85(2):437–446.

8. Galper S et al. Prognosis after local recurrence after conservative surgery and radiation for early-stage breast cancer. *International Journal of Radiation Oncology, Biology, and Physics* 2005; 61:348–357.

9. Gilliland MD, Barton RM, Copeland EM. The implications of local recurrence of breast cancer as the first site of therapeutic failure. *Annals of Surgery* 1983; 197:284–287.

10. Slavin SA, Love SM, Goldwyn RM. Recurrent breast cancer following immediate reconstruction with myocutaneous flaps. *Plastic and Reconstructive Surgery* 1994 May; 93:1191.

11. Borner M et al. First isolated locoregional recurrence following mastectomy for breast cancer: Results of a phase III multicenter study comparing systemic treatment with observation after excision and radiation. *Journal of Clinical Oncology* 1994; 12:2071.

12. Hortobagyi G. Can we cure limited metastatic breast cancer? *Journal of Clinical Oncology* 2001; 20(3):620–623.

13. Halverson KJ et al. Locoregional recurrence of breast cancer: A retrospective comparison of irradiation alone versus irradiation and systemic therapy. *American Journal of Clinical Oncology* 1992; 15:93–101.

14. Recht A et al. Regional nodal failure after conservative surgery and radiotherapy for early-stage breast carcinoma. *Journal of Clinical Oncology* 1991; 9:988.

15. Seidman AD. Sequential single-agent chemotherapy for metastatic breast cancer: Therapeutic nihilism or realism? *Journal of Clinical Oncology* 2003; 21(4):577–579.

16. Hortobagyi GN. Can we cure limited metastatic breast cancer? *Journal of Clinical Oncology* 2002; 20:620–623.

17. Falkson G et al. Survival of premenopausal women with metastatic breast cancer: Long-term follow-up of Eastern Cooperative Group and Cancer and Leukemia Group B studies. *Cancer* 1990; 66:1621.

18. Chia S et al. The impact of new chemotherapeutic and hormonal agents on the survival of women with metastatic breast cancer in a population based cohort. *Proceedings of the American Society of Clinical Oncology* 2003; 22:6a.

19. Giordano SH et al. Is breast cancer survival improving? *Cancer* 2004; 100(1):44–52.

20. Hamaoka T et al. Bone imaging in metastatic breast cancer. *Journal of Clinical Oncology* 2004; 22:2942–2953.

21. Hillner BE et al. Update on the role of bisphosphonates and bone health issues in women with breast cancer. *Journal of Clinical Oncology* 2003; 21:4042–4057.

22. Patchell RA et al. A randomized trial of surgery in the treatment of single metastases to the brain. *New England Journal of Medicine* 1990; 322(8): 494–500.

Chapter 21

1. Slamon D et al. Addition of Herceptin (humanized anti-HER2 antibody) to first line chemotherapy for HER2 overexpressing metastatic breast cancer

(HER2+/MBC) markedly increases anticancer activity: A randomized, multinational controlled phase III trial. *American Society of Clinical Oncology Proceedings* 1998; 17:98a.

2. Comen EA, Robson M. Poly(ADP-ribose) polymerase inhibitors in triple-negative breast cancer. *Cancer* J 2010 Jan-Feb; 16(1):48–52.

3. Howell A et al. Comparison of gulvestrant versus tamoxifen for the treatment of advanced breast cancer in postmenopausal women previously untreated with endocrine therapy: A multinational double-blind, randomized trial. *Journal of Clinical Oncology* 2004; 22(9):1605–1613.

4. Robertson JF et al. Fulvestrant versus anastrozole for the treatment of advanced breast carcinoma in postmenopausal women: A prospective combined analysis of two multicenter trials. *Cancer* 2003; 98(2):229–238.

5. Osborne CK et al. Double-blind, randomized trial comparing the efficacy and tolerability of fulvestrant versus anastrozole in postmenopausal women with advanced breast cancer progressing on prior endocrine therapy: Results of a North American trial. *Journal of Clinical Oncology* 2002; 16:3386–3395.

6. Ellis MJ et al. Lower-dose vs. high-dose oral estradiol therapy of hormone receptor-positive aromatase inhibitor resistant advanced breast cancer: A phase 2 randomized study. *Journal of the American Medical Association* 2009; 302(7):774–780.

7. Farquhar C et al. High dose chemotherapy and autologous bone marrow or stem cell transplantation versus conventional chemotherapy for women with metastatic breast cancer. *Cochrane Database Syst Rev* 2005 Jul; 20(3).

8. Von Minckwitz G et al. Trastuzumab beyond progression in human epidermal growth factor receptor 2-positive advanced breast cancer: A German breast group 26/breast international group 03–05 study. *Journal of Clinical Oncology* 2009 Apr 20; 27(12):1999–2006.

9. Valachis A et al. Bevacizumab in metastatic breast cancer: A meta-analysis of randomized controlled trials. *Breast Cancer Res Treat* 2010 Jan 9.

10. Lipton A et al. Pamidronate prevents skeletal complications and is effective palliative treatment in women with breast carcinoma and osteolytic bone metastases: Long-term follow-up of two randomized, placebo, and controlled trials. *Cancer* 2000; 88(5):1082–1090.

11. Hillner BE et al. American Society of Clinical Oncology 2003 update on the role of bisphosphonates and bone health issues in women with breast cancer. *Journal of Clinical Oncology* 2003 Nov 1; 21(21):4042–4057.

12. Spiegel D. *Living Beyond Limits: New Hope and Help for Facing Life-Threatening Illness.* New York: Times Books, 1993.

13. Tobin DR, with Lindsey K. *Peaceful Dying.* Reading, MA: Perseus, 1999.

Index

A-bomb, 141–142, 143
Abortion, 153, 393, 394
Abraxane, 507, 598–599
Abscesses, 88–90
Absolute risk, 129
Accelerated partial breast radiation
  (APBI), 479
Actiferous sinus, 11
Acupuncture, 80, 274, 440, 442,
  529–530, 557
Adenocarcinoma, 29, 295(table)
Adjuvant therapy
  duration of, 491–492
  Herceptin, 358
  lifestyle changes, 359–360
  local recurrences, 473–474
  mortality rate reduction and survival
    estimates, 347(table)
  neurological metastases, 594
  oncologist referral affecting choice
    of, 325
  procedure and drugs, 493–499
  targeted therapies, 353–355
  weighing treatment options,
    344–348
Adriamycin, 287, 349, 350, 500, 503,
  506, 516, 607
Affirmations, 526–527
African Americans
  basal carcinomas, 316
  BRCA 1 and BRCA 2 mutations,
    168
  breast cancer incidence statistics,
    131(table)
  inflammatory breast cancer, 380

postmenopausal cancer around the
  world, 137
risk factor variations, 140–141
statistical risk evaluation, 192
*After Breast Cancer: A Commonsense
  Guide to Life after Treatment*
  (Schnipper), 267
Age
  adjuvant therapy benefits, 346
  basal carcinomas, 316
  breast cancer incidence statistics,
    131(table)
  breast physical exam, 246–247
  cancer around the world, 137
  cancer in elderly women, 395–396
  cancer in very young women, 388–
    392
  cysts, 67
  DCIS recurrence, 374
  fibroadenomas, 73, 74–75
  flap procedure and, 461
  hereditary breast cancer, 113
  increasing risk of cancer, 140
  inflammatory breast cancer, 380
  local recurrence after breast
    conservation, 579
  mammogram frequency, 249, 253
  nipple discharge, 92–93
  radiation-induced cancer, 141–142
  relative and absolute risk, 129,
    132–133, 132(table)
  survival estimates with and without
    adjuvant therapy, 347(table)
  See also Menopause
Aggressiveness of cancer, 295–296, 298

Sarcoma, 488, 548
Sartorius, Otto, 88, 186
Sauter, Ed, 187
Scar tissue
  flap procedures, 461
  infiltrating ductal cancer, 293–294
  local recurrence, 579–583
  mammography, 215–216
  mastectomy incision, 441
  silicone implants, 54–55
Schain, Wendy, 269
Schnipper, Hester Hill, 267, 269
Scoliosis, 34, 143
Screening tests
  breast physical exam, 246–247
  breast self-examination, 37–38, 243, 245–246
  early detection, 241–242, 243–244
  evaluating tests, 242–245
  frequency recommendations, 242–254
  goals of, 248–249
  metastatic disease, 307–310
  PET scanning, 232–233
  physical and emotional reaction to, 257–259
  See also specific tests
Second cancers, 505, 548, 579
Segmental mastectomy, 422. *See also* Lumpectomy; Partial mastectomy
Seidman, Andrew, 583
Selective estrogen receptor modulators (SERMs), 202, 204, 511, 557
Sensations
  artificial nipple, 41
  breast sensitivity, 30–31
  cyclical breast pain, 77–83
  loss after partial mastectomy, 429–430
  lymph node surgery, 420
  nipple sensitivity after breast reduction, 49, 51
  radiation-induced sensitivity, 486
  reconstructed breasts, 448
  total mastectomy, 436
Sentinel node biopsy
  cancer in both breasts, 387
  DCIS treatment, 374–375
  in elderly women, 396

  localization of lesion, 424–425
  locally advanced breast cancer treatment, 378
  lymphedema and, 544
  men with cancer, 399
  Paget's disease of the breast and, 384
  pathology report, 299
  procedure, 414–417
  purpose and procedure, 338–340
Seroma, 419
Serotonin, 500
Sesame seeds, 196
Sexuality
  bras and, 29
  breast anatomy and function, 13
  breast exploration, 32
  breast sensitivity and, 31
  chemotherapy side effects, 504–505
  choosing mastectomy, 262–263
  relationships after treatment, 564–568
  vaginal dryness, 559–561
Shalala, Donna, 629
Shapiro, Susan, 617, 625–626
Shark cartilage, 532
Shaw, William, 48, 450
Side effects
  cyclical breast pain treatment, 81
  follow-up after treatment, 538
  implants, 53–59, 455, 464
  MRI, 230
Side effects, chemotherapy
  appetite and sense of smell, 502
  bone loss, 514, 552–553
  "chemo brain," 505, 549–551
  fatigue, 508
  GCSF, 494–495
  hair loss, 503–504
  long-term, 439–440, 505–508
  metastatic disease, 608
  nausea and vomiting, 500–501
  premature menopause, 502–503
  sexual problems, 504–505
  supplements reducing, 529
  weighing treatment options, 349
  weight gain, 501–502
Side effects, hormone therapy
  aromatase inhibitors, 511–513
  bone density, 514–516, 552–553

About the Authors

Susan Love, MD, MBA, is an author, surgeon, researcher, entrepreneur, and mother. She is Clinical Professor of Surgery at UCLA, President of the Dr. Susan Love Research Foundation, and a founder and Director of the National Breast Cancer Coalition. She is the author of *Dr. Susan Love's Breast Book,* one of the first books for the lay public that explained the scientific information and options for treatment in an accessible manner. Updated every five years, it has been termed the "bible" for women with breast cancer by the *New York Times.* Her second book, *Dr. Susan Love's Menopause and Hormone Book* was the first to sound the alarm about the dangers of long-term use of hormone replacement therapy in post-menopausal women. She served a six-year term as a presidential appointee to the National Cancer Advisory Board and continues to advise both for profit and not-for-profit organizations regarding breast cancer and women's health. In addition to her media appearances, speaking, and political activities, she dedicates her time through her foundation to performing innovative collaborative research and developing resources for other researchers to find the cause of breast cancer. Most recently she has been responsible for the Love/Avon Army of Women (www.armyofwomen.org), a new online appoach to linking women who are willing to participate in studies to the scientists who need them and the Health of Women Study in collaboration with a team at City of Hope and CaBIG of the National Cancer Institute. Her website, www.dslrf.org is a place where women can find out how to become part of the solution as well as find answers to all their health care questions. She shares her home in Southern California with her wife, Helen Cooksey MD, their daughter Katie, and their companions, two dogs, two cats, and eight fish.

Karen Lindsey is the author of *Divorced, Beheaded, Survived: A Feminist Reinterpretation of the Wives of Henry VII; Friends as Family;* and *Falling Off the Roof;* and co-author of *Dr. Susan Love's Menopause and Hormone Book* and, with Dr. Daniel Tobin, *Peaceful Dying.* She has co-authored *Shelter from the Storm: Caring for a Child with a Life-Threatening Condition,* with Drs. Joanne Hilden and Daniel Tobin. Her articles have appeared in *Ms., The Women's Review of Books, Sojourner, International Figure Skating,* and many other publications and anthologies. She teaches women's studies at the University of Massachusetts/Boston, and writing and literature at Emerson College.